AF518283

Basic and Molecular Genetics

The Authors

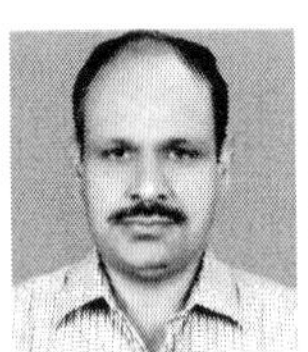

Dr. Arun Kumar Tomar is presently holding the position of Head, Division of Animal Genetics and Breeding for the last four year and Director ICAR-Central Sheep and Wool Research Institute, Avikanagar, via Jaipur, Rajasthan. He did Ph.D. (Animal Breeding) from CCS, HAU, Hisar, B.Sc. (Ag.) and M.Sc. (Ag.) in A.H. and Dairying from J. V. College, Baraut, Bagpat (U.P.). He was selected as Scientist in the discipline of Animal Genetics and Breeding of A.R.S. (ICAR) through All India Competitive Examination conducted by A.S.R.B. He was posted and joined as Scientist (Animal Genetics and Breeding) at C.S.W.R.I. Avikanagar (Rajasthan) in 1995, and subsequently promoted to the post of Senior Scientist and Principal Scientist (A.G.B) at Project Directorate on Cattle, now ICAR-Central Institute of Research on Cattle, Meerut (U.P.). He was selected on the post of Head (AGB) where he is working at present. He has published some books and booklets and many research papers and has experience of editorial work in the capacity of Assistant Editor of Research Journals. Dr. Arun Tomar has been awarded "Dr. Rajendra Prasad Award-2017" for his book "Unnat Bhed Palan 2016" in native language hindi.

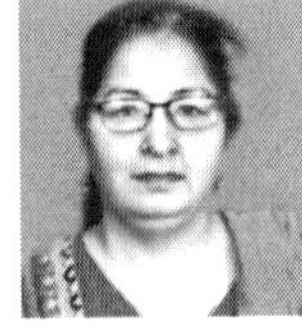

Mrs. Archana Tomar is M.Sc., B.Sc. (Genetics), B.Ed. from Kurukshetra University, Kurukshetra (Haryana). She is presently engaged in teaching work, U.P. Govt. Education Department, Gaziabad. She has 12 years experience of teaching work.

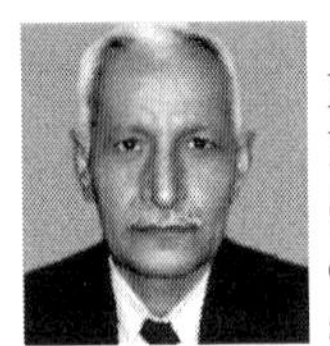

Professor Sukhvir Singh Tomar is Ph.D. (A.G.B.) from N.D.R.I., Karnal. He did B.Sc. (Ag.) and M.Sc. (Ag.) in A.H. and Dairying from J.V.College, Baraut, Bagpat (U.P.). He started his career as Lecturer, J.V. College, Baraut (Meerut) in 1965 and subsequently at P.A.U, Hisar campus in 1967. Later on in 1975, he joined ARS of I.C.A.R. as Scientist (AGB) at C.S.W.R.I. and subsequently worked as Senior Scientist and Principal Scientist (A.G.B.) at I.C.A.R. - N.D.R.I., Karnal from where he was retired in 2005 having 40 years of research experience making significant contribution in the area of Animal Breeding Research and teaching experience to B.Sc., M.Sc. and Ph.D. Classes. Dr. Tomar has published about 300 research articles and 3 text books during the tenure of his service life. He has long experience of about 28 years as Editor of Research Journal and guided a number of M.Sc. and Ph.D. students. He has made notable contribution in research in the area of Animal Breeding, particularly pertaining to threshold characters, replacement rate, selective value, and other aspects of sire evaluation at earliest possible age. He is still actively engaged in research and publication work. Dr. Sukhvir Singh Tomar was awarded "SARC outstanding Authorship in Science and Technology Award 2011 for making significant contibution in research and his excellent efficiency in teaching work through publishing his books."

First two authors have already published three books on the subject during 2014 -16. The first book "*Animal Genetics and Breeding*" covered the syllabus prescribed by Veterinary Council of India for B. V. Sc. and A.H. of Indian Agricultural Universities. The two books "*Genetics of Livestock Population*" and "*Sustainable Livestock and Poultry Breeding*" covered both theory and practical exercises as per syllabus prescribed for post-graduate classes in the discipline of Animal Breeding in the country.

Basic and Molecular Genetics

Arun Kumar Tomar

Archana Tomar

Sukhvir Singh Tomar

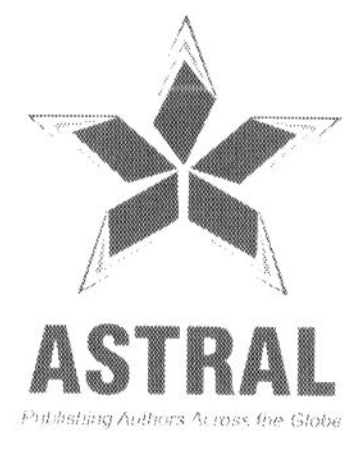

2025

Daya Publishing House®

A Division of

Astral International Pvt. Ltd.

New Delhi – 110 002

© AUTHORS

ISBN 978-93-5124-871-2 (HB)

First Published, 2018

Reprinted 2025

Publisher's Note:

Every possible effort has been made to ensure that the information contained in this book is accurate at the time of going to press, and the publisher and author cannot accept responsibility for any errors or omissions, however caused. No responsibility for loss or damage occasioned to any person acting, or refraining from action, as a result of the material in this publication can be accepted by the editor, the publisher or the author. The Publisher is not associated with any product or vendor mentioned in the book. The contents of this work are intended to further general scientific research, understanding and discussion only. Readers should consult with a specialist where appropriate.

Every effort has been made to trace the owners of copyright material used in this book, if any. The author and the publisher will be grateful for any omission brought to their notice for acknowledgement in the future editions of the book.

All Rights reserved under International Copyright Conventions. No part of this publication may be reproduced, stored in a retrieval system, or transmitted in any form or by any means, electronic, mechanical, photocopying, recording or otherwise without the prior written consent of the publisher and the copyright owner.

Published by : **Daya Publishing House®**
A Division of
Astral International Pvt. Ltd.
– ISO 9001:2015 Certified Company –
4736/23, Ansari Road, Darya Ganj
New Delhi-110 002
Ph. 011-43549197, 23278134
E-mail: info@astralint.com
Website: www.astralint.com

Digitally Printed at : **Replika Press Pvt. Ltd.**

All the editions by the authors are great tribute to lovely memory of

Ch. Lal Singh
F/O Prof. (Dr.) Sukhvir Singh Tomar and

dedication to his significant and unforgettable contribution for the family, whole heartedly donation to the Educational Institutions, and inspiring his son to adopt teaching as a profession.

Preface

The ***genetics*** is a new subject of 20th century stemmed on the work of Mendel (1822 – 1884) who formulated the Laws of Heredity in the year 1866. However, his laws of inheritance remained hidden and came into existence with the beginning of 20th century with the rediscovery of these Laws after reviewing and recognizing their significance by three scientists in the year 1900 and coining the term *genetics* for the study of heredity and variation by William Bateson in the year1906. Thereafter, there has been tremendous progress and improvements in this field from phenotypic level of gene expression to molecular level (*replication, transcription* and *translation* of genetic material in the form of DNA and RNA as well as *new molecular techniques*). These tremendous advancements during 20th century made by various scientists has emerged a new branch of science called *genetics*.

Considered the need of the day to compile the entire subject matter related to *"Mendelian Genetics and Molecular Genetics"* in a single volume to meet the requirement as per syllabus of Post Graduate programme of Animal Genetics and Breeding taught in State Agricultural Universities in India. The related subject matter has been collected and compiled from different published sources covering the theoretical aspects and practical numerical problems and exercises, arranging and presenting the entire subject matter in a simple and illustrative language. The subject matter of *Genetics and Molecular Genetics* in this book has been covered in 3 parts comprising 27 chapters.

The *first part* covered *"Mendelian* or *classical genetics"* in 11 chapters dealing with introduction to genetics, sources of genetic variation, heredity and environment, Mendelism, Chromoomal theory of inheritance, Exceptions to Mendelism [Multiple alleles, gene expression (action) on phenotypic level, Linkage of genes and crossing over], Sex determination and sex controlled inheritance. The *second part* is of the book covered *"Molecular genetics"* in 14 chapters on microbial genetics, genetic material (DNA) and its molecular structure, changes in its structure (mutation), and replication of DNA; Gene expression at molecular level (transcription and translation), Regulation of gene expression in prokaryotes and eukaryotes, Gene manipulation techniques and applications. The last *III part* covered *"Genetic Statistics"* which included 2 chapters on the probability and Chi-square testing of discrete variable.

This book on ***"Genetics"*** has been written to fulfill the hope and requirement of post-graduate students, teachers and of those intend to appear and pass the competitive examinations on All India basis like SRF, NET and ARS conducted by ASRB (ICAR), UGC and UPSC. However, the originality of subject matter is hereby not claimed by the authors but with lots of thanks to the original workers and earlier authors on different subject matter.

The authors are highly thankful to Dr. Sunderason, Dr. R.M. Acharya, Dr. A.L. Chaudhary, Dr. R.N. Singh, and Dr. S.B. Basu for their valuable guidance, kind cooperation, suggestions, and helping in different ways. Smt. Shakuntla Tomar, Dr. Ajay Kumar Tomar, Dr. Amit Kumar Tomar and other family members of the authors also deserve our thanks for their helping attitude, consistent encouragement and kind cooperation from all corners at every step.

The authors also welcome the readers to point out the mistakes that are likely to occur and to give suggestions for further improvement of the book.

Dr. Arun Kumar Tomar

Archana Tomar

Prof. Sukhvir Singh Tomar

Contents

PART 2: MOLECULAR GENETICS

ANNEXURES

Part 1

Mendelian Genetics

Chapter 1
Introduction to Genetics

Sexuality is the most important, main, and the prime phenomenon of living world, also the source of creating the genetic variability and forms the basis of genetics as well. There is sex dimorphism having male and female as two sexes mostly. However, in rare cases, a third sex called intersex or neutral gender is found which form the sex polymorphism.

Sexual reproduction is observed in most of the living organisms wherein the union of two sex gametes as a result of mating of the individual of both sexes produces a new living organism. Sexual reproduction is the main source of genetic variability. This variability reflected in phenotype is the *beauty of nature*, of *economic importance* for improvement in performance traits, brings *identity to individuals* in a population, and also of biological or *evolutionary significance* to evolve new species.

Sexual reproduction give birth to a new living individual (progeny) arises from a pre-existing two similar individuals which are known as parents and these parents themselves had arisen from the earlier pre-existing two individuals (called as grand- parents which are four in number), and so on. Thus, each living individual has the ability to produce its similar (own) type of new individuals and so there is continuity of being produced a new living individual of next generation of its parental type.

1.1 BIOLOGICAL ESSENCE OF SPECIES

The species has been considered as a base or unit of biological classification. The reason is the existence of the diversity among the individuals of any one species to the extent that they are dissimilar in various physical and other traits but they can reproduce successfully due to which they share common gene pool and hence there is no genetic isolation among them. On the contrary, there is reproductive isolation among the individuals of any two species and hence they have genetic isolation. This type of diversity among the individuals of two species is a basic and essential factor to the recognition of the species (***speciation***). This is the reality and base of "***biological essence of species***" to consider the species as a ***unit of biological classification***.

1.2 TWO MAIN TENDENCIES OF A SPECIES

The individuals of a species show two main peculiar tendencies/characteristics. The first is the tendency of *"like begets like"* in each species and second tendency is the existence of *discrete groups within a species*.

- ☆ *LIKE BEGETS LIKE:* Despite the fact of diversity of life, all the individuals of a species have the tendency to look alike because they have the physical characteristics similar and unique to those of their own species to which they belong. Therefore, having these unique physical characteristics they can be recognized and identified, and grouped as the individuals of that particular species. This tendency of having similar physical characteristics by the individuals of a species is due to the reason that organisms of a species give rise to the individuals of their own type *viz.* women give birth to human babies, cat to kittens, dogs produce the dogs, pea seeds will grow pea plants, wheat seeds to wheat plants, mango tree gives rise to mango tree, *etc.* Thus, a newly produced living individual has the characteristics similar and common to its species. This tendency is what is called ***"like begets like"***.
- ☆ *DISCRETE GROUPS IN A SPECIES:* In spite of the tendency of "like begets like" in a species, the different individuals of a species having some of the similar physical characteristics to large extent, also show dissimilarities to various extent. The similarities and dissimilarities among the individuals of a species form the distinct groups within a species. Thus, the species in spite of a basic unit of biological classification, each species is further divided into sub-species, breeds/races/eco-types or demes (local populations)/strains/lines/herds of cattle and buffaloes/flocks of sheep, goat, and poultry/varieties of plants throughout the world.

This second tendency of discrete groups among the individuals belonging to a particular species (breed, herd/flock/strains/lines) is that they differ from each other to the extent that each and every individual is unique and ***no two individuals are identical***, how closely related they are, except identical twins and clones. Therefore, any two individuals related either through the descent (direct relatives, parent offspring) or as the collateral relatives (full sibs, half sibs, cousins, etc), they resemble each other only to some extent, and hence the resemblance is not exact. This implies that there is also the *tendency of differences* among individuals of similar heredity besides similarities. The related individuals thus have the similarities and also the differences among themselves in their characteristics.

However, there is no reproductive isolation among these sub-groups of a species and the mating occurs within them (between the individuals of sub-groups of a species) as a requirement of sexual reproduction. Thus, the individuals of a species belonging to any sub-group but living in a locality may mate together and reproduce. Thus, there is gene exchange among them and hence there is no genetic isolation. Moreover, there is gene exchange more frequently among the individuals residing in the same locality compared to the individuals of the same species located distantly. Thus, the individuals of a species residing in the same area share more genes in common due to the gene exchange among themselves but may differ in gene frequencies of the gene pool of other sub-populations of the same species residing distantly.

The variation within a species can be categorized as:

(i) *Group variation*: The individuals of different breeds within a species, lines and herds/flocks of a breed form different groups and differ from each other in most of their characteristics. These variations are called as group variation (*breed variation, herd variation and line variation,* sire line etc).

(ii) *Individual variation*: The closely related individuals, even of the same sire-dam families, show variations among themselves. This variation among individuals of the same group is called as the individual variation.

(iii) *Within individual variation*: The phenotypic values for any quantitative trait recorded on an individual at different times are different. The variation between records of the same individual taken at different times is called within individual variation or intra individual variation.

1.3 RESEMBLANCE AND DIFFERENCES AMONG RELATIVES

The phenomenon of "like begets like" is the unique ability and universal. It is the result of transmission of *genetic material* or *hereditary material* (genes, the parts of DNA) by the descent (parent) to their descendents (progeny). The transmission of genetic material is accomplished through the process of sexual reproduction which involves gamete formation by meiotic cell division, mating of animals of opposite sex and union of gametes of opposite sex (fertilization). The genetic material transmitted is contained in the reproductive cells (germ cells, called gametes), embodies the necessary information required to guide the formation of a newly produced living individual of the species own type, development of its various characteristics similar to its own species, performing various life activities to carry out biochemical reactions and physiological functions, and maintenance of its life.

The genetically related individuals resemble to each other, though this resemblance is not exact or perfect. The animals produce their progenies that resemble to their parents. The progeny may resemble to either one of the two parents or may have combined features of both the parents. Thus, parent-offspring (direct relatives) and other family members related by descent (collateral relative's *viz.* brothers, sisters, uncles, *etc.*) have resemblance to each other. Therefore, every succeeding generation has similarity (resemblance) to the preceding one as well as among its members of the same generation.

However, it is also a fact that the resemblance is up to a certain extent rather than exactly the replication of the same characteristics and hence the succeeding generation is never a replica of the preceding generation. Every individual show similarity in some respects but differs in others to its direct or collateral relatives. Therefore, the living individuals of genetically related group show some similarities and also have differences as well among themselves.

1.4 MECHANISMS INVOLVED FOR GENETIC DIFFERENCES AMONG RELATIVES

The genetic material passed on (transmitted) by the parent to all of the progenies is similar to produce "like begets like" within a species as well as to produce similarities (resemblance) among relatives. However, at the same time, the genetic material passed on to the progeny is not exactly identical but differ in some way to produce dissimilarities (differences) observed even among close relatives.

The differences in genetic material transmitted even among close relatives are caused by the following genetic processes discussed in detail in next chapter number 2.

(*i*) ***Existing genetic variations***: There exist already the differences in genetic material (genes) which have arisen due to existence of *genes in pairs* at all loci in every diploid individual, existence of *multiple alleles* at a locus, existence of the *number of gene loci* (polygenes) affecting a character, and existence of *sex chromosomes*.

(*ii*) ***Newly arisen genetic variation***: Some of the genetic variations arise a fresh due to change in genetic material caused by *chromosomal aberrations* and *gene mutation*, changes resulting from *genetic segregation and redistribution of genes* as a result of crossing over between homologous chromosomes, change resulting from *recombination of genes* (combining genes as a result of zygote formation by the union of maternal and paternal chromosomes after fertilization takes place), change occurring from *gene action* or expression resulting from new gene combinations *viz.* additive and non additive gene action.

Chance events: The phenomenon of ***crossing over*** by exchanging homologous parts of chromosome to cause genes segregation is a chance event because it is not certain that which portion of chromosome will have crossing over, with what rate the crossing over will occur and further which half of the total DNA content will go into which of the two gametes formed by meiotic cell division.

Further, the consequence of **fertilization** as a result of the union of two sex gametes from mating of two parents forming zygote is also not certain but also a random process and hence a chance event. Thus, all the genetic phenomenon (known as the genetic segregation and recombination), involving mutual crossing over of some homologous parts of chromosomes causing genes segregation in gametes and union of gametes of opposite sex on fertilization forming zygote and resulting recombination of genes are all chance events.

All these genetic mechanisms, of ***crossing over*** (gene segregation), ***halving nature of inheritance*** and **sampling nature of inheritance** (genetic recombination) on fertilization to form zygote, produce the gene combinations which are different (causing genetic differences) among progeny and parents, among the different progenies of same parents (full sibs and half sibs, the collateral relatives) and among other collateral relatives. Therefore, all these above genetic phenomenon cause the genetic differences among relatives. This explains the phenomenon of *genetic dissimilarities among relatives* besides the effects of mutations and of the environmental factors.

The mystery of similarities and differences among relatives had been solved in the beginning of 20th century and new branch of biological science, called as *Genetics* has emerged which deals with all these mysterious phenomenon and it has gained tremendous advancements.

1.5 SCIENCE OF GENETICS

The term genetics was coined by William Bateson (1906) from a Greek word gen which means 'to become' or 'to grow into' or *'to generate'*. Thus, he defined genetics as for the ***study of heredity and variation***. The heredity involves the genetic material (genes) and its transmission from one generation to the next. The variation includes the differences observed within each species. The differences among individuals of a species are hereditary as well as environmental in origin.

The hereditary differences are called genetic differences which are brought by two ways (mentioned under section 1.4 and discussed in detail in chapter 2). The heredity, the genetic material (genes) determines the basic pattern of a character and the environment modifies the development of a character to different degrees. The heredity and variation have the significant role in the formation of new species that are reproductively isolated. The production of new species is called as the *speciation* and a part of the evolution.

Geneticists consider that the genetics is a branch of biology which is the study of various aspects of life. But in the last century there had been fast and tremendous developments into the study of the transmission and molecular aspects of the genetic material and *genetics* has now grown into a separate subject. Pai (1974) in his book "Foundations of Genetics" had rightly considered the genetics as the study of life. He argued that besides heredity, all the characteristics like reproduction, response to environmental stimuli, evolution and the activities to carry out biochemical reactions and physiological functions that characterize the living being from the non living ones are genetically controlled. All the aspects of life (covered under biology) are genetically controlled. The subject matter of *genetics* is the genetic control of different aspects of life. In this context, it would be better to call the ***genetics*** as the upper level or ***synonym of biology***. *There is end of life when the genes stop functioning or start improper functioning.* Therefore, the term genetics should be considered as the synonym or parallel to the biology rather than its branch. Accordingly, the time has come to mention at this place that Genetics has its two following main branches –

- ***Botany***: The study of various apsctes of plant life, and
- ***Zoology:*** The study of various aspects of animal life.

Sexual reproduction: Genetics is obviously based on the *sexual reproduction of organisms* which is important for a geneticist for several reasons.

- ☆ *First* is that the man, higher animals and plants reproduce by this process.
- ☆ *Secondly,* different forms of life occur on earth due to sexual reproduction because it leads to variation in characters (through fusion of male and female gametes), sometimes lead to the formation of new species (speciation) and also form the basis of evolution due to variations. There will be no exchange of genes between members of the species without sexual reproduction. Thus, new gene pool will not be formed and also there may be end of life under changing environment. The sexual reproduction generates innumerable genetic combinations through crossing over depending upon the number of heterozygous loci and independent assortment of gametes. The chromosomal differences between opposite sexes have fostered genetic differences during evolution.
- ☆ *Thirdly,* it provides better opportunities for understanding the mechanism of inheritance than asexual reproduction, for the reason that the different individuals can be mated/crossed and their consequences can be studied though successive generations.
- ☆ *Fourth,* the small size, précised organization and activity of reproductive cells (sperms and ova) and the product of their fusion (zygote) are considered a remarkable method of organic multiplication. The eggs are little larger than sperms as they store materials for early development. These minute and organized materials (gametes) form the physical basis for the transmission of inherited qualities and are called the *germ plasm.*

1.6 LEVELS OF GENETICS

The study of the principles of inheritance (heredity) in animal species including physical and chemical basis of inheritance (how the characters are transmitted or inherited from parents to offspring) showing similarities and differences based on the outcome of the individual mating as well as the mating in a population is the subject matter of ***animal genetics***. Therefore, the animal genetics is broadly studied mainly at two levels primarily on the basis of the levels of mating and their outcome:

1. First Level of Genetics - At Individual Level

This includes the *classical genetics,* and *molecular genetics* including *genomics.* The meanings of these branches of genetics are given below:

(*i*) ***Classical genetics*** was the main genetics prior to the discovery of the structure of DNA. The classical genetics is studied by analyzing the outcomes of crosses between different strains and the inheritance of trait differences are used to identify the genes. This is because the trait differences are explained and ascribed due to different alleles *viz.* tall vs short pea plant studied by Mendel. The structure and behavior of chromosomes, pattern of inheritance (nature of the genetic material to control the traits), chromosome mapping by linkage analysis, and change in genetic material at chromosome level are subject matter of classical genetics.

(*ii*) ***Molecular genetics*** *was* entered as a new field of genetics after the discovery of the structure of genetic material (structure of DNA). The analysis of gene structure (DNA sequencing), gene functions (replication, expression through protein synthesis, and mutation of genetic material), and gene manipulation (Recombinant DNA technology, cloning, transgenesis, *etc.*) are now studied at molecular level.

(*iii*) ***Genomics*** is a very new concept in molecular genetics dealing with the study of genomes regarding their structure (mapping and sequencing – *structural genomics*), manipulation after examining the products of gene expression (*functional genomics*), and comparative study of genome (*comparative genomics*).

2. Second Level of Genetics - At Population Level

This includes the *applied genetics viz. population genetics* by analyzing the variability, and *animal breeding* by exploiting the variability for genetic improvement.

(*i*) **Population Genetics:** Individuals of a population have different alleles of a gene as well as different alleles of many genes. As a result the genetic makeup of different individuals differs from each other. Thus, it is required to determine the frequencies of specific alleles in a population and the changes in gene frequencies occurred over time (generation). The change indicates the evolution. Population genetics is the study of variation of both types (genetic and environmental) at population level along with their partitioning into different components based on the outcome of the mating using the biometrical techniques.

(*ii*) ***Animal breeding*** is the application of the principles of animal genetics and population genetics using biometrical techniques to exploit genetic variation for the improvement of animals.

1.7 PHYSICAL AND CHEMICAL BASIS OF INHERITANCE

The present knowledge of genetic mechanisms to transmit the hereditary characteristics from generation to generation has arrived from the following discoveries, known as the ***milestones of genetics***:

(i) Physical Basis of Inheritance – Chromosome Theory of Inheritance

– Bridge of inheritance:

- ☆ *Phenotypic level studies* (**Mendelism and its exceptions:** patterns of transmission of phenotypes to next generation),
- ☆ *Cellular level studies* (Cell theory - cell division and sexual reproduction),

(ii) Chemical Basis of Inheritance – Gene Structure and Functions - Genomics

- ☆ *Molecular level studies* (**Watson and Crick Model of DNA** - molecular structure of genetic material), and
- ☆ *Genomics (mapping, sequencing, and functions of genome –* ***Human genome project*** *launched in 1990 under the Directorship of Watson, James).*

(I) Mendel (1822-1884) Laws of Heredity

Mendel made unique contribution to the knowledge of genetics at phenotypic level. He grew the pea in monastery and studied the inheritance pattern of seven traits. He demonstrated that hereditary factors (now called genes) are discrete entities without being admixing in the hybrid plant, occur in pairs (now called alleles) in each individual, one factor of each pair comes from each parent, follow the law of segregation, and the hereditary factors assort independently during their transmission.

Sutton and Boveri (1902-04) ***Cytological basis of heredity*** (Mendelian inheritance at cellular level): The process of transmitting the genetic material by the parents to the offspring through sexual reproduction for maintaining the genetic continuity from one generation to the next is called as the ***bridge of inheritance.***

The cytological basis states that the chromosomes occur in pairs in somatic cells, carry the hereditary factors (genes) which also occur in pairs, divide exactly and are distributed equally in daughter cells due to their segregation during cell division (meiosis), one member of each pair of chromosome is paternal in origin while the other member is maternal in the fertilized ovum which is the result of fertilization (union of egg and sperm) and give rise to the new individual.

In other words, it is the ***physical basis of inheritance*** which includes the genetic material, its particulate nature and distribution in chromosomes, chromosome theory of inheritance, and its transmission from parents to offspring by the process of cell division (meiosis) and fertilization.

(II) Watson and Crick Model of DNA Structure (1953)

The DNA model proposed by them helped to understand the ***chemical basis of heredity*** (at molecular level) by which the genes express themselves. The chemical structure of the genetic material (nucleosome concept or DNA structure) and the DNA function (replication and protein synthesis) form the *chemical basis of inheritance.*

The ***chemical basis of inheritance*** enunciates that:

- ☆ Genes carry genetic information (in the form of purine and pyrimidine nitrogen bases in the DNA molecule – ***molecular structure of gene***),
- ☆ Genes may change in their chemical composition through change in one or more of the nitrogen bases to create new arrangement of sequence of bases in DNA molecule (***mutation – evolutionary function of gene***).
- ☆ Genes must duplicate (***DNA replication - genotypic function of gene***) itself with great precision (double strand DNA structure and the separation of the two strands of the helix),

- ✩ Genes translate the genetic information to develop the characteristics of the individual (***phenotypic function of gene – gene expression***), *and*

(III) Human Genome Project Initiated in 1990 for DNA Sequencing

It was a world wide project collaborating scientists in many different countries to determine the sequence of nucleotide pairs in human DNA. The complete set of chromosomes as haploid or monoploid, of an organism is called ***genome.***

1.8 FUNCTIONS OF GENETIC MATERIAL

The above mentioned chemical basis of inheritance can also be viewed and explained in terms of the **functions of genetic material.**

The genetic material is the DNA in all cellular organisms. The DNA is composed of a sugar, a phosphate and nitrogen containing bases (Purines and Pyrimidines) and it is a double stranded molecule. This genetic material (DNA) performs its functions through its exact replication (DNA replication) in transmitting its exact copies to different cells during development of the organism and to the every new organism produced by sexual reproduction, rare change in its structure due to error during replication (gene mutation), and protein synthesis to carry out the different activities of an organism. Therefore, the genetic material must have the following three essential functions:

- ✩ ***Evolutionary function of gene (Gene Mutation):*** The DNA must be able to change (***mutation***) so as the organism can adapt to the changing environment. The change in genetic material (mutation) occurs during DNA replication due to incorporation of new nucleotide in place of the original one. The DNA replication is extraordinarily accurate process, though not perfect. Sometimes there is incorrect incorporation of nucleotides in the replicated DNA chain. This disrupts the information encoded in genes.
- ✩ ***Genotypic function of gene (DNA replication):*** The DNA *m*ust be able to ***self duplication*** (replication). This function is required so that its exact copies are transmitted to different cells during development of the organism and to the every new organism produced by sexual reproduction. The DNA replication is exact extraordinarily and this process like others is also catalyzed by the enzymes.
- ✩ ***Phenotypic function of gene (Gene expression):*** The DNA must ***have information*** to direct cellular activities and other functions of the organism (development, carrying out all the life activities, and behavior). The information is encoded in nucleotide sequences of DNA molecules of the genome. The genetic information contained in the DNA flows from DNA to RNA to protein. This flow of information is the ***gene expression*** which is the synthesis of proteins specific for a specific life activity. Such a process of flow of information is known as ***central dogma of molecular biology*** and accomplished in two stages of *transcription* (DNA to RNA) and *translation* (RNA to protein).

The traditional or conventional animal breeding programmes to bring genetic improvement in animal production since domestication involved selection and mating systems based on performance recording and cross-breeding, form the traditional biotechnology. During the last three decades, newer technological breakthrough in the field of reproduction, genetics and related aspects (nutrition, health care) have opened the new area of animal improvement. These new techniques using biological systems or their substances at molecular (gene) level are the areas of modern biotechnology.

1.9 APPLICATIONS OF GENETICS

The knowledge of genetics has been proved to be of great and vital importance to the mankind having deep impact on the socio-cultural aspects besides helping in improvement of domestic animals and agricultural crops.

1. ***Improvement of animals***: The knowledge of genetics has made a significant contribution in the improvement of different livestock and avian species like cattle, buffaloes, sheep, goat, pigs, poultry *etc.* The animal breeders have exploited the knowledge of genetics by conducting various experiments related to breeding systems and selection to make use of the existing genetic variability. This has increased in development of new breeds for higher production of milk, meat and egg and it has come out with white revolution. The domestic animal species are now quite different in their appearance, behavior and productive performance from their wild ancestors.

2. ***Improvement of agricultural crops:*** Like improvement of livestock and poultry production, genetics has made also the notable contributions in making improvement and development of new high yielding varieties of food crops and horticultural crops *etc.* The disease resistant varieties of crop plants have been developed with the knowledge of genetics. The green revolution for improvement of yield of crops and fruits is the outcome of the applications of the genetic principles. It is not only the improvement in the quantity but the quality of food has also been improved *viz.* seedless varieties with higher juice percentage in orange *etc.* have been developed.

   A number of crop species have been descended from wild grasses. Wheat cultivation was started 10,000 years ago in the Middle East. The progenitors of modern cultivated wheat were the low yielding grasses grown by the ancient people of Iran, Iraq, Syria, and Turkey. Modern cultivated wheat (*Triticum aestivum*) has been evolved as a hybrid of at least three different species of low yielding wild grasses. This triple cross wheat of modern days has the chromosomes of each of its progenitors of three species and hence it is really a ***genetic amalgamation*** of the genomes of three different species of grasses. The first event of evolution of wheat was the production of a hybrid species as a crop plant which was improved by selection as the civilization advanced and then interbreeding of this hybrid with a third species, producing a triple-hybrid that proved better for agriculture and human consumption. Thus, the present day varieties of wheat have been descended from triple hybrid plants. The triple-hybrid wheat is superior to its ancestors due to larger grains, easy cultivation and that too in a wide range of conditions. Wheat has become now-a-days one of the major food crop throughout the world for about more than a billion people, having thousands of varieties with an annual production of about 60 MMT (million metric tons) in the world, and accounting about 20 percent of the food calories of entire human population.

The corn has also been developed from its ancestor wild grass (teosine). Likewise, the breeders have developed high-yielding varieties of many other cultivable crops like rice.

The efforts are now being made continuously to design schemes to change the genetic makeup to incorporate particular alleles responsible for economic characters like grain yield, disease resistance, etc through the application of the techniques of molecular genetics. The plants and animals whose genetic makeup has been changed by introduction of foreign genes are called "***genetically modified organisms*** (GMOs)". The ***BT corn*** and ***BT cotton*** developed in United States are the examples. The BT corn contain gene from bacterium *Bacillus thuringiensis.* The gene incorporated in BT corn is toxic to many insects. The people are though reluctant to consume genetically modified food. Many crop and livestock genome sequencing projects are in progress.

3. ***Application in medical science***: Every character has its genetic base and likewise most of the diseases in men are inherited like diabetes, haemoglobin abnormalities, hemophilia, tuberculosis, colour blindness, blood pressure and other heart troubles, some types of blindness and deafness, idiocy and some genetic defects. There is long list of diseases which are caused by mutant genes which cause metabolic abnormalities. The present day knowledge of genetics has helped to develop the techniques of genetic surgery and genetic engineering for correcting various disorders. The frequency of genetic defects can also be reduced in a population by use of the principles of genetics.

   A large number of inherited human disorders have been identified. The cytogenetics is of applied significance in medical science to allow the study of association of *chromosome abnormalities* with disease conditions.

   The physicians have been trained in genetics and they have learned to diagnose the genetic diseases using family data and to predict the probabilities of inheritance of a particular disease. The *genetic counseling* has also been started to examine the patients, interviewing the relatives, and analyzing the vital statistics on births, deaths, and marriages. The *genetic counselor* assess the risk and make a forecast about the birth of a normal or abnormal child and this work require the knowledge of probability, statistics, and genetics.

   The molecular genetics provide ways to detect mutant genes in individuals through *diagnostic test based on DNA analysis* and to treat diseases. The diabetic patients were given earlier the insulin obtained from animals (pigs) but now the human insulin is manufactured on industrial scale in bacterial cells that carry the human insulin gene.

Likewise is the case of human growth hormone (HGH) which is also manufactured in bacterial cells. This hormone is given to those children who carry mutant alleles of this hormone and cannot produce sufficient amount of this hormone for their proper growth.

The molecular genetics techniques are also used as *human gene therapy* to treat diseases. The gene therapy involves inserting healthy, functional copy of a particular gene into the cells of an individual carrying mutant allele of that gene to compensate the faulty gene. Although gene therapy has not been successful to cure cystic fibrosis (respiratory disorder) by introducing CF gene into lung cells but some success has been done in *treating immune system and blood cell disorders* by introducing normal genes into bone marrow which later differentiate into immune cells and blood cells.

4. ***Application in solving legal disputes:*** The blood group in men is genetically controlled. Likewise, the DNA finger printing has genetic base as the DNA of two individuals in not identical. This knowledge is helpful in solving many legal issues like dispute parentage, divorce, legal estate to convict the guilty and to exonerate the innocent, authentic claims to inheritance, to identify the dead, *etc.*

5. ***Removal of misconceptions:*** The knowledge of genetics has helped to understand the reality of some false beliefs which prevailed worldwide in human society, like blood relation and blood relatives, blood will tell, bloodline and a very bad phrase "bad blood' being used in the society. The knowledge of genetics has made it clear that it is not the blood but it is DNA of reproductive cells (gametes) which is carrier of genetic information and transmitted from parents to offspring. Thus blood has nothing to do with all these phrases.

6. ***Genetics to serve society:*** The advancement in technology in basic science has shaped the lifestyles, modern societies, the manufacturing and service industries, provided food and health care. The genetics has provided business opportunities in biotechnology industry like pharmaceutical industries, diagnostic tests, provide service to DNA profiling.

Chapter 2

Variation in Populations

There is gradual change in everything of universe even there is a change in the relative positions of stars and planets, in the boundaries of continents and oceans, in the structure of social groups, in the climate too, and change in the various characteristics of plants and animals are not exception. Thus, it is true that variation is the only invariable law and beauty of nature. The change in plants and animals is must so as they adapt themselves and survive longer under changing environmental conditions otherwise it is not possible.

It has been discussed in previous chapter that in spite of the tendency of "like begets like" in a species, each and every individual in a species is unique and ***no two individuals are identical***, how closely related they are, except identical twins and clones. There are discrete groups even among relatives within a species showing the individual variation.

2.1 TYPES OF VARIATION

The variation may be classified according to the type of cell in which the variation occurs. The cells may be somatic or somatogenic and germinal or blastogenic and the variation produced are called *somatic variation* and *germinal variation*.

(1) Somatic or Environmental Variation

The variation arises in somatic cells due to environmental factors is called *somatic variation or environmental variation*. These variations are not inherited by the parents to their offspring but acquired by the organism during its life. Such characters are called *acquired characters*. The somatic variation may be caused by -

☆ *Environment:* The environment includes the factors like light, temperature, habitat, food, humidity, air pressure, enemies which affect markedly the form and functions of all living beings and such variations are called environmental variation.

☆ *Use and disuse of organs*: The use and disuse of any part or organ of the body affects the various characters by better development for particular organ like *exercise* affect the muscle strength, *domestication* has affected different characters, *e.g.* lion in zoo is weak than living in forest, *civilization* has made weak the teeth of modern civilized man who can take only soft cooked food compared to old uncivilized man who had strong teeth to masticate the hard and coarse food, and *singing* practice develops the vocal organs due to constant use. Likewise some people become left handed or even some may write with foot as they use these organs since childhood.

Conscious efforts: The conscious efforts of man which may produce somatic variation include *castration* by damaging the testes; *mutilation* by cutting organs like horns, pinnae, and tail; varied styles of hair, beard and moustache through barber's skill; *growing of nails* particularly by women; *small feet* by wearing tight shoes in Chinese; by using tight garments and belts by European women. Likewise the *education* makes a man more civilized, *slender waists* for better understanding, and tolerance, *etc*; *learning an art* makes a person perfect in particular field (*swimming, tailoring, dancing, driving, cycling, knitting, typing, etc.*), development of some *good or bad habits* cause somatic variation; and *trimming* of plants to give some shape by human.

(2) Germinal or Genetic Variation

These variations are due to change in germ cells and hence- these are transmitted to next generation. This chapter has been particularly devoted to this type of variation.

A number of *techniques to detect the genetic variation* among individuals of a population are available. These are the prediction and measurement of response to selection, measurement of inbreeding depression with its converse heterosis, protein gel electrophoresis to show variation in protein structure, and DNA sequences which show genetic variation.

2.2 GENETIC VARIATION IN NATURAL POPULATIONS

There is ample information available about the variation in populations. The variations in the phenotypes of different characteristics of organisms are caused by the underlying genetic variation. These variations can be detected and documented not only in the phenotypes of different characteristics of organisms but also related to the variation in chromosomes differences, amino acid differences in proteins synthesized by genes, and variability in nucleotide sequences of gene at molecular level.

2.2.1 Variation in Phenotypes of various Characters

The phenotypic variations in various characteristics (phenotypic traits and blood groups) of organisms have been described within many species. There is a long list of characters showing the phenotypic variability among organisms of various species. Some of the examples of phenotypic variability can be cited regarding the phenotypic variations in:

(i) Coat colours in mammals *viz.* cattle, horse, sheep, cat, rat (mice), dog;

(ii) Colours and patterns of the wings of butterflies and moths;

(iii) Colour bands and coiling patterns of the shells of landsnails;

(iv) Eye colour and eye shape in *Drosophila;*

(v) Comb colour and comb pattern in poultry, *etc.*

Such phenotypic, differences in phenotypic characteristics are known as ***polymorphisms*** (Greek word, meaning "many forms") which have underlying genetic basis.

The research works carried out in laboratory through breeding experiments on *Drosophila* collected from natural populations have shown that progeny characteristics are associated with mutant alleles. The examples of mutant genes responsible for eye colour and body colour in this species have been documented. The mutant genes were found responsible for white eye in place of red eyes (wild type) and yellow body colour instead of gray body colour (wild colour).

The analysis of blood data through pedigree analysis and population sampling have also shown polymorphisms, particularly for the blood types determined by antigens on the surfaces of cells. The studies on antigens have indicated that the different antigens are produced by different alleles and hence these alleles are polymorphic. For example, two antigens identified for Duffy blood-typing system are encoded by two different alleles of a gene locus located on chromosome number 1 and these alleles were denoted by Fy^a and Fy^b. The analyses of this blood group data in different human populations have indicated significant differences in the frequencies of the two blood groups among human populations of England, South Africa, and Korea (Cavalli-Sforza, L. L. and Adwards, A. W. F., 1967). They found that both blood groups are equally frequent and hence common among the people of England ($Fy^a = 0.42$ and $Fy^b = 0.58$) whereas only one each of the two blood group alleles was common in the area of southern Africa ($Fy^b = 0.94$) and Korea ($Fy^a = 0.99$).

2.2.2 Variation in Chromosome Structure

The variation in chromosome structure (polymorphisms) can be easily observed in the polytene chromosomes taken from salivary glands of *Drosophila* at larval stage. This is done by analyzing the banding patterns in the polytene chromosomes. The changes in the banding patterns of polytene chromosomes can be examined by breeding the *Drosophila* in laboratory to produce larvae. Such experiments have been carried out by Theodosius Dobzhansky and his collegues for more than 25 years on several species of *Drosophila*, the most important among which were *D. pseudo-obscura, D.persimilis,* and *D. Miranda* found in North America. In third chromosome of *D. pseudoobscura* natural populations, they had identified about 17 different arrangements of the banding patterns with each arrangement having one or more inversions in most common banding pattern. The Standard banding pattern (ST) in natural populations of coastal area of California and in northern Mexico was most frequent (48 to 58 percent of third chromosomes); the Arrowhead (AR) arrangement was found to the extent of 88 percent of chromosomes in Arizona, Utah, and Nevada; and Pike's Pied (PP) arrangement was observed up to 71 percent of chromosomes in Texas. Further findings have indicated significant seasonal and year variation in these arrangements. They had suggested that balancing selection had been important to maintain these polymorphisms of chromosomes in natural populations.

2.2.3 Variation in Protein Structure

The genetic variation in amino acid differences in proteins of natural populations have been detected using the protein gel electrophoresis technique by Lewontin, R.C. and Hubby, J.L. (1966) in *Drosophila* and by Harris, H (1966) in humans. This technique differentiates between different forms of a particular protein based on their movement rate through electrophoretic gel. The different forms of a protein show fast and slow movement and controlled by different alleles of the same gene locus. Thus, the individuals having different alleles are identified and this helps to estimate the allelic frequencies. The electrophoretic polymorphisms have been shown by ¼ to 1/3 of all genes that encode soluble proteins and about 12 – 15 percent of individuals within a population are heterozygous for a given polymorphic gene. The amount of genetic variability within a population is reflected conveniently from the proportion of polymorphic genes and proportion of heterozygous individuals.

Ingram, V. and colleagues (1957) showed that the sixth amino acid of the β-globin chains of sickle-cell haemoglobin was valine instead of glutamic acid found at this position in normal haemoglobin of adult human. A codon changes from GAA (glutamic acid) to GUA (valine) and thus valine is incorporated instead of a glutamic acid residue, resulting in production of another protein (abnormal protein, Hb S) and another phenotypic expression of the character (anemia, known as sickle-cell anemia).

2.2.4 Variation in Nucleotide Sequences

The DNA sequence can now be analysed to study genetic variation. The polynucleotide sequences are compared for their length. Martin Kreitman (1983) conducted analysis of nucleotide sequences in different populations of *Drosophila melanogaster* to study variability in the gene controlling alcohol dehydrogenase (*Adb*). He sequenced from different populations 11 *Adb* genes which contain 4 exons and 3 introns, catalogued the differences among these sequenced *Adb* genes, and found altogether 43 nucleotide positions as polymorphic. The majority of them were in noncoding regions of the *Adb gene* (introns or untranslated region) and in the DNA near this gene. However, the coding sequences had also some polymorphisms but only one of these polymorphisms had amino acid differences in the *Adb* polypeptide at position 192. This difference was in *lysine* versus *threonine* at this position having different mobility of the *Adb gene*. The rate of moving was faster for the polypeptide with lysine than with threonine. The rest of the nucleotide differences in the coding sequence of the *Adb gene* have no effect on the amino acid sequence of the polypeptide and hence showed ***silent polymorphism***.

Now-a-days, it is not difficult to get DNA sequences to observe genetic variation. The polymorphisms in DNA structure can be detected by sequencing cloned or PCR-amplified DNA region of interest and carrying out the sequencing of DNA products by machine. This sequence data can be analyzed by computer to identify variation among individuals to asses the level of variation in functionally different parts of DNA (exons).

Another way to know the variation at molecular level is the *gene chip* technologies. These techniques allow the screening of the single nucleotide polymorphisms (SNPs) which are present every 1-2 kb of genomic DNA. Many different genomic DNA samples may be analysed and many SNPs can be detected on a single chip by using these technologies.

2.3 SOURCES OF GENETIC VARIATION

There are different sources of genetic variation within the individual as well as among the individuals of a species. The genetic variation are thus present at individual levels, called the primary level of genetic variation and those present at population level, called the secondary level of genetic variation.

2.3.1 Primary Level of Genetic Variation

There are some genetic factors which shape and change the genetic structure of the individual. These are the ultimate sources of genetic variation at *individual level.* These can be classified as:

- ☆ Chromosomal variation that are already existing as well as those newly arising in newly arisen individual (Section 2.3 below), and
- ☆ Extra chromosomal variation (called cytoplasmic inheritance) as discussed in section 2.4 below.

2.3.2 Secondary Level of Processes causing Genetic Variation

There are genetic variations at *population level.* These processes change the genetic structure of population rather than of the individual. The different factors that change the genetic structure of a population are:

- ☆ Population size (Random genetic drift),
- ☆ Mating systems (Inbreeding and outbreeding), and
- ☆ Evolutionary forces (Selection, mutation, and migration).

These processes are the subject matter to study as a subject called *"Population Genetics"*. These are capable of molding the genetic make up of a population into new species in conformity with the environment and ecology of species.

The genetic variations produced by either level of process are ultimately fixed. The isolating mechanism either geographical or reproductive helps in the fixation of genes.

2.4 CHROMOSOMAL VARIATION

The hereditary material of all living beings is present in the nucleus of the cell. The greater part of the heritable variation has been traced to differences in nuclear genes. The *chromosomal variation* includes the existing genetic variation, variation arising from segregation and recombination of genes during meiosis, variation within individual arising from gene action and the future variation caused due to change in genetic materials.

2.4.1 Existing Genetic Variations

There exist already the differences in genetic material (genes) which have arisen due to the followings:

(i) Existence of genes in pairs at all loci in every diploid individual,

(ii) Existence of two or multiple alleles at a locus,

(iii) Existence of the number of gene loci (polygenes) affecting a character, and

(iv) Existence of sex chromosomes.

The two or more alleles (multiple alleles) of a locus may or may not be similar but different in structure and produce different phenotypes if different in structure.

2.4.2 Newly arisen Genetic Variation

Some of the genetic variations arises a fresh due to the followings:

(i) Chromosomal aberrations

(ii) Gene mutation,

(iii) Gene segregation

(iv) Recombination of genes on zygote formation

(v) Gene action or expression *viz.* additive and non additive gene action

1. Gene Present in Pairs

The genes are present in pairs on the chromosomes found in the nucleus. The two alleles at a locus may or may not be similar but different in structure and produce different phenotypes if different in structure. The differences between genes at the same locus result variation in genotype. The proof that the genes are present in pairs at a particular locus is evidenced by the existence of heterozygotes for that locus. The mating of heterozygous individuals at a locus (Aa × Aa) produces 3 genotypes, 25 per cent (1/4) of the total will be homozygous for each of the extreme genotype (AA, aa) while the rest 50 per cent will be heterozygous.

The genetic variation is demonstrated by the fact that three genotypes are produced by mating two heterozygous individuals for a locus. Thus a wide variety of genotypes are present in a population of animals. Differences among genotypes give rise to the genetic variation in a species with respect to a quantitative trait.

2. Multiple Alleles

The number of multiple alleles at some loci are also present in the population and this also gives rise to genetic variation. These multiple alleles are all different in their structure and hence produce different phenotypes. The number of multiple alleles at one locus of cattle has been recorded as many as 300. The numbers of multiple alleles vary at different loci.

3. No. of Genes at each Chromosome

The exact number of gene loci on a chromosome in any species of farm animals is not known. With two genes, segregating independently, 6.25 per cent of the F_2 individuals (1/16 of the total individuals) will be homozygous for each of the extreme genotypes (AA BB, aa bb). When 4 genes are segregating only one individual in 256 (1/256 or 0.39 per cent) will be homozygous for each of the extreme genotype and rest will be heterozygous. This reduces the chance of extreme genotype and thus heterozygosity is more. In this way, with the increase in number of gene loci affecting a trait, the genetic variation is created.

The two alleles at a locus differ in their frequencies. The traits affected either by one or many gene pairs may vary in a population because of the differences in the frequency of two alleles at a locus and at several different loci.

An individual heterozygous for only one gene pair (*Aa*) produces two types of gametes (*A* and *a*). The individual heterozygous for *n* pairs of genes produces genotypic combinations in the progeny equal to $(10^n)^2$. This results in innumerable combinations of genes producing great diversity due to sexual reproduction and allows more chances of suitable and desired selection.

The ***number of different kinds of gametes*** produced by heterozygous individual for ***n*** pairs of genes are 2^n that are distributed according to the coefficients of binomial expanded to the nth power $(½ + ½)^n$. The ***number of genotypes*** produced in F_2 will be 3^n which will be distributed among homozygote and heterozygote as:

No. of genotypes = No. of homozygote + no. of heterozygote

$$3^n = 2^n + (3^n - 2^n)$$

The ***number of phenotypic classes*** in F_2 generation will be 2n + 1 and the ratio of phenotypic classes in F_2 generation as $[2n!/k!\,(2n-k)!]\,(½)^{2n}$. The ***k*** is the number of contributing genes in the genotype. The number of phenotypic classes of quantitative traits increases in arithmetic way with an increase in the number of gene pairs (n) on the assumption that the genes are segregating independently with additive and cumulative effects, having equal gene frequencies and unaffected by environment.

4. Sex Linked Genes

The simple autosomal variation or autosomal inheritance was discussed assuming that both the parents (male and female) contribute equally to the genotype of the progeny and it is considered as simple pattern of inheritance. Besides the autosomes, the sex chromosomes have some genes which affect certain traits.

The parents for sex linked genes do not contribute equally to the offspring. In mammals and Drosophila the females transmit a *random* of X chromosome to her offspring regardless of the sex of offspring while the males transmit the X chromosome to the female progeny and Y chromosome to the male progeny. Therefore, the female progeny receive equal inheritance from both parents for sex linked genes but the male progeny receive the genes only from their mother. The reverse is true in those species in which the males are homogametic and females heterogametic. The recessive white eye mutation was the first sex linked gene (X^W) found in Drosophila and it was a mutant form of the wild (and dominant sex linked) gene for red eye (X^W). For the sex linked single locus trait with two alleles, the females produce 3 genotypes *viz.* $X^+ X^+$, $X^+ X^W$, $X^W X^W$, while the males produce only two genotypes *viz.* $X^+ Y$ and $X^W Y$, and thus providing 3 genotypic values (a, d, -a) by females and 2 values (a,-a) by the males.

The reciprocal crosses involving autosomal traits (the traits controlled by genes present on autosomes), produce equal results. But for sex linked traits governed by genes present on sex chromosome (X or Z chromosome) the different results are produced by reciprocal crossings. When the sex linked recessive allele is present in the male parent, the reciprocal cross results in the disappearance of the trait in the F_1 but reappears if males of the F_2. This is called as criss-cross or skip type of inheritance which characteristics the sex linked genes.

5. Variation from Gene Mutations

Gene mutation or point mutation is a process by which new alleles of a gene are produced. The mutation occurs due to change in DNA during its replication. The DNA replication is an essential process of producing another copy of DNA which is exactly similar to the original DNA. The formation of a new allele is the result of amino acid substitution.

The mutation changes one allele into another one at a locus. This new allele is different in structure and function as well to the origin. The process of changing or converting one allele (say, A) into another one (say, a) at the locus is known as mutation. When two or more alleles are present at a locus, it is taken that either of the allele has arisen or produced by mutation from the other. Thus different alleles at a locus (say, for example, A, a, a′, A′ *etc.*) arise only due to mutation. The mutation is the only source of new allele (s) at a locus. The existence of two or more alleles at a locus produces genetic variation which gives rise to new genotype and hence new phenotype to the individual. The rate of gene mutation is very low and varies for individual loci, chromosome and species.

6. Changes in Number and Structure of Chromosome (Chromosomal Aberrations)

Besides the gene mutation, changes in chromosomes either in their structure or number have been observed. The chromosomal changes have been exploited by plant breeders to produce new variety or species whereas in farm animals the chromosomal changes are of evolutionary significance. Cytological studies have revealed two types of changes in chromosomes, namely numerical and structural.

The *numerical change* is the change in the actual number of chromosomes which involve change in entire set of disomic chromosomes called the *euploidy viz.* Haploid (n), Diploid (2n), Polyploid (triploid. (3n), tetraploid (4n), pentaploid (5n)), and the change that involve only single chromosome within a set called the aneuplody *viz.* Nullisomic, (2n-2), monosomic (2n-l), polysomic (trisomic *2n+1*, tetrasomic 2n+2, pentasomic 2n+3.).

Second is the *structural change* which means the loss, gain or rearrangement of particular section of chromosome. Thus there is a change in the number or arrangement of the loci within the whole chromosome complex. In general, these changes have been classed as deficiencies (deletions) which represent a loss in chromosomal material or duplications which represent the gain of a section of a chromosome in excess of the normal amount, rearrangement of the genetic material with the same amount of genetic material. The rearrangement is of two type *viz.* inversion and translocation. The frequency of chromosomal aberration is very low and hence it is not a common cause of genetic variation in animals.

Chromosomal aberrations are brought to light by discrepancies in the breeding behaviour of those individuals affected with these changes. This results in the appearance of variable offspring in the formation of new linkage relations, or in disturbances of the normal expected Mendelian ratios *etc.* These changes are found to have close correspondence with the chromosomal changes as evidenced by cytological studies. The chromosomal theory of inheritance is strongly supported by this close correspondence.

In some situation a portion of a chromosome becomes inverted resulting the reversion in the gene order. This is called inversion. The inversion may happen due to the chromosome becoming looped and breaking of the chromosome with healing of the ends in reversed order. Thus the order of gene is changed. Sometimes the broken pieces of a chromosome become attached to a non-homologous chromosome and this is known as translocation.

7. Gene Segregation (Crossing Over)

The Chromosomes are present in pairs and hence the alleles (genes) at each pair of chromosome are also present in pairs at the homologous chromosome. There is exchange of the parts of homologous chromosomes and *segregation of genes* during meiosis which is a requirement of gamete formation in sexually mature animal of both the sexes. This process of exchanging the parts of homologous chromosomes is called the crossing over. After the process of crossing over is completed the homologous chromosomes are divided equally in two daughter cells called as the gametes. This process of crossing over produces two types of the gametes (parental and recombinants) and the genes present on homologous chromosomes are segregated in two gametes having half of the total DNA in each gamete. These gametes contain one chromosome of each pair of homologous chromosome and this contains half the number of chromosomes. This half number of chromosomes is called as haploid dose of chromosome. These newly formed chromosomes, after crossing over, have combination of gens different from the original (parental) chromosomes.

8. Recombination (Redistribution of Genes)

This is the primary source of genetic variation with immense potential. The chromosomes are present in pairs. The two members of each chromosome pair are homologous (similar in size and shape). Those two members of each chromosome pair segregate (separate) from each other during meiotic cell division to form two gametes each containing half the members of chromosomes present in parental cell. The two gametes from opposite sex are united at fertilization to form zygote that gives rise to a new living individual. The segregation and recombination of chromosomes create a very great possibility for the formation of different genotypes in progeny generation. The possibilities of forming new genotype are unlimited owing to the presence of hundreds of gene loci on each chromosome. This produces genetic variability in each succeeding generation. The new genotypes give rise to new phenotype. This makes practically impossible to produce any two progeny (individual) by any pair of parents to have identical genetic makeup. The recombination of genes results when the zygote is formed as a result of the chromosomes coming together from the uniting gametes. One of the two chromosomes of a pair goes to each of two gametes formed during the process of meiosis. These two gametes will be different from each other because of some heterozygous loci on the chromosome pair. The other factor of producing different gametes is the crossing over phenomenon during meiosis. In different primary germ cells of the same animal, many types of gametes are formed due to crossing over because several loci are heterozygous. The mating of two heterozygous animals for a single locus, for example, will produce two gametes by each parent with three different genotypes in the progeny as shown below:

Parents genotype	Aa	X	Aa
Gametes	A and a	↓	A and a
Progeny genotypes	AA,	Aa,	aa

Similarly, if the two mated individuals are heterozygous for two loci, four different types of gametes will be formed by each parent with nine different genotypes in the progeny as shown below

Parents	Aa Bb		X	Aa Bb	
Gametes	AB and Ab		↓	aB and ab	
Progeny	AABB	AABb	AAbb	AaBB	AaBb
-Genotypes	Aabb	aaBB	aaBb	aabb	

If two animals were heterozygous for three pairs of genes eight different types of gametes will be produced by each parent *viz.* ABC, ABc, AbC, Abc, aBC, aBc, abC, abc with 27 different genotypes in the progeny. Thus the kinds of gametes and the progeny genotypes will depend upon the number of loci and the type of genes on each locus (homozygous or heterozygous). This can be illustrated with the help of the following example, considering 5 loci for each of the two parents as:

Male	Aa	bb	CC	Dd	EE
Female	Aa	Bb	cc	DD	EE

In this case the number of genotypes in the progeny will be 3 at the A locus (AA, Aa, aa), 2 at B locus (Bb, bb), I at C locus (Cc), 2 at D locus (DD, Dd) and 1 at E locus (EE) making a total number of genotypes in the progeny as $3 \times 2 \times 1 \times 2 \times 1 = 12$. Thus 12 genotypes (full brothers or sisters) are possible to be produced from this type of mating. All the progeny from this mating have identical pedigree, but their genotypes will be different ranging from AA Bb Cc DD EE to aa bb Cc Dd EE. Thus the full brothers or sisters will differ greatly if the capital letters denote the desirable alleles and the smalls as undesirable. It can thus be concluded that the identity of pedigree does not mean the identity of inheritance, because the parents are heterozygous for some pairs of genes and practically heterozygosity is mostly prevalent except among highly inbred lines.

In the above examples only 1, 2, 3, 5 pairs of genes were considered. The exact number of genes located on each chromosome is not known exactly. The number of genes is in hundreds on each chromosome and the numbers of pairs of chromosomes vary from 19 in swine to 30 in cattle and goat. Taking the cattle as an example there would be a total of 6000 genes considering 100 genes on each chromosome. Thus each parent will transmit 3000 genes.

For a simple locus heterozygous on each of n chromosome pairs, there will be 2^3 possible numbers of gametes from each parent and 3^n progeny genotypes by mating individuals with heterozygous genes on each chromosome pair. Considering the case of cattle for 3000 gene pairs (hypothetical), and assuming that all combinations were possible due to the independent assortment and crossing over, there will be 3^{3000} different progeny genotypes. Even if it is assumed that the linkage is complete in all chromosomes, there will be $2^{30} = 1073741824$ different recombination of complete chromosomes. This indicates tremendous amount of genetic variation from recombination, and provides a proof of any two full brothers or sisters and parent offspring being different from each other.

On mating each parent transmits only one of the two gametes (carrying only half of the total DNA) to each of its progeny. These form the new combinations of existing genes. The whole process of crossing over, segregation of chromosomes and the combination of the chromosomes at fertilization is called as the genetic recombination. This genetic recombination though creates no new gene but put (arrange) the genes into new combinations and hence produces genetic variability that give to the phenotypic variability in new generation.

9. Types of Gene Action

Variation in Gene expression- The greater part of the genetic variation (heritable variation) is mainly attributed to the differences in genes effect. The differences in genotypes give rise to the variation of two kinds *viz.* additive effects of genes, in the form of differences between homozygotes which is heritable and fixable component of variation, and the second is the interaction effect of genes depending on the special properties of heterozygotes which is not heritable.

(*i*) *Additive Gene Action*: The effect of substituting one allele for another at any of the loci (average effect of gene substitution) forms the main and basic type of genetic variation.

(*ii*) *Non-Additive Gene Action*: The entire genetic variation is not additive type and fixable. The interaction between genes present on the same locus or on different loci occurs to produce the genes combination effects. The gene interaction is indicated when a gene produces a different effect in the presence of other gene than in its absence. The interaction is of two types depending upon the location of genes on the chromosome *e.g.* the interaction between genes which are alleles (present on the same locus) or between genes which are not alleles (present on the different loci). The first type is called the allelic or intra-allelic interaction. The examples are the dominance, incomplete or partial dominance and over-dominance.

The second type (interaction between genes which are not alleles) is called the non-allelic or inter-allelic interaction commonly referred as the epistasis. The genes which are not alleles may be present on different loci of the same chromosomes or of different chromosome. The genes at one locus influence the effect of gene at another locus. Therefore, it is the interaction of two or more pairs of genes that are not alleles.

The gene interaction causes only a small part of genetic variation as evidenced from the partitioning of genetic variance.

(*iii*) *Multiplicative gene action* - Some genes act in a multiplicative way forming a geometric series such as 2, 4, 8, 16 representing the contribution of 1, 2, 3, 4 active alleles, respectively. The effect of multiplicative genes increases in a multiplicative increment and form a geometric series rather than in arithmetic or additive increment (which is in case of additive gene action). For example, the geometric mean of 1.4 and 3.6 = 1.4 x 3.6 = 2.24 forming the geometric series 1.4, 2.2, 3.6, 5.7 .... which is increasing by a multiple increment of 0.6. The arithmetic mean of 1.4 and 3.6 is (1.4 + 3.6)/2 = 2.5 forming arithmetic series 1.4, 2.5, 3.6, 4.7 which is increasing by an additive increment of 1.1. Some examples of multiplicative gene action are known in tomato for mean fruit weight.

2.5 EXTRA-CHROMOSOMAL VARIATIONS

These variations involve the plasmatic factors called as plasma genes or cytogenes or plasmids (cytoplasmic factors). The ***cytoplasm*** is the protoplasm of a cell outside the nucleus in which cell organelles (plasmids, mitochondria, golgi body, etc) reside or all living parts of the cell except the nucleus. The inheritance (hereditary transmission) controlled by cytoplasmic factors (cytoplasm or cytoplasmic structures *viz.* plasmid characters in plants) rather than the nuclear genes is called as ***cytoplasmic inheritance*** or extra-chromosomal inheritance. The cytoplasmic factors do not contribute to genetic variation in metric traits. Therefore, the variation in metric traits due to cytoplasm is not important.

The DNA present in nucleus is the genetic material and is the store house of genetic information for most of the characteristics. The chromosome complement in the male and female individual is the same and the genes from male and female parents contribute equally to the genetic constitution of the progeny. Based on equal contribution of two parents to progeny generation, the reciprocal crosses between homozygous parents should give the similar results in terms of producing the progeny of identical phenotype except the sex linked inheritance.

However, the studies have shown that some *extra-nuclear genes* or DNA molecules are also present outside the nucleus in the cytoplasm. Thus, the genetic information exists in the cytoplasm also. The female parent contributes more cytoplasm to the zygote, it is expected that there should be differences in the results of reciprocal crosses for the characters having cytoplasmic control. If the reciprocal crosses differ, it would be due to the maternal effect as a result of contribution of cytoplasm. This is the *criteria for testing the role of cytoplasmic inheritance.* The possible role of cytoplasm in the inheritance of certain characters was suggested by Sangers and his colleagues in 1950's. The inheritance of certain characters in *Chlamydomous* is controlled by non-chromosomal genes and hence the inheritance is independent of chromosomal genes. It was found that in these cases the cytoplasm has self perpetuating hereditary factors which are formed of DNA. The factors of cytoplasm are called plasmon or plasmagenes.

The *cytoplasmic DNA* has been indentified by autoradiography, electron microscopy, Feulgen staining, and density gradient centrifugation. The DNA is present in plastids of plants and algae, and mitochondria of both plant and animal cells. These cell organelles in plants contain their own DNA and protein-synthesizing apparatus. The electron microscopy have shown that cytoplasmic DNA is thinner than the protein covered DNA rnolecule of eukaryotic nuclear chromosome and have thin fibrous appearance believed to be naked nonhistone DNA like that found in prokaryotes. The DNA present in chloroplasts and mitochondria is double stranded which replicate semi-conservatively. The chloroplasts of certain algae contain circular DNA.

The characters showing cytoplasmic inheritance have *maternal influence.* This is because most of the cytoplasm of the zygote is contributed by the female gamete and moreover if there are some hereditary units present in the cytoplasm, these are expected to be transmitted to the progeny.

The cytoplasmic inheritance and or maternal effects are indicated from the followings:

- ☆ The characters controlled by cytoplasmic inheritance show differences between the results of reciprocal crosses. The reciprocal crosses produce the progeny of different phenotypes.
- ☆ The characteristics of the mother are exhibited by the progeny for such characters. Thus, the genotype of the mother determines the phenotype of the progeny rather than genotype of the progeny.
- ☆ Such characters do not show segregation like nuclear born genes.

The expression of certain characteristics of the progeny is not due to their own genotype but is influenced by their maternal parent. In mammals, the mother may affect the development of their offspring through egg cytoplasm as well as through the intra-uterine environment *viz.* maternal effect on the birth weight via maternal nutrition, embryonic defects caused by maternal diabetes. The maternal effects are taken when the mother contributes to the phenotypic expression of her progeny besides that being produced from nuclear borne genes.

The ***maternal effect*** is also taken as a trait controlled by a gene of the mother but expressed in the progeny. Such a gene whose product acts in the progeny of the female who carries the gene is called the ***Maternal-effect gene***. The inheritance controlled by extra-chromosomal (cytoplasmic) factors that are inherited through the egg is called the ***Maternal- inheritance***.

Causes of Maternal Effects

The maternal effects may arise in one or other of the following manners-

1. Maternal Environment

(*i*) *The maternal nutrition* in mammals produces the maternal effects. The example is the birth weight. The heavier dams produce heavier progeny because of the better and adequate nutrients supply to the foetus. The reciprocal crosses have shown that birth weight is a maternal trait, because the birth weight of the progeny deviates from mid parent value towards the birth weight of maternal breed (Tomar, 1979).

(ii) *Seedling characters* in plants show maternal effects which are diminished with increasing age, *e.g.* radio sensitivity in the tomato (first true leaves and second leaves), length of first seedling leaf in the rye grass, juvenile traits (characters expressed in early age) of sexual offspring.

The cytoplasmic inheritance differs from the maternal effects in the sense that the effects of plasmagenes do not disappear after one generation but persist as long as such plasmogenes are capable to self perpetuation.

2. Cytoplasmic Factors

The following are some of the examples of maternal effects with *cytoplasmic factors:*

(i) *Maternal effect for* ***shell coiling in snail*** (*Limnaea pegera*- water snail): In snails, there are two types of cleavages depending on the direction of coiling and these are genetically controlled. The first type is known as dextral coiling in which the coiling is clockwise (shell coiled towards the right), found in most of the cases and controlled by dominant gene (D) so that dextral is DD. The second type is known as sinistral cleavage (coiling) in which coiling is counter clockwise (shell coiled towards left), found in some cases and controlled by recessive allele (d) so that sinistral is dd. Thus normal dextral are normal while sinistrals are mutants. The two alleles of a gene pair are inherited as per Mendelian laws. However, the action of any genetic combination is expressed only in the next generation after the one in which a given genotype is found. It is important that the type of coiling produced from reciprocal crosses is determined by the genotype and not by the phenotype of the female parent.

In the reciprocal crosses, the heterozygous genotype Dd may be dextral as well as sinistral and this depends on the genotype of the female parent. In a similar way, if the genotype of the female parent is dominant (Dd), the dd genotype will turn in dextral coiling. Thus the phenotype of the female parent does not have any effect on the phenotype of the progeny but it is the genotype of the female parent which decides the coiling pattern of the progeny. Therefore, the coiling character is determined by the gene of the mother and not by the individual's own gene. The results of reciprocal crosses can be summarized as under:

(a) Dextral female (DD) x Sinistral male (dd): All the F_1 snails (Dd) have dextral coiling because of dextral mother. Also all the F_2 progeny have dextral coiling irrespective of their homozygous recessive genotype (dd) that are supposed to develop sinistral coiling with genotype dd. But the dd genotype of F_2 snail develops dextral coiling because the F_1 mother was dextral (Dd).

(b) Sinistral female (dd) x Dextral male (DD): All the F_1 progeny (Dd) developed sinistral coiling, though they were heterozygous and should have develop dextral. This was because the genotype of mother was sinistral (dd). All the F_2 developed dextral coiling irrespective of their recessive genotype (dd) supposed to develop sinistral. This was because the F_2 progeny were produced from F_1 mother having genotype as Dd (dominant gene for dextral).

(*ii*) *Maternal effect of* ***pigment production in eyes of flour mouth*** *and in water flea:* The normal eye colour is dark due to dominant gene, in both these invertebrates. The pigment production in eyes depends on a pair of nuclear born gene showing dominance relation between two alleles. The dominant gene (A) produces a substance known as *kynurenine* which produces pigment (causing production of dark eyes) whereas the recessive allele fails to develop the pigment. In this case, the gene A produces a pigment precursor, kynurenine which is involved in pigment synthesis and restored in the cytoplasm of the eggs (ova). In flour moth, the gene A is dominant to produce darkening of skin producing dark eyes. The recessive gene a fails to develop pigment and the eyes are red. A cross of recessive female (aa) with heterozygous male (Aa) produce only half of the larvae which show dark pigment in the eye while the reciprocal cross (Aa female with aa male) produces all larvae with dark eyes.

(*iii*) ***Respiratory deficiency*** *in yeast* (Sacchoromyces cerevisiae): In the presence of sugar glucose, the growth of yeast is slow (producing very small size colonies, called petites) because they are unable to utilize oxygen in the metabolism of carbohydrates. This respiratory deficiency in yeast prevents growth on carbon source and prevents them (petite) from producing spores. The petites mated with normal yeast cells produce three petite varieties. (a) *nuclear or segregational petites* which follow Mendelian segregation; (b) *neutral petities*, caused by an extra chromosomal factor because they follow non- Mendelian behaviour, produces only wild type ascospores and colonies and the petite trait never appears, in further generation; (c) *suppressive petities* which suppress normal respiratory behaviour in crosses with normal strains, and segregate in a manner different from chromosomal genes.

(iv) ***Slow and normal spore germination*** *trait in fungus* (Neurospora): The reciprocal crosses of two stains of fungus with slow and normal germination produce different results. The slow germination trait persists when each generation is backcrossed with normal germination strain. Such type of inheritance is possible if the cytoplasm carries some hereditary units for the expression of a character.

(v) ***Male sterility*** *in plants*: There is pollen failure in many flowering plants which results in male sterility, like wheat, maize, onion *etc.* In these plants, the fertility is controlled to some extent by cytoplasmic factors. The male sterility in corn which is caused by the failure of pollen to develop properly (the sterility factor is not present on chromosome) is the example of cytoplasmic inheritance. The male sterility in maize is controlled by cytoplasm. If the female parent is male sterile, the F_1 progeny will also be male sterile. This is due the reason that cytoplasm was of the female parent male sterile.

(vi) ***Plastid inheritance*** *in four o'clock and corn:* There are three types of leaves and branches in four O'clock plant depending on the presence of plastids *viz. full green leaves* having chloroplast, *white* (pale leaves and branches) with no chloroplast and the *variegated branches* (mixed green white) with leucoplast in white area and chloroplast in green area. The colour of the progeny depends on the branch colour of female parent and is due to the production of chlorophyll by the plastids (chloroplast) present in cytoplasm. The chlorophyll pigment of chloroplast is related to photosynthetic prepared food. The leucoplast cannot perform photosynthesis and the pale parts take food from green parts. Similarly, is the inheritance of the character (Iojap) with contrasting strips of green and white colours on leaves of a maize plant.

3. Transmission of Pathogens and Antibodies

Via prenatal blood supply or by post natal feeding (*Infective particles*): The followings are the examples of cytoplasmic inheritance:

(*i*) *Inheritance of* ***kappa particle*** *in Paramecium* (*Protozoa*): Some cytoplasmic factors are not self perpetuating and disappear unless replaced by the effect of a nuclear gene. Thus, there is a relationship between a nuclear gene and a cytoplasmic factor. The Kappa particle in paramecium is reproduced in the presence of a nuclear gene (K) in some strains of protozoa (paramecium). Kappa seems to be an infective particle with a hereditary continuity of its own. The kappa particle produces a toxin substance (paramecin) which is toxic to the strains not having kappa (sensitive strain). The kappa particle is produced by a dominant allele.

(*ii*) *Inheritance of* ***sigma particle*** *in Drosophila:* There are certain characters for which the cytoplasmic characters are transmitted by infection *e.g.*

sensitivity of CO_2 in a strain of Drosophila. The sensitivity factor is carried by the cytoplasm of the egg. Injection of body fluid from a sensitive fly into a non-sensitive fly can induce sensitivity. This sensitivity to CO_2 is inherited on a maternal basis called infective heredity.

(*iii*) ***Breast tumour*** *in mice:* The maternal effect by way of transmission of pathogen through parental blood supply or post-natal feeding is evident in case of development of *mammary cancer or breast tumour in mouse.* The cross fostering experiment showed that the development of mammary cancer is responsible to carry the factor. It is found to be maternally transmitted or having cytoplasmic inheritance. Recent studies have shown that this character is developed through mother's milk, known as milk fever, as a result of the presence of some virus in milk.

Chapter 3

Heredity and Environment

There had been controversies in early days regarding the relative importance of heredity and environment. It is now clear that both are important. The potentiality of an individual is determined by heredity (genetic constitution) called as genetic potentiality which is achieved by the proper environment. The control mechanism for differentiation, organization, and growth in living beings responsible for the development and carrying out the living activities are dependent on both the genetic and environmental factors. The development of living system is so complex to understand all the possible steps involved in the expression of any one characteristic.

Some genes do have their consistent effect to produce the phenotypic effects under all sort of environmental diversities but other genes respond differently and the phenotype appears as a result of close-knit interaction or cooperative result of many factors. For the development of a character neither genes nor environmental influences can be solely responsible but it is their cooperative result and one or the other factor may have negligible effect. Thus, both heredity and environmental influences work together for the development and expression of a character via many individual steps involving interaction between the genotype and environment. The gene action is affected by biological and physical factors in the environment. Some of the examples of modification of action of major genes in different environments have been given in this chapter.

3.1 RELATIVE ROLE OF HEREDITY AND ENVIRONMENT

Environmental dependence of genotypes has been covered here mainly for the modification of expression of major genes in relation to change in environment. A number of characters can be enlisted with the relative influence of variability in hereditary or in environmental factors acting upon them.

(1) In some cases the environment may be more effective and the heredity, being similar in all the individuals, may not have any effect in the variation of the character. The example of *measles* fits beautifully in this category, in which everyone inherits susceptibility to it but its occurrence depends entirely on the environmental contact of the individual with the causative agent.

(2) There is a second category of characters which are more affected by the heredity and no environment of sufficient potency can alter the expression of genes present and responsible for. The *ABO blood groups* in human are remarkably stable in most environments to which the human beings are subjected. The gene for antigen A always produce antigen A in the cells regardless of environmental influences and the antigen A is not developed in the absence of gene producing it. There are only a very few environmental conditions, such as the *disease leukemia*, which change the blood type of a particular person.

(3) There is third category of characters in which the variations are found due to both the heredity and the environment. The body weight and other *quantitative characters* have genetic component but are more influenced by the diet of the individual and other environmental factors.

Susceptibility to *diphtheria* is dependent on a simple gene and immunity by its dominant allele. But for the contraction of the disease, infection with the causative agent is necessary. The individuals with inherited immunity (resistance) to diphtheria would not have the disease upon infection to the bacillus but with inherited susceptibility would develop it. Therefore, the heredity has the variable effect in this case. In another situation, the individuals with inherited susceptibility to disease will have the disease on exposure to the pathogen but unexposed individuals will not have. This is the case of variable effect of environment.

This leads to the confusion because in one case the diphtheria was the result of hereditary influence but in another it may be concluded that environment was responsible. Further, an example may be taken when a person is made artificially immune to diphtheria (by means of toxin antitoxin) in spite of the inherited susceptibility. However, it does neither mean that he does not inherit the susceptibility nor that he will not transmit the susceptibility. The assumption of the heredity and the environmental effect for a condition cannot be invalidated by the fact that a causative agent is known for a condition nor that the condition can be changed or cured. On the other hand, it does not mean that a genetically determined abnormality cannot be controlled by the requisite environmental manipulation. Thus, all the characters are limited by hereditary and environmental effects realizing that the heredity is a relative term, when the variation in the character is caused mainly by differences in the genetic makeup of the individual.

The different behavior of similar genotypes in different environment is the basic fact of gene action. However, this never means that the gene might have been changed but it may be that the reactions controlled by the gene are influenced by the environment. High temperature promotes the chemical reactions more rapidly than a low temperature. There may be cited a number of examples of conspicuous inherited characteristics which are influenced by the environmental conditions.

3.2 ENVIRONMENTAL FACTORS AND EXPRESSION OF MAJOR GENES

The environmental factors controlling the qualitative characters may be external environmental factors which affect the population as a whole and the internal environmental factors which affect at individual level.

(I) External Environmental Factors

The various external environmental factors affecting the expression of major genes are the temperature, sunlight, nutrition, and cultural conditions.

1. Temperature

The temperature can play a very significant role in gene expression. Chemical reaction proceeds more rapidly at high temperature than at low temperature. The basic developmental effect of many genes is to control the rate of specific reaction and a change in temperature can be expected to have an effect on development. It is not necessary that the genes act during the temperature effective period but the gene may have its action earlier and the period may coincide with an embryological process at the time of utilization of gene product. It may also be possible that a substance required for the gene action is produced during the temperature effective period.

The temperature influences the *coat colour* in Himalayan rabbit and Siamese cats which are born white but later develop black pigment at the extremities like paw (feet), nose, ears and tail. The animals develop no colour at birth because they have the body temperature of the mother in *utero*. The dark colour is developed, as the animals grow, at the extremities where the temperature is somewhat lower than body temperature. The black pigment (melanin) responsible to produce colour in skin is genetically controlled. The gene responsible for black colour causes the production of an enzyme which is necessary for the formation of a black pigment. However, this enzyme is produced at slightly low body temperature than at normal temperature. The enzyme is inactivated at high temperature. Therefore, the black pigment is formed only on the extremities of the body (nose, ears, feet and tail) where the temperature is relatively lower than main parts of the body which are white in colour.

A strong temperature effect has been shown on the formation of melanin pigment responsible for development of black colour. The experiment with Himalayan rabbit indicated that shaving off the fur from the animal and keeping the animal under changed temperature results in change of colour. If the environment (temperature) is changed, after removing the dark fur, by keeping the animal under warm condition, the white fur grow instead of dark fur. On the other hand, if the white fur is removed and the animal is kept under cold condition, the fur grown is black. Thus, the phenotypic expression of the genes (for pigment formation) depends on the temperature at the time of fur growth.

The *development of wings* in Drosophila is also influence by temperature. The gene affects the organs of Drosophila to develop into wings in 35 per cent individuals raised at high temperature (25° C) and it cases a reduced penetrance from 35 to only 1 per cent if the flies are raised at low temperature (17° C).

The *number of facets in Bar-eye mutation* is another character in Drosophila affected by temperature. The rearing of Drosophila at high temperature has been found to develop *Bar eye* compared to that reared at low temperature. The number of facets decreases in Bar-mutation with the increase in temperature from 15° C to 31° C, while for an allele of Bar-mutation, known as *Infrabar,* the number of facets increases with the increase in temperature. Temperature changes during the period from 90 to 97 hours after fertilization influences the Bar eye in Drosophila. The eyes of Drosophila have about 50 facets at 35° C during this period and about 150 facets at 25° C compared with 700 to 800 facets for wild type.

The *Bristle formation* in Drosophila is also influenced with the changes in temperature at any time throughout larval and pupal stages.

Likewise, the phenotype of the *shibire* (a Japanese word indicating paralysis) mutation in Drosophila is an example. The shibire flies are viable and fertile at normal temperature of 25° C, but they are sensitive to a sudden shock. The shibire flies fall to the bottom of the culture if the culture is shaken but they not only fall to the bottom of the culture but also die if the culture is kept at a slightly high temperature 0f 29° C. This shows that flies with shibire mutation are temperature sensitive because the mutant allele for shibire phenotype is lethal at slightly higher temperature but viable at normal temperature. Such a behavior of shibire flies can be explained the mutant allele produces a partially functional protein at normal temperature but this protein becomes nonfunctional at 29° C.

The small water insect, Daphnia, commonly found in ponds, show temperature sensitivity to their *survival*. They survive at 20° C and die when the temperature goes to 27° C. On the other hand, a mutant type of this water flea survives and thrives in warmer temperature (25° C - 30° C) and dies at low temperature (20° C).

2. Sunlight

The sunlight has also been found to change the expression of genes. The ability of genes to express themselves in relation to sunlight is more evident in plants. The light provides energy and is essential for growth and development of all plants. The plants grown in dark do not develop chlorophyll and therefore appear as albino, although they have genes for chlorophyll.

Hypersensitivity to sunlight is heritable trait in Southdown sheep. The liver of the affected individuals fails to function properly and the by-product of metabolism (Phyllaerythrin) is not excreted but starts accumulating in bloodstream and skin whereby activated by sunlight, causing the *eczema to develop on face and ears* which may become fatal if the animals are exposed to sunlight. But the animals are free from symptoms if kept indoors away from sunlight and allowed to graze during night hours.

Cancer eyes of Hereford cattle is believed to be inherited and provoked (frequently developed) in areas of intense sunshine, developed in younger animals maintained on high plane of nutrition and more incidence in white eyed than in pigmented eyelid cattle.

The *face freckling* (spotting) occurs among the people of certain genotypes exposed to sun. The potentiality to produce freckles was acted upon by sunlight to produce different phenotypic extremities. Few freckles were developed on the face of a girl who worked indoors as compared to many freckles developed on the face of its identical twin girl who worked out in the sun.

3. Nutrition and Culture Conditions

The nutrition (food) has many functions providing energy and material necessary for structural functions. Any living individual cannot show its full genetic potential in lack of nutrition.

The change in physical environment (diet) may leads to a change in the expression of genotypes. The diet rich in amino acid, phenylalanine in the children with recessive genotype (***pp***) develop a disease called ***phenyl-keton-urea* (PKU).** The clinical impact of this disease can be reduced by keeping the children having recessive genotype (PKU homozygous) on a low phenylalanine diet after birth.

The appearance of *yellow fat in rabbit* depends on two factors – one is the recessive gene in homozygous condition (yy) and second is inclusion of green vegetable in the diet (xanthophylls). The yellow fat disappears if the diet is devoid of green fodder. An enzyme found in the liver control the process of breakdown of certain yellow compound (Xanthophyll) of the green diet. The breakdown of Xanthophyll to colourless derivatives does not occur when the rabbit lacks the enzyme and the Xanthophyll is stored as such in the animal's fat giving it yellow colour. Thus, the difference between white and yellow fat rabbits is caused due to the presence or absence of enzyme. The allelic alternatives Y and y determines the presence or absence of the enzymatic function. A single dose of Y allele is sufficient to produce enzyme needed to breakdown all the Xanthophyll eaten by the rabbit. The genotype yy produce white fat on a Xanthophyll free diet. Therefore, the genes determine the potentialities which ate exploited by the environment under which the genes perform their functions.

Abnormal abdomen in Drosophila (irregular abnormal segments) is affected by environment (culture condition). This abnormality is caused by a gene but abnormality is developed in the flies which hatched first when the culture bottles are moist and it is not expressed in the flies which hatched later or grown in bottles having less moisture, even the flies carry the gene. Thus, the environment is the determining factor in the expression of gene to develop the character (abnormality, in this case).

The *crooked calf* (deformities of front legs) are developed by feeding lupine and high level of lead during pregnancy or feeding of diet low in manganese.

The *Cyclopean malformed lambs* (single eye centrally located) can be produced by feeding the weed *veratum californicum* during early pregnancy.

(II) Internal Environmental Factors

There are various internal environmental factors which influence the expression of major genes. These factors include hormones, age of the organism, and chemical environment.

1. Hormones

The hormones are also important in this respect. The genes for growth cannot express themselves due to lack of growth hormone produced by anterior pituitary gland. A gene has been reported to cause *dwarfism in mice* through failure of the production of growth hormone.

The phenotypic differences between two sexes are observed in reproductive structures, secondary sexual characteristics, growth pattern, and behavior of each sex. These sex differences are associated either with different sex chromosomes present in two sexes (sex-linked traits) or due to different sex hormones that results the expression of genes differently in two sexes (***sex limited traits and sex influenced traits***). The detail discussion on these characters has been given in chapter 7.

2. Age of Animal

It is well known that gene expression is age specific. The genotype of every living being is determined and fixed at zygotic stage, remaining unchanged throughout the life. However, the phenotypic changes in many characters occur in all organisms according to their age. Some genes express themselves early in embryonic life, some exert their effects at birth, some a few weeks after birth, some other express themselves at different ages of later life (younger age/sexual maturity, old age) of the organism.

The followings are the ***examples of age specific gene expression*** –

- ☆ *Short tail in sheep* is an inherited condition for which the genes express early in embryonic life at the time of bone formation;
- ☆ The genes for the formation of *blood group antigens* express in early embryonic life;
- ☆ The effect of *eye colour* genes in humans starts a few weeks after birth and not at birth;
- ☆ *Alkaptonuria* (darkening of urine- an abnormality) starts at birth;
- ☆ *Infantile amaurotic idiocy* starts at 4 – 6 months of age;
- ☆ *Vitamin D – resistant rickets* starts at 1 year of age;
- ☆ *Muscular dystrophy* starts at 2 – 5 years of age;
- ☆ *Hereditary baldness* at 25- 35 years of age and
- ☆ *Diabetes mellitus* and *Huntington's chorea* (nervous disorder – a progressive mental deterioration) develop over a wide range of age from 30 – 60 years.

The genes for semen production, appearance of moustaches and beards in males; breast/udder development, ova production, milk production and egg production in females; growth of puberal hair in both males and females starts expressing with sexual maturity, *etc.* However, in all these cases, the genes responsible for the expression of these characters are present at zygotic stage but their expression (visible effects) depends on the age of organism.

3. Chemical Environment

To speak of gene activity without specifying a particular environment has no meaning. There are a number of situations/examples of modification of gene expression in the absence of proper substrate/chemical environment of genes.

The *diabetes mellitus* is inherited in humans but it is not manifested unless the person consumes a large amount of carbohydrate over a long period of time and the pancreas is overloaded by sugar accumulation. The sugar level is controlled by the pancreatic hormone, *insulin* in normal condition but in diabetes the sugar level is not properly regulated, causing high blood sugar level and excretion of sugar in the urine leading to a change in body metabolism from the use of sugar for energy to the excessive use of fatty acids. The consequence is the coma and death of the diabetic patient.

Scrotal hernia in Swine though heritable but it is influenced by the maternal effect.

3.3 PHENOTYPIC STABILITY (CANALIZATION) AND ENVIRONMENT

The stability means a constant state and hence the genetic stability refers to imply a constant state for a population genome. The phenotypic stability is the consequence of stabilizing selection (selection of individuals near the mean of population). The tendencies for a constant state in development are of fundamental importance to maintain a uniform phenotype with genetic variability in secrete form (*hidden genes, known as* ***cryptic genetic variability***). Some buffered ontogenetic sequences of events in development are responsible for the steady state.

The phenotype is an end product of development via diverse genetic pathways. Each species has the phenotypic uniformity and adaptive norm. An individual has the capacity to develop itself, through the internally buffered sequences of processes, and counteract the upsetting tendencies of environmental stresses. This capacity of counteracting the environmental stress is called the ***development buffering*** *or flexibility*. The developmental buffering makes the individual react to the environmental change by switching from its normal developmental path to an alternate path which in turn helps the individual to develop unimpeded by environmental stresses. The stability for population genome is promoted by stabilizing selective mechanisms and genetic interactions. The basis of stabilizing selection is the superiority of heterozygote due to the gene interaction. The heterozygote are well buffered to withstand environmental variability and hence able to live successfully in a wider range of environmental conditions than homozygote. Therefore, the heterozygote has the advantage to show superiority even in the stress condition. A biochemical basis for superiority of heterozygote was proposed by Haldane (1954) suggesting that if homozygote controls only a single protein form (allozyme, globin, *etc.*), the heretozygote allows two forms which could function in more diverse environmental conditions. Thus, heterozygote shows greater stability having wider range of enzyme activity over temperatures compared to that of either homozygote at that temperature. Therefore, hereozygote have more homeostatic (buffering) adjustments than homozygote.

Waddington (1957) coined the term ***canalization*** to the developmental buffering of genotype-environment interaction during growth or to a balance between a flexible ontogenetic process and inflexible final phenotype, so that there is maximum fitness in a wide variety of environment. This makes the phenotype to develop unimpeded (without obstruction) by environmental stress or by underlying genetic variability. He described the canalization as one of the products of stabilizing selection which eliminates the homozygotes which are sensitive to the potentially disturbing effects of environmental stresses. This leads to fixation of alleles in homozygous balanced state and reduction of genetic variance but the genetic variability is present in a balanced state.

The high degree of uniformity is shown by various characters particularly which are associated with fitness *e.g.* wing shape and body proportions in insects have usual very small variability and are important for survival in nature. The absence of phenotypic variability can be taken in the absence of genetic variability but this is not true. The reason for uniformity lies in the fact that the development of phenotype for canalized characters (having uniformity and developmental buffering) is caused by interactions between many genes so that a minor change in one gene usually has little or no effect on the phenotype. The development system is therefore said to be buffered or canalized.

Very rare events like mutation or heat stroke (environmental stress) upset the canalization (buffering) and cause a change in the normal phenotype. The environmental stress disrupts the development of the normal phenotype by exposing the hidden polygenes to selection. Thus the polygenes (with minor effect), which exist but cannot express their effects on the phenotype (called as hidden genes causing cryptic genetic variability), start showing their effect due to environmental stress and cause a change in the normal phenotypes and a new phenotype is produced.

The presence of canalization (buffering capacity against variability – secret/hidden/cryptic genetic variability, which comes into expression under environmental stress) can thus be detected by giving environmental shock which disrupt the phenotype during development and by selecting such genotype which differ from normal phenotype. If the normal phenotype is upset by environmental stress or in the presence of a mutant gene and the new phenotype start showing inherited differences by exposing the underlying genetic variability (which already exists as hidden) it then indicates the existence of canalization (buffering) for the phenotype. This canalization (buffering) of phenotype is upset by environmental stress or in the presence of mutant gene by exposing the expression of hidden polygene to environmental stress.

Selection and canalization: Waddington (1953) produced cross-vein-less wings (like sex linked mutant trait) in *Drosophila melanogastator* flies by subjecting them to environmental shock. The continued environmental shock treatment each generation to the crossveinless flies and breeding such flies separately produced the new phenotypes (crossveinless) in the selected lines in high frequency with the phenocopy treatment (environmental stress). More interestingly, the new character (crossveinless wings) appeared in some flies without treatment. This indicated that new phenotype is caused by numerous genes whose effects were exposed by phenocopy treatment. Thus, selection after phenocopy treatment appears to change the primary expression of the genotype and also changes the zone of canalization (buffering) of phenotype. Milkman (1961) also obtained the similar effect of heat treatment on cross-vein-less character.

The genotypes for their sensitivity to particular environment can be detected by use of environmental stress or by incorporating major gene mutation (like bar eye or scute). The underlying genetic variability which can modify a character can be exploited by selection up to selection limit. The selected phenotype may be retained as an *"assimilated"* genotype even after removing the environmental stress or removing major gene (Waddington, 1961).

The selection limit (plateau) is attained with continued selection leaving no genetic variability and the homozygosity is reached for all the genes controlling the trait under selection, though reverse selection is effective to the control level. Similar is the effect of inbreeding to reduce heterozygosity to a certain level beyond which further decrease in heterozygosity does not occur. Therefore, genetic variability is maintained in a population in spite of the effects of all the forces acting to reduce the genetic variability. Lerner (1954) termed this phenomenon as the *genetic homeostasis.* This can be defined as the capacity of the population to maintain genetic equilibrium in variable environmental conditions by favouring heterozygotes in natural selection. In other words, it is the ability of a genotype to withstand (oppose) environmental fluctuations. The genes which appear in homozygous state due to selection may have their pleiotropic effect on fitness to reduce viability. This resist to a further increase in homozygosity and hence the population maintains genetic variability. This is the *population homeostasis*.

The genetic homeostasis involves both individual resistance and population resistance (buffering) which results in consistent performance of a population and may not be associated with heterozygosity or homogeneity. The overall action of the genetic system under environmental conditions decides the maintenance of a state of equilibrium and the integrated physiological processes during the course of development decides the mechanism of genetic homeostasis. The genotypes which have the capacity to make physiological adjustments for stability of development in various environments are called as *homeostatic genotypes*. Thus, the stability of a genotype in various environments is the property of homeostatic genotypes. *Homeostasis* thus denotes the power of an organism to hold the physiological processes within normal limits in spite of varying external conditions.

3.4 PHENOCOPY: ENVIRONMENTALLY INDUCED PHENOTYPE

The environment has its effect to the extent that one of the environments permits the expression of a genetic character while other environment does not permit the expression of the same character. Response of the genotype to the environmental conditions gives rise to the characters of organisms and sometimes the characters are changed due to changed environmental condition in the same way as they are changed when a gene mutates. Thus, change in environment sometimes induces non-hereditary phenotypic change which is similar to that caused by mutation. This non-heritable environmentally induced modification in phenotype resembling the phenotype of a known mutant gene is called "***phenocopy***". This is the environmental change in phenotype resembling the phenotype of a different genotype. Thus, the phenocopy is the production of same phenotype by two genotypes under changed environment.

Such induced change may persist for the life of the individual and it may also persist in the progeny or may disappear in next generation. The production of phenocopy depends on the strength of environmental change to modify the effects of genes. There are some examples of G-E interaction in qualitative characters to illustrate the concept.

It is assumed that that the environmental agents sometimes affect certain chemical reactions which are similar to mutations and results in similar end products. To determine the inheritance of a phenotypic change, appropriate crosses are made and the difference between mutation and phenocopy is tested.

The term phenocopy was coined by Goldschmidt (1935). He subjected the larvae of Drosophila for short interval at different periods of development cycle to higher than normal temperature (35° C). This resulted into several phenocopies of wing abnormalities indistinguishable to genetic mutants of vestigial (vg) series.

Waddington (1953) subjected the Drosophila to environmental shock which produced flies *lacking cross-veins wing*, similar to that caused by a sex-linked mutation, but this was non inherited phenocopy.

There are some phenocopy producing agents, drugs and treatments. The *diabetic symptoms* in genetically normal people appear due to specific environmental changes like infection, injury or removal of pancreas in humans. This is the phenocopy of diabetic individual of genetic origin. Similarly, the phenocopies of normal individuals can be produced by treating with insulin the diabetic patient that inherits diabetes. The diabetes in humans and animals seems to be a hereditary disease. A patient is unable to metabolize the glucose properly. Consequently, the glucose level in the blood stream becomes high to the extent of its excretion with the urine, finally causing death. The maintenance of blood sugar level is under the control of insulin produced by the pancreatic gland. The insulin prevents the occurrence of diabetes. The diabetes develops only when the insulin production is inadequate for a long time by the over consumption of carbohydrate. The insulin treatment does not permit the diabetes to develop.

The diabetes in animals may also be induced by introducing antibodies against an individual's own insulin, by pituitary and thyroid hormone and by chemicals such as alloxan; and in all these conditions the effects are not inherited but are only environmentally induced.

The normal *body colour in Drosophila melanogaster* is brown with its variant yellow colour. If the normal larvae with normal genotype for brown body are raised on diet containing silver salt (silver nitrate), they develop yellow colour like the yellow mutant but give rise to brown in normal environment.

The Himalayan *albino rabbits* have black colour on feet, ears, nose, and tail but the remaining body is white. If the rabbits are shifted to cold place after cutting of white hairs (from white parts), the black hairs appear instead of white hairs.

The phenocopy of *creeper trait* (shortened limbs) caused by genes in poultry can be produced with phenocopy treatment by injecting boric acid into chick eggs.

Landauer (1948) produced phenocopies of several mutations in the fowl with *skeletal effects*. He injected eggs of normal genotype with insulin before incubation or during development. This resulted in rumpless phenocopies if treatment was given in early stages up to 72 hours, shortening of limb (micromelia) if injected on 5th and 6th day, and other abnormalities of skull and upper beak similar to that of several mutant genes. The insulin effects are accompanied by hypoglycemia (a symptom of carbohydrate metabolism) after the establishment of circulation. An injection of nicotine amide counteracts the effect of insulin by way of acting as a coenzyme in cell respiration. The rumples phenocopies were also produced in chickens with normal genotype by mechanically shaking the eggs at a critical period and also by treating the embryos at 48 hours of age with *sodium methyl arsenite*. These chemicals produce shortened limbs similar to a dominant mutation called "creeper". These are two mutations in chicks causing rumpless abnormality characterized by the absence of caudal vertebral and tail structures including muscles, feathers and oil secreting gland which supply oily secretion to the feathers. Both the mutations have the same end product but differ in their nature of inheritance – one being dominant and the other recessive with low penetrance, location (*i.e.* they are not alleles and also not closely linked), and also differ in structural details, chemical composition of bones and embryonic development.

The mouse kept at reduced atmospheric pressure during pregnancy produce the offspring lacking regions of the urogenital system similar to that of a mutant gene (Danforth short tail).

Human *limb abnormalities* including complete absence of hands and feet (acheiropody) are rare and inherited in some families. A serious effect of sleep inducing drug (thalidomide) by pregnant ladies result in limb defects and the eye defects following measles during pregnancy resemble to hereditary abnormalities of limbs and eyes. The sleep inducing drugs produced their effect on skeletal formation of the foetus at the time of formation of limb buds and the babies are born with shortened limbs giving a flipper like appearance called phocomelia. Thalidomide has similar effect in mice, monkeys and rabbits. The dietary changes and atomic bomb testing were assigned as the cause of these sudden increases in phocomelia in early seventies of 20th century in German. Irradiation induced several skeletal and neurological anomalies resembling in genetically produced phenocopies.

3.5 VARIABILITY IN GENE EXPRESSION

Besides above types of gene action, some other types of gene expression indicate that the pathway between a genotype and its phenotypic expression (Phenotype) is modified which may be due to some environmental factors or due to some factors in genetic background. Such factors have been found in resulting modification of Mendelian original phenotypic ratios. The penetrance and variability of genes for some characters are the phenomenon of such examples.

3.5.1 Penetrance

This is the ability of a gene to be expressed phenotypically in only some individuals of the population. The penetrance of a gene is the frequency (percentage) of expression of a trait in the population. Thus, *the degree (percentage)* or ability *of phenotypic expression of genes in the population is known as penetrance.* When a gene produces a constant phenotypic effect, it is said to have 100 per cent penetrance (complete penetrance). The dominant genes express themselves in all the individuals carrying that gene and have 100 per cent penetrance in homozugous dominant as well as in heterozygous individuals while the recessive gene could properly be said to have zero penetrance unless it is present in homozygous state. In such cases the structural genes fail to produce expected phenotypic ratio. Thus, penetrance may vary from zero to 100 per cent. The penetrance may thus be complete or incomplete.

The trait has *incomplete penetrance* when the individual having the appropriate genotype (homozygous or heterozygous state) does not show the trait. The ***polydactyly*** (presence of extra to normal number of fingers and or toes) in men is an example of incomplete penetrance. The poydactyly is controlled by the presence of a dominant gene (P) arisen as a *dominant mutation* whereas its recessive allele (p) in homozygous condition (pp) governs the normal number of fingers on each limb. The presence of dominant allele in all heterozygote (Pp) should produce polydactyly but it does not hold true in all cases and some of the individuals are not polydactylous, indicating that the allele is penetrant but to a lesser degree.

The ***fragile X syndrome*** is the second most common form of an inherited mental retardation in humans, caused by a dominant X-linked mutation (expanded CGG trinucleotide repeats on X chromosome) with incomplete penetrance since about 20 percent of hemizygous males and about 30 percent of heterozygous females do not show this disorder.

The other examples of penetrance are *Blue scleroties, stiff little finger, diabetes insipidus and multiple exotoses* (cartilaginous tumours of the long bones) in human which are governed by single dominant genes but with reduced penetrance.

The *blue sclera* anomaly had a penetrance of 90 per cent and it is expressed by a blue discolouration of the white (sclera) of the eye and by bristtleness of the bones.

In several of the pedigrees the *diabetes* skip (an individual whose father or mother had the condition and some of whose children are also affected, but one individual remains unaffected). The diabetes mellitus develops only in those individuals of the twins who take more carbohydrate foods (starch and sugars) in their diet.

The penetrance of dominant gene for *multiple exotosis* is lower than 75 per cent in women but considerably higher in men. The penetrance may be equal or unequal in the two sexes.

Eye cancer (*retinoblastoma*) and some forms of *colon cancer* appear to be inherited as simple dominant conditions, though they show incomplete penetrance and variable expressivity.

The obstruction of the orifice of the stomach (*pyloric stenosis*) is due to a recessive gene with some reduction in penetrance in boys but much more reduction in girls. The trait becomes sex-limited when the penetrance is completely reduced in one sex.

The expression of the D allele in horses for coat colour is remarkably constant with few exceptions where the D allele fails to produce the usual phenotypic effect (Palomino – a dilute colour in the heterozygous condition Dd or in the presence of at least one B). A mare with genotype aa Bb Dd was found black and not Palomino by Castle and King (1959) and when it was mated with a chestnut stallion (a- bb dd), it produced a palomino foal. Thus, the black mare had gene D but failed to produce any phenotypic expression (palomino) which indicated that the D allele in this case has low penetrance or no penetrance.

The gene for *coat colour in guinea pigs* exhibits complete penetrance. The recessive gene for wing character (vestigial wings) in *Drosophila* has complete penetrance.

The environment besides the genotype of the character also influences the phenotype of the character. Thus, the expression of the genes depends on environmental conditions as well as on genetic background of the character. A particular character is produced as a result of the interaction between genotype and environment.

The lethal genes show differences in their pentrance and expressivity, showing broad range of effects. They may have complete lethality to complete viability. However, semilethal do not cause definite lethality.

3.5.2 Expressivity

The degree of effect produced by a penetrant genotype is known as expressivity. The term expressivity is used for a condition when a trait is not manifested uniformly among the individuals that show it. Thus, expressivity is the ability of a gene to express itself uniformly in all the individuals with same genotype. The genes may have uniform or variable expressivity. A gene that expresses itself uniformly in all the individuals carrying the gene, has uniform variability, *viz.* Mendelian characters.

However, some of the characters show the range of different phenotypes. The expressivity represents merely an *expansion of penetrance* in the visible range. When a penetrant character (controlled by a gene) *show individual variation*, it means the gene is having variable expressivity. Thus, the gene in one individual may produce its effect to a lesser degree but to a greater degree in another individual. *The expressivity is the variable degree of gene expression among different individuals carrying this gene.* Thus, a character may be penetrant but it may be quite variable in its phenotypic expression in different individuals.

Variation in the expression of genes for tail length in sheep has been observed. The *length of the tail* varies from almost normal to a condition where a part of the spinal column may be missing.

Another example is the *"snorter' dwarfism in beef cattle* which vary from very small animals that die soon after birth to those which attain normal size surviving for several years of age.

In human, the well known example is of variable expressivity is *juvenile cataract of the eye* (Lutman and Neel, 1945) due to a dominant gene whose expression may vary from a *slight milkiness of the lens to dense opacity.*

A dominant gene is associated with an "allergic diathesis" with various manifestations in different individuals as asthma, vasomotor rhinitis, atopic dermatitis or hay fever (Schwartz, 1953).

Further observations regarding the *polydactyly in human* indicated that this condition is not present in all the four limbs, but it may be observed either in one hand and not in the other or it may be in the hands and not in the feet. Thus, although the gene (P) which controls the trait is present in the individual and have shown its effect (penetrance) but with varied expression within the individual itself. *This variable effect of a penetrant genotype within the individual is also called the variable expressivity.*

The dominant *lobe eye mutation* in Drosophila shows variable expressivity among individuals because the phenotypic expression of this mutant allele is extremely variable from tiny compound eyes to large *lobule* eyes and also other phenotypes between these extreme phenotypes for lobe eyes. There is full range of different phenotypes in flies heterozygous for the mutant allele.

Viability is another example of variable expressivity. The sub lethal alleles in homozygous recessive condition also varied in their phenotypic expression and thus they are not fatal to all the individuals before sexual maturity. Some lethal genes have their variable effect from complete lethality to sterility if the genotype survived to sexual maturity. Thus, the viability is another ontogenetic manifestation of a gene. Some genes do not affect the life span, some others result into sterility if the individual survive to sexual maturity, others definitely reduce the chances of living and still others are lethal in homozygous state.

The expressivity of a gene (genotype) is influenced by the environment. The identical twins raised on different diets attain different height. The exposure to childhood disease to an individual of the twin also affects the expression of adulthood characters.

The variable expressivity, like partial dominance, can be explained by modifying genes and or by environmental influences.

Chapter 4

Mendel's Laws of Heredity

Gregor Johann Mendel was born in 1822 in a poor farmer family in a place now in Czechoslovakia. He could not fulfill his desire of proper education due to his poverty and hence went to Augustinian monastery at Brunn. He was appointed a priest in 1847 and subsequently sent in 1851 for training in physics, mathematics and natural sciences to the University of Vienna. He became a teaching monk after his return to Brunn in 1854 and started his experiment in 1857 on garden peas (*Pisum sativum*) in the monastery garden. The discoveries made by Mendel were published in 1866 in the proceedings of the Natural history Society of Brun, where he worked.

Mendel was the first and pioneer worker to discover the law of heredity and hence called the *"**father of genetics**"*. He died in 1884. But his paper remained unnoticed till 1900, when it was rediscovered by 3 Botanists, namely Hugo de Vries in Holland, Carl Correns in Germany, and Eric von Tschermak-Seysenegg in Austria when they worked independently and searched the literature in support of their own theories of heredity and they found that Mendel had already made the analysis 35 years ago. Mendel's findings were accepted.

William Bateson, British botanist, published English translation of Mendel's German Text in 1902 what he called Mendelism – the principles of Dominance, Segregation, and Independent Assortment. Later in 1909, he published a book *Mendel's Principles of Heredity*. His book contained the results of breeding experiments on different plants and animals. He coined the term ***genetics*** to the study of heredity. He took this word from the Greek word meaning "to generate".

4.1 MENDEL'S EXPERIMENT

Mendel's experiment has been given here in terms of the plant he has selected with reasons in favour of selection, the characters under study, the crosses made, the experimental findings, and the conclusions made by him.

(i) Materials of Mendel's Experiment – Plants Selected

Mendel's selected garden pea (*Pisum sativum*) for his research. There had been the following reasons to select the pea plant for the study:

- ✰ The peas were easily available in a wide array of different forms and colours,
- ✰ The plants were easy to grow and took only a single growing season to have one generation,
- ✰ Pea was a sexually reproducing, self fertilized (unisexual – having both male and female organs on the same plant), and diploid plant (having chromosomes in pairs, called homologous chromosomes, responsible for two alternate forms of the same character). The pea plant has a reproductive peculiarity that the petals of its flowers close down and prevent the entry or exit of pollen grains. This compels self-fertilization and produces highly inbred strains. Thus, there is little or no genetic variation among succeeding generations and hence ***true breeding strains***. The male organs are called anthers which produce pollens (sperms – male gametes) whereas the female organs called ovary which produces eggs (ovum – female gamete).The ovary is at the bottom of the pollen tube (pistil) while on the top of the pistil is the stigma which is a sticky part so as to receive pollen grains in cross pollination. He used selfing as a technique in his experiment and for cross fertilization experiment it was easy to emasculate and to cross fertilize, and to study the inheritance of both the forms of each character included in his experiment,
- ✰ Pea had many sharply defined inherited characters each with two alternate appearances (phenotypes or characters having clear cut differences), and
- ✰ Mendel studied the inheritance pattern of one character at one time (***monohybrid cross*** – plants differing in one character) as well as two characters (***dihybrid cross*** – plants that differed in two characters) and kept records.

(ii) Plant Characters Studied

Mendel had a collection of many different true-breeding strains of pea. Each stain was distinguishable by a particular characteristic. He had chosen 7 characters individually and crossed two varieties each having different appearances of the character. These seven characters in garden peas were:

Characters		*Phenotypes (Dominant or recessive)*
Seed characters:	(1) Form of ripe seeds	Round or wrinkled surface
	(2) Colour of seed	Yellow or green
	(3) Colour of seed coat	Gray coat or white coat (Violet flowers or white flowers)
Pod characters:	(4) Form of ripe pods	Full (inflated) or wrinkled (constricted)
	(5) Colour of ripe pods	Green or yellow
Stem characters:	(6) Length of plant	Tall (6-7 ft) or dwarf (¾ - 1 ft)
	(7) Flower position on stem	Axial or terminal flowers (along stem on its top)

4.2 MONOHYBRID AND DIHYBRID CROSSES AND MENDEL'S LAWS

The results of Mendel's experiment on garden pea have been illustrated taking monohybrid cross for one character (Seed shape - round verses wrinkled) and dihybrid crosses for two characters together (Seed shape - round verses wrinkled; and seed colour – yellow and green). The monohybrid cross has been shown in proving the law of dominance and segregation while dihybrid cross has shown to prove independent assortment of genes.

4.2.1 Monohybrid Crosses and Mendel's Laws

Mendel made the ***monohybrid cross.*** This was a cross in which only one character was under study at a time. The cross fertilization between two varieties differing in their height (tall and dwarf plants) was done by avoiding selfing so as both the distinguished appearances (phenotypes) of the same character were united in hybrids. The male organs (pollen - anthers) were removed from one variety before their maturation and used pollen to the stigma. Thus, hybrids (F_1) were produced. These hybrid seeds (F_1) were shown next year. The original pure breed plants **(*parental strains*)** used for hybridization were called the parental generation denoted by the letter ***P*** whereas their offspring were referred as ***first filial generation or*** F_1 (hybrids) from a Latin word meaning "son" or "daughter". The succeeding generations descended from this cross (F_1) by self fertilization were called F_2 ***generation*** and so on.

It was observed that the F_1 plants grown were uniformly tall. The dwarf character did not appear in F_1 in any experiment irrespective of the way the experiment was done (reciprocal cross). Mendel was interested to know the genetic makeup of these tall plant hybrids (F_1) and so he allowed self fertilization among the F_1 plants. He recorded the results on plant height and observed that there were two types of progeny (tall and dwarf plants) among F_2. Thus, the dwarf character reappeared in F_2 generation. Out of total 1064 F_2 plants, he observed 787 as tall and 277 as dwarf, in a ratio of about 3:1.

Appearance of dwarf phenotype in F_2 plants afforded the evidence that the F_1 hybrids are capable to produce dwarf plants and they had a hidden factor to produce dwarf which did not appear in F_1 generation. The similar results were obtained for all of the rest 6 monohybrid crosses (disappearance of one phenotype of each character in F_1 generation, reappearance of the same phenotype in F_2 generation that remained hidden in F_1 generation). The conclusion from the experimental findings was that there were entities "hereditary determinants or factors" and each adult pea plant had two factors, one from each parent, for each characteristic. These Mendelian factors were later called as genes by a Danish plant breeder (Wilhelm Johannsen, 1909) and the two alternative form of gene as ***alleles,*** *e.g.* dominant and recessive forms of gene. The gene responsible for recessive phenotype was called as ***allele*** by Johannsen, W. (1909) from the Greek word "of one another". Mendel concluded that the ***genetic factors (genes) are present in pairs***. The parental varieties had two identical copies of a gene producing two different appearance of the characters. These are called now as ***diploids*** and ***homozygous.*** It was interesting to note that reciprocal crossings did not change the results and gave identical results.

Out of two alternate forms of character of parental variety, only one appeared in F_1. The reciprocal crosses gave identical results. The F_1 hybrids are not exactly intermediate in appearance between the two parental varieties but resemble to one of the two parental characters for all the seven crosses. Thus, only one phenotype of the character appeared in the hybrids (F_1) and the other disappeared. The character which expressed itself unchanged in the hybrid (F_1) was called as ***dominant character*** whereas that which was not expressed (remained hidden or latent) in the hybrid (F_1) was called as ***recessive character***. The hybrid zygote had two different alleles, each from two parents. Such a hybrid having two different alleles of a gene pair was called ***heterozygote.***

The character which disappeared or remained hidden (recessive) in F_1, reappeared in F_2, but its frequency was as low as about ¼ of the total progeny in F_2. The dominant and recessive phenotypes among the F_2 plants were observed in a ratio approximately of 3:1. Mendel also proposed that the two copies of genes are reduced to one copy during gamete formation as a result of meiosis. Thus, the gametes carrying a single copy of a gene are haploid.

The next conclusion made by Mendel was that the diploid gene number would be restored in the zygote as a union of opposite sex gametes on fertilization. He found that the inheritance of two pairs of genes was independent to each other.

Mendel noted that self fertilization of F_2 plants with recessive character (wrinkled seed, rr) always bred true. On the other hand, the self fertilization of F_2 plants with dominant character behaved differently in the way that some of them breed true and others did not. The plants which did not breed true produced two types of plants- some with dominant characters (smooth or round seed, RR) and others with recessive character (wrinkled seeds, rr) in a ratio of 3:1. Thus, F_2 individuals were of two types- one of pure producers, made up of identical genes (homozygote, RR and rr; *homo* means the same) and others of hybrid or mixed

Parents	(P_1) Smooth	x	(P_2) Wrinkled
	RR	↓	rr
F_1 (cross of P_1 x P_2)		Smooth (hybrid), Rr	
F_2 (selfing of F_1)			

Male gametes	Female gametes R (½)	r (½)
R (½)	RR (¼)	Rr (¼)
r (½)	Rr (¼)	rr (¼)

Results of F_2 progeny:	3 Smooth : (RR, Rr)	1 Wrinkled (rr)
F_3 (selfing of F_2)	($^1/_3$ breed true : + $^2/_3$ hybrid)	All breed true

Figure 4.1: Monohybrid Cross Showing Law of Dominance and Law of Segregation of Alleles.

producers (heterozygote, Rr; *hetero* means different). The cross can be shown as under for seed form (shape):

The hybrid plants (heterozygote), which did not breed true and produced two types of plants with dominant and recessive characters, must contain factors (genes) for producing both the phenotypes of the character (*viz.* seed shape), one each for dominant (round) and recessive appearance (wrinkle). Likewise, the true breeding plants must also have two genes because pure lines are expected from each type (RR and rr) upon their self fertilization. Mendel realized that these results could be possible only if two genes of a pair remained distinct in the hybrid without changing their identity, in the hybrids, and the hybrids possess both types of parental factors (dominant and recessive) which produce two types of plants.

The situation discussed above is possible only if the two factors (R and r) responsible for the two parental types (round and wrinkle) segregate (separate) from each other during gamete formation and one gamete carries gene (R) for dominant character (round) while other gamete carries gene (r) for recessive character (wrinkle). Thus, there are two kinds of equally frequent pollen (R and r) and two kinds of equally frequent eggs (R and r). Therefore, members of a given pair of gene (R and r) segregate (separate) from each other during gamete formation, into equal numbers of gametes. The recessive gene (r) expresses itself in F_2 generation. Mendel called to this reappearance of the parental recessive character (wrinkle) as the segregation (separation) of the members of a given pair of gene (R and r). It is known as the principle of segregation.

The genes exist in pairs in the cell of the individual located on the paired chromosome (homologous chromosomes). The two members of a gene pair are now called, *alleles* of a single gene. These alleles of a single gene segregate (separate) from each other during gamete formation (anaphase of the first meiotic division). The paired chromosomes are separated by moving towards the opposite poles of the cell. There is physical separation of homologous chromosomes and this segregates the alleles from each other. Eventually these segregated chromosomes go to the daughter cells so that each gamete receives one copy of all the chromosomes containing one gene of each pair (called alleles).

The genes are consequently not blended or mixed to each other in the hybrid, but they preserve their identities and transmitted unchanged in hybrids, segregate at the time of gamete formation and reappears in the offspring. This stability of genes and their segregation and transmission in unchanged condition between cells and generation is termed as ***purity of genes*** or gametes. The two alleles (dominant and recessive) of a gene pair remain together through generations without permanent influence on each other.

Mendel's Law of Inheritance (Monohybrid Crosses)

On the basis of Mendel's work on garden pea and his findings on monohybrid crosses, the following laws of inheritance were formulated:

- ☆ The genes are present in pair,
- ☆ One gene is dominant on its allele (Law of dominance),
- ☆ The two alleles of a gene pair segregate from each other during gamete formation (Law of segregation), and

(1) Law of Paired Factors

From the evidence of F_1 and F_2 results it was clear that there were two forms of every character and hence there were two determining agents (factors or now called genes) responsible for each form of the character (trait). This showed that genes or factors were in pairs and it is sometimes referred to as ***law of paired factors.***

(2) Law of Dominance

The appearance of one form of a character could be hidden in F_1 but not destroyed/modified because it reappeared again in F_2. This is due to the interaction of genes (Alleles) present on the same locus. The two alleles of a gene pair interact in such a way that one allele hide (conceal) the presence (effect) of another allele. The allele which can express phenotypic itself in the heterozygote as well as in homozygote is called a dominant gene or ***dominant character*** whereas the gene (allele) whose expression remains hidden in F_1 and can only express itself in homozygote is called a ***recessive character*** (factor or gene). This phenomenon by which one form of character appears and the other alternate form remain hidden, though the factors for both the forms of character are present, is called the ***dominance*** and referred as ***law of dominance***. The phenomenon of dominance is very common but it is ***not universal.***

The reappearance of a recessive/hidden character in F_2 was a disproval to the theory of blending inheritance and hence it was a notable observation to the hereditary theory.

Importance of Dominance

The phenomenon of dominance is of practical importance. The mutant alleles are recessive and detrimental to the organism while the dominant alleles produce normal character. For example, idiocy in man is caused by a recessive mutant gene besides being caused by other factors. Thus, a man with heterozygous genotype is normal without showing any sign of idiocy but carrier for idiocy allele. Therefore, the marriage of two heterozygous parents will produce some idiot children, in spite of the fact that none of the parent showed any sign of idiocy.

(3) Law of Segregation

This law tells about the transmission of characters from one generation to the next. According to the laws of inheritance, an allele is transmitted even it was not expressed in the parent generation due to its presence in heterozygote state and its recessive nature of not expressing in heterozygote state. The basis of this law is based on the genes being present in pairs on homologous chromosomes which are separated during meiosis.

The ***homologous chromosomes*** or ***homologous genes*** are those that have evolved from a common ancestral chromosome or gene, respectively. The homologous (chromosomes or genes) can be categorized as orthologous and paralogous. The ***orthologous*** (genes) are those homologous present in different species whereas the ***paralogous*** (genes) are those homologous present within a species.

Therefore, *the segregation of the alleles of a single gene from each other is called the law of segregation. The law of segregation is based on the separation of homologous chromosomes during anaphase of the first meiotic division. This law of segregation is applied universally.*

4.2.2 Dihybrid Cross and Law of Independent Assortment of Genes

Mendel also made the ***dihybrid cross*** involving two characters. For example, the plants producing yellow and round seeds were crossed with plants producing green and wrinkled seeds. Such a cross was made with the objective to study whether the two traits are inherited together or independently. The yellow and round seeds were dominant because these characters were appeared in F_1 seeds. Mendel also self fertilized these F_1 plants, recorded the results on seed colour and shape of the seeds obtained from F_2 plants. The experiments were repeated for several times and generations. The ***reciprocal crossings*** were also made.

(4) Law of Independent Assortment

This law of Independent Assortment states that *the segregation of alleles of two or more loci is independent of each other into two gametes at the time of gamete formation and hence they are transmitted independently into the progeny.*

Combining two sets of results in a single dihybrid cross for two different pairs of genes affecting two different characters (round vs wrinkled seeds and yellow vs green cotyledons), Mendel found that the two pairs of genes behaved independently of one another. Each pair of genes was segregated/assorted independently in two gametes in a manner that other pair of genes was not there. This means that the chance for a plant to have smooth or wrinkled seeds do not interfere with the appearance of another character *viz.* cotyledon colour (yellow or green). Thus, the appearance of one character (seed shape) was independent of the appearance of other character (seed cotyledon colour). Mendel called it as the law of independent assortment, due to independence of these two pairs of genes in segregation during meiosis for gamete formation.

The independent assortment of gametes for two or more pairs of genes is also based on the anaphase separation of chromosomes containing alleles during meiosis. From Mendel's law of segregation, it is known that:

R gametes = r gametes = ½; and

Y gametes = y gametes = ½

The results of a di-hybrid cross for two pairs of genes among F_2 progeny can be illustrated for independent assortment of two pairs of genes as under:

Parents **Round - Yellow** X *wrinkled - green*

RR YY *rryy*

↓

F_1 Hybrid **Round – Yellow**

Rr Yy

F_2 Female gametes (ova or eggs)

		¼ RY	¼ Ry	¼ rY	¼ ry
Male gametes (sperms)	¼ RY	**Round Yellow** RRYY	**Round Yellow** RR Yy	**Round Yellow** Rr YY	**Round Yellow** Rr Yy
	¼ Ry	**Round Yellow** **RR Yy**	Round green RR yy	**Round Yellow** **Rr Yy**	Round green Rr yy
	¼ rY	**Round Yellow** Rr YY	**Round Yellow** Rr Yy	***wrinkled Yellow*** ***rr YY***	***wrinkled Yellow*** ***rr Yy***
	¼ ry	**Round Yellow** **Rr Yy**	Round green Rr yy	***wrinkled Yellow*** ***rr Yy***	***wrinkled green*** *rr yy*

Figure 4.2: Showing Law of Independent Assortment of Genes.

Significance of Independent Assortment

Two new combinations of genes in a dihybrid cross are produced. Likewise, the F_2 progeny of trihybrid cross show six new combinations and so on it goes on increasing with the polyhybrid crosses. This knowledge of producing new combinations due to independent assortment of genes helps the breeder to produce and breed new combinations of useful characters. The independent assortment of genes is not universally applied.

4.3 TESTS OF HOMOZYGOUS AND HETEROZYGOUS DOMINANT

Mendel used two types of tests to distinguish between homozygous and heterozygous dominants. These were self-fertilization and back cross (test cross).

An individual heterozygous for one pair of gene (R and r) is called *monohybrid* and a cross of two individuals that are heterozygous for one pair of gene is called a *monohybrid cross*. This is the cross between two pure breeding individuals which differ from each other only in one character and the resulting hybrid is called monohybrid. The *dihybrid* or *polyhybrid* crosses are the cross between two pure breeding individuals which differ in two or more than two characters, respectively.

(i) Self Fertilization

The self fertilization of dominant individuals produces individuals only with dominant character. On the contrary, the self fertilization of heterozygous individual produces two types of individuals- one type are those having dominant character and other type are those having recessive character, in a ratio of 3 dominants: 1 recessive. Therefore, the appearance of recessive character from self fertilization of hybrid individuals (heterozygous) or from self fertilization of homozygous recessive individuals indicated that the plants which produced two types of plants were heterozygous. These crosses can be illustrated taking dominant gene as R and the recessive gene as r:

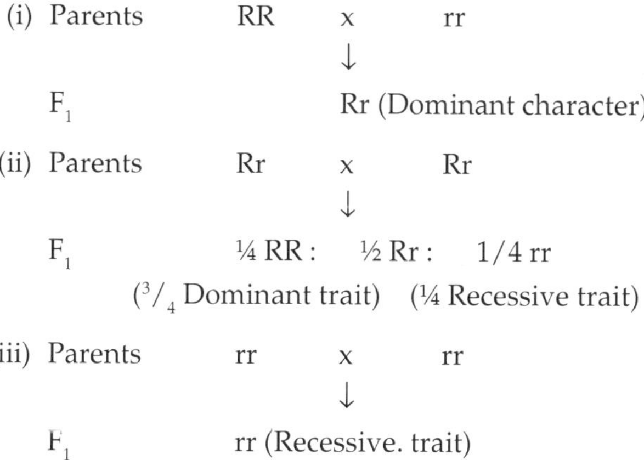

(ii) Back Cross or Test Cross

The crossing of heterozygous progeny (Rr) with any one of its parent (dominant, RR or recessive, rr) is called as *back cross* whereas the *test cross* is a form of back cross when the heterozygous progeny (Rr) is mated to a recessive homozygous parent (rr). A breeding test performed to determine the genotype of an individual with dominant phenotype is called the *testcross*. The test cross is performed by mating of the individual under test (dominant phenotype) with a recessive homozygote. The crossing of homozygous dominant individual with homozygous recessive individual produces all the progeny with dominant character as:

RR x rr

↓

Rr (Dominant Phenotype)

The *test cross* (Heterozygous x Recessive homozygous) results in a 1:1 ratio of dominant and recessive phenotype as:

Parents	Rr	x	rr	
		↓		
	Eggs (female gametes)			
		r	r	
Pollen (male gametes)	R	Rr	Rr	(All with dominant phenotype)
	r	rr	rr	(All with recessive phenotype)

The results of test cross provided very useful information in providing a tool for *determining the type of gametes produced by the parents* and therefore, the recessive back cross is often referred to as a *test cross*.

The backcross of hybrid F_1 with homozygous dominant parent produces all progeny with dominant phenotype and hence cannot be taken as a test cross. This has been shown as under:

Parents	Rr	x	RR	
		↓		
Progeny	RR, RR: Rr, Rr			(All with dominant phenotype)

Therefore, recessive back cross (test cross) has great importance because it produces identical phenotypic and genotypic ratios.

4.4 APPLICATIONS OF MENDEL'S LAWS OF HEREDITY

The Mendel's laws of heredity have their great significance. These principles have founded a new subject called genetics. The classical genetics is rooted in Mendel's discovery and stem on these laws of inheritance founded by Mendel. The Mendelian laws are applied to predict the outcome of different types of crosses, provided the genetic basis of the character is known. There are ***three procedures to predict the outcome of crosses***. The two methods are based on the systematic calculation of all the zygotic genotypes or phenotypes whereas the third method involves a mathematical approach.

(1) Punnet's Gametic Checkerboard Method or Punnet's Square Method

This method is applied for one or two pairs of genes. In this method all the gametes likely to be formed are written. The gametes equally formed in both the sexes. The gametes of one sex are written on one side while the gametes of opposite sex are written on second side. A British geneticist, R.C. Punnet gave this method. This can be understood for one pair of genes (R and r) as shown in Figure 3.1 and for 2 pairs of genes in Figure 3.2.

(2) Branching Method or Fork Line Method

There is also alternate method called *branched* or forked-line method to represent different combination used to obtain F_2 ratio by drawing branched diagram and then using the product rule considering the two monohybrid cross *i.e.* Rr x Rr and Yy x Yy operating together. If one allele of a gene pair is dominant, it results in a 3:1 ratio from both the monohybrid cross. Both the pairs of genes being independent, each monohybrid allele will segregate and will combine with any of the other. It can be shown as:

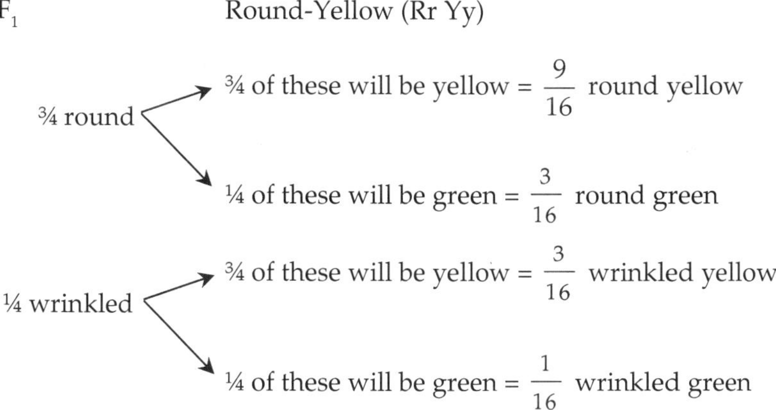

(3) Probability Method – Mathematical Approach

The laws of probability are used here because the gene segregation is like that of an event of coin tossing.

(i) Single Gene Pair

The probability of producing dominant allele (R gamete) is ½ and the probability of producing gamete containing recessive allele r will also be ½ from a heterozygous parent. It can be said that these are the frequencies of two types of gametes produced by the heterozygous parent (Rr) and used to predict the outcome of crossing two heterozygote parents (Rr x Rr). See Fig 3.1 here for a cross Rr x Rr. Both the heterozygotc will produce two gametes with equal frequencies (probabilities) of ½. Any of the two gametes of either sex can combine with either gamete of opposite sex. Therefore, the chance that male gamete with dominant allele (R) will combine/fertilize the female gamete containing dominant allele (R) will be ½ x ½ = ¼. This chance is the combined probability or frequency of uniting male gamete with female gamete, both having dominant allele obtained by multiplying the two probabilities because two gametes are produced and united independently. The chance or frequency or probability of producing recessive homozygote (rr) is ½ x ½. But the probability of producing heterozygote zygote is ½ because the heterozygote is produced in two ways. The dominant allele (R) may be either from male or female and likewise the recessive allele may be either from male or from female. In both the cases the probability is ½ × ½ = ¼. The total probability will be ¼ + ¼ = ½. The probability distribution of the genotypes formed from heterozygous mating will be:

RR = ¼, Rr = ½, rr = ¼

As per the law of dominance, the probability of progeny having dominant phenotype will be ¼ + ½ = ¾ and that of recessive phenotype will be ¼. Thus, the F_2 ratio as per Mendel's law is 3:1. This has come true by this method of probability.

(ii) Two Gene Pair

(See Figure 3.2) This method of probability is applied by taking one gene at a time when there are two or more genes under consideration. The frequencies or probabilities are obtained by considering the law of dominance and law of independent assortment. The combined probability for more than one gene pair is obtained by using both the rules of probability *viz. multiplication rule* for independent or equally likely events and the *additive rule* for mutually exclusive events which do not occur together or simultaneously.

Half of the half R gametes will contain Y gametes (*i.e.* ½ Y of ½ R = ¼ RY, another half of R gametes will contain y (*i.e.* ½ y of R = ¼ Ry), and likewise half of r gametes will contain Y (½ Y of ½ r = ¼ rY) whereas other half of r gametes will contain y gametes (½ y of ½ r = ¼ ry). Therefore, dihybrid F_1 individuals produce 4 types of gametes in each of the two sexes in equal proportions *viz.* RY, Ry, rY, ry. Consequently, the probability of forming 4 gametes being (by product rule):

R and Y = ½ × ½ = ¼ RY; R and y = ½ × ½ = ¼ Ry

r and Y = ½ × ½ = ¼ rY ; r and y = ½ × ½ = ¼ ry

Again the product rule of probability will be applied during zygote formation, because any gamete is free or independent to unite with any gamete of opposite sex. Thus the probability of the zygote with RRYY will be ¼ RY × ¼ RY = 1/16 RRYY and likewise will be the probability for all the 4 × 4 =16 combinations of zygotes.

The F_2 ratio closely fit the 3:1 ratio of crosses involving single pair in which dominance occurs. Both set of results are combined in a dihybrid cross, when each gene pair acts independently. Therefore, if a seed has a ¾ chance to be round (smooth) with a ¾ chance of being yellow cotyledons, its chance of being both round and yellow at the same time in a dihybrid, will be ¾ × ¾ = 9/16 and likewise the ratio of each phenotypic combination may be obtained by multiplying the probabilities of the individuals phenotype. A phenotypic ratio of 9:3:3:1 among the F_2 progeny is obtained as:

¾ round × ¾ yellow = $\frac{9}{16}$ round-yellow

¾ round × ¼ green = $\frac{3}{16}$ round-green

$\frac{1}{4}$ wrinkled × $\frac{3}{4}$ yellow = $\frac{3}{16}$ wrinkled-yellow

$\frac{1}{4}$ wrinkled × $\frac{1}{4}$ green = $\frac{1}{16}$ wrinkled-green

The above phenotypic ratio among F_2 progeny can be obtained algebraically based on product rule of probability of two independent events. The gamete combination of one parent is multiplied with that of other parent as:

$$(\tfrac{3}{4} + \tfrac{1}{4})(\tfrac{3}{4} + \tfrac{1}{4}) = (\tfrac{3}{4} + \tfrac{1}{4})^2$$

$$= (\tfrac{3}{4})^2 + 2[(\tfrac{3}{4})(\tfrac{1}{4})] + (\tfrac{1}{4})^2$$

$$= \frac{9}{16} + \frac{3}{16} + \frac{3}{16} + \frac{1}{16}.$$

(iii) More than Two Gene Pairs

This method of probability to predict the outcome of a cross involving more than two alleles is applied on the same basis taking one gene at a time. The Punnett square method is not a better approach for prediction of the outcome of a cross involving more than two allele. In such a complicated case of more than two gene pairs, the probability method is a better method to use for predicting the outcome (results) of a polycross. Some of the situations are considered below:

(*a*) *The combined probability of producing recessive homozygous of either type (AA BB CC DD or aa bb cc dd) for 4 different genes when each gene is assorting independently:* Such individuals are called as *quadruple recessive homozygote.* This will be obtained by considering one gene at a time. The probability of homozygous for either allele of gene pair is ¼. Therefore, the combined probability for all the 4 gene pairs will be = ¼ × ¼ × ¼ × ¼ = 1/256.

(*b*) *The combined probability of homozygous progeny for all the 4 genes*: This will be obtained by considering both types of homozygote for all the 4 gene pairs (Dominant homozygote, AA BB CC DD; and recessive homozygote, aa bb cc dd) considering one gene at a time. There are 2 types of homozygote (dominant and recessive) and the frequency of both types of homozygote are half of the total progeny (¼ AA + ¼ aa = ½). Therefore, the probability or frequency of the homozygous progeny of both the types for all the 4 gene pairs will be ½ × ½ × ½ × ½ = 1/16.

(*c*) *Combined probability of recessive phenotype for either one gene pair in a dihybrid cross (AaBb x AaBb):* First step is to know the number of genotypes producing this type of progeny. In a dihybrid cross, 3 genotypes will be homozygous recessive for one gene pair. These genotypes are A – bb, aa B -, and aa bb. Now the probability of each of the 3 genotypes will be estimated. The probability of A – bb genotype will be ¾ × ¼ = 3/16; of aa B – genotype will be ¼ × ¾ = 3/16; and of aa bb genotype will be ¼ × ¼ = 1/16. Now totaling the probabilities of all the 3 genotypes will be 3/16 + 3/16 + 1/16 = 7/16.

4.5 REASONS FOR REMAINING UNNOTICED THE MENDEL'S LAWS FOR 35 YEARS

Mendel's discoveries remained unnoticed for 35 years during 1866 to 1900. There had been certain special reasons for long delay in recognition to Mendel's work.

(1) Mendel had chosen discontinuous characters and many biologists were concerned with the problems of evolution to study the gradual changes in continuous variation. The concept of inheritance of continuous variation was not proved with Mendel's law.

(2) Mendel's law could not be proved with other organism by him and Nageli, the famous botanist who worked with hawkweed, *Hieracium* and failed to achieve a demonstration of segregation. It was because the hybrids between two different varieties in this organism arise directly from diploid tissue in the ovary without fertilization of gametes and thus some of the embryonic tissues will have exactly the same genetic constitution as its maternal parent and will not thus segregate for different characters among its offspring.

(3) Mendel's findings indicated that there was constancy of hereditary factors among generations *i.e.* the factors do not change but expressed themselves in new and different combinations among the offspring. The constancy of hereditary factors was unacceptable to those biologists who were interested for a source of variability in evolution.

(4) Mendel's preoccupation with probability events and mathematical ratios was an unfamiliar approach to biology.

(5) The physical basis of heredity (in terms of nuclear and chromosomal division) was not known.

(6) Mendel's results were published in an obscure periodical of limited circulation.

(7) Mendel was by then having trouble with the administration of monastery of which he had become the abbot (head) and hence could not work further.

4.6 BASIC MONOHYBRID CROSSES

The cross between two purebreds (homozygote) is called a *parental cross* or the *P_1 cross*. The progeny produced from parental cross is heterozygous and called as the first *filial* or F_1 *generation*. The progeny produced from mating of two F_1 individuals are called the F_2 *generation*.

An individual heterozygous for one pair of gene (having two different alleles at a locus, Aa) is called a *monohybrid*. Here, the mono refers one pair of gene and the hybrid means heterozygous or heterozygote having different genes. Thus, the two alleles at a locus are different in a monohybrid individual. A cross of two individuals which are heterozygous for one pair of gene is called a *monohybrid cross*.

There are *six types of monohybrid crosses:* These six crosses can be classified as:

(i) Crossing of Homozygote

Three crosses involve the crossing of homozygote of either type (AA × AA, aa x aa, and AA × aa) and each of the three crosses produces only one kind of progeny *viz.* the *first cross* (AA × AA) will produce all progenies with genotype AA, the *second cross* (aa × aa) will produce all the progenies with genotype aa, and *third cross* (AA × aa) will produce all progenies with genotype Aa. It can thus be concluded that a cross between any two homozygote (as the above three crosses) will produce all the progenies of only one kind having the same genotype.

(ii) Crossing of Homozygote with Heterozygote

This involves two crosses (Aa × AA and Aa × aa, say *cross number 4 and 5*) which are similar in that one of parent is heterozygote (Aa) and other parent is homozygote (either any of the two homozygote, AA or aa) and both the crosses will produce two types of progeny (heterozygous and homozygous) in equal proportions. [The cross Aa × AA will produce ½ Aa : ½ AA whereas the other cross (Aa × aa) will produce ½ Aa : ½ aa]. Moreover, the genotypes of two kinds of progenies in both the crosses are identical to those of the parents. The second type of cross (say lat cross number 6) involves the crossing of both the heterozygous parents (Aa × Aa). The last cross (heterozygous mating) produces three types of progeny in the ratio of ¼ AA: ½ Aa: ¼ aa.

(iii) Heterozygous Mating

This last cross of heterozygous mating (*cross no. 6 = Aa x Aa*) is special with respect to illustrate the segregation of genes in gametes during meiosis (the two members of each pair of homologous chromosomes are distributed into a separate gamete) and recombination of genes in the zygote in all possible combinations as a matter of chance. This is called the *law of segregation and recombination* which is the first law of genetics. This law was discovered by Mendel and hence the subject of the expression of phenotypic ratios due to segregation and recombination of genes is referred to as *Mendelian genetics.*

EXERCISES

3.1 As per the findings of Mendel on garden pea, round seed shape (R) was dominant over the wrinkled (r). Predict the genotype of the parents from the following results:

Parents	*Progeny*	
	Round	*Wrinkled*
(i) Round × Round	85	0
(ii) Round × Round	118	39
(iii) Round × wrinkled	90	0
(iv) Round × wrinkled	82	78
(v) Wrinkle × wrinkle	0	60

3.2 A highly inbred strain of mice with black fur was crossed with another inbred strain having gray fur. It was found that all the offspring had black fur. Predict the results of interbreeding the offspring.

3.3 A true breeding pea variety with tall plants and grey seed coat was crossed with another true breeding variety with dwarf plants and white seed coat. The F1 progeny results showed that all of them were tall with grey seed coat. The backcrossing results with dwarf white parent strain indicated 62 tall gray, 59 tall white, 57 dwarf grey, and 60 dwarf white. Whether two pairs of genes assort independently?.

Answer: Yes.

3.4 Predict the results of the following crosses of peas based on Mendelian observations when (i) a true breeding tall variety was crossed with dwarf variety, (ii) the self fertilization of F_1 progeny obtained from above cross, (iii) Back cross of F_1 progeny with both of their parents.

Answer: (i) All tall (ii) ¾ tall, ¼ dwarf (iii) all tall (iv) ½ tall and ½ dwarf

3.5 *Red feather colour* in pigeon is caused by dominant allele R and *brown colour* by recessive allele r. Another pair of gene controls the feather pattern, the *checkered pattern* being governed by dominant allele (C) and *plain pattern* by recessive allele (c). The birds of a true breeding checkered – brown strain are crossed with the birds of true breeding strain of plain red colour. Predict the phenotypes of the progeny produced and what phenotypes and in what proportions will appear the progeny from inter se mating of the progeny.

Answer: CC rr × cc RR = All F_1 will have genotype CcRr and hence their phenotype wiil be checkered, red. Among F_2 progeny, 9/16 will be checkered, red (C-R-): 3/16 plain, red (ccR-): checkered brown (C- rr): 1/16 (cc rr)

3.6 Black fur in rabbit is controlled by dominant allele B while the recessive allele produces brown fur. Another independently assorting gene pair controls the fur length, long fur being under the control of dominant allele, L while its recessive allele l controls the short fur (rex). A cross was made between a homozygous rabbit having long brown fur with a rabbit having short black fur. The F_1 offspring were intercrossed. What proportions of the rabbits with long black fur will be heterozygous for both genes.

Answer: Among the F_2 progeny 9 genotypes will have black long fur. These genotypic ratio are 1 (BB RR): 2 BB Rr: 2 BbRR: 4 BbRr. Thus, 4/9 of the rabbits with long black fur will be heterozygous for both genes.

3.7 The following crosses were made:

(i) AA × aa (ii) AABB × aabb (iii) AABBCC × aabbcc

Give the general formulae to predict the expected number of F_1 gametes, F_2 genotypes and phenotypes. What will be the expected number of F_1 gametes, F_2 genotypes and phenotypes from the above crosses?.

Hint:	F1 gametes	F2 genotypes	F2 phenotype
General	2^3	3^n	2^n
(i)	2	3	2
(ii)	$2 \times 2 = 4$	$3 \times 3 = 9$	$2 \times 2 = 4$
(iii)	$2 \times 2 \times 2 = 8$	$3 \times 3 \times 3 = 27$	$2 \times 2 \times 2 = 8$

Where, n = number of genes

3.8 Gray colour mice crossed with white mice (albino) produced all gray progeny. The F_2 population was produced by *inter se* mating of F_1. There were found 202 gray coloured and 70 white mice. Draw a diagram of the crosses and suggest the type of inheritance this colour character had based on these results. Test your hypothesis.

Chapter 5

Chromosome Theory of Heredity

Functions of chromosomes are to carry genes from parents to offspring (vehicle of heredity), role in sex determination, undergo mutation and play role in evolution, and help the cells to grow, divide and maintain itself by protein synthesis.

5.1 GENES ARE LOCATED ON CHROMOSOMES

- Parallelism between chromosomes and Mendelian factors.

The chromosomes are considered as the physical bases of heredity. They contain the units of inheritance, now called as *genes* but which were earlier called as Mendelial factors or determinants. The chromosomes (*genome*) are capable of transmitting the hereditary material (genes - DNA) to the next generation. The evidence in support of this chromosomal theory of heredity (genes are located on the chromosomes) requires:

- ☆ The mutant allele should define a gene,
- ☆ The chromosome should be distinguishable morphologically, and
- ☆ The pattern of gene transmission should be reflected by the chromosome behavior during reproduction. This means that the behavior of chromosome during meiosis provides the physical basis for the segregation and independent assortment of genes.

The chromosomes have DNA which is universally accepted as the genetic material to carry genetic information from parent to offspring. The chromosomes, being the carriers of genetic material (genes), are known as ***vehicles of heredity*** as they transmit the genetic material from one generation to the next.

Walter S. Sutton (1902) proposed *'Chromosomal Theory of Heredity'* showing the *parallelism between chromosomes and Mendelian factors* indicating that chromosomes are the vehicles of heredity.

(i) Two identical sets of chromosomes are present in each diploid cell, one each from each parent. The chromosomes behave as per expectation of heredity to make equal contribution of both the parents as a result of meiosis,

(ii) The chromosomes contain Mendelian factors (genes). The evidence comes from chromosome behavior at the time of gamete formation during meiosis (DNA replication), in terms of the mechanism of segregation, and independent assortment of characteristics.

(iii) The chromosomes are able to retain their structural uniqueness and individuality, unless there is a change (chromosomal aberration and mutation), and the changes are associated with the transmission of changed characters.

5.2 EVIDENCE OF CHROMOSOME THEORY OF HEREDITY

(I) Genes are Linked to Chromosomes - Experimental Evidence

Morgan, T. H. from America found the *Drosophila melanogaster* as the most suited organism for conducting genetic studies for the reasons of its quick and prolific reproduction, least costly to rear, and having only few number of chromosome (only 2n = 8 = 4 pairs of genes/chromosome) including one pair of sex chromosome which were morphologically different and distinguishable from each other as well as from autosomes. The two members of sex chromosomes in female fruit flies were ***homozygous*** (XX) which were equal in size and shape whereas the male flies were ***hemizygous*** [one of the two members of sex chromosome was longer (X) having genes than the other (Y) having no gene].

The inheritance of a sex-linked trait in *Drosophila* gave the first experimental evidence that the meiotic behavior of chromosomes is the basis of Mendelian principles of segregation and independent assortment of genes.

Morgan, T. H. (1909) conducted an experiment on *Drosophila melanogaster* (Fruit fly) and studied the inheritance of white eyes. He found the transmission of the mutant condition (white eye colour) in a male fly in association with sex. He correlated the inheritance of that gene with the transmission of the X chromosome during reproduction. This suggested that the gene for eye colour was present on the X chromosome. The following crosses were made:

Parents	$W^+ W^+$		x	$W\ Y$	
	(Red-eyed)		↓	(white-eyed)	
F_1	$W^+ W$			$W^+ Y$	
	(Red-eyed)		↓	(Red-eyed)	
F_2 progeny:	$W^+ W^+$	$W^+ W$		W^+Y	WY
	(Red)	(Red)		(Red)	(White-eyed)

On crossing the wild-type red eyed female fly with a mutant white eyed male, all the F_1 offspring were red eyed. This showed that white eye colour was recessive. On *inter se* mating, four genotypic classes of eye colour of F_2 progeny were produced, each class with different combination of genotypes for sex chromosomes (2 genotypes among females: $X^{W+} X^{W+}$ and $X^{W+} X^W$; and 2 genotypes among males: X^{W+} Y and X^W Y). All the F_2 females were red eyed but half of the male F_2 were red eyed and other half F_2 males were white eyed. This type of inheritance suggested that

- ☆ Eye colour was linked to sex chromosome (X) and hence the gene for eye colour was present on X chromosome but not on Y, and
- ☆ Also that two eye colour phenotypes were due to two different alleles of the sane gene.

Morgan repeated twice his experiment's hypothesis that the gene for eye colour in *Drosophila is X-linked* (present on X-chromosome):

In *one experiment* heterozygous females (red eyed: $X^{W+} X^W$) were crossed to white eyed males (X^W Y) and found that half of the progeny of each sex were red eyed and another half were white eyed.

First experiment

F_1	$W^+ W$		$W\ Y$	
	(Red-eyed) ↓		(White-eyed)	
F_2	$W^+ W$	$W\ W$	$W^+ Y$	WY
	(Red)	(White)	(Red)	(White)

Second experiment

P	WW		$W^+ Y$	
	(White-eyed) ↓		(Red-eyed)	
F_1	$W\ W^+$		$W\ Y$	
	(Red)	↓	(White)	
F_2	$W\ W$	$W\ W^+$	$W\ Y$	$W^+ Y$
	(White)	(Red)	(White)	(Red)

In the *second experiment*, he crossed homozygous white eyed females to red eyed males and observed that all the F_1 daughters were red eyed ($X^{W+} X^W$) whereas all the F_1 sons were white eyed (X^W Y). But on crossing these F_1 progeny, half of the progeny of each sex were white eyed and other half were red eyed.

The experimental findings showed that the eye colour mutation allele was present on the X chromosome and that gene was inherited along with the X chromosome during reproduction. This was then the conclusion that a gene for eye colour was physically located on X chromosome.

Morgan (1910) proposed the mechanism of *sex linkage* for white eye in Drosophila and gave the concept of linear arrangement of genes on chromosomes and supported the chromosome theory of inheritance.

(ii) Abnormal Chromosome (Non-disjunction) and Chromosome Theory

Bridges, C.B., one of the students of Morgan secured proof of the chromosome theory of inheritance showing that exceptions to the rules of inheritance could also be explained by chromosome behavior.

Bridges repeated the above second experiment of Morgan by crossing white eyed females to red eyed males. The results of F_1 progeny of this cross were as per expectation (red eyed females and white eyed males) with exception that few females were white eyed and few males were red eyed. All the exceptional males were found sterile but the exceptional females (white eyed) were fertile because they produced many progeny on crossing to normal red eyed males, progeny produced were white eyed daughters and red eyed sons in large numbers. These exceptional F_1 females also produced exceptional progeny.

Bridges gave the explanation that the exceptional F_1 females had been produced due to abnormal chromosome behavior during meiosis in the females of parent generation. Normally the X chromosome in these females should have been separated (disjoin) from each other during meiosis but they could not be separated and hence produced female gamete with 2 X chromosomes or no X chromosome at all. The results of this cross with X chromosome non-disjunction responsible for abnormal progeny can be shown as:

Parents	$X^W X^W$	X	$X^{W+} Y$
	(White eye)	↓	(Red eye)
F_1	$X^W X^{W+}$		$X^W Y$
	(Red-eyed)		(White-eyed)

F_2 progeny:

Female gametes

Male gametes (Normal)	X^W	$(X^W X^W)$ (Abnormal) Diplo- X ovum	O (Abnormal) Nullo – X ovum
X^{W+}	$X^{W+} X^W$ Red eye female	$X^{W+} (X^W X^W)$ Meta-female (Usually dies)	$X^{W+} O$ Red-eyed - sterile (Exception)
Y	$Y X^W$ White eye male	$Y (X^W X^W)$ White-eye (Exception)	Y O (Fertile) dies

The non-separation of 2 X chromosome during gamete formation would have been resulted a zygote with an abnormal number of sex chromosomes on fertilization of such abnormal female gametes by normal sperms. The non-disjunction female gametes containing either 2 chromosomes or no X chromosome unite with normal sperm having either X chromosome or Y chromosome to produce 4 types of zygote. As a result, XXY zygotes develop into female with white eye colour, the XO zygotes develop males with red eye colour and cold not produce progeny (sterile) whereas the YO zygotes die. Also the zygotes with XXX chromosomes with red eye colour will die.

Fertilization of abnormal female gamete ($X^{w}X^{w}$) with normal sperms (X^{W+} bearing) produced meta-female or super female ($X^{W+}X^{w}X^{w}$). These super females had anatomical abnormalities and hence these were weak and sickly, usually dies, whereas the fertilization of another abnormal female gamete (O, called null X) with normal sperm (Y bearing) produced YO zygote which were inviable (dies) due to the absence of X chromosome.

These exceptional results were due to abnormal chromosome behavior during meiosis (gamete formation) as a result of non-separation (disjunction) of 2 X chromosome in the female parent. Bridges called this abnormality as ***non-disjunction*** which occurred in the formation of female abnormal gamete ($X^{w}X^{w}$: Diplo - X ovum) by not separating the 2 X chromosomes ($X^{w}X^{w}$), leaving the other female gamete without X chromosome (O: Nullo – X ovum).

The above results gave strong view that genes are located on chromosomes and that Mendel's laws can be explained by the behavior of chromosome during reproduction. The chromosome theory of heredity stand proved.

The results proving that the genes are located on chromosomes are of great significance. On this basis of chromosome behavior during reproduction (Meiosis – gamete formation) the Mendelian principles of segregation and independent assortment can be explained.

5.3 MENDEL'S PRINCIPLES BASED ON CHROMOSOME THEORY

The cytogenetics which is a twin science comprising ***cytology*** (study of cells) and the ***genetics*** (study of heredity) through the discovery of genes provided evidence that the genes play significant role in sex determination. Wilson Edmund Beecher was a cytologist, showed interest to study the behavior of chromosomes in sex determination, and he was the first to investigate the differences in the chromosomes of two sexes. The sex differences were found to be confined to a special pair of chromosomes called sex chromosomes. Morgan, a geneticist and a friend of Wilson, discovered a gene that gave different phenotypic ratios in males and females. This enabled Morgan to hypothesize that this gene was located on one of the sex chromosomes. Bridges, C., one of the students of Morgan proved true the Morgan's hypothesis of location of gene on sex chromosomes that are visible structures within the cells. This helped the geneticists to explain the Mendelian principles of inheritance in terms of chromosome behavior during meiosis.

The chromosome theory of heredity has indicated that the genes are located on chromosomes. This theory has made it possible to explain the Mendelian principles of inheritance based on chromosome behavior during meiosis.

(i) Law of Segregation

The homologous chromosomes pair during the first meiotic division (chapter 9). These homologues come from different parent of opposite sex. The crossing of mother homozygous for an allele A for gene loci on this chromosome (AA) and the father homozygous for *a* for the same gene (aa), the progeny produced will be heterozygous of the genotype (Aa). During the anaphase of the first meiotic division, the paired chromosome separate and move to opposite poles of the cell. The separation of two homologous chromosomes segregates the alleles from each other and moves to the different daughter cells. This shows that segregation law of Mendel is based on the separation of homologous chromosomes during anaphase of the first meiotic division.

(ii) Law of Independent Assortment

The separation of anaphase chromosome is also the basis of the principle of independent assortment. This can be proved by taking a dihybrid cross (*Aa Bb*) for the two gene loci present on two different pairs of chromosomes. This dihybrid (*Aa Bb*) was produced by crossing of *AA BB* female with *aa bb* male, assuming tnat two pairs of genes are located on different pairs of chromosomes. The two pairs of genes are equally likely to be present in coupling or repulsion phase. In both the situations, the alleles A and B will move to the same pole with a 50 per cent chance or they may move to another pole with 50 per cent chance. The same is for the movement of *a* and *b* alleles. On reducing the chromosome number at the end of meiosis, half the gamete should contain a parental combination of alleles (AB or ab), and half should contain a new combination (Ab or aB). Thus, there will be 4 types of gametes in equal proportion. The equal gamete frequency is a result of the independent behavior of the two pairs of chromosome during first meiotic division. This is the proof of random alignment of different pairs of chromosomes at metaphase.

Chapter 6

Multiple Alleles

Mendel's fundamental experiment on garden pea contributed to basic knowledge about the unit nature of inheritance of characters which are inherited without change or dilution through generations. Mendel found F_2 ratio of 3:1 for monohybrid crosses and 9:3:3:1 for dihybrid crosses as a result of segregation of two different alleles for one and two pairs of gene, respectively among which one allele was dominant and the other was recessive. These F_2 ratios were called as Mendelian ratios. Mendel's laws of inheritance were confirmed following the rediscovery of Mendel's work in 1900 with other organisms.

6.1 CAUSES OF MODIFICATION IN MENDEL'S GENETIC RATIOS

Post Mendelian findings did not show the appearance of the phenotypic ratios as per Mendelian rules (Mendelian ratios) but some modified ratios were observed without following Mendelian rules of heredity and it was observed for both the monohybrid as well as the dihybrid crosses. These modified phenotypic ratios could not be explained by the presence of only two alleles for a gene pair among the population and by law of dominance at one locus. When the normal phenotypic ratios based on law of inheritance (Mendelian ratios) were not obtained it was but natural to think of other possible mechanism of inheritance to explain these modified phenotypic ratios.

The *phenotype is the expression of genes* (*genotype*) in such a way that the gene expression can be observed or measured. The genes are found to express themselves phenotypically in different ways. There are a number of *causes of variation in gene expression*. The gene expressions, based on modified phenotypic ratios, have been explained on the basis of the followings:

- Multiple allele system -Presence of more than two alleles for a gene pair,
- *Gene interaction:* Gene action which includes additive and non-additive gene action (interaction),
- *Lethal gene* has effect on modification of phenotypic ratios,
- *Environmental dependence of genotype:* Some genes produce their effects by interacting with *environmental agent,*
- *Linkage of genes* present adjacently on the same chromosome,
- *Sex controlled inheritance*

This chapter deals with the multiple allelic system; in the next chapter (number 5) have been discussed the different ways of modification of phenotypic expression of genes due to different types of gene action controlling the characters affected by one or more pairs of gene and the effect of lethal genes in modifying the phenotypic ratios and environmental dependence of genotype. The effect of linkage phenomenon of genes on modification of phenotypic ratios has been discussed in the subsequent chapter number 6 and the sex controlled inheritance has been given in chapter 7.

6.2 MULTIPLE ALLELES

Mendel gave the concept that the genetic factors or determinants now called genes exist in no more than two forms (states). This concept given by Mendel had to be modified on the discovery of genes with three, four, or more alleles.

Before a discussion on multiple alleles, it is necessary to understand the meaning of the two terms *viz.* locus and alleles.

Loci

The location (position or site) of a gene on a chromosome is called the *locus* (loci-plural). Thus, every gene has a locus on the chromosome. This was first described by Mendel that the factors (now called as genes) are present in pairs. Mendel called the genes as the factors. Therefore, an individual has only two genes at a locus and called as *diploid*. Therefore, maximum two genes are present at corresponding positions on homologous chromosomes of diploid individual.

Alleles and their Types

The two genes present at a locus of homologous pair of chromosomes may be identical in their structure or they may not be identical but both the genes are present at the same locus affecting the same character. These different forms of the same gene (in terms of different structure) found at the same locus on homologous chromosomes are called *alleles.* There are thus three points to consider a gene as an allele *viz.* the two genes are different in structure, present on the same locus on homologous chromosome and affect the same character. The word *allele* has been taken from Greek word meaning "of one another" because the alleles are alternate forms of a gene. The dominant and recessive forms of a gene are called alleles.

Consider an example of a particular gene present at the same locus (called as locus A) affecting a trait. There will be present two genes at this locus in an individual. These two genes in an individual may be identical in structure or not. If both the genes at this locus A are identical in their structure, the two genes may be written as AA or aa and the individual will be called as *homozygote* to have homozygous genotype (AA or aa). The homozygote produces only one kind of gamete *viz.* the individual with genotype AA (homozygote) will produce two gametes, each having the same allele (A) and the second homozygous individual with genotype *aa* will produce two gametes, each having the same allele (*a*). If the two genes at this locus are different in structure, one of the two genes will be written as A and the other gene as *a* and the individual will be called as *heterozygote* to have heterozygous genotype (Aa). These two genes (A and a) are called as alleles of each other, because they are the alternate forms of the same gene (being differing in structure) but they are present on the same homologous locus on the homologous chromosome affecting the same character. The heterozygote (Aa) produces two gametes of different types having different alleles, one gamete will have the allele A and the second gamete will have the allele *a*.

Suppose the character is the presence or absence of horns (called as polled condition). One of the two genes present on the same locus will develop the horns in a cow while its allele which differ in structure (alternate form of that gene which cause a cow to develop horn) will cause another cow not to develop horns and hence the cow will not have horns (called as polled). It has been observed that the alleles causing the absence of horn in a cow is dominant, designated by the capital letter P whereas its alleles which causes the horn to develop is recessive, designated by the small letter p.

Isoallele

Different forms of a gene that produce the same phenotype or very similar phenotype in homozygous state are called *isoalleles.* The whites in *Drosophila* of different origin are not alike. The hybrids are not alike which are produced by crossing of separate strains of whites to those that carry one of the intermediate allele (as eosin). The varions were observed in dilution of eosin colour.

Sub-allele

The genes from different strains are not exactly alike (Stadler) and show different distribution of the pigment. Such alleles are called as *sub-allele.* For example, Rr series for the purple aleurone and purple plant colour in maize behavelike a compound gene.

Pseudogene

An inactive but stable component of a genome resembling a gene and apparently derived from active genes by mutation. The multiple alleles at a given locus may not be mutants but they occupy different loci in close proximity in a chromosome. These are closely linked genes and called *pseudoalleles.* These pseudoalleles influence the expression of normal genes and show position effect. For example, the normal eye colour of *Drosophila* is red with some other shades like pink, apricot, white, *etc.*

The F_1 hybrids from crossing apricot with white are intermediate and hence prove two alleles.

Later on, Lewis (1951) observed some red flies among hybrid flied when crossing ove is increased in the vicinity of white locus. This shows that red coloured flies are the resultant cross-overs. He thus concluded that apricot and white are not alleles but reside at adjacent loci and hence pseudoalleles which suppress the expression of normal gene.

These alleles may arise by mutation on normal locus at adjacent locus in different chromosomes of the same pair and that there is no possibility of crossing over between them. Thus, *there is close relation between close linkake and allelism.* Therefore, the series of multiple alleles showing white, apricot and red colours may be actually the example of close linkage. Another example in *Drosophila* is the mutation of vestigial and antlered mutations which have occurred on two separate loci close to each other so as there is no crossing over between them. Thus, the normal, vestigial and antlered phenotypes have the genotypes as ++, vg vg and an an, respectively.

Concept of Multiple Alleles

During post Mendelian era, it became known that more than two alternate forms of a gene (alleles) occurred in population. The normal allele is called as *wild allele* while the newly formed allele is called as the *mutant*. The newly arisen allele (*mutant*) is produced from normal existing gene as a result of change in chemical structure of normal gene. This change is called *mutation* which is very rare. The mutation may occur several times in a gene and so several forms of the same gene may be produced. A large numbers of alleles at a locus are thus expected to be present but in different individuals of the population. Only two alleles can exist in a single individual because there are only two locations on a pair of homologous chromosomes. Therefore, the genes may exist in different allelomorphic states having two or more forms (alleles) but more than two forms of a gene (alleles) will be present in different individuals of the population. *This situation of existing more than two allelic form of a gene at a given locus in the population is called a multiple allelic system or series and the alleles are called as the multiple alleles.* When more than two alleles control a character, it is said that the character is controlled by multiple alleles.

The identity of a new mutation is tested by a simple test providing that the new mutation is recessive. A cross is made to combine the new recessive mutation with recessive mutations of known genes. The hybrid progeny producing a mutant phenotype indicates that a new mutation has arisen. But in case the hybrid progeny show a wild phenotype, it does not indicate the mutation. However, this test detects only the recessive mutation and the dominant mutations cannot be tested in this way.

Functional Relationship among Multiple Alleles

This relationship is studied by producing heterozygote with different multiple alleles by crossing homozygotes. This can be understood with an example of multiple allelic series producing variant coat colours in rabbits taking here only 4 alleles of the c gene by combining them in different kinds of heterozygotes *viz.* c^hc, c^{ch} c, c^+ c, c^{ch} c^h, c^+ $c^{h,}$ and c^+ c^{ch}.

The dominant recessive relations among these 4 alleles producing coat colour in rabbits can be studied by these heterozygotes. Among these, the wild type allele c^+ is completely dominant over all the other alleles in the series and produces wild colour (full colour, agauti colour – coloured hairs throughout the body). The *chinchilla* allele (C^{ch}) is partially dominant over the *Himalayan* (C^h), and *albino* alleles (c). The *Himalayan* allele is completely dominant over the *albino* allele. The dominance hierarchy among alleles is based on the phenotypic effect the alleles have on the character, coat colour. Thus, the dominance hierarchy (dominance relations among 4 alleles) is written as: $c^+ > c^{ch} > c^h > c$.

The *c* gene controls a step in black pigment formation in the fur. The wild type allele (c^+) produces coloured hairs on complete body. The *Himalayan* (c^h) and *chinchilla* (c^{ch}) alleles partially functional in producing some coloured hairs in the fur, whereas the albino allele (c) is not functional at all and hence does not produce any colour in the hairs of the fur. Such completely *nonfunctional alleles* are said as ***null*** or ***amorphic*** (Greek word meaning "without form") and these alleles are almost always completely recessive. *Partially functional alleles* are said to be ***hypomorphic*** (Greek word meaning "beneath form). These are recessive to the alleles that are more functional, including the wild type allele. Such mutant allele (*hypomorph*) has less expression than a wild-type allele.

Symbols for Genes and Multiple Alleles

There are different conventions to symbolize the genes and their mutations. Mendel denoted the genes by using letters, starting with A and proceeding further through the alphabets. William Bateson was the first to symbolize the genes by using the first letter of the word that was used to describe the phenotypic effect of the gene.

The mutant trait that deviates from the ancestral type is usually chosen the basis for the symbol of gene. The multiple allelic system/series are indicated (written) by the dominance hierarchy of alleles. The dominant allele to all others in the series is distinguished by capital letter, the recessive to all others in the same series is designated by the small letter and the intermediate alleles between these two extremes will be designated by some superscript with a small letter. The true breeding individuals are homozygous for different alleles of a gene controlling a character, *e.g.* plant height. The allele for dwarf is recessive and hence symbolized by the lowercase letter *d* and the allele for tallness of the plant which is dominant is symbolized by the corresponding uppercase letter ***D***. Thus, the letter used to denote the alleles of a gene is usually taken from the word that describes the recessive trait (d, for dwarf).

However, sometimes the mutant allele is dominant. In this case of dominant mutant allele, the nomenclature is to name the gene after the phenotype it produces. The example in this case may be taken for naming the gene responsible for controlling the length of tail in mice. The mutant allele discovered was found responsible to cause shortening of tail in heterozygote. Therefore, the dominant mutant allele was symbolized by the capital letter (uppercase letter) T, representing the tail length.

Secondly, in case of designating the multiple alleles of a gene, it is customary in genetics nomenclature, that the genes are often named after the mutant allele which produces the most abnormal phenotype. This is thus the naming of a gene after recessive allele, because most mutant alleles are recessive. The different alleles are distinguished from each other by superscripts. Thus, the multiple alleles of coat colour series in rabbit will be written in dominance hierarchy as $C > C^{ch} > C^{h} > c$.

There is another way to represent the wild type allele by a superscript plus sign after the letter used to represent the gene, like C^{+}. There is another practice that the letter is omitted and only the plus sign is used. Thus, C^{+} may be written simply as +.

6.3 CHARACTERISTICS OF MULTIPLE ALLELES

The multiple alleles of a series occupy the same locus on the homologous chromosome. In diploid individuals only two alleles of the multiple series are present in the cell of an individual. The crossing over does not occur within the alleles of a same multiple allele series because only two forms of a gene are present at homologous locus in an individual. They influence the same character but each allele has its different manifestation. Thus, they carry the same function but having different degree of efficiency.

The wild type allele (normal gene) is nearly always dominant over all the mutant alleles while the other mutant alleles in the series may show dominance or co-dominance among themselves or there may be an alternate phenotypic effect. The crossing of mutant with mutant produces mutant type and not the wild type. The two members of an allelic series are governed by the principle of segregation and recombination.

6.4 THEORY OF MULTIPLE ALLELES

There are following three theories about the multiple alleles

- ☆ Mutation theory
- ☆ Pseudoallelism (Close linkage among genes), and
- ☆ Heterochromatin theory of allelism.

The ***mutation theory*** of the origin of allelomorph has been widely accepted. Under the concept of multiple alleles, it has been postulated on the basis of mutation theory of allelomorphs that no crossing over occurs between alleles of a multiple series.

Pseudo-alleles Theory

Some gene loci may be so closely located and linked to each other that they are inherited together with minimum chance of crossing over. Such genes, undoubtedly different genetically, may behave like the alleles of the same gene and by mistake may be taken as multiple alleles. Such genes occupying two separate loci but having close linkage and hence very rare chance of crossing over, often inherit together are called pseudo-alleles (Lewis, 1951). Thus, *the pseudo-alleles are two closely linked genes and affect the expression of normal gene showing position effect.* Lewis conducted experiment on inheritance pattern of a sex linked character, the eye color, in

Drosophila. The normal eye colour is red which is wild type but with other shades of eye colour like, pink, apricot, cherry, buff, pearl, eosin, white. These were considered to form a multiple allelic series. The experiment of Lewis showed that red flies are cross over and therefore he concluded that apricot and white are not actually the alleles but they are pseudo-alleles occupying adjacent loci.

On the other hand, Pontecorvo (1958) had considered the *pseudo-alleles* as the different mutational and recombination sites within the same gene and thus the gene was regarded as sub-divisible defined by functional properties. Recombination through crossing over may also occur within such a gene rather than only between the genes. This functional gene has been termed as cistron (Benzer, 1957). The pseudo-alleles are functionally related and closely linked to inherit together most often. The mutant loci are so close to the normal allele that crossing over between them is not possible. The red, apricot and white colour which appear to form multiple allelic series are actual examples of (pseudoalleles) close linkage because red hybrids are produced when crossing over is greatly increased. In this context it needed to change the classical concept of gene that a classical gene may consist of more than one functional unit or cistron.

The alleles which produce the same phenotypic effect in homozygous state, nevertheless differ, are called as iso-alleles. Some genes behave as though it was a compound gene. Stadler had found that these genes are not exactly alike and called as sub-alleles.

Heterochromatin theory is another theory of allelisms. This theory states that the heterochromatin is brought next to genes by the chromosomal breakage and rearrangement and suppresses the expression of genes. There is evidence that position effects in maize are sometimes due to the transposition of very minute invisible fragments of heterochromatin.

6.5 EXAMPLES OF MULTIPLE ALLELES

The presence of multiple alleles has been found on autosomes as well as on sex-chromosomes.

Coat Colour in Cattle

Three colour patterns in cattle are governed by 3 alleles at a locus in a dominance hierarchy of alleles as $S^h > S > s$. These three colour patterns are as:

- ☆ $S^h S^h$ = Hereford pattern (white-face, white underside of body and top of neck),
- ☆ S S = Angus breed (solid colour, with no white spot),
- ☆ s s = Holstein breed of cattle (white spotting).

A fourth allele at this locus (S^c) has also been reported. This fourth allele produces the colour-sided pattern in Pinzgauer breed of cattle (Dutch). The colour-sided pattern contains the presence of coloured hairs on head, neck and sides of body, and a white strip extends from withers down the neck and behind the animal, continuing along the underline to the brisket. The gene, S^C is co-dominant over allele

S^h, thereby the heterozygote ($S^h S^c$) shows both patterns (Hereford and colour-sided pattern) and this allele is completely dominant over other two alleles (S and s).

The four alleles have been fixed in these different four breeds in homozygous state, as mentioned above. The crossbreeding results (crossing of four breeds in different combinations) on colour of purebred animals of these different four breeds, their F_1 and F_2 progenies have indicated that these 4 alleles producing different colours are located on the same locus and hence these four alleles are the multiple alleles. The combinations of these 4 alleles produce the following phenotypes with 10 genotypes as indicated below:

Homozygous	Heterozygous	Phenotypes
S^hS^h	$S^h S, S^h s$	Hereford pattern (white-face)
S S	Ss	Solid colour (Angus)
$S^c S^c$	$S^c S, S^c s$	Colour-sided (Duch cattle, Pinzgauer)
–	$S^h S^c$	Colour-sided and white-face
s s	–	Holstein spotting (white)

Coat colour in Horses: The coat colour patterns in horses are controlled by genes at several loci (see next chapter, under modifying genes). One colour series is controlled by at least three or four alleles. The 4 alleles with dominance hierarchy are: A′> A > a′>a. The 4 phenotypic classes (colour patterns) produced are:

- ✰ Wild type (bay colour with no markings, controlled by allele, A′);
- ✰ *Bay pattern* (black colour mane, tail and lower parts of legs with rest of the body usually of brown or reddish brown in colour, controlled by the allele, A);
- ✰ *Seal brown* which is similar to black except that lighter brown or tan hair over the muzzle and ears, and the flank area (controlled by the allele, a′); and
- ✰ *Black* hair on whole body (controlled by the most recessive allele in homozygous state, aa).

The four colour patterns with genotypes are shown here:

Phenotypes	*Genotypes*
Wild type	A′A′, A′A, A′a′, A′a
Bay pattern	AA, Aa′, Aa
Seal Brown	a′a′, a′a
Black (Solid colour)	a a

Some reports had shown that the wild allele (A′) is not present at this locus and hence only three alleles (A, a′ and a) control the three colour patterns.

Coat Colour in Mice

The multiple allelisms are also shown by coat colour of mice and cat as well as in various insects and plants. The coat colour in mice is determined by two series of multiple alleles.

The *albino series* comprises 4 alleles producing grey coat colour by normal allele represented by the + sign and others are albino (a), medium light grey (a^m), and extreme light (a^e) showing all the 3 alleles recessive to normal allele.

The second is the *black locus* but located on different chromosome. In this series the normal is the gray colour allele with multiple alleles of this series are those of producing black (b), yellow (y), grey body with light belly (G^L) and black body with light belly (b^L). The light belly colour is recessive to grey and also to the black (b) but the yellow of this series is dominant to all the effects of alleles.

There is another explanation about the series of multiple alleles controlling coat colour in mice:

Agouti locus with lethal effect: The agouti locus produce full colour and it has 5 alleles (A^y, A^W, A, A^t and a) in the series. The gene for yellow (A^y) is lethal in homozygous condition ($A^y A^y$) in embryonic stage and hence the yellow colour is produced from heterozygous state with one yellow allele. The progenies produced from mating of yellow mice are 2/3 yellow: 1/3 non-yellow (*gray brown* or *agouti*). The individuals (mice) with homozygous genotype for yellow colour (A^yA^y) dies in embryonic stage. Thus, the phenotypic ratio is modified. The allele A^y does not show complete dominance to other four alleles in this series which show dominance hierarchy as: $A^W > A > a^t > a$. Sometimes, the dominance hierarchy among alleles is considered as: $A^y > A^W > A > a^t > a$. These alleles in this series produce yellow (A^y gene in heterozygous state), white belly agouti, solid agouti (full colour), black with tan belly, and non-agouti (black), respectively. The gray-brown colour which is wild type colour is known as *agouti* colour.

Albino locus: Another coat colour in mice is produced by the *albino* locus, having 5 alleles, present on different chromosome. The albino allele is mutant of the gene (C) controlling the production of melanin in the hair, skin and eyes. The 5 alleles with dominance hierarchy are $C > C^C > C^h > C^e > c$. These 5 alleles produce full colour, Chinchilla, Himalayan, extreme dilute colour and albino phenotypes, respectively, when in homozygous state as well as in heterozygous state with other alleles (recessive alleles) of dominance hierarchy.

Coat Colour in Rabbits (Rodents)

One type of coat colour in rabbit is called albino series and governed by 6 alleles at a locus. The alleles are designated in order of dominance hierarchy as C (full colour) $> C^d > C^{ch} > C^l > C^h > c$. The 6 alleles produce 21 genotypes but only 6 phenotypic classes (6 types of skin colour) as under:

Colour phenotypes	*Genotypes*
1. Full colour or *agouti* or *wild colour*	CC, $C C^d$, CC^{ch}, $C C^l$, CC^h, Cc
2. Chinchilla (Silver gray)	$C^{ch} C^{ch}$, $C^{ch} C^l$, $C^{ch} c^h$, $C^{ch} c$
(i) Dark chinchilla	$C^d C^d$, $C^d C^{ch}$, $C^d C^l$, $C^d C^h$, $C^d c$
(ii) Light chinchilla	$C^l C^l$, $C^l C^{ch}$, $C^l c$
3. Himalayan white	$c^h c^h$, $c^h c$
4. Albino (pure white) or *colourless*	c c

The coat colour of wild type rabbit is known as *agouti or full* colour. Agouti is the wild colour and the allele for agouti is usually dominant, represented by capital letter C. These animals have banded hairs, being gray near the skin, followed by a yellow band and finally a black band or brown tip.

The *chinchilla* rabbits appear silver grey (diluted agouti) due to the optical effect of black and gray hairs. They lack yellow pigment. The allele for chinchilla shade is represented by C^{ch}. There are dark as well as light shades of chinchilla.

The allele for *Himalayan* (Russian) is represented by c^h. This coat colour pattern is white except for black extremes of ears, tail, feet and nose.

There is no pigmentation in *albino* rabbits and their eyes remain pink due to lack of pigment in iris of eyes. The albino allele is represented by the small letter c.

Coat colour pigments in Dogs: It is controlled by 3 alleles at a locus with dominance hierarchy of $A^s > A^y > a^t$ and produces 3 colours with the genotypes as:

Dark pigment	$A^s A^s$, $A^s A^y$, $A^s a^t$
Tan colour	$A^y A^y$, $A^y a^t$
Spotted pattern like	$a^t a^t$
(tan and black, tan and brown)	

Coat Colour in Foxes with Lethal Effect

There are three alleles controlling the coat colour in domestic foxes which show co-dominance and the two alleles are lethal in embryonic stage. The three alleles are represented as: W, w and p. The alleles w and p have lethal effects both in homozygous (ww and pp) and in heterozygous state (wp), resulting death at embryonic stage or at the most within a few hours after birth, in few cases. Three coat colours are produced. These are silver fur (WW), white-faced silver (Ww), and platinum colour (Wp). It is important to note that white-faced silver and platinum colours are produced from heterozygous genotypes. The lethal effect of w and p alleles modifies the phenotypic ratios resulting from certain mating *viz.* Ww x Ww, and Wp x Wp.

Eye Colour in Drosophila

The ***normal eye colour*** in Drosophila is red which has its variant colours. There are probably 12 alleles present at a locus on X chromosome for this system and produces several phenotypes. The white eye color was probably one of the first mutant allele known in this insect and subsequently different alleles producing different colour shades are designated as below:

Phenotype	Genotype	Phenotype	Genotype
Wild type Or Red	W	Honey	w^{h}
Coral	w^{co}	Buff	w^{bf}
Blood	w^{bl}	Tinged	w^{t}
Eosin	w^{e}	pearl	w^{p}
Cherry	w^{ch}	Ivory	w^{i}
Apricot	w^{a}	White	w

The wild type (red) colour is completely dominant and white is completely recessive to all other alleles in the series. Each allele in the series except w produces pigment but with less intensity in the series as indicated above between the eye colour of parental homozygote.

Wing Size in Drosophila

The Character wing size in Drosophila is controlled by 3 multiple alleles *viz.* L^{+}, L^{vg} and L^{a} with dominancy hierarchy as $L^{+} > L^{vg} > L^{a}$. The normal wing size or wild type is long represented by the allele L^{+} and dominant to other two alleles. The allele L^{vg} in homozygous condition produces vestigial wings and the allele L^{a} produces antlered wings.

In Drosophila, there are some ***wing abnormalities*** ranging in size from no wing to normal wings. These abnormalities producing gradations in the amount of wing are also controlled by multiple alleles when associated with certain gene combinations *viz.* normal wings being produced by the allele Vg^{+} whereas no wing condition is produced by the allele Vg^{nw} in homozygous condition. The others are small stump (Vg), narrow strap like wing (Vg^{st}), notched (Vg^{no}), and nicked (Vg^{ni}). The wild type allele (Vg^{+}) is dominant over other members of the series with dominance hierarchy as $Vg^{+} > (Vg^{st}=Vg^{no}=Vg^{ni}=Vg^{nw}=Vg)$.

Shell Colour of Land Snail

The colour pattern is due to 3 alleles at a locus showing dominance hierarchy as Brown > pink > yellow. Thus the yellow colour is most recessive. The 3 alleles can be represented as B, P, Y, respectively for the three colours in descending dominance. The three phenotypic classes of colours with their genotypes will be produced as:

Brown	BB, BP, BY
Pink	PP, PY
Yellow	YY

Plumage Colour in Mallard Duck

The trait is dependent on 3 alleles with their dominance hierarchy as $M^{r} > M > m$ and produces the following 3 phenotypes with their genotypes as:

Restricted mallard pattern	M^rM^r, M^rM, M^rm
Mallard	MM, Mm
Dusty mallard	mm

6.6 MULTIPLE ALLELES IN HUMANS

(i) Blood Groups in Man: Dominance and Co-dominance

The phenomenon of the exception of simple dominance, called co-dominance, is shown by human blood types.

The mixing of blood from two persons is not always safe. The introduction of blood tansfusion sometimes cures the patient but sometime kills. The reason is the differences in blood proteins of different persons. There are two types of substances in the blood which are known as ***antigens*** or *agglutinigens* present in RBCs and ***antibodies*** or *agglutinins* that occur in plasma. A person having an antigen in his BCs his plasma then has natural antibodies against the other antigen. Thus, a person who has antigen –A in his RBCs, his plasma will have antibody ***b***. There is reaction between antigen and antibody which results agglutination (coagulation). The antigen – antibody have lock and key system in their reaction. However, now it has been shown that antigens A and B ar not proteins but these are mucopolysaccharides (sugar + amino acids) and have a mol. Wt. of 3000,000.

On the basis of the presence and absence of antigens and antibodies, the people have 4 types of blood groups known as ABO blood group system in human population.

- ☆ Person of blood group A have ***antigen A*** in the RBCs and ***antibody b*** (anti B) in their plasma,
- ☆ Person of blood group B have ***antigen B*** in the RBCs and ***antibody a*** (anti A) in their plasma,
- ☆ Person of blood group AB have ***antigen A*** and ***B*** in their RBCs but no ***antibody*** in their plasma,
- ☆ Person of blood group O have no antigen in the RBCs but have both ***antibodies a and b*** (anti A and B) in their plasma.

This blood group system is genetically controlled by 3 alleles (A, B, O) at a locus. This is the well *known example of multiple alleles* in humans is the ABO blood group system.

The allele O is taken as normal allele whereas the alleles A and B represent two dominant mutations which have occurred on the same locus and represent co-dominance between them and both these alleles (A and B) are dominant over O. This is the mixture of co-dominance and dominant alleles. These blood groups are inherited in simple Mendelian fashion.

The 3 alleles form 6 genotypes *viz.* AA, AO; BB, BO; AB; and OO in the population. The heterozygous mating between blood group A and B (AO x BO) can produce children of all the blood groups. As a result of interaction among three alleles the following 4 blood groups (phenotypes) are produced from 6 genotypes as:

Blood groups	A	B	AB	O
Genotypes	AA, AO	BB, BO	AB	OO

The blood group A has ***4 subgroups*** (A_1, A_2, A_3, A_4) determined by separate alleles, among which $A_1$is more common and dominant to others. The A_2, A_3, A_4, alleles occur usually in combination with A_1 and rarely found in homozygous condition The A_1, is dominant to A_2, and so on. The reaction with B-serum is the basis of subgrouping.

Use of ABO Blood Groups

The discovery of ABO blood group system has been proved very useful to mankind in medico-legal aspects. It helps in solving the:

- ☆ Legal problems of disputed parentage,
- ☆ Problem of illegitimacy and the disputed cases of claimants to estates, and
- ☆ Problem to identify the persons in criminal proceedings.

Testing ABO Blood Groups

The coagulation test to ascertain the blood group is conducted. Antisera-A and antisera-B are taken either on slide or in test tube and adding a drop of given blood in each tube or on each slide. Now thorough mixing is done and observations are made as under:

(i) Coagulation of blood in tube A with antisera –A indicates that the blood group is A.

(ii) Coagulation of blood in tube B with antisera –B indicates that the blood group is B.

(iii) Coagulation in both the tubes indicates that the blood is of AB group.

(iv) No coagulation in either of the tube indicates the blood group is O.

The RBCs of blood group O persons have no antigen on their RBCs and hence not clumped by the serum of any blood group. Thus, such person can donate blood to the persons of blood group but may take blood from person of his own blood group. Therefore, the persons with blood group O are called ***universal donors***.

The serum of blood group AB has both antigens (A and B) and does not cause clumping of RBCs of any group. Thereforre, these persons may take blood from the persons of all the blood groups and hence called as ***universl recipients*** but can give blood to the persons of their own group. However, after the discovery of Rh factor the terms are not applicable. The persons of blood group A and B may take and give their blood to their own groups and also can give blood to persons of blood group AB and receive blood from persons of blood group O.

Donor's Blood Group	*Recepients Agglutinate the Blood of*				*Can be given to*	*Can receive Blood from*	*Remark*
	O	*A*	*B*	*AB*			
O	–	–	–	–	O, A, B, AB	O	Donor
A	+	–	+	–	A and AB	O and A	–
B	+	+	–	–	B and AB	O and B	–
AB	+	+	+	–	AB	O, A, B, AB	Recipient

(ii) Rh Factor in Humans

Landsteiner and Wiener (1940) discovered Rh factor from rabbits immunized with blood of monkey, *Macaca rhesus*. On injecting the blood of rhesus monkey into guinea pig produced the antibodies which would agglutinate the RBCs of all rhesus monkeys. This was an indication that monkey's RBCs contain a particular antigen which was designated as Rh. The guinea pig serum was used to test the human blood and it was observed that some person's RBCs were clumped while others were not clumped. Thus, it was the conclusion that some persons have the antigen similar to that found in rhesus monkeys and these were designated Rh^+ while others do not have this antigen and hence designated as Rh^-. The genetics of this antigen has indicated that Rh^+ is dominant over Rh^- character. This Rh factor in human has been found of great significance in child birth.

The Rh^- woman becomes sensitized by carrying an Rh^+ child from her Rh^+ husband. This is because some of the cells of Rh^+ embryo may mix into her blood during pregnancy. The first child from this type of genetic makeup is always normal but the RBCs of the foetus in second pregnancy are damaged because of passing through the placenta the antibodies in the blood of mother. This disease is called as ***erythroblastosis foetalis*** characterized by anemia due to damage of RBCs in the foetus and jaundice is the ultimate result because the blood vessels in the liver become clogged with damaged cells and bile is absorbed by the blood. This ultimately causes death of foetus before birth or soon after birth. In case of delivery of Rh^+ child, the mother is given injections of rhogam (preparation of anti-Rh antibody obtained from immunized donors) if the foetal Rh^+ cells are present in her blood. The rhogam forms a coat around foetal RBCs in mother's blood. This stops the availability of Rh^+ antigen to stimulate mother's circulation and there is no formation of antibodies.

There are more than two Rh blood groups determined by a series of *multiple alleles* according to Wiener while Fisher putforth the theory of *pseudoalleles* closely linked together so as they are inherited together as a block.

(iii) Haemoglobin Polymorphism in Human

The normal haemoglobin is determined by the allele A, sickle cell haemoglobin by the allele S (which causes the RBC to be sickle under reduced oxygen tension and causes haemolytic anaemia becoming fatal before the age of 20). The individuals with a third haemoglobin C in homozygous condition produce mild anemia with hemolysis. All the 3 haemoglobin are produced by 3 alleles present at a locus and all the 3 alleles have co-dominance relationship. Thus 6 genotypes are produced resulting into 6 phenotypes as:

AA, SS, CC, AS, AC and SC.

(iv) RBC Acid Phosphatase Enzyme

In man is controlled by 3 alleles at a locus with co-dominance among all the 3 alleles, designated as A, B and C producing 6 genotypes and 6 phenotypes.

Blood Groups of Farm Animals

There are some multiple allelic systems in farm animals affecting blood groups.

Sex-linked Multiple Alleles

The multiple alleles are also present on sex-chromosomes. The *feather colour of pigeons* is an example of sex – linked multiple alleles. Three alleles have been reported at a locus on Z chromosome. The three alleles can be designated as A, B, and b, producing ash red, blue and chocolate feather colours, respectively. The three alleles have the dominance hierarchy as: A > B > b. In pigeon, the males are homogametic (ZZ) and the females are heterogametic (ZW). The genotypes in two sexes and feather colours can be shown as:

Genotypes		*Phenotypes (feather colours)*
Males (ZZ)	*Females (ZW)*	
AA, AB,	Aa A (W)	Ash red
BB, Bb	B (W)	Blue
Aa	a (W)	Chocolate

6.7 IMPORTANCE OF MULTIPLE ALLELES

The presence of multiple alleles is general and has proved very important. The multiple alleles have their significant contribution in the analysis of genetic problems like reverse genetic approach.

NUMERICAL EXERCISES

6.1 If a man belongs to blood group B, his wife to blood group A, can they produce the children of all the four blood groups? Give your answer with full support.

[**Hint**: If both parents are heterozygous, they can produce the children of all blood groups]. This can be proved by making such a cross between AO and BO.

6.2 A young man and a girl, both having AB blood group, are married to each other. Find out the possible blood groups of their children.

6.3 A child having blood group O is claimed by two pairs of couples. The first couple belonged to blood group A whereas the husband of second couple belonged to blood group O and his wife to blood group AB. Give your decision that to which pair of couple the child belonged.

[**Hint:** The child must belong to the first pair of couple having blood group A]

6.4 A child had blood group O, his father had blood group B and his mother belonged to blood group O. Find out whether this child was really of this couple.

[**Hint**: There is 50 per cent probability of the child to belong to this couple provided his father is heterozygous B blood and her mother of O group. Make a cross and check.]

6.5 The crossing of coloured rabbit (full colour, agouti) with albino (pure white) produced the progeny in 1:1 ratio of coloured: albino whereas the crossing of colored rabbit with Chinchilla (silver grey) produced ½ coloured: ¼ Chinchilla: ¼ Himalayan. What were the genotypes of the parents in these crosses?

Chapter 7

Gene Action

I. Allelic Interaction (Additive Gene Action)

The existence of genes, to play their role in controlling a character, is inferable only from the expression of genotype in the form of a phenotype (character). The expression of a gene is different in the presence or absence of another gene present on the same or different locus. This is the basis of variation in gene expression (action or effect) which is of different types. The gene expression to produce phenotype is of two type *viz.* additive gene action and non-additive gene action (gene interaction).

7.1 ADDITIVE GENE ACTION (AGA) - LACK OF GENE INTERACTION

The *additive effect of genes* means the individual effect of genes which is independent of the presence or absence of another gene(s) and hence it is produced without being interacting with another gene(s) of the same gene pair or of another gene pair. This implies that the effect of a gene is not affected by the presence or absence of another gene. The important aspect of additive gene action is that each gene is contributing gene, adding some value to the character and the effect of each allele is considered to be arithmetically equivalent and additive or cumulative, for which these genes are called as additive or cumulative. The additive effect of gene either increases or decreases the phenotypic value (phenotype) on a linear scale of measurement.

The term additive gene action is used for explaining the effect of polygenes or minor genes affecting the economic characters in farm animals. This type of gene action leads to the population mean to be changed by replacement of a gene with another gene. The additive gene action merely implies an increasing or decreasing effect of a gene on the phenotypic value of a trait. Thus, the gene effect is expressed as the change in population mean due to the introduction of a gene. The amount of change in population mean attributable to gene substitution is called the average effect of gene. The gene influencing a trait by adding some amount to the phenotypic value of the trait is called favourable or positive allele while the gene which decreases the phenotypic value is called the unfavourable or negative allele or neutral gene. This is the actual meaning of additive gene action that the presence of each allele either adds or deducts the genetic value by one unit.

In additive gene action, there is no sharp distinction between genotypes, but many gradations are present in between the two extreme phenotypes. The skin colour inheritance in human may be taken as an example of the additive gene action (Davenport's theory). In this type of inheritance some genes are called the *contributing genes* which make their contribution in darkening of the skin, genes A, B, *etc.* whereas the genes *a* and *b*, etc make no contribution in affecting the skin colour and hence are called as neutral genes for their no contribution to skin colour. Therefore, the genotype *aabb* is called as the *residual genotype* which has no contributing gene. In this type of gene action, no gene is dominant or recessive and hence this indicates *lack of dominance* or *lack of epistasis*.

Additive type of gene action is most important in influencing most of the characters of farm animals which are of quantitative in nature (measured in metric units). The examples are production of milk, wool, egg, meat, growth rates and body weight, quality traits of milk, meat, fleece, egg. These traits are polygenic in nature.

7.2 NON-ADDITIVE GENE ACTION (NAGA)

The *non-additive gene effect* means such an effect of gene which is produced in the presence of another gene of the same locus or of different loci and hence the gene produces its effect after being interacting with another gene. Thus, the non-additive gene effect is dependent on presence of another gene and hence a gene produces its effect when combined and interact with another gene. In this type of gene action, the addition of a gene to the genotype does not add an equal amount to the phenotype. Thus, it is called as non-additive gene action (NAGA) which is the nonlinear expression of genes, also called as the *gene interaction* or gene combination effect which is of the following two types.

7.3 ALLELIC INTERACTION

The allelic interaction occurs when the genes interact with their own allele. This is also called as intra-allelic interaction. The example is the *dominance* which may be complete, incomplete or partial and over-dominance. The allelic interaction depends on the expression of heterozygous genotype. The phenotypic expression of heterozygous genotype is variable. It may be either similar or different to varying degree to the phenotypic expression of either homozygote. The example of similar phenotypic expression of heterozygote to either homozygote is the dominance whereas the examples of phenotypic expression of heterozygote different to homozygote to varying degrees are the incomplete or partial dominance and over-dominance.

(1) Dominance or Complete Dominance

The dominance arises when the phenotypic expression of heterozygous genotype is similar to either of the homozygous genotype. The allele of a gene pair is called as *dominant* if it expresses itself in the heterozygote by inhibiting the expression of another allele. The allele whose expression is masked/inhibited is called *recessive allele*. This phenomenon is called as *dominance*. When the dominance is complete, identical phenotypes are produced by the heterozygous individuals and by dominant homozygous individuals as:

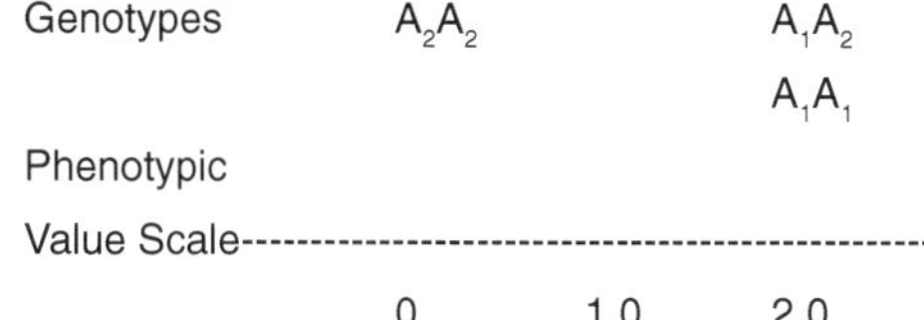

Figure 7.1: Dominance Model.

The phenotypic ratios of monohybrid crosses among F_2 progenies with complete dominance are 3:1, *i.e.* [3 (dominants):1 (recessives)]. The examples of traits showing complete dominance, in different species are:

Species	*Characters*	*Dominant Phenotype*	*Recessive Phenotype*
Cattle	Horn	Polled (No hornPP, Pp)	Horns (pp)
	Ear notch (Ayrshire)	Notch (NN, Nn)	Normal (nn)
	Colour	White face	Coloured (solid)
		Solid colour	Irregular white spotting
		Black hair coat	Red hair coat
		Red	Yellow (light red)
	Hoof type	Cloven hooves	Mule feet
Sheep	Coat colour (wool)	White wool (Bb, Bb)	Black wool (bb)
	Fleece type	Hairy fleece	Wooly fleece
	Eye colour	Brown	Blue
Swine	Coat colour	White	Black
	– do –	Black hair	Red hair (Hampshire)
	Foot condition	Mule footed (MM, Mm)	Cloven hoof (mm)
	Ear	Erect	Drooping
Poultry	Plumage colour	White	Coloured
	Comb shape	Rose comb (RR)	Single comb (rr)
		Pea comb	Single comb
	Feathers on legs	Feathered (FF, Ff)	Clean legs (ff)
	– do –	Normal feathers	Silky feathers
	Feathers colour	Coloured	White
	– do –	Black feathers	Red feathers
	Skin colour	White skin	Yellow skin

Species	*Characters*	*Dominant Phenotype*	*Recessive Phenotype*
Horse	Hair colour	Black hair coat	Chestnut or sorrel
		Bay	Black (non-bay)
		Smooth hairs	Curly hairs
	Movement	Trotting	Pacing
Turkey	Coat colour	Bronze (RR, Rr)	Red (rr)
	Feather condition	Normal (HH, Hh)	Hairy (hh)
Rabbit	Hair length	Short (LL, Ll)	Long (ll)
	Hair colour	Black hair (BB,Bb)	white hair (bb)
	Hair morphology	Normal	Wuzzy- unkempt
Drosophila	Body colour	Gray (b'b', b'b)	Black-ebony (bb)
	Eye shape	Lobe shaped (LL, LL')	Oval (L'L')
	Eye colour	Red (S'S', S'S)	Sepia (SS)
	Wing size	Normal (vg'vg', vg'vg)	Vestigial (vg vg)
Guinea pig	Coat colour	Black (BB, Bb)	White (bb)
	Hair length	Short (LL, Ll)	Long (ll)
	Coat texture	Rough (RR, Rr)	Smooth (rr)
Fox	Coat colour	Red (BB, Bb)	Silver black (bb)
	Body Size	Normal (DwDw, Dwdw)	Dwarf (dw dw)
	Behaviour	Normal (VV, Vv)	Waltzing (vv)
	Tail shape	Kinkled (KK, Kk)	Normal (kk)
Dog	Body colour	Dark (solid)	Albino (White spotting)
	Hair colour	Red hair	Yellow hair
	Hair size	Short	Long
	Hair texture	Wire haired (WW, Ww)	Smooth hair (ww)
	Deafness	Normal (DD, Dd)	Deaf (dd)
	Ear	Erect (EE, Ee)	Drooping (ee)
	Barking	Barkness (BB, Bb)	Silence (bb)
	Tail	Stumpy	Normal
Cat	Hair length	Short	Long hairs
	Hair colour	Black	Brown hairs
	Skin colour	Tabby	Black or blue
		Colour	White
		Agouti	Non-agouti

(2) Co-dominance (Independence of Allele Function)

The co-dominance implies that the two alleles at a locus are independent in their functioning to produce the phenotype in the heterozygous individuals. This exception to simple dominance arises when a heterozygote shows characteristics found in each of the associated homozygote. Thus, neither allele is dominant or even partially dominant over the other. This is also called as lack of dominance. The co-dominance occurs when the two alleles at a locus do not show dominance-recessive relation in their expression but both the alleles are capable to express them phenotypically in the heterozygous condition and the phenotype is a mixture of the phenotypic traits produced by either of the alleles in homozygous condition. The co-dominance differs from additive gene action in the sense that the effect of co-dominant alleles is not the additive though both alleles express themselves in heterozygous condition.

The co-dominant alleles are not shown by the upper- and lowercase letters like the dominant recessive alleles but these (co-dominants) are represented as superscripts of the first letter of the name of discoverer or by the upper case letters of both the alleles, as M and N. The MN blood group was discovered by Karl Landsteiner and hence the M allele is written as L^M and N allele as L^N.

The co-dominance of alleles modifies the F_2 phenotypic ratios of monohybrid crosses from 3:1 (with complete dominance) to 1:2:1, *i.e.* [1(dominant homozygote):2 (heterozygote):1 (recessive homozygote)]. The examples showing co-dominance for qualitative traits are as under:

(i) Cattle: *Coat colour in Shorthorn cattle*: The character coat colour in Shorthorn breed of cattle is controlled by one pair of gene which shows co-dominance to produce hair colours on the body. The two alleles are denoted as R and W which produce three different coat colours *viz.* Red (RR), White (WW) and Roan (RW). The heterozygous animals (RW) had a different colour of the body called as *roan* which is admixture of red and white hairs on the body. The heterozygous mating produce red, roan and white offspring in 1:2:1 ratio and thus the phenotypic and genotypic ratios are equal and similar. Both the alleles (R and W) have their effect in heterozygous condition and hence called as co-domonant alleles which do not prevent the effect of each other. Thus, the dominance was lacking or absent.

Body size of Hereford cattle: The body size of Hereford breed of cattle is controlled by one pair of gene denoted as N and C. These two alleles produce animals of three different sizes *viz.* normal size (NN), dwarf size (CC) and comprest dwarf size (NC) which is intermediate. The mating of comprest dwarf animals produce the animals in the ratio of 1 Normal (NN): 2 Comprest (NC): 1 Dwarf (CC). The mortality rate is high among dwarfs (CC) and it is impossible to mate them with normal to produce comprest as the *dwarfs* do not survive to maturity, having lethal effect.

The examples of genes expressing like co-dominance in other species are as under:

Species -	*Characters*	*Homozygote 1*	*Heterozygote*	*Homozygote 2*
(ii) Sheep -	Wool quality	Normal(N′N′)	Medulated (N′N)	Hairy (NN)
(iii) Guinea pig -	Coat colour	Yellow(YY)	Cream (YW)	White(WW)
(iv) Poultry -	Feather morphology	Normal (NN)	Mild Frizzle (NF)	Frizzle (FF)
	Feather colour	Black	Blue	White

(v) Drosophila -	No. eye facets	800 (B′B′) Normal	250-500 (B′B)	60 (BB)
	Eye colour	Red eye	Pteridine (reduced pigment)	Sepia colour
(vi) Goat –	Ear size	Long ears	Medium	Short
(vii) Swine -	Body colour	Black	Black and Red spots	Red

The blue Andalusion fowls, arise from the combination of alleles for white and black feathers, is not a true breeding variety. The blue Andalusian fowl, exhibiting codominance between black and white feather colour alleles, is in real sense a fine mosaic of black and white areas that appear to be blue.

(viii) The *coat colour in horse* show lack of dominance. The *palomino* horses (copper or golden colour) never breed true due to heterozygosity for colour genes (Cc). The palomino are produced from mating of *Chestnut* (full colour, CC) or Sorrels (which are homozygous for one of the alleles) with pseudo albino or white *Cremello*, the light cream colour (cc) which are homozygous for another allele (Castle, 1948).

(ix) The *sickle cell disease in humans* is characterized by severe chronic anemia, retarded physical development and pains in joints, muscle and abdomen. This disease is the result of a gene, S, when homozygous (SS) and is almost fatal without exception. The homozygous individuals (SS) had all the RBC in their blood of grossly abnormal form (sickle shape), instead of the normal round shape, due to deprivation of access of oxygen to the blood. The heterozygous individuals are healthy but having some RBC as sickle shape and all of the cells can be sickled by oxygen deprivation though a greater reduction in oxygen tension will be required than in persons of SS genotype. In normal persons (AA) only haemoglobin A is found in the RBC. The genotype AS produce both types of haemoglobin (A and S). In this case neither gene affects the expression of other gene. The heterozygote has seldom anemia (mild). The SS individuals seldom survive to reproduce and usually die of anemia. The heterozygote (AS) are more resistant to malaria than normal AA persons.

(x) The *human blood groups* (MN system and ABO blood systems) show co-dominance. The genes M and N are co-dominant for MN group whereas the genes A and B are co-dominant for ABO system.

The blood testing for M-N blood group is done by agglutination test. One serum called anti-M recognizes only the M antigen on human blood cells while another serum called anti-N recognizes only the N antigen on these cells. The production of M and N antigens on cells is under the control of a gene locus with two alleles. One allele allows the M antigen to be produced while the other allele allows the production of N antigen on the cell. Homozygote for M allele (MM) produce only the M antigen and the homozygote for the N allele (NN) produce only the N antigen whereas the heterozygote individuals having both the alleles (MN) produce both the antigens. These two alleles are said to be codominant because both the alleles contribute independently to the phenotype of the heterozygote for this locus.

(3) Incomplete or Partial or Semi Dominance

This is the invariable expression of co-dominant alleles, when the dominant allele does not completely mask the expression of its recessive allele. In this case, the phenotypic value of heterozygote is different from either of the two homozygotes but somewhere in between to them.

A heterozygote has its phenotype different from that of either homozygote. The best example of incomplete or partial dominance relation among alleles is the flower colour in the ***snapdragon*** (*Antirrhinum majus*). There are two pure varieties which are homozygous for different alleles of a colour determining gene locus. One homozygous variety produces white colour flowers while the second pure variety produces flowers of red colour. On crossing these two pure varieties, the flowers of F_1 hybrid had pink colour. Thus, the production of flowers of another colour was an evidence of the fact that none of the allele is either dominant or recessive for producing flower colour.

Geneticists have explained that the intensity of pigmentation depends on the amount of a product of colour gene. Therefore, the allele responsible for producing red colour of flowers had incomplete or partial dominance over the allele producing no colour (white flowers). The allele producing no colour is therefore designated by the lower case letter *w*while the allele producing red colour is designated by the uppercase letter *W*. Therefore, the allele *W* produces a product responsible for red colour whereas the intensity of red colour in terms of the amount of pigmentation is reduced in the presence of *w* allele in heterozygous condition (Ww). The flower colour of heterozygous plants is thus diluted from red to pink colour because the heterozygous flowers have only one dose of the colour producing gene (W) whereas the homozygous plants (WW) have double dose of the colour allele (W) and hence the homozygote for colour gene will produce flowers with more intensity of pigmentation for red colour. The heterozygote (Ww) will thus produce less intense colour (Pink) in their flowers. This partial dominance is also said as ***semi dominance.*** The word ***semi*** is a Latin word meaning "half" and thus making half dominant and hence called semi-dominant.

The partial dominance in quantitative terms indicates that heterozygote is not exactly at the midpoint of the phenotypic value of two homozygotes, whereas the incomplete dominance indicates that one allele is more dominant than the other.

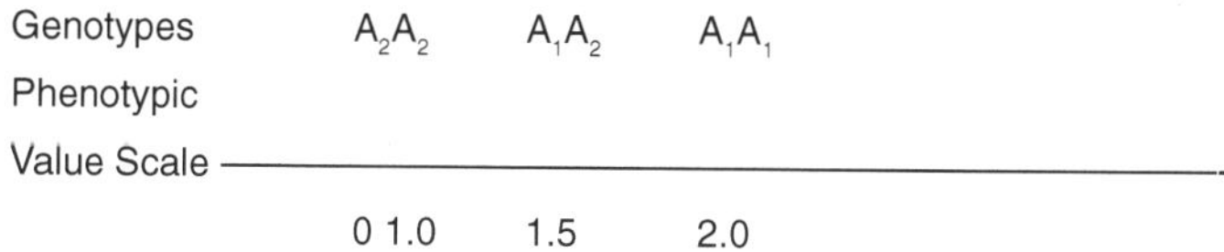

Figure 7.2: Incomplete Dominance Model of Gene Action.

However, irrespective to the term used for this type of allelic interaction, it is important to note that the expected phenotypic ratios of monohybrid crosses should be 1:2:1, similar to co-dominance, instead of 3:1 expected with complete dominance.

(4) Over-dominance

The over dominance is also allelic type interaction and is indicated when the phenotypic value of heterozygote is superior to either of the two homozygote.

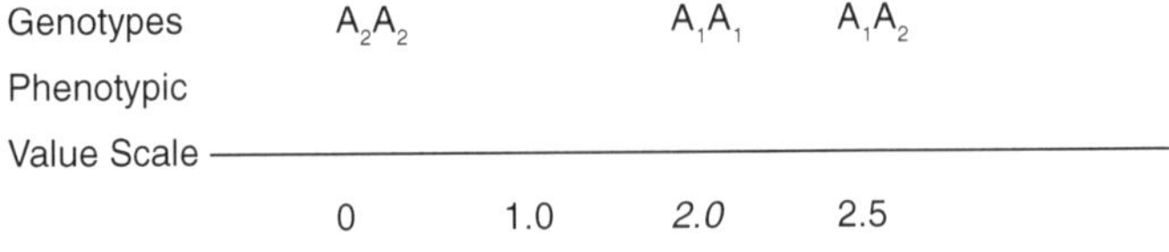

Figure 7.3: Over Dominance Model.

This is a type of gene action as a result of which the progeny is superior to either of the parent. The gene is a complex organic molecule. Therefore, a chemical reaction between two alleles (A and a) may be different and greater than the reaction between AA or aa. Thus, genes in heterozygous state enter into some kind of interaction whereby a greater net result is produced than the genes in either of the homozygous condition and this makes the heterozygous individual to be superior to either of the homozygous.

As a result of this type of gene action, the heterozygous individuals pass through unfavourable environmental conditions more successfully than the homozygote because "A" allele may respond more favourably to one type of environment and "a" allele to the different environment. Thus "Aa" condition produces more favourable results than AA or aa condition.

The phenomenon of overdominance is illustrated in the inheritance of a particular *blood type in rabbit* (*RBC antigen*) where 2 alleles are responsible: One allele produces one antigen and the second allele produce second antigen, and a different third antigen (which was not present in either homozygous) was produced in the homozygous individuals.

The *human haptoglobin* (*binding haemoglobin*) is another example. The two homozygote produce 2 haptoglobins which are proteins and the heterozygote produce a third (not present in either of the 2 homozygote) plus these 2 haptoglobins which are produced in the 2 homozygous individuals.

The phenomenon of overdominance, besides the allelic interaction, may probably involve many pairs of genes (non-allelic) affecting the same character. In case of polygenic inheritance, the effect of any one pair of genes may be rather small but the combined effect of many pairs result in a considerable advantage to the heterozygote and the combined effect of many loci is greater than the sum of the total effect of the additive effect of genes. The expression of hybrid vigour by crossing certain lines, strains, or breeds could be a result of over-dominance together with dominance and epistasis. Heterozygote are at advantage because of the combined effect of many pairs of genes brought together rather than the small effect of any one pair of gene.

These types of gene action (allelic interaction) are all varied expressions of dominance and do not differ too much except in overall effects and the interrelationship among them may well be illustrated by taking a hypothetical example as under. The value of A is taken as 5 units and of a = 2 units.

Type of Gene Action	*AA*	*Aa*	*aa*
Lack/absence of dominance (Additive)	10	7	4
Complete dominance	10	10	4
Partial/incomplete dominance	10	8	4
Overdominance	10	12	4

(5) Lethal and Sub-lethal Genes (Pleiotropic effect of genes)

It has been recognized that most of the mutations are recessive which are detrimental (deleterious) to the organism. There are many detrimental genes in farm animals. However, some mutation are beneficial like polled trait in cattle is beneficial to man but such beneficial mutations are few.

The detrimental genes have been defined and classified depending on the time and extent of their effect (drastic effect) on the organism. The mutant allele may affect the vigour or vitality of the individual at any age of the individual. Accordingly, *the detrimental genes* are classified into three types *viz.* detrimental or non-lethal (called as sub-vital genes), semi-lethal (or sub-lethal) and lethal genes.

Sub-Vital Genes or Non-Lethal

This group of detrimental genes express themselves to some extent only in reducing the vigour and vitality of the individual, and thus they can escape to be detected.

Lethal Genes

Second group of detrimental genes cause death of the individual and called *lethal genes.* The effect of lethal genes starts from gamete formation resulting in *prenatal death* (before birth) at zygotic stage or embryonic (foetus) stage during pregnancy or *peri-natal death* at the time of birth or soon after birth within few hours or *post-natal death* in early life (young age). However, a number of genetic and non-genetic (environmental) factors may be responsible for death. The genetic cause of death is due to genes which are incompatible with development and these genes are called lethal genes. ***Yellow*** is lethal in mice, ***creeper*** lethal in chickens, lethal in cattle (like ***bull dog calf***), ***brachyphalangy*** (short fingers), ***sickle cell anaemia*** in man, ***Huntington' chorea*** in man (muscular failor, mental retardation and finally death), ***epiloia*** lethal in man is caused in heterozygous condition (dominant lethal) and causes mental defects, tumours and abnormal skin growths. The lethal genes may be dominant lethal, recessive or conditional.

Semi-lethal or Sub-lethal Genes

Third group of detrimental genes causes death of individuals but sometime at later age of life and called as *semi-lethal* or *sub-lethal genes*. The semi-lethal or sub-lethal genes also cause some death losses in animals *e.g. dwarf condition* in Hereford cattle produced by mating of comprest with comprest. The dwarf animals are born alive but die before sexual maturity.

Abnormalities and lethal genes are mostly recessive in inheritance caused by one or more loci. However, in some cases the recessive is not complete but the gene has its phenotypic effect in heterozygous state. The heterozygote are sometimes more desirable than homozygous normal *e.g.* Dexter breed of cattle, infertility in Swedish dairy cattle due to *gonadal hypoplasia* is hereditary but is correlated with high milk production with higher fat content.

The mode of expression of lethal genes is that they being mostly recessive or partial dominant must be in homozygous condition to have their full effect. The frequency of recessive genes which are either detrimental or sub-lethal is very low in the population and they appear in homozygous state only through inbreeding. This is one of the reasons that inbreeding is avoided. However, when the frequency of lethal or detrimental genes is high in the population, they are produced without inbreeding.

Increased rate of inbreeding results the recessive lethal to come into play and thus inbreeding leads to higher death losses in the young ones from conception to birth or up to weaning age. Inbreeding is thus very important to discover the recessive mutations particularly for the mutations resulting in defective development in which the heterozygote does not have selective advantage.

Sickle cell disease in humans is caused by a gene in homozygous state (ss). This gene has its drastic effect to result in death. Such genes are called lethal genes. The fully dominant lethal allele arises occasionally by mutation from a normal allele and majority of mutations are recessive in their effect. However, the dominant lethal have more effect in a population because they are fatal to both dominant homozygous as well as to heterozygous individuals. The completely recessive lethal gene have their effect only in homozygous condition, but some of the recessive lethal alleles also exhibit a distinctive phenotype without lethal effect when present in heterozygous state *i.e.* in a co-dominant system. Such genes result in the modification of Mendelian ratios if they kill the organism before birth, or before hatching in poultry or before germination in plants.

Dominant Detrimental/Lethal Genes

The examples of dominant detrimental/lethal characters are as under:

The *creeper condition in fowl* is due to a dominant gene (Cc) which has an effect on the vitality when homozygous (CC). The creeper birds are always heterozygous (Cc) because the cross of creeper with creeper produce 2:1 ratio of creeper to normal. The normal birds are recessive homozygous (cc), the creepers with short and deformed legs and wings are heterozygous (Cc) and the dominant homozygous (CC) birds die before birth.

Hairless condition in Mexican dogs is produced by the heterozygous condition (Hh). The homozygous recessive dogs (hh) are normal whereas puppies homozygous for H allele (HH) are usually born dead with abnormalities of mouth and absence of ears. Thus, heterozygous creeper (Cc), normal (cc), and homozygous dominant (CC) is lethal.

The *coat colour in mice* is controlled by genes located at about 24 or more loci and some of these genes also affect skeletal growth and development of certain body tissues. The heterozygous yellow mice (Yy) survive but the dominant yellow mice (YY) die during pregnancy. The yellow colour gene is dominant (Y) and lethal over non-yellow. Thus, heterozygous yellow (Yy), non-yellow (yy), and homozygous yellow (YY) is lethal.

The gene for *coat colour (platinum) in foxes* is dominant and lethal. The homozygous dominant foxes with platinum colour (PP) die before birth and the mating of heterozygous platinum foxes (Pp) produce platinum to silver progeny in 2:1 ratio instead of 3:1. The silvers are homozygote recessive (pp).

The *gray colour in sheep* is due to a partially dominant gene. The homozygous gray sheep (GG) have defect of digestive tract (abnormal abomasum) and die during embryonic stage or within few months after birth. The heterozygous gray sheep (Gg) survive. The black colour sheep are homozygous recessive (gg).

Pelger anomaly of rabbit (abnormal WBC number segmentation) is expressed in heterozygous state of two alleles (Pp) and the normal individuals are homozygous recessive (pp). The homozygous dominant genotype (PP) causes grossly deformed skeleton causing death before or very soon after birth.

Polydactyly in cattle (extra toes on one or all feet) is most probably controlled by dominant gene. Such animals show lameness and hence undesirable. The gene is thus detrimental.

The *umbilical hernia in cattle* (Holstein-Friesian) appears at the age of 8-20 days, persists up to 7 months age, is limited to male calves and controlled by a dominant gene.

Brachyphalangy (shortening of middle joint of one or more fingers) also called *brachydactyly* and the *thalesemia* in man are dominant characters which cause lethality before sexual maturity in heterozygous individuals. The homozygous individuals for thalessemia have severe anemia (thalessemia major) and die before maturity, heterozygote have mild anemia (thalessemia minor).

Huntington's chorea in human is a disease, caused by a dominant gene and results in progressive degeneration of the nervous system. This causes death after about 30 years of age. This disease is caused by the dominant latent lethal (sub lethal) gene, having its effect after sexual maturity, getting a chance to reproduce.

(ii) Recessive Detrimental/Lethal Genes

There are some alleles which are lethal in homozygous recessive state. The followings are some of the examples of recessive detrimental/lethal characters:

Amputated condition (absence of legs) in *Swedish Friesian cattle* is caused due to a recessive lethal gene. The calves are still-born or die soon after birth. The mating of normal with normal produces an amputated calf which is usually dead at birth.

The *parrot beak in Shorthorn cattle* (abnormal lower jaw with impacted molar teeth): The gene in heterozygous condition shows no detectable sign of gene's presence and the cattle are normal. The gene in homozygous recessive condition result the still-born calves or they die after birth within one week and they have parrot beak.

Hairless and semi-hairless cattle are the two characters which are due to recessive gene. Another character *snorter dwarfism in Angus and Hereford cattle* is semi-lethal. The dwarfs have difficulty in breathing for which the term *snorter* is used. The gene is actually semi-dominant and has some effect in heterozygous condition.

Bull dog in cattle is recessive lethal (semi-dominant lethal). The heterozygous (Dd) are Dexter type showing the effect of lethal gene having short leg. The homozygous dominant (DD) cattle are known as Kerry type having long size legs. The homozygous recessive (hh) produces a lethal bull dog calf (*achondroplasia*).

Syndactylism (having one toe in place of two, on one or more feet) has been reported in Holstein-Friesian cattle and is probably controlled by a recessive gene.

White heifer disease has been reported in *Shorthorn* heifer with constricted hymen, missing of anterior vagina and cervix and rudimentary uterine body is probably a sex limited recessive character.

Short vertebral column is due to a recessive gene. The calves are still-born or die soon after birth.

Prolonged gestation of 310-315 days in cattle seems to be due to a lethal recessive gene.

Parrot mouth dwarfs has been reported in *Southdown sheep*. This is due to semi-lethal recessive gene, killing all lambs within a month of birth.

Amaurotic idiocy is a recessive hereditary abnormality causing death within the first few years of life in homozygous recessive state. This condition is characterized by mental and physical retardation, abnormal lipid metabolism and total blindness. The heterozygous individuals are normal, indicated that the allele causing the defect is recessive.

Tay Sach's lethal in young children causes death. It is recessive lethal.

Conditional lethal: The normal gene in a particular environment may become lethal as a result of change in environment.

A recessive gene in poultry causes feathers to break off and the chickens homozygous in homozygous state of the gene are featherless. These chickens survive in relatively warm environment but they die when temperature falls below optimum.

The *Drosophila* flies survive normally at a temperature at 16.5 °C but at high temperature of 25 °C they starts dying.

Balanced lethal system: It is the condition when both homozygotes die leaving only the heterozygous phenotype. Such systems are known in mice, *Drosophila*.

NUMERICAL EXERCISES

Monohybrid Crosses: Complete Dominance

7.1 Black wool in sheep is dominant over white controlled by one pair of gene(B). A black sheep was mated with a white ram. Estimate the percentage of black F_2 progeny. What will be the expected mating among F_2 progeny?

7.2 Abnormality of eyelid in human is controlled by a pair of gene with complete dominance. A woman and her father had eyelid abnormality called *ptosis* (difficulty in opening eye lids completely) but her mother had no problem. Find out the possible genotypes of all the 3 people and the proportion of children to be born if this woman with eye abnormality marries with a man with normal eyes.

7.3 Black colour in guinea pig is dominant over white. Find out the expected genotypes of a black male and black female if their mating resulted into 9 black and 3 chocolate guinea pigs, and the mating of a black male with chocolate female produced 5 black and 5 chocolate offspring.

7.4 Grey colour is dominant over black in fly. The F_2 progenies of a cross resulted into 400 offspring, out of which 300 were grey and rest were black. What were the genotypes of both males and females of parent generation?.

7.5 The barking in dogs during training is governed by a singe gene pair (B) expressed in two forms as barking which is dominant and silent expression of the trait. Another trait is erection or dropping of ears which is also governed by single gene pair (E) and erection of ears show dominance over dropping ears. A heterozygous erect eared barker was mated with dropping eared silent nature. Give the genotypes of the mated pair and find out the ratio of progeny with different phenotypes.

Codominance

7.6 The coat colour in Andalusian fowl (black and white) is controlled by one pair of gene with two alleles (B and W) and the heterozygous genotype at this locus (BW) produces blue coat colour which is a mixture of black and white hairs. Work out the genotypic and phenotypic ratio in F_2 progeny and name the type of gene action.

7.7 The coat colour in Shorthorn cattle (red and white) is governed by single locus two alleles (R and W). The red colour cattle have RR genotype while those of white colour have WW genotype. The crossing of cattle with these two coat colours produce F_1 cattle with roan colour (a mixture of red and white coloured hairs called as roan colour. Find out the results of F_2 generation and interpret the results. Is it possible to develop a breed of cattle that would transmit consistently the roan colour ?

7.8 The ear size in goats is controlled by two alleles at a locus, the long ears and short ears in size are due to homozygous genotypes for the two alleles, respectively while the heterozygote at this locus produces goats for medium size ears. Interpret.

7.9 The yellow guinea pigs breed true, whereas the mating of yellow with cream colour produces yellow and cream coloured progeny in equal ratio. What type of inheritance (gene action) is involved? What is the colour of heterozygote guinea pigs? [Answer Co-dominance and Cream colour].

7.10 A pair of dominant alleles controls the palomino colour. Two homozygote produce *chestnut* (CC) and *white* (cc). Predict the phenotypes from the following crosses, assuming large random mating population: (i) White mated with white, and with chestnut (ii) Chestnut x chestnut, (iii) palomino crossed with palomino, chestnut, and white.

Lethal Alleles

7.11 The trait hairless in dogs results from heterozygous genotype (Hh) and the normal condition is due to a recessive gene in homozygous condition (hh) while the dominant homozygous state (HH) is lethal in embryonic stage. Predict the phenotypes from mating of hairless dogs with normal dogs, and inter se mating of hairless dogs.

7.12 In poultry, the creeper condition results from heterozygous genotype (Cc), the homozygous recessives (cc) are normal whereas the homozygous dominants (CC) are died in embryonic stage.

7.13 *Pelger anomaly of rabbit* (abnormal WBC number segmentation) is expressed in heterozygous state of two alleles (Pp) and the normal individuals are homozygous recessive (pp). The homozygous dominant genotype (PP) causes grossly deformed skeleton causing death before or very soon after birth. (a) Whether it is possible to produce a litter with all progeny to be pelgers? (b) Taking the average litter size at weaning as four, what is the expected litter size from a mating of pelgers with pelgers? (c) Predict the average litter size at weaning from mating of pelgers with normals.

Answer: (a) It is not possible because only the pelgers can be produced from a cross of both homozygote (PP x pp) and the dominant homozygote (PP) die before reproducing.

(b) Three. This is because the mating of pelgers with pelgers produces the progeny in a genotypic ratio of of 1 PP: 2 Pp: 1 pp. The genotype PP is lethal before weaning and hence the average litter size at weaning is expected to be three. (c) Four. This is because the mating of pelgers (Pp) with normal (pp) will produce 2 pelgers and 2 normal.

Chapter 8

Gene Action II. Non-Allelic Interaction (Epistasis)

The epistasis is similar to the dominance but it occurs when the character is influenced by many pairs of gene and these genes interact with their non-alleles (other pairs of genes) present on other loci of the same chromosome or of other chromosome. This is also called as inter allelic interaction and generally known as *epistasis* (when one pair of gene influences the expression of another pair of gene). The epistasis is the result of ***interaction between the products of non-alleles*** and hence called as non-allelic interaction which is of several types. The *epistasis* (means act of stopping) is the interaction between non-allelic genes Present at separate loci) in which one gene masks (Inhibits or suppress or stops the expression of other gene. The gene suppressing the other gene is called ***inhibiting or epistatic factor*** and the gene whose effect is suppressed is called ***hypostatic.*** It is similar to dominance and recessiveness but for the two gene pairs located on separate loci. Thus, epistasis involve intergenetic inhibition while dominance involved intra-allelic gene inhibition.

The epistasis involves the interaction between genes that are not alleles and hence present on separate loci. Thus, the genes at one locus interact with genes at another locus to produce a character that cannot be produced by either locus acting independently. In other words, the genes at one locus modify the expression of genes at another locus. In this type of inheritance, the effect of one gene does not add directly to the effect of another gene to influence the phenotype but the phenotype is the result of interaction of genes at two or more loci.

Thus, an *epistatic factor* (*gene*) is one which prevents a gene other than its allele from exhibiting its normal effect on the development of the character and the gene which is being prevented from exhibiting its normal effect in the development of the character due to the epistatic gene is known as *hypostatic gene*.

It is not known to certain that in what manner the genes may act to influence the quantitative traits but some kind of epistasis have been observed and reported for qualitative characters.

8.1 EPISTASIS AND ITS TYPES

There is different types of gene interaction (epistasis) for two gene pairs, when each gene pair assorting independently. The different types have been given here.

Classical Ratio for Two Gene Pairs

As the epistasis involves the interaction between two pairs of gene, it is essential to have the knowledge of dihybrid ratios, so as to know whether the epistasis is present or not and that too which kind of epistasis is present. This needs to know the classical dihybrid ratio expected from dihybrid crosses, based on complete dominance between alleles at both the loci. The classical dihybrid F_2 ratio was observed in garden pea for yellow-green and round-wrinkled characters. The F_2 ratio depends on the dominance recessive relationship between alleles at two loci. The F_2 phenotypic classical ratio with complete dominance at each of two loci was 9:3:3:1 (yellow round: yellow wrinkled: green round: green wrinkled):

	AA BB	AA bb	aa BB	aa bb
	2 AA Bb	2 Aa bb	2 aa Bb	
	2 Aa BB			
	4 Aa Bb			
Total =	*9 (A - B -)*	*3 (A – bb)*	*3 (aaB -)*	*1 (aabb)*

The different types of epistasis may or may not modify the above phenotypic classical ratios of 9:3:3:1. The numbers of phenotypes in classical ratios for dihybrid cross are four whereas these may be four or less than four in case of epistasis. The appearance of less than four phenotypic classes is the evidence of epistasis. Two or more phenotypic classes of the classic ratios are combined together as a result of epistasis, if the numbers of phenotypic classes are less than four. Broadly speaking, the epistasis which modify the classical ratios (9:3:3:1) can be grouped in two categories *viz.* simple statistics and duplicate epistatis.

The phenotypic ratios as a result of epistasis of different types between two gene pairs are modified in different ways as shown below:

8.2 SIMPLE EPISTASIS

The simple epistasis is when the genes at one locus modify the expression of genes present at second locus. Thus epistasis is only in one direction and the genes at second locus have no effect on those at first locus. The examples of simple epistasis are dominant epistasis and recessive epistasis. In simple epistasis only two genotypic classes of the classical ratios are combined, producing three phenotypic classes. This is one way epistasis, being of two types, *viz.* recessive and dominant epistasis-

(1) Recessive Epistasis (9:3:4)

This is ***supplementary gene inheritance*** or recessive epistasis. ***It is epistasis due to recessive gene.*** There is complete dominance at both gene pairs (two independent pairs of dominant genes). Either gene in homozygous state (bb and cc) is epistatic to dominant gene at other locus. *They interact in such a way that one dominant gene produces its effect irrespective of the presence of other. The second dominant when present changes the expression of the first one but only in the presence of the first one.* In other way, *one gene in homozygous recessive state (cc) is epistatic to both the alleles of other gene pair (B and b).* The combination of both the genes in dominant condition (A- B-) produces another phenotype. The F_2 ratio becomes as 9:3:4.

Many species of mammals have albino gene which exhibit recessive epistasis. The dominant gene C controls the production of pigment melanin, but the recessive gene in homozygous condition (cc) fails to produce enzyme that produce melanin and hence causes albinism. The recessive homozygous genotype (cc) at the C locus masks the expression of the alleles at another locus (B and b).

The example of this type of gene action is ***coat colour in rabbit***. The black hair colour is dominant over brown. The inter se mating of F_1 dihybrid progeny (BbCc) produced 3 coat colours among the F_2 progeny as:

9 Black (B - C -): 3 Brown (bbC -): 4 Albino (B - cc and bbcc)

Another example of recessive epistasis is ***coat colour in rat (guinea pigs)***. On crossing black mice with albino mice, the F_1 dihybrid produced are Agouti (Bb Cc). On inter se mating of F_1 dihybrids, the F_2 individuals are 9 agauti: 3 black: 4 albino as -

F_2 progeny 9 (B – C -): 3 (bbC -): 4 [(B - cc) + (bb cc)]

= 9 Agouti : 3 Black : 4 [3 Albino + 1 Albino]

The agouti colour pattern has colour bands in a way that the hairs are of grey colour near the skin, followed by yellow band and finally black or brown at the tip of hairs. The agouti colour gene is A whose effect is masked by recessive genotype at other locus (bb). The mice with bb genotype mask the effect of colour gene A- and produces black coat.

The dominant allele B in the absence of C produces albino mice (BB cc and Bb cc). The dominant allele C in the presence of dominant allele B produces agouti colour. Thus two independent pair of alleles interact to produce the coat colour in a way that one dominant (B-) produces its effect (albino) in the absence of C (cc-homozygous recessive) but the gene C can produce its effect (to produce agouti) only in the presence of other gene (B-). Therefore, these two pairs of genes are called as supplementary genes.

(2) Dominant Epistasis (12:3:1)

This is also called *inhibitory factor inheritance*. There is complete dominance at both gene pairs. The dominant epistasis occurs when a dominant gene at one locus interacts to suppress or modify the expression of genes at second locus. Therefore, the *dominant gene of one pair (A) is epistatic to both the alleles of other pair (B and b).*

When A is epistatic to B and b, the F_2 ratio becomes as 12:3:1. In this case, the two phenotypic classes (A –B – and A – bb) of F_2 progeny expressed similarly.

The examples are ***coat colour in dogs*** as well as *in cats* which appeared as 12 white: 3 black: 1 brown and *colour of summer squash* appeared as 12 white: 3 yellow: 1 green. In pigs white coat colour appears to be dominant due to the action of epistatic gene ***I*** which prevents the formation of pigment. The other gene B which is hypostatic produces black coat while its hypostatic allele **b** produces brown coat colouronly when gene **I** is recessive. The dominant gene **I** stops to function and produce white colour.

The dominant gene B produces black colour. The gene A produces white colour and masks the effect of colour gene (B). Thus, B produces black colour but in the absence of A because the gene A is epistatic to B and b. White dogs carry colour gene (B) that are inhibited from forming colour in the hair due to the presence of gene, A. The individuals in F_2 generation appear in 12:3:1 ratio as under:

P	AA BB (White)	x	aa bb (Brown)	
		↓		
F_1		Aa Bb (white)		
F_2	12 [9 (A – B -) + 3 (A – bb)]:		3 (aaB -):	1 (aabb)
	= 12 [9 white + 3 white] :		3 Black:	1 Brown

The brown dogs (aa bb), lack the gene for black colour (B), therefore, brown in colour, because they also lack the inhibitor (epistatic) gene A. Such genes are often called as *inhibitors*.

8.3 DUPLICATE EPISTASIS

These are both ways epistasis. The duplicate epistasis act in both the directions, the genes at both loci interact simultaneously and the phenotypic classes are reduced to two except in one case of duplicate interaction (incompletely duplicate epistasis) in which there are three phenotypic classes. These are of the following four types –

(1) Duplicate Dominant Epistasis (15:1)

This is called ***duplicate genes.*** *The dominant gene at one locus (A) is epistatic over dominant gene of other locus (B and b) and vice versa (B is epistatic to A and a).* The dominant allele at one locus (A) is epistatic to its non allele (B and b) whereas the dominant allele at other locus (B) is epistatic to its non allele (A and a). Thus, the dominant alleles of both the loci produce the identical phenotype by masking the manifestation of genes of other pair. The ratio appeared as 15:1.

The examples are the presence and absence of ***feathers on the shanks of legs in poultry*** (15 feathered: 1 clean shank with genotype aabb); *bursa seed capsule shape* (15 triangular: 1 oval shape).

The black Langshan breed of chicken has feathered shanks whereas most of other breeds have no feathers on shanks (clean shanks). The crossing of feathered shank poultry (AA BB) of Black Langshan breed with clean shank poultry (aa bb) of Buff-rock breed (Plymouth Rocks) produced all feathered F_1. The inter-se mating of F_1 produced the following results:

15 [9 (A – B -) + 3 (A –bb) + 3 (aaB -)] : 1 (aabb)

= 15 [9 Feathered + 3 Feathered + 3 Feathered]: 1 clean

The presence of dominant genes at either locus as well as at both loci causes the feathers to grow on the legs whereas the double recessive genotype (aabb) results absence of feathers on the legs.

(2) Duplicate Recessive Epistasis (9:7)

This is also called ***complementary gene action***. In this type of epistasis, the recessive gene at both loci in homozygous condition masks the effect of dominant combination of both loci. Thus, *aa is epistatic to its non alleles (B and b) and bb is epistatic to its non alleles (A and a)*. In this case, the last three phenotypic classes of classical ratio expressed similarly and hence show similar phenotype. The F_2 ratio appeared as 9:7. *The genotypes having recessive homozygous genotype for either gene locus as well as for both gene loci produce identical phenotypes.*

Fowl colour: There exists a locus controlling white feathers in poultry. The recessive genotype at this locus (aa) produces white feathers while A gene produces colour. Homozygous white Silkie fowls mated to homozygous white Plymouth fowls produce F_1 birds which are all coloured, and a ratio of 9 coloured: 7 white is obtained among F_2 offspring. The F_1 individuals, Aa Cc, have both the genes, A and C, necessary for the production of colour while the parents with genotype AA cc and aa CC, have only one gene, either A or C. Therefore, the presence of recessive genes for either locus in homozygous condition produces white.

Deafness (Deaf-mutism) *in human* also shows this type of gene action because recessive genes of both pairs (aa and bb) mask the manifestation of dominant genes of other pair *i.e.* aa is epistatic to B and b whereas bb is epistatic to A and a. Both the deaf parents have only one gene either A or B but the F_1 getting both the genes A and B have normal hearing capacity. Interaction between dominant genes A and B results normal hearing and speech. A person is deaf-mute if homozygous for either of the two recessive alleles. Thus, dominant alleles of both pairs are required for normal hearing. Among F_2 offspring, 9 normal: 7 deaf individuals were produced.

9 (A –B -): 7 [3(A – bb) + 3 (aaB-) + 1 (aabb)]

Human hearing = 9 Normal: 7 deaf

Fowl colour = 9 coloured: 7 white

(3) Dominant and Recessive Epistasis (13:3): Inhibitory Factor Inheritance

In this type of epistasis one dominant combination at one locus is epistatic over one recessive combination at other locus. The *dominant allele at one locus (A) is epistatic to both alleles of other locus (B and b) whereas the homozygous recessive genotype of other locus (bb) is epistatic to both the alleles at other locus (A and a)*. In other words, the dominant gene at one locus and the recessive gene at second locus are mutually epistatic. Thus, *the dominant allele of one gene pair in homozygous (AA) and heterozygous condition (Aa) as well as the recessive homozygote of another gene pair (bb) produce the same phenotype.* In this case, the 1st, 2nd and last phenotypic classes of classical ratios expressed similarly and hence show similar phenotype. The ratio become as 13:3.

Feather colour in chickens is an example of this type of epistasis. There are two white breeds (white leghorn and white Plymouth rock) in poultry. White plumage of white leghorn is dominant over coloured variety and the white plumage of white Plymouth is recessive to coloured variety. Bateson and Punnet (1908) crossed White feathered Leghorn (IICC) with White Plymouth Rock (iicc) having white feathers and obtained white feathered F_1 progeny. Among F_2 progeny, the white and coloured individuals appeared in a 13 white: 3 coloured individuals.

There may be present an inhibiting factor which prevent the development of pigment even when it is present. The **I** is inhibiting factor and i is recessive allele; **C** is the colour factor for pigment then the white is produced when both colour and inhibiting factors are present ((***IC***) but when both are absent (***ic***) and when the colour factor alone is absent (***ccII or ccIi***).

The F_1 birds having Ii Cc genotype are white in colour with coloured tips. The F_2 birds presented the usual dihybrid genotypic ratios with phenotypic ratios as:

13 [9 (A –B -) + 3 (A – bb) + 1 (aabb)]: 3 aaB -

or 13 [9 (I – C -) + 3 (I - cc) + 1 (iicc)] : 3 ii C-

= 13 [9 white + 3 white + 1 white] : 3 coloured

All the F_2 individuals having inhibitor gene in its dominant allelic form (II, Ii) or cc were white whereas the individuals lacking I allele but having CC or Cc genotype were having coloured feathers. The gene I is the inhibitor and C is the colour gene whose expression is inhibited by I. Thus, the gene C fails to develop colour (melanin) because the gene I modifies (inhibits) the expression of gene C. The coloured gene (C) in its homozygous recessive state (cc) does not allow the melanin to be produced and hence produce white. The genotype cc is epistatic to any genes for colour. This type of epistasis is termed as "Dominant and recessive epistasis" because dominant gene I is epistatic to C, c and the recessive gene (c) of other pair is epistatic to I, i. This is also called as the *inhibitory factor inheritance.*

(4) Incompletly Duplicate Epistasis (9:6:1)

There is complete dominance at both gene pairs. The interaction between both dominants produces new phenotype. This is also called as *duplicate genes with cumulative effect.* In this type of epistasis, the recessive genotype for either pair of gene masks the manifestation of dominant genes of other pair to a certain extent. There is incomplete masking of recessive combination of both loci on dominant combination of both loci. The genotype aa is partially epistatic to its both the non alleles (B and b) and bb is epistatic to its both the non alleles (A and a). Thus this type of interaction occurs *when the dominant condition at both locus produce one phenotype (= 9/16); the dominant condition at either locus (but not at both) viz. A-bb (= 3/16) and aaB- genotypes (= 3/16) produce identical (same) phenotype;* and the absence of any dominant gene at either locus (aabb = 1/16) produce a separate phenotype. In this case, the two middle classes expressed identical phenotype. The ratio appeared as 9: 6:1.

The example is coat colour pattern in Duroc swine (9 red: 6 sandy: 1 white). There is one sandy coloured race of Duroc swine having red swine (AA bb) and white swine (aa BB). On crossing them produce F_1 (Aa Bb) with red colour. The F_2 offspring having at least one A and one B gene are red, lacking both A and b are white, and having at least one A with 2 b's or at least one B with 2 a's are sandy.

F_2 offspring 9 (A – B -): 6 [(3 A – bb) + 3(aaB -)]: 1 (aabb)

= 9 Red : 6 [3 Sandy + 3 Sandy)] : 1 white

In this type of epistasis, the dominant gene at either gene pair produce sandy colour, dominant gene at both loci produce red colour and absence of dominant gene at both loci produces white colour.

8.4NO MODIFICATION OF RATIOS BY EPISTASIS (COMPLEMENTARY OR COLLABORATIVE GENE ACTION)

The above examples of characters have been given the controlled by two gene pairs showing epistasis and modifying the dihybrid classical ratios of 9:3:3:1 among F_2 (with dominance recessive relation between alleles of both gene pairs). However, there are some examples of gene interaction (epistasis) wherein the classical dihybrid ratios among F_2 are not modified. Such examples of epistasis of two pairs of genes influencing the same character of comb shape in chickens and coat colour in rats can be cited. The two gene pairs interact but do not modify the phenotypic ratio of 9:3:3:1.

Certain factors cannot express themselves except in the presence of some other factor or the modification of their expression may be due to the presence of some other factor.

(i) Comb Shape in Chicken

Domestic breed of chicken have different comb shapes. The birds of Wyandotte have *rose comb;* Brahmans and Cornish breeds have *pea comb;* Leghorn, Langshan and white Plymouth Rock breeds have *single comb*. The gene R produce rose comb, P produces pea comb. Both are dominant over single comb. Both R and P together produce a new phenotype (Walnut comb) by complementing the effect of each other or by their collaborative effect.

When rose comb fowls (RR pp) were mated to pea shape comb fowls (rr PP), the F_1 was produced with another type of comb, Walnut shape (Rr Pp). When the Walnuts (F_1) were mated *inter se,* the four types of comb shape were produced among the F_2 progenies. The F_2 results were as under:

RR PP	RR pp	rr PP	rr pp
2 RR Pp	2 Rr pp	2 rr Pp	
2 Rr PP			
4 Rr Pp			
= 9 Walnut:	3 Rose:	3 Pea:	1 Single

Neither single nor walnut comb was present in the original parental lines. The F_2 results indicated the followings-

- ✰ The normal F_2 ratio (9:3:3:1) was obtained which suggested that two pairs of genes are involved and that dominance recessive relation exists between each of two pairs of alleles.
- ✰ The ratio also suggested that F_1 walnut comb shape chickens were dihybrids (RrPp).
- ✰ Two more phenotypes (Walnut and Single) appeared in F_2 which are the result of interaction of two gene pairs. The phenotypic class representing a ratio of 1:16 indicated that the single comb type is the result of the combined effects of two pairs of recessive genes (rr pp). The phenotypic class representing a ratio of 9:16 indicated that walnut shape is the result of at least one dominant gene at each of two loci (R - P -).
- ✰ It is clearly an interaction between non-alleles, because none of the comb type can be explained based on one pair of genes. The two genes R and P are non-allelic but they were dominant on their alleles (R over r and P over p). These two dominant genes responsible for rose comb and pea comb interacted to produce walnut comb, similar to the co-dominant alleles and the absence of both dominant genes (rr pp) resulted in a different phenotype as single comb. Therefore, non-allelic genes acting in this manner are called *co-epistatic genes or complementary.*

Comb shape in poultry is thus governed by two pairs of genes with complete dominance at both gene pairs. New phenotypes are produced by interaction of dominants at both gene pairs (walnut shape) as well as by interaction of both homozygous recessives (single shape) in contrast to supplementary gene action. Both rose (Wyandott) and pea (Brahman) comb shape is dominant to single (White Leghorn) shape comb.

The homozygous Walnut may be produced by inbreeding and selection, because R and P are apparently located on different chromosome pairs. But if R and p (and like manner r and P) had been located on the same chromosome (not allowing the crossing over) it would have been impossible to obtain a homozygous strain of Walnut comb.

(ii) Coat Colour in Rats

The yellow rats were mated to black rats, all the F_1 progeny were gray in colour. The *inter-se* mating of F_1 gray colour, produced the F_2 progeny of four colours in a ratio of 9 (gray): 3 (black): 3 (yellow); 1 (cream). The F_2 results in this case are explained on the same logic as was used to explain the epistasis involved in the inheritance pattern of four comb shapes in poultry above.

The complementary action of genes is another expression of gene interaction and the characters of economic importance are affected by this type of gene action, and usually many gene pairs are involved, if the characters are of a quantitative nature and in that case the expression is less clearly marked than in the above example.

(iii) Umbilical Hernia in Swine

This trait is at least stimulated by 2 independently inherited factors. Three inbred lines A, B and C in swine have no umbilical hernia. The crossing of inbred line A either with inbred line B or C produce all the crossbred progeny having umbilical hernia. The F_1 from both crosses were culled for umbilical hernia and inbred, and in both the cases the hernias disappeared from the lines in 2 generations. The conclusion was that line A carrying a factor potent for hernia which expressed itself when introduced in the genetic environments provided by B and C lines. The cross between line B and C did not develop hernias.

8.5 MODIFYING GENES

In addition to the different types of epistasis mentioned above, there are other types of gene action. The inheritance of coat colour in some species of domestic animals suggests that the inheritance of some characters is not as simple as explained above. A mutant gene expresses itself in a background of normal alleles at all other loci. All genes have a dual effect - one is that they are necessary for the well being of the individual and if a portion of these genes is lost, it leads either in improper development of the individual or results in its death.

The *modifying genes* are those that modify the effects of genes present on other locus controlling a character. For example, take the inheritance of coat colours in mammals. The pigment melanin is the basic requirement of all colours in animals. This melanin is of two types *viz.* black (*Eumelanin*) and red melanin (*phaeomelanin*). These two pigments are modified by genes at several loci. These genes affect the synthesis of pigments and associated enzymes as well as the distribution and location of pigment granules in the skin, and hair to produce various shades of colours.

(i) Eye Colour in Drosophila

It is due to a single factor (gene pair), but in addition to this, seven other factors (genes) that cause modifying effects have been identified. The gene *w* for white eye prevents the colour development in homozygous condition in females (w/w) and in hemizygous condition in males (w/y). The other genes are necessary, though not for the production of white eye but for the normal development of fly in which the white eye can be expressed. The interruption at white locus of the *w* mutant inhibits the development of pigment which results in a white eye.

(ii) Coat Colours in Mammals

Regarding coat colour inheritance, the wild colour is known as agouti which is a familiar colour in wild rats, mice and rabbits. The agouti is produced by a dominant gene (A-) whereas its recessive condition (aa) produces non-agouti which is usually black unless modified by other genes. The agouti series has other alleles in different species. The mechanism of production of melanin pigment from the amino acid tyrosine involving the catalytic action of an enzyme (tyrosinase) under the control of a gene (C) and the absence of the production of enzyme (Tyrosinase), causing the deficiency of melanin under the control of a recessive allele in homozygous condition (cc) resulting in albinism has been explained in chapter 10 under the article *"How genes function"*. The melanin is a brown or black pigment.

The 3 basic genes for colour in wild animals are A, B and C. The C is dominant gene which produces melanin pigment in the hair and skin. Its recessive allelomorph c in homozygous condition (cc) results in albinism. The gene B is another dominant gene which produces black pigment with C. The gene B's allelomorph in homozygous state (bb) changes the black colour to brown, which is less completely oxidized melanin pigment. The gene A is dominant gene which modifies the expression of B and C so as to produce agouti or wild coat pattern. In the domestic horses, it modifies the action of B and C to produce bay colour.

At albino locus A, there are some other alleles which act as the production of variable amount of *tyrosinase* and result in production of modified phenotypes. The two coat colour phenotypes in rabbits and rats may be cited here. These are the *chinchilla* (gray colour which is diluted agouti colour) and *Himalayan* (white with black extremities of the body *viz.* tail, feet, and neck).

At locus B, the genes decide the type of melanin (*Eumelanin* - Black or brown; or *phaeomelanin* - red or yellow) depending on other modifying genes present at locus E. The modifying effect cause the series of colours from black (dominant extreme) to red or yellow (recessive end of series).

At locus D, the genes cause clumping of pigment granules which leads to a decrease in light absorption and dilution of colour. The dilution gene may be dominant or recessive.

The examples of coat colour inheritance in different mammalian species are -

(1) Coat Colour in Cattle

The coat colour in HF cattle (white spotting) is due to a single pair of gene but the coat colour varies from almost white to almost black having black spots of varying size. The indication that the modifying genes are responsible for the expression of the genes for spotting comes from the successful selection for spot size in either direction. The variation in white spotting in Holstein cattle occurs to the extent that some cattle have very little amount of white that they are almost all black while others are almost white. All these indicated that white spotting is modified by genes present at several loci.

Yellow colour in Guernsey cattle is due to a recessive gene when homozygous (cc) which dilutes the red colour but does not affect black. The black (B -) is dominant over red (bb). The Angus cattle are black and do not carry the dilution gene (BB CC). Hereford cattle are of genotype bb CC whereas the Guernsey cattle are of the genotype bb cc.

(2) Coat Colours in Horses

There are a number of loci which control and modify the coat colours in horses. The effect of genes at locus A has already been discussed in chapter three on multiple alleles. This locus (A) determines the variability in expression of black pigment (aa) to its full to remain limited to only some parts (black colour mane, tail, legs with red body, called bay). The *black* (aa) is recessive to bay (A -). The *bay like* pattern (brow or reddish body with black markings on mane, neck and foot) has also been reported by some workers to be due to the presence of another allele, A^t which is dominant over A and *a* alleles. The *seal brown*, which is modified black with light brown areas on muzzle, eyes, legs and flanks, is said to be controlled by another allele at this locus (A^l) which is recessive to A but dominant to the allele *a*.

The shade of melanin (black or brown) is determined by the genes at locus B. The dominant allele (B) produces black, except as restricted by A - whereas the homozygous state of recessive (bb) produces *chocolate brown*.

The gene at locus C is the only allele in horses (c^{cr}) known as cream dilution gene which is codominant and partially epistatic to ee. The term *cremello* is used for this cream dilution. The homozygous dominant (CC) expresses the colours as determined by genes at other loci (A, B and E). The heterozygous state (Cc) results in *palomino* due to partial dilution (modification) of red or yellow pigment but does not affect the black melanin. The *chestnuts* (reddish colour) and *sorrel* (light red) are diluted to the *palominos* (Copper or golden colour, with lighter mane and tail than rest of body).

The genes at locus E further influence the type of melanin (black or brown) which needs the presence of gene E whereas its recessive homozygous state (ee) restricts the expression of black and brown so that red or yellow (phaeomelanin) is produced on the whole body (including mane, tail and legs) and causes the reddish colour (light or dark shade), called as *chestnut*. The light shade is called *sorrel.*

The gene at locus D, causes dilution of colour in horses (called as dilution gene which reduces the intensity of all pigmentation). The gene D in the homozygous condition (DD) combined with bb results in type A albino and the DDBb genetic state results in type B albino. Neither of the above one are, however, true albino; the true albino condition can result only from the presence of cc genes. The buck skin or dun colour is produced by the DdBb genetic state and the *Palomino* colour (copper or golden) from the Ddbb genetic state. These colour patterns can be shown as:

Colour patterns	*Genotypes*
Albino type A	DD bb
Albino type B	DD Bb
Dun colour	Dd Bb
Palomino	Dd bb

The genotypes for five coat colours in horses can be written as:

Coat colours	*Genotypes*
Black	aa B – E –
Chocolate brown	aa bb E –
Bay with black points	A – B – E –

Bay with brown points	A – bb E –
Chestnut - any genotypes having ee:	A – B – ee,
	A – bb ee,
	Aa B – ee, and
	aa bb ee

The gray and roan patterns are also exhibited in horses with inter spread of white hairs with coloured hairs. The proportion of white hairs in genetically gray horses is progressively increased with increase in age, some breeds of horses have no coloured hair in older age. The gray is dominant (G -) to non-gray (gg). The situation of the presence of white hairs in roan horses is different than gray pattern, in that the proportion of white hairs in roan horses is not changed with progressive increase in age, as in case of gray horses. The roan pattern is usually absent on the head and feet compared to body. Some reports have indicated that roan gene (R) is partially dominant or co-dominant with lethal effect in embryonic stage when homozygous (rr).

(3) Coat Colour in Cats

The coat colour in cats is of *tabby pattern* which consist black stripping on a yellowish-gray background (similar to agouti which is full colour). The agouti pattern (full colour) is due to dominant gene at the A locus (A -) whereas the homozygous genotype at this locus (aa) produces black. There are three different tabby patterns *viz. Mackerel tabby* which is like wild pattern, found in mongrel cats; *blotched tabby* which consists irregular stripping than mackerel tabby; and third tabby is that which has *no stripping* except in small amounts on the leg and tail, found in Abyssinian breed. Three alleles in a dominance hierarchy of $T^a > T > t$ are responsible for three kinds of tabby. The allele T^a controls the tabby of Abyssinian breed, T controls Mackerel tabby and t controls blotched tabby (most recessive trait to other two tabby).

A dominant gene at B locus (B -) is necessary for the expression of black (aa). The recessive gene at B locus in homozygous state (bb) produces brown or chocolate. The recessive gene at B locus (b) is epistatic to aa. There are references indicating that a third allele which is recessive to b allele produces milk chocolate colour which is lighter brown.

Two alleles at C locus produce two popular colour patterns. The allele C^b in homozygous condition (C^b C^b) produces a brownish body colour due to reduced intensity of black with darker extremities than body and the eyes being sometimes blue. This is found in Burmese cats. The second allele (C^S) in homozygous state as C^S C^S produces almost white body with dark extremities as in case of Himalayan rabbits and this colour pattern is found in Siamese cats. Further, these two alleles are co-dominant and hence the heterozygote (C^b C^S) produces an intermediate phenotype. However, both these alleles are recessive to C (responsible for full colour expression determined by genes at other loci).

There is absence of true albino colour in cats like horses and dogs, though white cats are produced by a dominant gene (W -) at another locus, in which the genotype ww produces non-white phenotype. The eyes of these cats may be blue, yellow or odd-coloured. This gene is an example of pleiotropic effect on hearing ability, as half of the white cats are deaf. The white hairs are the result of the failure of the production of melanin due to a dominant inhibitor gene (I).

A dominant gene (S -) at another locus seems to control the irregular white spotting in cats, known as piebald spotting pattern. The piebald is a dominant trait.

Another locus in cats is found responsible for dilution of colour. The full colour is produced by D – whereas the recessive dilution gene (d) when homozygous (dd) dilutes the colours. The black is diluted to blue and yellow to cream colour.

A *sex-linked locus* with co-dominant alleles exists in cats. This locus produces black, yellow and tortoise coat colour, as explained in chapter number 6.

(4) Coat Colour in Dogs

About 10 gene loci have been reported to affect the coat colours in dogs.

The locus A (agouti series) has four alleles with dominance hierarchy as $A^y > a^w > a^t > a$. All these four allele, are observed in German Shepherds and respectively, produce cream or gray-coloured body with a brown or light brown saddle ($A^{y)}$; cream or gray-coloured body with a black saddle (A^w); black and tan colour (called as bicolor, A^t), the black varying from a black saddle to black on whole body except the points as seen in many Dobermans, the tan colour is an intense (reddish tan rather than the light tan or cream) with genotype (A^y– or A^w -) and the last solid black in homozygous state (aa).

The black or brown eumelanin (Chocolate) depends on the genes at B locus. The black is determined by aaB- and brown by aabb. The recessive gene for brown (b) is epistatic to *aa.* The dominant gene at E locus produces *eumelamin* (Black or brown) whereas the recessive homozygous genotype (ee) causes the *phaeomelanin* (red or yellow) to be produced and ee is epistatic to aa, B -, and bb. These results the following body colours in dogs-

Solid black	aa B - E –
Solid brown (Chocolate)	aa bb E -
Red or reddish yellow with dark nose and lips	aa B - ee
Yellow or golden with pink nose and lips	aa bb ee

The genes at C and D locus result in dilution of colours. The dominant gene C produces full colour. Another gene at C locus (*Chinchilla,* c^{ch}) modifies the *phaeomelanin* that changes tan to cream colour, and red and yellow to light yellow and golden colours. But the allele c^{ch} does not affect the *eumelanin* like the cream dilution gene producing *palomino* in horses.

The gene at locus D in homozygous recessive state (dd) affects the production of melanin of both types. The black is diluted to blue and the effect of dilution of yellow is similar to chinchilla dilution, described for C locus. The recessive gene *d* has an effect like *dun* dilution in horses, though in horses it has dominant effect.

The *piebald pattern* (irregular spotting) also exists in dogs, produced by recessive state (ss) and the dominant gene S produces an effect of absence of spotting. The amount of spotting varies from very little white to the complete white. The recessive condition of a gene at W locus (ww) results in all-white dogs with pigmented eyes.

The progressive graying with age has also been observed in dogs, similar to that in horses and controlled by a dominant gene (G).

Two other loci (T and M) have also been found associated with white. The small pigmented spots (ticks) on white background appear due to dominant gene T. The amount of white in the coat is increased by a co-dominant gene M in heterozygous state (Mm), producing a pattern of dilute and intense patches, called *merle* whereas the homozygous dominant condition (MM) produces almost all-white coat with pale blue eyes and pleiotropic effects including blindness, deafness and some structural abnormalities of the eyes.

(5) Coat Colour in Mice

In mice, white spotted pattern behaves as a single recessive to self coloured coat but spotted mice range from nearly self coloured to nearly all white. The variations are attributed, for the most part, to modifying genes which affect the white spotting.

8.6 INHERITANCE OF MORPHOLOGICAL CHARACTERS IN POULTRY

The qualitative traits are controlled by one or two pairs of genes with their major effect and most of them are not affected by environment. Most of these characters in poultry are related to morphological features. The native (chickens) as well as the English, American, and Mediterranean breeds of fowl have great variability in morphological traits controlled by major genes. These variations are due to some of the major gene effects which have caused the adaptability to varying environments. The followings are the examples:

(1) Body Size: Dwarf Gene

The dwarf gene (dw) in poultry is *sex-liked recessive* reduces the body size by 10 – 30 per cent and has an effect on reduction in metabolism, increase in fitness and disease tolerance.

(2) Plumage Pattern (Distribution)

The feathers in poultry are known as plumage. The variations have been observed in development, distribution and texture of plumage.

(a) *Fast and slow feathering:* The plumage pattern is mono-factorial. The birds of some breeds (Mediterranean) are fast feathering whereas Asiatic, English and American breeds are slow feathering. Slow feathering gene (k) is a *sex-linked dominant* causing delay of feathering with side effect on reduction in fat deposition and protein requirement, increases heat loss and delay the immune response mechanism.

(b) *Necked and frizzle feathering:* Some breeds have no feathers on the neck (*Necked neck*). Some breeds have *frizzle feathers* while others have *normal feathers*. Both necked neck and frizzling genes are autosomal. The necked gene (N) is *incomplete dominant* with direct effect on loss of neck feathers and secondary feathers and its indirect effect to increase convention ability and fitness but reducing the hatchability. The frizzle gene (f) causes curling of feathers and reduced feathering with side effect of improving the convection ability.

(3) Plumage Colours

The black pigment melanin is not thoroughly distributed in the feathers and this creates variation in feather colours. The different colours of plumage are white, black, red and blue and the genes controlling plumage colours are *autosomal*. The white plumage colour is breed specific character. It is used to identify the breeds and varieties within breed and to study the type of gene action.

(i) ***White*** plumage is *dominant* in White Leghorn but recessive in White Plymouth Rock.

(ii) ***Black*** plumage is *recessive* to white in White Leghorn but dominant to white in all recessive white breeds.

(iii) ***Red*** plumage colour is found in Red Leghorn, RIR, New Hampshire and Red Sussex. The inheritance pattern of Red plumage seems to be *multifactorial* in view of the variation in intensity of red colour.

(iv) ***Blue*** plumage is present in Andalusian breed in a heterozygous state and shows *co-dominance.*

(v) ***Buff*** plumage is controlled by autosomal gene. This gene for buff plumage present in some breeds/strains is *dominant* to recessive white but it is recessive to black plumage gene.

(vi) ***Columbian*** colour pattern of plumage is found in Columbian Leghorns, Columbian Plymouth Rocks and Light Sussex. This colour pattern is due to a dominant sex-linked gene, **S** (silver) and an autosomal gene which inhibits the spread of black on neck, wings and tail, while the recessive gene **s** produces gold colour.

(vii) ***Barred*** plumage is controlled by *sex-linked gene*, present in Barred Plymouth Rocks and dominant to non-barring. This gene is helpful in sexing of chicks at hatching time. The mating of RIR or New Hampshire cocks to Barred Plymouth Rock hens produce males all having bright yellow shank and head spot markings but the female chicks have black shanks and are solid black in down colour without head spot.

(4) Comb Types

The comb is a fleshy growth on head of the fowl and more developed in males than females. There are four major comb types *viz.* Pea, Rose, Single and Walnut, though Duplex and Breda comb are also found.

(i) The ***pea comb*** is a kind of triple comb resembling three small combs lying side by side of which the middle is the highest. The pea comb gene is dominant and causes the compact comb size with side effect to improve the convection ability.

(ii) The ***rose comb*** is solid comb, flat on top, covered with small regular points with spike.

(iii) The ***single comb*** has 5 to 7 points and a blade moderately thick and smooth. The point of comb is the spike on the blade of single comb.

The Pea and Rose type are considered dominant over Single comb. But actually the relationship of Single comb is not of dominant-recessive type with Pea or Rose comb, it is of epistatic type because the genes for Pea (P) and Rose comb (R) are present on different chromosomes. Thus, it is better to say that Single comb is hypostatic and the Pea and Rose comb genes are epistatic.

(iv) The ***walnut comb*** is the result of complementary effect of Pea and Rose comb when combined. Thus, two pairs of genes produce all the four types of comb in such a manner that the birds with genotype rr P- produces Pea comp, R- pp produces Rose comb, rr pp produces Single comb and R- P- produces Walnut comb. This is called ***complementary gene action*** producing the F_2 ratio as 9 Walnut, 3 Pea comb, 3 Rose comb and 1 Single comb.

(*v*) ***Duplex comb*** is controlled by a pair of gene having two alleles showing incomplete dominance. This type of comb is found in Polish breed.

(*vi*) ***Breda type*** **comb** is controlled by a pair of alleles (B and b) having dominance recessive relationship and found in Dutch breed (Breda). The females with b gene have no comb whereas the males show only two papillae.

(5) Skin Colour

The skin colour genes are autosomal and show dominance recessive relationship. The domestic fowls have mainly the yellow and white skin colours, found mostly in American and European breeds. The white skin and shank colour is dominant (W) over yellow skin and shank colour (w). The deposition of carotenoid pigment xanthophylls produces yellow colour. The dominant gene W does not allow the transfer of xanthophylls pigment in skin, beak and shanks and hence these are of white colour. The melanin colour pigment caused by melanin gene causes dark skin and when combined with xanthophylls pigment causes green or nylon colour of shank and beak and this form the breed characteristic of Polish Greenleg and Sicilian Buttercups as well as of native breed Khadaknath. The Silkie breeds have dark blue colour.

(6) Earlobe Colour

The earlobe is fold of the skin just below the ear in fowl. The earlobe colour is also used for identification of different breeds, though this character is considered to be polygenic in chickens. Some sort of relationship has been observed between the colour of earlobe and eggs laid by the birds. The Meditarranean breeds have white earlobes and produces white eggs whereas the breeds having red earlobe produce brown eggs with exception of Dorking and Red caps having red earlobes producing white eggs and Araucana breed with red earlobe produces blue eggs. The earlobe is bluish in Khadaknath and Silki breeds.

Blood Group Systems in Chickens

The blood group genes are present on autosomes. There has been reported 13 blood groups in poultry which are A, B, C, D, E, H, I, J, K, L, N, P and R. These blood groups show independent segregation except A and E groups which are closely linked. The study of blood groups helps in identifying the pedigree, besides the association of some blood groups with disease resistance and susceptibility. The blood group B is a marker for major histocompatibility locus and blood group C for minor histocompatibility locus.

8.7 PLEIOTROPIC GENE ACTION

A gene may influence many characters like that a character is influenced by many genes (polygenic character). The phenomenon of affecting many phenotypes (characters) by a gene is called ***pleiotropy.*** This word has been taken from Greek language in which the pleiotropy means *"to take many turns"*. There can be cited a number of example of pleiotropic gene action.

Male sterility and weak pulmonary function in *human* are caused by a gene. The sickle cell gene in homozygous condition causes abnormal shape of RBC (sickle shape) also reduces the O_2 carrying capacity of blood, causing anemia and finally become fatal to the animal. A mutant gene for coat colour also causes sleepiness.

The gene for *PKU in humans* is also an example of pleiotropic gene action. The recessive mutation of the gene causes the toxic substance to accumulate in the brain leading to mental impairment. The synthesis of melanin pigment is also interfered by this mutant allele. The PKU patients frequently have light brown or blond hair (lightening the hair colour). The disease phenylketonurea (PKU) in human also produces a number of abnormal phenotypic traits or symptoms (syndrome) *viz.* short stature, mental retardation, widely spaced incisors, pigmented patches on the skin, and excessive sweating. The PKU patients have compounds in their blood and urine that are absent or rarely present in normal persons. Such multiple effects (pleiotropic effect) result from inter-connections between the biochemical and cellular pathways under gene control.

The mutation affecting *Bristle formation in Drosophila* is an example. The gene responsible for the shape and length of bristle also affects the health and fertility. There are long smoothly curved bristles on the head and thorax in wild type flies. The flies homozygous for the singed bristle mutation have short and twisted bristles (like as if scorched). Thus, the wild type, singed gene product is required for proper formation of bristles. It is also needed for the production of healthy and fertile eggs. This is because the homozygous females for certain singed mutations are completely sterile and lay flimsy ill formed eggs which never hatch. But these mutations have no adverse effect on male fertility. It can thus be concluded that singed gene controls many phenotypes for the formation of both bristles and eggs in females and the formation of bristles in males.

The recessive gene for vestigial wings in *Drosophila* also affects structure of reproductive organs, reduction in the egg production, reduction in longevity, and the bristles on the wings.

A gene in a Sahiwal heifer was observed for *athelia* (no teats) with reduced birth weight and subsequent body weight, late puberty, and reduction in viability resulting death before reproductive age (Tomar, *et al.*, 1982).

Pleiotropy as a Cause of Genetic Correlation among Quantitative Characters

The pleiotropy is the property of gene and said to be the most important cause of genetic correlation. The effect of some genes may be synergetic or antagonistic. The synergetic effect means that the gene affects two or more characters in the same direction *i.e.* the gene may increase or decrease the value of two or more characters causing positive correlation whereas the antagonistic effect means that they affect the two or more characters in opposite direction i.e they may increase the value of one trait and decrease the value of other trait causing negative correlation. Therefore, the pleiotropy may not be necessarily causes an appreciable amount of correlation and the magnitude of correlation due to pleiotropy depends on the direction of their effect. The genetic correlation caused by pleiotropy is similar in magnitude and direction in any population and does not change in random mating population over generations. It is difficult to identify and measure the pleiotropy as a cause of correlation but it can be imagined *viz.* the genes responsible for growth also increase the stature or size and weight of the animal and it is interpreted that such genes cause a correlation between these traits. Likewise, the genes affecting the digestion or absorption of nutrients may affect the growth and other traits like production of milk, wool, eggs, meat or work efficiency.

EXERCISE

8.1 The birds with feathered shanks (Lagshan, Brahama breeds) were crossed with the birds with clean shanks (Cornish, Minorca, Australorp breeds). All the F_1 had feathers on shanks. In F_2 progeny of 325 birds, 19 birds were fond clean shank. What was the type of gene action responsible for expression of this character?.

Solution: Feathered birds in F_2 = 325 – 19 = 306.

Assuming two gene interactions, there will be 16 genotypic classes.

Therefore, 1/16 part of 325 = 325/16 = 20.31.

The ratio of 306 feathered birds based on 16 genotypes will be = 306/20.31 = 15.06

The ratio of feathered to clean shank birds is 15:1

This ratio of 15:1 indicates duplicate dominant recessive epistasis.

8.2 The genotype AABB produces red phenotype whereas the double recessive genotype produces white phenotype. The recessive homozygous genotype at either gene loci (aa B- and A- bb) produces a third phenotype (sandy). What will be the phenotype of F_1 generation?. Also find out the phenotypic ratios in F_2 generation and name the type of gene interaction.

8.3 The pea comb shape in poultry is dominant (P -) over the single comb shape (pp). Another trait feather colour is due to co-dominance of a pair of alleles producing black (BB), white (bb) and blue (Bb) feathers. In a brood from white hen with pea comb shape, it was observed that 2 birds were blue pea comb, 4 were white pea comb, 2 were white single comb and 1 bird was of the phenotype blue feathers with single comb. (a) Predict the genotype of the hen and the cock. (b) Among the 4 white pea comb progeny, how many are expected to be heterozygous for pea comb gene (c) If each of the four white pea comb progeny are used in a test cross and each produced at least one progeny with single comb, how many of these four progeny are expected to be heterozygous.

Answer: (a) The genotype of the hen is bb Pp and of cock will be Bb pp. This is because the mating with these genotypes will produce the four types of progeny in a ratio of 2: 4: 2: 1.

(b) The four white feathers and pea comb progeny from above cross (Bb pp x bb Pp) will be of genotype bb Pp and all the four will be heterozygous for pea comb gene.

(c) The test cross will be mating of double recessive (bb pp) with the given genotype (bb Pp). This cross produces at least one progeny with single comb and hence all the original four progeny are expected to be heterozygous.

8.4 A dominant gene (S) produces short hair in rabbit and the recessive allele (s) causes long hairs. The pelger anomaly is caused as detailed in question numbe 4.14. Predict the phenotypic ratios among several litters from mating of heterozygous short-haired pelgers among themselves at weaning.

***Answer*:** The genotype of short-haired pelgers would be Ss Pp. The alleles for length of hais show dominance-recessive relationship and hence will produce 3 short hair: 1 long hair whereas the alleles causing pelger anomaly are dominant lethal (PP) causing death upto soon after birth and hence will produce the 2 pelgers: 1 normal. Therefore, the combined segregation and recombination will produce the progeny at weaning as:

[3 (short): 1 (long hair)] x [2 (pelgers): 1 (normal)] = ?

Chapter 9

Linkage and Crossing Over

This chapter deals with two processes of linkage and crossing-over, effect of linkage on normal gene segregation, and the importance of linkage in modifying the normal phenotypic ratios among progenies.

9.1 THEORIES OF LINKAGE

There had been some landmarks before the chromosome theory of linkage was developed by Morgan, T. H. (1911).

Sutton's Theory (Sutton, 1903)

The presence of more than one pair of genes on the same chromosome pair is possible if the number of genes exceed to the number of chromosomes in the cell of an organism. This was made clear first time by Sutton (1903) who proposed the theory that chromosomes are the bearers of the hereditary units (genes). According to Sutton-Bovery hypothesis, the number of chromosomes in any organism is considerably less than the number of genes (Mendelian factors). Under this situation, large number of genes will have to be located on one pair of chromosome. Therefore, it is likely that all the genes present on each pair of chromosome may transmit in groups rather than singly.

Theory of Coupling and Repulsion (Bateson and Punnet, 1906)

After rediscovery of Mendel's law in 1900 by 3 Scientists, the law of independent assortment was tested by Bateson and Punnet (1906) by making a dihybrid cross between two varieties of sweet pea. They found a different ratio than reported by Mendel among the F_2 progeny. The proportions of parental type progenies were higher and new combinations (recombinant types) were lesser than expected on the basis of independent assortment of genes. Such deviated results are logically possible if the gene pairs failure to segregate and assort (distribute) independently, and also if more than one pair of genes are present on a chromosome with an association or link between different gene pairs. They developed a theory of *"Coupling and repulsion"* to explain their results, depending upon the dominant and recessive genes coming from one parent (coupling) or from two parents (repulsion).

Morgan's Concept

The genetic and cytological studies together have produced the modern picture of chromosome organization. The landmark in this respect has been the study made by Morgan, T. H. (1909) to demonstrate that the gene for white eye in *Drosophila* was located on the X chromosome. He stated that *coupling* and *repulsion* concepts putforth by Bateson and Punnet (1906) is the two aspects of the same phenomenon to which he called ***linkage***.

Chromosome Theory of Linkage

Morgan and Castle have proposed chromosome theory of linkage. They stated that the genes showing linkage are located on the same chromosome (attached to one another much like beads on a string), assumed a linear model of chromosome organization, linked genes show no recombination but remain in original combination during their transmission to the progenies, and the distance between the linked genes is inversely proportion to the strength of linkage.

Morgan's student, Sturtevant, A. H. (1911) constructed the world's first chromosome map and invented the procedure for chromosome mapping. He analyzed the data from the experimental crosses with *Drosophila* making the linkage as the base that genes on the same chromosome should be inherited together.

9.2 LINKAGE

The two or more pairs of genes residing in the same chromosome and transmitting together are said to be *linked* and the phenomenon is said to be *linkage*. Thus, *the phenomenon of existence of numerous pairs of genes on the same pair of chromosome and their inheritance together is called linkage.* Such linked genes present on a chromosome form a *linkage group*. The numbers of linkage groups correspond to the chromosome numbers in haploid individuals and to the numbers of chromosome pairs in diploid organisms. Sturtvant used the linkage as the basis of mapping procedure. This was due to the reason that the linked genes are physically attached to the same chromosome and hence should be inherited together.

Expectation

Dihybrid individual produces two types of games *viz.* parental and recombinant types, in equal proportion, when there is independent assortment of two pairs of genes. The linkage and crossing over result in deviation of the production in the proportion of parental and recombinant gametes. The Mendelian dihybrid ratios of F_2 cross and of testcross are modified. This has been explained on the basis of experimental findings here -

9.2.1 Linkage Causes Deviation in Dihybrid F_2 Cross

Bateson and Punnet (1906) worked on the inheritance of two characters (flower colour and length of pollen grains) of sweet pea. They crossed a variety of sweet pea having red flowers and long pollen grains (RR LL) with another variety that had white flowers and round (short) pollen grains (rr ll). They found that flower colour and pollen shape are controlled by separate gene pairs with dominance of red flower and long pollen grain over the alleles for white colour and round pollen. They made a dihybrid cross of red-long and white-round. The F_1 hybrids were heterozygous for red-long (Rr Ll). These F_1 were selfed to produce F_2 progeny. The results of F_2 generation were 583 red long (parental), 26 red round (recomb.), 24 white long (recom.), and 170 white round (parental). These results of F_2 progeny were in a ratio of 24.3: 1.1: 1: 7.1 and hence clearly a deviation of normal classical F_2 dihybrid phenotypic ratio of 9:3:3:1 as was proposed by Mendel.

Another cross was made by them in confirmation of the deviated normal classical F_2 dihybrid phenotypic ratios, with different combination of characters. The red-round plants (RR ll) were crossed with those having white flowers and long pollens (rr LL). The resulting dihybrid F_1 were again had red flower and long pollen. On crossing the F_1s, it was again observed the deviation of normal classical F_2 dihybrid phenotypic ratio.

In both the crosses, they found that the F_2 progeny with parental combination were in higher proportions and the recombinants occurred in lesser proportion than expected on the basis of independent assortment of two pairs of genes.

The cross in which the dominant genes at both loci come from the same parent (one chromosome) was said to be in *coupling phase* and the cross that include two dominant and recessive genes from different parents was said to be in *repulsion phase.* Thus, linkage relationship is of two types *i.e.* coupling phase and repulsion phase. Accordingly, purple-long x red-round cross illustrates the coupling phase whereas the purple-round x red-long cross illustrates repulsion phase. These two terms (*coupling and repulsion*) are used to distinguish the two possible arrangements of two pairs of genes on a single pair of homologous chromosome.

9.2.2 Linkase Causes Deviation in Dihybrid Test Cross

Morgan (1910) worked on the inheritance of two characters (eye colour and wing length) of Drosophila. He selected the flies differing in two different characters controlled by two pairs of gene, one pair affecting the eye colour (Purple, pr and red, pr′) and the other pair affecting the wing length (vestigial, vg and long, vg′). The red eye colour and long length of wing were normal and hence taken as wild type. The red eye colour is dominant over purple colour and the long wing gene is dominant over vestigial gene.

The first cross was that of coupling phase. *The second cross* was that of the repulsion phase when each of the two parent was homozygous for only one of the two dominant gene pairs. The resulting dihybrid F_1 females were *test crossed* with double recessive homozygous males, in both the crosses. The results obtained were drastically different than Mendelian prediction of 1:1:1:1 test cross phenotypic ratio.

9.2.3 Conclusion of the Results of F_2 Cross and Test Cross

It was evident from the results obtained from F_2 and test cross that the coupling as well as the repulsion phase relationship of genes gave similar trend of results in F_2 and test cross data. The similarity in both the crosses *viz. F_2 cross and test cross* (both coupling and repulsion relationship) was that *parental type progenies* produced were in *higher proportions* than *recombinant types.* Based on the deviation of results, Morgan replaced the Bateson theory of *coupling and repulsion* with *linkage and crossing over.* Morgan found that coupling and repulsion are two aspects of a single phenomenon to which he called as *linkage.*

The term *linkage* was defined as the tendency of genes present on the same chromosome (linkage group) to enter the gametes in parental combinations (tendency of genes to remain together during the process of inheritance) whereas the tendency of genes, residing on the same chromosome, to enter the gametes in the combinations other than those of parents (recombinants *i.e.* new combinations) was defined as *crossing over.*

The ***theory of linkage*** states that:

- The tendency of genes to remain in their parental combination is due to their presence on the same chromosome,
- The parental combinations of linked genes remains unchanged during the process of inheritance, and
- The genes on a chromosome are in a linear arrangement. The distance between linked genes on a chromosome is variable and decides the strength of linkage.

The deviation from the test cross ratio (1:1:1:1) and the F_2 ratio (9:3:3:1) based on independent assortment of genes indicated that two pairs of genes do not assort independently and are not located on different pairs of chromosomes but must be present on the same pair of chromosome. Morgan explained that the higher frequency of parental type progeny in either test cross or F_2 generation might be due to the presence of two pairs of genes on the same pair of chromosome, because the different pairs of genes being located on the same pair of chromosome are always transmitted together having come from the same parent (linked genes). This explains partly why the parental gene combinations remain together and occurred in higher proportions. When the two pairs of genes are located on the same pair of chromosome and are inherited together (linked group), there should have been no recombinants. These results neither follow the independent assortment law nor show linkage phenomenon but fall between the two. In other experiments also the recombinants occurred in almost all the cases, with few exceptions. Now, the matter is to explain the production of recombinants that how they occur (the process by which the recombinants occur) when there is a linkage between the genes. This means that some process is taking place in the formation of recombinant gametes during meiosis so as to produce the intermediate results between linkage and independent assortment of genes. The process which forms the recombinant gametes and produces the intermediate results is the *crossing over.*

9.3 RECOMBINATION AND CROSSING OVER

The linkage of genes was not taken as an absolute phenomenon by early geneticists (Bateson and Punnet, Morgan and his students, *etc.*) on the basis of their experimental data. The results of their experimental data have shown that the genes present on the same chromosome may be separated during meiosis and form new combination of genes (as discussed above). This phenomenon was called ***recombination***. Morgan postulated that recombination of linked genes is accompanied through a process by which the homologous chromosomes exchange parts (Johanssen, 1909). This process of physical exchange of parts between homologous chromosomes was called ***crossing over.***

The event of crossing-over occurs between non-sister chromatids of homologous chromosomes at the time of synapsis during late prophase and metaphase of first meiotic cell division when duplicated chromosomes have paired. This involves actual exchange of chromosome material. Each of the four chromatids goes into separate gamete to form four gametes. The two gametes carry the gene combinations identical to the parents and other two gametes are produced by crossing-over and hence called as crossover gametes or ***recombinants***. These two recombinant gametes on fertilization produce two recombinant phenotypes which are different from parental phenotypes. These recombinant phenotypes are the result of crossing over. The percentage of recombinant is also referred to as the percentage of crossover which is simply the number of recombinant phenotypes expressed as a percentage of the total number of progeny.

Conditions of the Recombinants to Occur

The recombinants can result either due to independent assortment when the two gene pairs are present on different chromosomes or due to crossing over when the genes are present adjacently and linked to each other on the same chromosome. Thus, there are two types of recombinants:

(i) *Inter chromosomal recombination* which arises from the genes located on different pairs of chromosomes assorting independently. The frequency of recombinants in this case is always ½ or 50 per cent of the total gametes produced in a test cross.

(ii) *Intra chromosomal recombination* which arises from the genes located on the same chromosome by the process of crossing over during meiosis. The frequency of recombinants in this case is less than 50 per cent. This frequency provides very useful genetic information to provide genetic variability and to know the relative position of two or more genes located on the same chromosome (linkage or genetic map).

9.4 ILLUSTRATION OF CROSSING OVER

The phenomenon of crossing over can be illustrated by genetic studies involving crosses and by cytological proof.

(i) Genetic Studies

The genetic crossing over was first considered a consequence of the exchange of parts between two homologous chromosomes. The phenomenon of crossing over provided the most reasonable physical mechanism for recombination of genes to occur between the members of a linkage group. The assumption of crossing over was based on the fact that the recombinants are actually produced by the exchange of chromosome segments between homologous chromosomes for the genes located on the same chromosome. The results of genetic studies showed crossing over (exchange of parts between homologous chromosomes) because it was the only possibility of recombinants being produced. Therefore, in order to produce recombinants between two different allelic pairs located on the same chromosome pair, crossing over must occur between the loci of genes involved.

(ii) Cytological Proof of Crossing Over

The cytological proof of crossing over was demonstrated by Stern (1931) in Drosophila, and Creighton and McClintock (1931) in Mize. There were faced some difficulties to prove crossing over cytologically. The main difficulty was to demonstrate the physical exchange of parts of homologous chromosomes because the members of a pair of homologous chromosome are not visible clearly from each other due to their identical appearance. Secondly, the four chromatids are identically coiled around each other during crossing over. Moreover, the crossing over cannot be seen in living cells.

The experimental results obtained by Stern (1931) on *Drosophila* and Creighton and McClintock (1931) in Mize gave evidence that crossing over causes recombination.

(a) Stern Experiment

Stern (1931) recognized the value of cytological marker for demonstrating crossing over. He obtained female *Drosophila* whose both of the two X- chromosomes had structural abnormalities – each of the two X chromosomes has one abnormality. A portion of Y- chromosome was attached to one of the two X- chromosomes while the second X chromosome had another distinguishing feature composed of two equal fragments, each with its centromere (the X- chromosome being broken into two pieces). These two abnormalities (one each in two X chromosomes of female fly) lead to the recognition of these two X-chromosome from each other based on two abnormalities as well as from normal X- chromosome. The female *Drosophila* carrying these two abnormal X - chromosomes (one with attached X with a part of Y chromosome and other with broken piece) as distinct cytological markers and genetically heterozygous for carnation (light) eye colour (recessive to normal eye colour) and bar eye shape (small eye, a dominant eye shape over normal wild type) were crossed with males of carnation eye colour and normal eye shape (wild shape of eye).

The results were recorded on genetic aspect (linkage and crossing over) as well as cytological aspect (chromosome appearance). Examination of the chromosomes of the progeny whose phenotypes showed genetic recombination indicated that genetic recombination was followed as a consequence of appropriate exchange of identifiable chromosome segment.

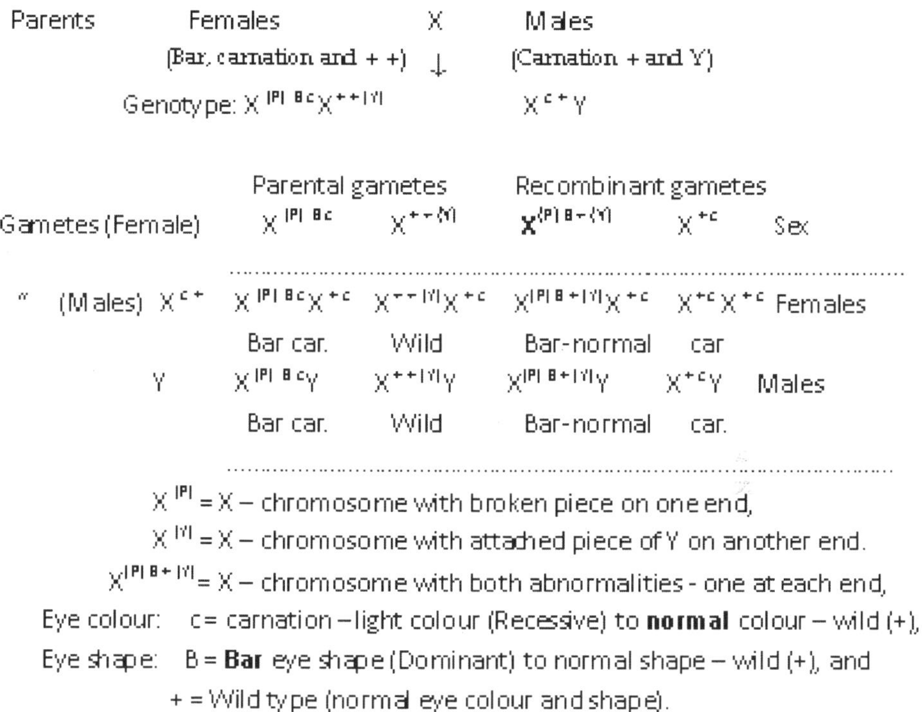

Figure 9.1: Stern's Experiment (*Drosophila*) for Cytological and Genetic Evidence of Crossing Over.

The two abnormalities (broken piece and attached piece, wild type) present on two different X-chromosomes can only come together on one member of a pair of chromosome if crossing over takes place between two X chromosomes containing two abnormalities in female *Drosophila*. He found that the parental types determined genetically (Bar, carnation and + +; wild type) always had parental chromosome configuration (Bar, carnation flies) having bar, carnation and + + (wild type) flies. On the other hand, the chromosome of the recombinant progeny had new chromosome arrangements, with Bar + and + carnation. Carnation, is a recessive mutant eye colour (c) to wild type red colour (C) whereas the bar shape eye (small or narrow, B) is dominant over wild type normal eye shape (b). Thus, the genetic, physical and cytological crossing over was established.

To demonstrate the crossing over with chromosome exchange, it is thus important to have chromosomes which are cytologically different in which the crossing over occurs. The above experiment showed relationship between genetic and cytological crossing over, and that cross over was a result of physical exchange.

(b) Creighton and McClintock Experiment

Harriet Creighton and Barbara McClintock (1931) studied homologous chromosomes 9 in maize. One of these two homologous chromosomes was normal while the second chromosome had two cytological abnormalities one at each end. The abnormal chromosome has a heterochromatic knob at one end while there was a piece of a different chromosome (8 th) at other end. Thus, one member of the pair of chromosome number 9 had two marker genes. Further this abnormal chromosome was heterozygous for two loci (C for coloured kernel or aleurone and wx for waxy texture of kernel or endosperm) while its partner homologous chromosome which was normal having no abnormality was heterozygous for these two loci (c, for colourless kernel or aleurone – outermost layer of the endosperm in a seed; and Wx, for statchy texture of kernel or aleurone). They made a testcross (heterozygous Cc wx/c Wx of coloured starchy phenotype, with a recessive homozygous, c c wx wx of colourless waxy phenotype) and examined the recombinant progeny.

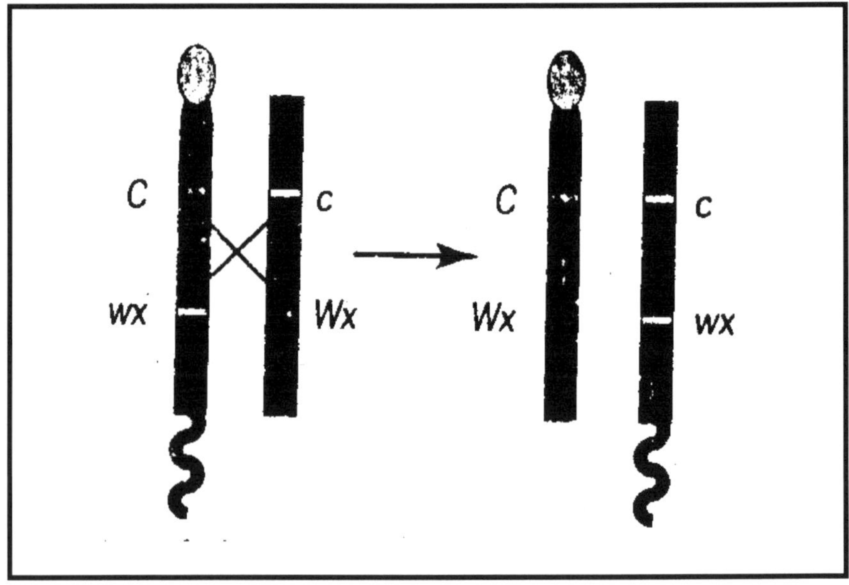

Figure 9.2: Creighton and McClintock's Experiment on Maize.

The results of the cross indicated that two recombinant gametes produced had C Wx and c wx recombination of genes on two members of chromosome 9. They found that each member of the chromosome pair number 9 had only one abnormality after recombination of genes (gamete formation) - one member had knob with C Wx genes and the second member had another abnormality (a piece of chromosome number 8) with c wx genes. It was thus evident that such a recombination of genes (C Wx and c wx) with only one abnormality on each of two members of homologous chromosome 9 was the result of a physical exchange (crossing over) between the two members of homologous chromosome 9. Therefore, it is an *evidence that crossing over causes recombination.*

(iii) Molecular Mechanism of DNA Recombination – Genetic Control

The homologous DNA molecules recombination involves the products of many genes. These gene products play their role in crossing over and recombination by helping in-

- ✰ Chromosome pairing,
- ✰ Catalyzing the process of exchange (to cleave, unwind, and repair), and
- ✰ Rejoining the broken chromatid segments (strands of DNA).

The recombination is thus under genetic control. The recombination between homologous DNA molecules is the result of the material exchange through breakage of parental chromosomes and rejoining of the parts in new combinations, as explained above by two genetic studies. The crossing over has also been demonstrated by radiography and other techniques. The biochemical studies of *recombination-deficient mutants* of *E. coli* and *S. Cerevisiae* provided the base of the molecular details of crossing over because these mutations were deficient in various enzymes and other proteins required for recombination. Therefore, the recombination mechanism at molecular level has become clear from the combined results of genetic and biochemical studies.

Robin Holliday (1964) proposed a model of crossing over by a mechanism involving the breakage (cleavage), reunion, and repair of DNA molecules. His model explained most of the genetic data available on the subject. This was a *single-strand breaks model* involving only one of the strands of parental double helices.

The mechanism of recombination (called as genetic or DNA or chromosome recombination) starts by pairing of homologous chromosomes. Now there is cleavage (breakage) of single strand of each of the two parental DNA molecules by an enzyme endonuclease. The enzymes DNA helicases unwind the two strands of DNA in the region adjacent to the breaks (incisions) in single strands and with the help of single-strand binding proteins displace the segments of the single strands on one side of each cut from their complementary strands. Therefore, the strand displacement is completed by the activities of endonuclease which makes breaks in DNA and the DNA helicase which unwinds the two strands of DNA. The next step is the strand exchange. This reciprocal exchange process of DNA single strands between two DNA double helices is promoted by proteins, called RecA-type proteins which mediate the exchanges by binding to the unpaired strand of DNA. Finally, the cleaved strands are covalently joined (reunion) by the enzyme DNA ligase. Now the two recombinant DNA molecules are produced.

Jack Szostak and collegues (1983) had proposed the *double-strand break model* of crossing over in yeast. According to that model the recombination often involves a double-strand break in one of the parental double helices, instead of single strand break.

Gene Conversion

The genetic exchange between homologous chromosomes is not always reciprocal and called ***gene conversion***. In this process one of the alleles appears to have been converted to another allelic form. This gene conversion seems to the result from DNA repair synthesis associated with the breakage, excision, and reunion events of crossing over. In case of close linkage between genetic markers, the nonreciprocal recombination or gene conversion often occurs producing the segregating alleles in 3:1 ratio rather than 1:1 as per expectation. This is the most striking feature of gene conversion that the input 1:1 allele ratio is not maintained. The process involved in this may degrade the short segment of parental DNA and its resynthesis with template strand carrying other adjacent and linked allele.

9.5 CYTOLOGICAL BASIS OF CROSSING OVER

This was described by Johanssen (1909) through the formation of chiasma at the tetrad stage during spermatogenesis in Salamonders. He noticed that during meiosis at the time of pairing (***Synapsis***) of duplicated homologous chromosomes (*tetrads* or four-strands), two chromatids showed a cross-shape structure. This *cross-shape structure* of tetrads is called as ***Chiasma*** (plural- chiasmata). Thus, chiasma formation is probably the visible manifestation of crossing over. The chiasma becomes clearly visible during late prophase of the first meiotic division. At this time the paired chromosomes repel each other slightly having a close contact only at the centromere and at each chiasma. At this stage the number of chiasma may be counted accurately. The number of chiasmata is proportional to the length of chromosome.

The chiasma is a ribbonlike structure between synapsed homologues at the end of the first meiotic prophase, binding the chromatids along their length and facilitating chromatid exchange. Such a structure is called ***synaptinemal complex.*** Thus, the crossing over occurs between chromatids (tetrads) and not between unduplicated chromosomes. The crossing over is the physical basis of recombination (production of recombinant progeny).

9.6 MEIOTIC STAGE TO OCCUR CROSSING OVER

The crossing over between homologous chromosomes results to the production of recombinant gametes. This process of crossing over involves a physical exchange between the homologous chromosomes.

The crossing over (exchange event) occurs during the prophase of first meiosis, when duplicated chromosomes have paired. The cells near the end of the prophase of meiosis I give best cytological evidence of the occurrence of crossing over. During this stage the paired homologues repel each other slightly and the exchanges of parts between them are seen in the form of ***chiasmata.*** Thus, the crossing over has two observable outcomes *viz.* formation of *chiasmata* in late prophase as a result of pairing and duplication of chromosomes after which there is physical exchange of chromatid parts resulting recombination of genes on opposite sides of the crossover point. The second outcome of *recombination of genes* can only be observed in progeny generation on expressing the genes. The pairing of homologous chromosomes during meiosis is called ***synapsis***. The duplication of homologous chromosomes produces four homologous chromosomes, known as ***tetrad.*** The presence of tetrads during first meiosis is called a ***tetrad stage*** - four strands of homologous chromosomes.

The four products of meiosis (tetrads - two parental types and two recombinants) in the concerned breeding experiments is the genetic evidence of crossing over. This has given a strong proof that crossing over occurs at four-strand or tetrad stage called as ***chromatid stage***. Each of these four chromatids breaks at the point of crossover and reattach. The beaks in chromatids and their reattachment occur due to the action of enzymes acting on the DNA of the chromatids. Thus, there is formation of two recombinants and two parental gametes among a total of four. At any one point of crossover, only two chromatids are involved in crossing over while another two or any of the two chromatids may crossover at another point. This way there may be more than one crossover (double, triple, or quadruple crossovers). However, *no genetic recombination* occurs between sister-chromatids because they have identical genes.

The four different products of meiosis are possible if crossing over occurs at tetrad stage, because if the crossing over occurs at two strand stage, there would have been only two different products of a given meiosis (only two games with parental combination of genes) and hence there would have been no recombination of genes (no recombinant gamete) during gamete formation. This is an *evidence of crossing over as the physical basis of recombination.*

Kinds of Crossing Over

The Crossing over may be single, double or multiple depending upon the number of chiasmata formed. When only one chiasma is formed it results in single crossing over forming a single crossover gamete. This type is most frequent. Double crossing over results due to the formation of two chiasmata and it is less frequent type. The multiple crossing- over take place when more than two chiasmata are formed and it does not occur frequently.

Frequency of Crossing Over

The frequency of crossing over between two loci is expressed in terms of percentage of crossing over which is directly proportional to the distance between two loci. Thus the distance between two loci on a chromosome is indicated by the percentage of cross over. When two genes are located on a chromosome very close to each other, the frequency of their crossing over is less to produce cross over progeny. Sometimes the more closely located genes do not allow crossing over. In this case only parental types of progeny are produced due to linkage of genes and thus the frequency of crossing over is zero because no cross over progeny is produced. The percentage of crossing over is obtained from the data and helps to work out the relative distance between various loci on a chromosome which in turn determines the exact location of the genes on the chromosome. Thus it is of great significance because it helps in the construction of chromosome maps. The unit of crossing over is Morgan according to J.B.S.Haldane.

Factors Affecting Frequency of Crossing Over

The strength of linkage or the frequency of crossing over is influenced by genetic, physiological and environmental factors. These include intra-species variation (genotypes, chromosome structure and position of genes to centromere), differential effect of sex, temperature, chemicals and irradiation *etc.*

The ***gene mutation*** may affect the frequency of crossing over. In *Drosophila melanogaster*, a gene on 3rd chromosome (c 3 G) completely suppresses crossing over when homozygous in females but enhances recombination when heterozygous. Change in chromosome structure, *i.e.* order of genes on a chromosome (chromosomal aberration) in one pair of chromosome was found to increase the frequency of crossing over in other normal non-homologous chromosome.

The ***inversion of chromosome segments*** (rearrangement) greatly reduced recombination in heterozygote. The crossing over is usually inhibited near the breakpoints of a rearrangement, probably due to the reason that rearrangement disrupts chromosome pairing as a result of the selective loss of chromosome in the inverted region.

The ***genes located near the centromere*** show reduced crossing over and the position of genes relative to centromere of the chromosome can be changed by structural chromosomal aberrations. The crossing over is less frequent near centromere, at the tips of chromosomes and near another crossover. The crossing over is less likely to occur between the genes that are located relatively closer together on the chromosome and so recombinant gametes are less likely to be produced. On the other hand, a greater number of crossover gametes will be expected when linked genes are located relatively far apart on the chromosomes.

The ***sex*** has also effect on the frequency of crossing over. The crossing over in Drosophila males is negligible. Likewise, males of mammals also show little crossing over. But the crossing over does not occur in females of silk worm

The increase in ***age*** of the female of Drosophila is associated with decrease in the rate of crossing over to a certain age and thereafter it increases again in later age.

Deviation in ***temperature*** from 22°C in both the direction has been shown to increase the rate of crossing over in Drosophila.

The chemical composition of food, ***starvation, antibiotics*** and ***X-ray irradiation*** increase the crossing over.

Recombination under Genetic Control

The products of many genes have been demonstrated to be involved in recombination and its events. Different gene products are important in performing the different events involved in recombination. Thus, some gene products are involved in chromosome pairing, others in catalyzing the process of exchange of chromosome segments, and others in rejoining the broken chromatid segments. Thus, the recombination is under genetic control.

9.7 EXPECTED RATIOS WITH INDEPENDENT ASSORTMENT AND LINKAGE

The test-cross data as well as the F_2 data indicated the following three situations:

(i) Independent Assortment of Two Gene Pairs

This results in equal proportion of parental combinations and new combinations (recombinants), with further subdivision of both types of combinations in equal proportion resulting 1:1:1:1 ratio.

(ii) Linkage of Genes

The linkage of genes may be complete or incomplete, depending on the extent of crossing over:

- ✰ *Complete linkage between two gene pairs (No crossing over):* This results in only the parental types with both parental types in equal ratio.
- ✰ Incomplete linkage (Some *crossing over between two gene pairs):* This results in parental as well as in new combinations in unequal proportions, the parental combinations being higher than new combinations. This is the case of incomplete linkage or crossing over which results in 4 phenotypic ratios, two of each parental and new combination.

(1) Complete Linkage

It means no crossing over.

This is a rare phenomenon. The linkage is caused by linked genes being located on the same chromosome. Thus, the two or more genes located on the same chromosome should remain together in all cases to produce only the parental combinations and no new recombinants should be produced. This type of linkage is called as complete linkage which can be explained under the condition of no crossing over. This is only possible that the genes are so closely located in the same chromosome that they are always inherited together.

(*a*) ***Genes present of 4th chromosome*** in *Drosophila:* The example of complete linkage of genes was found for the genes present on 4th chromosome of D. *melanogaster:* The mutant carrying genes controlling ***bent wings*** and ***shaven bristles*** (bt svn/bt svn genotype). When these flies are crossed to normal flies (bt′ svn′/bt′ svn′), the F_1 produced are heterozygous for the mutant genes. The test cross progeny are either bent shaven or normal and thus only the original parental types progenies are produced without appearing any cross over (recombinant) types. This strong linkage among two genes was evident in both coupling and repulsion phase.

Studies have shown that crossing over is either absent or rare in male Drosophila and in female silkworm moth which are both hemizygous.

(*b*) ***Male Drosophila***: Morgan (1910) crossed the F_1 heterozygous female (for eye colour and wing size) with double recessive male (***purple eye-vestigial wings***, pr vg/pr vg). He obtained the parental as well as recombinants as obtained earlier. But when he changed the sex in the test cross *i.e.* F_1 heterozygous males were test crossed with double recessive females, the complete linkage was observed because no recombinants were produced. Thus the *linkage strength is different in the two sexes in Drosophila,* crossing over rarely or never occurs in the male.

Another example of complete linkage in this insect (Drosophila) can be cited. The gene for ***gray body colour*** (B) is dominant over its allele producing black or ebony body (b) and another gene for ***wing size*** resulting in long wing (V) dominant over its allele (v) producing vestigial wings. Morgan (1919) crossed gray bodied vestigial winged flies (Bv/Bv) with black bodied long winged (bV/bV). The F_1 were heterozygous having gray body long wing (Bv/bV). The test cross taking F_1 as male with double recessive female produced only two kinds of progeny which were of parental types with no cross over type. Thus the linkage was complete. On repeating this experiment in a way that the F_1's were female in test cross and the double recessive parent was male (black-vestigial), the test cross progeny produced had both parental as well as cross over types, the parental types were about 83 per cent and rest 17 per cent were cross over types. Thus, there is perceptible distance between the genes for black and vestigial which separates them. The cytological experiments of spermatogenesis in male have shown that homologous chromosomes undergo pairing

(c) ***Female silkworm moth***: A Japanese geneticist, Tanaka observed that there was no crossing over in female silkworm (*Bombyx mori*).

It was generalized based on above experiments that there was no crossing over in *hemizygous* sex but this notion failed because in most other organisms the crossing over has been found to occur in both sexes.

(2) Incomplete Linkage

It means that some crossing over takes place.

The complete linkage is very rare and the experimental results fall between complete linkage and independent assortment which means that some crossing over occurs that leads to incomplete linkage. The following examples can be cited for incomplete linkage:

Drosophila: Two pairs of genes on 3rd chromosome, hairy (h) which is a bristle mutant and approximated (app) which is a wing vein mutant, show linkage. Both genes are recessive to wild type. The test cross showed that there were 90 per cent parental types and 10 per cent recombinants. Similar results were obtained in coupling and repulsion phase.

Linkage in certain sex-linked characters in Drosophila have been observed *viz.* between white eyed and miniature wings; white eyes and yellow body colour; yellow body colour and cut wings. These genes are present on X- chromosome. The white eye and miniature wings are recessive mutants to normal eye (red) and normal wings size. Morgan (1911) reported 37.6 per cent cross over between these two loci for eye colour and wing size. The yellow body colour and white eye colour are both mutants to normal or wild type (gray bodied and red eye). The test cross data resulted in 1.5 per cent recombinants in both coupling and repulsion phase of linkage. The crosses involving yellow body colour and cut wings (a recessive mutant on X-chromosome) produced 20 per cent recombinants.

Poultry: The genes controlling the *Comb shape* and *length of legs* (short or normal) are reported to be linked. Rose comb (R) is dominant over single comb (r) whereas creeper (short legs) gene (C) is dominant over normal leg length (c). However, these two genes do not maintain their linkage completely, as the test cross data indicated that some recombinants were produced that were in lesser frequency (8.3 per cent) than the parental combinations (91.7 per cent).

Two other pairs of genes affecting *feather colour* (I, white and i, coloured, black) and *feather texture* (F, frizzle, and f, normal or smooth) are also linked (Hutt, 1933). The gene I was dominant inhibiting the expression of melanin pigment and the individual was white feathered. The test cross data indicated that the genes showed incomplete linkage both in coupling and repulsion phase. The recombinants produced were 18.2 per cent in coupling phase and 19.7 per cent in repulsion phase. A third loci affecting *head shape* (crested and non-crested) is linked with other two loci affecting the feather colour (black and white), and texture (frizzle and smooth).

The two loci which are sex-linked affecting *rate of feathering* (normal or slow and rapid feathering), and *plumage colour* (Silver and gold) are linked together, being present on sex chromosome. Rapid feathering and gold feathering are controlled by recessive genes in homozygous condition, respectively. A third gene locus affecting colour pattern (barred and black) is also present on sex chromosome. The barred (white bars on top of head, feathers are banded with bars of black on white background) is dominant (B) over black (b).

Mice: The genes for coat colour in mice (Black and Himalayan) and hair texture (freezy and normal smooth) are linked on the same pair of chromosome. Himalayan colour is recessive to full colour (black) and the frizzy hair coat is recessive to normal smooth hair.

Pigs: The genes for skin colour (Black and red) and for ear condition (erect and droopy ears) are linked together. The black is controlled by dominant gene while its recessive allele causes white hogs. The gene for erect ears is dominant over droopy ears. The Hampshire hogs are known to be homozygous for dominant genes at both these loci whereas the Duroc hogs are homozygous recessive for both pairs of genes.

Humans: The crossing over in sex-linked genes for ***haemophilia*** and ***colour-blindness*** was reported by Haldane. The linkage has also been observed for genes producing ABO blood groups and those producing nail-patella syndromes (dominant mutation - causing *abnormal nails* and *kneecaps*) reported by Renwick, J. H. and Lawler, S. D. (1955); and those between the genes for Rh blood groups and elliptocytosis, with around only 5 percent crossing over.

Factors affecting strength of linkage: The strength is affected b many physiological as well as environmental factors. The probability of crossing over is reduced with ***age***, thereby increasing the strength of linkage. The frequency of chiasma formation is increased at ***high temperature*** and hence the strength of linkage is decreased. Likewise, exposure to ***X – rays*** educes the strength of linkage.

9.8 LINKAGE DETECTION

There are two methods to prove/detect the linkage, based on above results. One is the *test cross* (back cross of F_1 with double recessive parent) and the second method is *F_2 data* obtained from *inter se mating of F_1.*

The ratios of different phenotypic classes obtained either from test cross or F_2 data are compared to the ratios expected on the basis of independent assortment. The significance of departure in the ratios from the test cross or F_2 with the normal expectation (based on I.A.) is tested by *chi-square test* (test of independence for linkage). Among these two tests of detecting linkage, the *test cross* is the most convenient method and used:

- ☆ For determining the linkage and
- ☆ To know relative position of the locus within the chromosome.

Indication of Linkage

In a test cross (Aa x aa), a dominant gene segregates from its recessive allele in the ratio of 1:1. Similar will be for segregation of second gene pair (Bb x bb). If the two gene pairs segregating independently (taking together) in the ratio r_1:1 and r_2:1, their joint segregation will be in the ratio r_1r_2: r_1: r_2: 1, producing 4 phenotypic classes [four combinations in equal ratio of 1:1:1:1 as a result of (1:1) (1:1)]. Thus, there will be 4 phenotypic classes in equal numbers in case of I.A. of two pairs of genes. The complete linkage is indicated if all the testcross progeny are of parental types only, whereas the linkage is incomplete if recombinants are also observed but in lesser frequencies than of parental types. The testcross ratios having fewer than 50 per cent recombinants suggest linkage.

The F_2 ratio for single gene pair (with complete dominance, A and a) is 3:1 and for two gene pairs (A,a and B,b) segregating independently will be 9:3:3:1 obtained from (3:1) (3:1). The deviation, from these F_2 ratios (9:3:3:1) based on independent segregation, will be due to linkage of genes. When the deviation in these ratios occurs due to linkage (either in a test cross or in a F_2 cross), the parental type progenies are always in greater numbers and the numbers of recombinants are fewer, depending on the strength of linkage.

Test of Linkage

The *linkage is tested* by *chi-square* (χ^2) *test* based on the observed numbers of 4 phenotypic classes (AB, Ab, aB and ab) considering their observed numbers (O) as: a_1, a_2, a_3 and a_4. The expected numbers (E) for joint segregation of two loci in the ratio 9: 3: 3: 1 will be, respectively as: $(\frac{9}{16})N$; $(\frac{3}{16})N$; $(\frac{3}{16})N$ and $(\frac{1}{16})N$. Where, $N = a_1 + a_2 + a_3 + a_4$.

$$a_1 = AB; \quad a_2 = Ab; \quad a_3 = aB; \quad a_4 = ab$$

$$16 = \frac{9}{16} + \frac{3}{16} + \frac{3}{16} + \frac{1}{16}$$

$$\chi^2_{\text{(Total)}} = \frac{\Sigma(O - E)^2}{E}$$ tested at 3 degree of freedom.

The above information on the observed numbers of all the 4 phenotypic classes can better be understood if arranged in a tabular form as given under –

A locus:

	A	a	Total
B locus: B	$AB = a_1$	$aB = a_3$	$R_1 = a_1 + a_3$
b	$Ab = a_2$	$ab = a_4$	$R_2 = a_2 + a_4$
Total	$C_1 = (a_1 + a_2)$	$C_2 = a_3 + a_4$	$N = (C_1 + C_2) = (R_1 + R_2)$

The total chi-square is partitioned into chi-square due to A locus, due to B locus and due to linkage, as under and each is tested at 1 degree of freedom.

$$\chi^2_{\text{(A locus)}} = \frac{(C_1 - 3C_2)^2}{3N} = \frac{(a_1 + a_2 \quad 3a_3 \quad 3a_4)^2}{3N}$$

$$\chi^2_{\text{(B locus)}} = \frac{(R_1 - 3R_2)^2}{3N} = \frac{(a_1 + a_3 - 3a_2 - 3a_4)^2}{3N}$$

$$\chi^2_{\text{(Linkage)}} = \frac{(a_1 \quad 3a_2 \quad 3a_3 + 9a_4)^2}{9N}$$

All the above 3 chi-square (χ^2) values are tested at 1 degree of freedom. The sum of all the 3 chi-square values will give the total chi-square.

[*See solved example 9.1*]

Square root method: The linkage may also be detected by *square root method.* The double recessive phenotypes among the F_2 progeny can be distinguished but the crossover percentage may not be known. In this case, the frequency of double recessive phenotype among F_2 progeny can be used to estimate the frequency of non-crossover gametes when the F_1 is in coupling phase and to estimate the frequency of crossover gametes when the F_1 is in repulsion phase.

Coupling phase: In coupling phase, the double recessives (aabb) will be one of the two parental types (AABB, aabb) and their (aabb) frequency will be half of the total parental types because other half will be double dominants (AABB). Let the frequency of 4 types of gametes be p for AB, q for Ab, r for aB and s for ab gametes. The probability of uniting two ab gametes to form double recessive (ab/ab), which are parental type, will be s^2. Therefore, *percentage of parental gametes*

$$= 2\sqrt{\text{Frequency of double recessive}}$$

For example, suppose the crossover percentage is 20, then parental gametes are expected be 80 percent (half of which, 40 per cent will be ab and rest half 40 per cent will be AB). The probability of uniting two ab gametes to form the double recessive genotype (ab/ab) will be $0.40 \times 0.40 = (0.40)^2 = 0.16 = 16$ percent. This is the frequency of double recessive. Thus, the percentage of parental gametes =

$$= 2\sqrt{\text{Frequency of double recessive}}$$

$= 2\sqrt{0.16} = 2 \times 0.4 = 0.80$ or 80 percent. Now if 80 percent are parental types, the other 20 percent must be recombinants.

Repulsion phase: In repulsion phase, the double crossover (aabb) will be one of the two recombinants (AABB, aabb) and its frequency will be half of the total recombinants. With the same logic, the probability of uniting two ab gametes to form double recessive, which are recombinants in repulsion phase, will be s^2. Therefore, the *percentage of crossover gametes.*

$$= 2\sqrt{\text{Frequency of double recessive}}$$

For example, with 20 percent crossover, 10 percent of the gametes are expected to be ab. Therefore, the probability of double recessive phenotype (ab/ab) $= 0.10 \times 0.10 = (0.10)^2 = 0.01 = 1.0$ percent. Thus, if 1.0 percent are double recessive, the

percentage of crossover gametes $= 2\sqrt{\text{Frequency of double recessive}}$

$= 2\sqrt{0.01} = 2 \times 0.10 = 0.20 = 20$ percent

The test cross over the F_2 has a special advantage that this cross provides simple ratio of 1:1:1:1 for comparison between the observed (from experiment) and expected (based on the hypothesis of I.A. of genes). But it is difficult to conduct a test cross than to get *F_2 progeny* by selfing of F_1 in some self-pollinating species, *e.g.* wheat. This is because the test cross requires emasculation in self –pollinating plants and cross fertilization from pollen of other plant (homozygous recessive). On the other hand, the F_2 plants are obtained easily from self fertilization of F_1 which requires only protecting the F_1 plants from foreign pollen. Therefore, when test cross is difficult to perform, it is easy to produce F_2 by selfing of F_1, but the F_2 ratios (9:3:3:1) are more cumbersome to handle than test cross ratio of 1:1:1:1.

In a dihybrid test cross data, the frequency of cross over directly estimate the percentage of crossing over and hence the strength of linkage. The percentage of recombinants equals the percentage of cross over and it is also taken as the distance between two gene loci.

9.9 IMPORTANCE OF CROSSING OVER AND LINKAGE

The crossing over occurs during meiosis and hence called as meiotic recombination and an essential feature of sexual reproduction. It is also called as genetic recombination because it creates new gene combinations by shuffling the genetic variation and hence it proves a potential evolutionary change. The new recombination may be as many as there are different gene pairs. The favourable mutations may come together by recombination. The new gene combinations formed by crossing over may be beneficial to the organism through increase in viability or fertility or other way. The new arisen combinations are expected to spread in a population and may become an essential and unique feature of some breeds/lines of a species. It thus increases the likelihood of variation among population and act as a potent force for generating variability.

The variation is a vital tool to evolutionary development. The numerous combinations caused by crossing over can be acted by natural selection. It is thus possible that favourable combination is created which may increase the economic and adaptive value of the individual and may give rise to evolve a new species. The favourable alleles of different genes may come together through recombination in one individual during evolution.

Secondly, the crossing over has shown that genes occur in organized linkage groups and in linear order. The frequency of cross over is constant and characteristic for any pair of linked genes under standard conditions. Thus, it helps to locate the position of more and more genes and to form the genetic or chromosome maps which represent the relative positions and distance of genes in each linkage group.

The plant breeders are always trying to produce new and useful varieties of plants of economic value by recombining genes through crossing of existing varieties. But this information is rarely utilized because some better gens are linked with bad genes (inferior genes) and therefore they are transmitted together to the progeny.

On the other hand, linkage has its own practical advantage in making a linkage group of some qualitative characters with quantitative characters. This association of qualitative characters which are easily recognizable with quantitative traits helps the breeder as an index of the linked quantitative characters for selection purpose, since the entire linked group is inherited together. These genes are called as ***marker genes***.

The linkage between genes reduces the possibility of production of recombinant gametes and hence reduces the genetic variability. The linkage association in farm animals between a qualitative and quantitative characters is not possible because so many genes are involved in affecting the quantitative characters and the expression of any single gene pair is very much weak (minor). Secondly, linkage relationship will have to be determined for each animal which vary among individuals. Moreover, it is difficult to differentiate the association among characters due to linkage or due to pleiotropic effect of the same gene or through a common physiological pathway affecting the two characters.

9.10 EFFECT OF LINKAGE

The linkage of genes has the following effects:

(i) *Linkage and classical F_2 ratio of dihybrid cross (9:3:3:1):* The two gene loci either in coupling phase (AABB and aabb) or in repulsion phase (AAbb and aaBB) will produce dihybrid F_2 ratio as 9: 3: 3: 1 without linkage. The percentage of recombinants in F_2 generation of a dihybrid cross is less with linkage than expected without linkage. The parental type F_2 progeny in coupling phase is expected to be 62.5 per cent based on [(9 + 1)/16] and the recombinants to be 37.5 per cent based on [(3 +3)/16], without linkage whereas in repulsion phase the proportion of two types of F_2 progeny is reverse, *i.e.* 62.5 per cent are recombinants and rest 37.5 per cent are parental types. The linkage of genes disturbs this ratio of parental and recombinants among F_2 progeny. The proportion of recombinants with linkage is reduced among F_2 progeny than expected ratio.

Similar tendency of lesser proportion of recombinants than expected (50: 50) is observed in test cross when the two gene pairs are linked.

(ii) *Linkage and epistatic ratios:* The classical F_2 ratio of 9:3:3:1 and the test cross ratio of (1:1:1:1) is modified due to epistasis. For example, the epistasis changed the test cross ratio into 1:1:2 combining two phenotypic classes without linkage. When the genes showing linkage are linked, the parental combinations are observed in greater numbers than recombinants. This indicates the linkage. This can be illustrated by an example of coat colour in rabbit as follows:

The black colour in rabbit is dominant over brown. The gene, B, responsible for black hair is dominant over its allele (b) which produces brown colour of hair whereas the albinism is a trait expressed by homozygous recessive genotype (cc) and the dominant allele (C) produces coloured hairs. The genotype CC and Cc produces pigment while cc produces albino. The cross of homozygous black rabbit (BBCC) with albino genotype (bbcc) produces hybrids (BbCc) with coloured hairs. The test cross made by crossing of F_1 heterozygote (BbCc) with homozygous recessive (bbcc) having albino colour will result into the following phenotypes with expectation as:

CcBb	:	Ccbb	:	ccBb and ccbb	
1	:	1	:	2	
(Black)	:	(Brown)	:	(Albino)	with no linkage

The ratio of 1:1:2 instead of 1:1:1:1 is caused by epistasis and hence the epistasis has modified the expression of the colour gene. The colour gene in homozygous state (bb) has modified the effect of the allele C and produced brown colour of the genotype Ccbb and the same allele in homozygous state (cc) has modified the effect of brown gene (B) in the genotype ccBb producing albino.

Now if the two loci are linked, the parental phenotype (black) appeared in greater number than the recombinants (brown). This indicates the linkage. The third phenotype (albino) cannot be properly classified as parental phenotype because the expression of colour gene is modified due to linkage. Thus, only the black and brown phenotypes are used for calculations to estimate the crossover percent.

(*iii*) *Linkage and sex linked genes*: The dihybrid, in a test cross, for sex linked gene, does not exist in homogametic sex as for autosomal linkage. This is the major difference produced by linkage.

(*iv*) *Linkage and pleiotropy:* The close or complete linkage produced the pleiotropic like effect. The complete linkage does not produce any recombinants whereas very close linkage produce some recombinants. It is required high number of test cross progeny to prodce one each of the two recombinants in the cross to reveal close linkage. The probability of crossing over between very closely linked loci is increased with higher numbers of progeny produced. Therefore, linkage is not important in farm animals compared to that in fruit fly. This is one of the problems associated with linkage studies of genes closely located.

9.11 CHROMOSOME MAPPING

The genes are located on chromosomes in a linear arrangement having their fixed relative position on the chromosome. The relative location (position) of different genes (loci) and the distance between the adjacent genes (loci) on the chromosomes is measured on different basis and shown in the form of a diagram of a chromosome. The graphical (diagrammatic) representation of genes on the chromosome indicating distance of genes between loci (called as *genetic distance* or *map distance*) and their relative position (location on a chromosome) from each other (called as *gene order*) in each linkage group (chromosome) is called as ***chromosome map*** and the process is known as ***chromosome mapping***. Thus, the distance of genes indicates the map distance that how far the two genes are located on the chromosome while the relative position of genes indicates the gene order (sequence of genes) on the chromosome.

The chromosome maps are constructed on different basis and accordingly called by different names. See section 23.6 and 23.7 for more details of the types of chromosome maps. These different chromosome maps are the –

- ☆ ***Genetic map*** is a diagram of a chromosome based on recombination frequencies (cM),
- ☆ ***Cytological map*** is a diagram of a chromosome based on differential staining (banding pattern) along its length, and
- ☆ ***Physical map*** is a diagram of a chromosome or DNA molecule with distances given in base pairs, kilo-bases, or mega-bases.

The genetic and cytological maps are co-linear but the genetic distances are not proportional to cytological distances.

(i) Map Distance or Genetic Distance

This is the distance between genes on a chromosome. The *crossing over* is a measure of *genetic distance*. Thus, the chromosome mapping is done by linked genes from their recombination as a result of crossing over. The numbers of crossovers occurring during meiosis allow the construction of the chromosome maps (*genetic map*). However, the counting of crossovers cannot be done directly due to the reason that the actual crossover events cannot be observed. The crossovers are thus estimated either by counting the chiasmata through cytological analysis or by the recombinant chromosomes through genetic analysis.

Sturtevant fundamentally considered that the genetic distance should have a direct relation with the number of crossovers between them. However, it is not an easy task to count the number of crossovers between the locations of any two genes because the chance of occurrence of crossing over may vary among cells due to a number of many independent opportunities for crossing over. The occurrence of crossing over may not take place in one particulat cell but in a large population of cells the crossover may occur several times (one, two, or more crossovers). Therefore, it is required to measure the average number of crossovers in a particular chromosome region so as the genetic map distance is based on average estimate rather than a single value. This average number of crossovers between genes is the genetic distance or map distance (distance between two genes on the genetic map of a chromosome).

The ***genetic length of a chromosome*** is the *average number of exchanges* on a chromatid at the end of meiosis. This can be understood from an example of the number of exchanges that occurred during meiosis on each of 100 chromatids that were recovered in gametes as:

Number of exchanges	0	1	2	3	4
No. of gametes	15	21	41	18	5
Frequency	0	0.21	0.41	0.18	0.05
Crossproducts (Exchange x frequency)	0	0.21	0.82	0.54	0.25

Total of crossproducts = 1.82 Morgan = 182 cM. = Average number of exchanges
= Genetic length of chromosome.

The *map distance* is represented in percentage of cross over (recombination) between loci along the chromosome. This is because the amount of crossing over, (percentage of crossover progeny produced), is proportional to the distance between two loci on a chromosome. This is based on the hypothesis formulated by Sturtevant (1913) that each gene has a definite position (locus) on its chromosome and the place for occurrence of chiasma (synapsis or pairing of chromosome for occurrence of crossing over) is a matter of chance and hence the frequency of crossover is proportional to the linear distance between genes on the chromosome. He thus suggested that the percentage of crossover can be used as a quantitative index of the gene distance on the chromosome. This helped in chromosome mapping. Thus, map distance is measured from the frequency of crossovers obtained either from test cross or F_2 data.

The map distance is measured in map units (***centiMorgan***, *cM*). 100 centiMorgans are taken as one ***Morgan.*** One percent recombination is equivalent to one map unit of length on the chromosome. The percentage of crossing over is constant between any two loci but it is different between different genes. The maximum percent of crossover cannot exceed to 50 percent and thus the relative length of any chromosome is 50 map units, represented as 50 cM or 0.5 M. Therefore, one map unit is 1/50 of the length of chromosome.

The map distance in terms of map units is helpful in only estimating the distance between two genes but it is not helpful in deciding the actual location of different genes on the same pair of chromosome.

(ii) Gene Order

The sequence of genes on the chromosome is the *gene order* which is linear. This information on actual location of different genes requires the relative distance between each of the two genes as well as other genes located on the same chromosome. The test cross involving three gene loci is required to know the actual position of different genes (sequence of genes on the chromosome).

The gene order is detected from *three-point cross* (trihybrid cross involving three genes in a cross at a time). In three point cross, three types of crossovers are possible *viz.* two single crossovers (crossover between first two genes, region I; between second two genes, region II) and double crossing over simultaneously between first two and second two loci, such as taking 3 loci A, B and C. The single crossover may occur between AB region (region I) in some chromosomes, between BC region (region II) in some chromosomes and double crossovers in some other chromosomes. The double crossovers results from the simultaneous crossing over in both the regions. This is referred to as the *multiple cross-over*. The test cross involving three points cross helps to reveal the occurrence of double crossovers. The comparison of double-crossover gametes to the parental gametes determines the linear order of genes on the chromosome. The genes in the double crossover gametes which have been transposed compared to the parental gametes are in the middle.

Assuming linkage, the parental type progeny are expected to be more frequent (more than 50 per cent) than any of the crossover types. Such results indicate an alternative to independent assortment of genes (*i.e.* linkage between genes).

9.12 METHODS TO ESTIMATE THE GENE ORDER

The gene order may be estimated by two methods which are the elimination method and the double crossover method.

(i) Elimination Method

This requires the computation of the frequencies of recombinants, taking two pairs of genes at a time and ignoring the third pair of gene. This can be illustrated citing the example of a trihybrid cross of fruit fly (*Drosophila*) performed by Bridges, C. B. and Olbrycht, T. M. (1926). They crossed the male flies having *crossveinless wing* (cv) with female flies having rough eyes (echinus gene, *ec*) and cut wing margin (ct). All these three characters are sex-linked and recessive to their normal (wild) type characters. Therefore, the F_1 flies were heterozygous normal (wild) for 3 characters.

The F_1 female should have produced 8 types of gametes in equal numbers but it was observed on backcrossing them with hemizygous recessive males (ec, cv, ct) that 8 types of F_2 progeny were not in equal proportions as shown here:

Phenotypes	*Genotypes*	*Observed Numbers*	*Types*
Crossveinless	+ cv +	2207	Parental
Echinus cut	ec + ct	2125	"
Echinus crossveiless	ec cv +	273	S.C.O. (I)
Cut	+ + ct	265	"
Echinus	ec + +	217	S.C.O. (II)
Crossveinless cut	+ cv ct	223	"
Scute Crossveinless cut	ec cv ct	3	D.C.O.
Wild type	+ + +	5	"

The frequencies of recombinants are computed taking two genes at a time as:

Steps	*Loci taken*	*Ignored*	*Parental Types*	*Recombinants*	*Freq. recomb.*
I	ec and cv	ct	2207+2125+217+223	273+265+5+3	546/5318
			(4772)	(546)	(0.102)
II	cv and ct	ec	2207+2125+273+265	217+223+5+3	448/5318
			(4870)	(448)	(0.084)
III	ec and ct	cv	2207+2125 +3+5	273+265+217+233	978/5318
			(4340)	(978)	(0.184)

The recombinant frequencies between two gene loci are the map distance between the respective two gene loci. The above results have indicated that crossing over has resulted the formation of 10.2 per cent gametes between Ec and Cv gene loci, 8.4 per cent gametes between Cv and Ct gene loci and 18.4 per cent gametes between Ec and Ct gene loci. Therefore, the gene distance between two respective loci was 10.2, 8.4 and 18.4 units. In addition to these, some gametes may be produced which contain both crossovers at the same time, called as *double crossovers* (D.C.O.) and this phenomenon is called *double crossing over*. However, D.C.O. progeny may be produced in few cases, the DCO gametes being least frequent than single crossover in two regions or parental combinations.

(ii) Double Crossover Method

The double crossover method depends upon identifying the double crossovers whose frequencies are expected to be least and that which of the three possible arrangements (sequences) of loci on the chromosome could produce the double crossover classes. It is important to note that production of *DCO type gametes depend on the gene order and the map distance between loci.* The method of DCO depends on:

- ✰ The estimation of DCO which are of least frequent type
- ✰ To know that which of the linear order of gene can produce the DCO genotypes.

The fundamental experiments on three point cross or trihybrid cross taking three sex-linked genes of fruit fly were conducted by Sturtevant (1921), Bridges and Olbrycht (1926), and others.

Two experiments on three – point crosses were conducted by Bridges and Olbrycht (1926) on Drosophila. *In one experiment* male flies (parental generation) having rough eyes (echinus, ec.) were crossed with female flies having scute bristles (absence of bristles, sc.) and crossveinless wings (cv). All these three characters were recessive to their normal or wild type characters so as the F_1 females were heterozygous normal for the three characters and hence the F_1 females produced 8 types of gametes in equal numbers.

In the second experiment, the F_1 flies were produced by crossing original parents (parental generation, P_1) having crossveinless male flies (cv) with female flies having echinus eyes (rough eyes, ec) and cut wing margin (ct, a sex linked recessive mutant gene). In both these experiments of three points cross, the original parents (P_1) were heterozygous.

Sturtevant (1921) conducted an experiment on Drosophila by crossing yellow (body colour, ***y***) carmine (eye, ***c***) females with forked (a bristle mutant gene, ***f***) males and the F_1 females were mated to yellow carmine forked males (***y c f***). Thus the original parents were ***y c +/y c +*** (female) and ***+ + f/y*** (male parent) and hence heterozygous. On the basis of the findings, the following conclusions were emerged-

(i) Parental combinations were more than 50 per cent of the total progeny (hence with highest frequency), the double crossover classes were least frequent (with lowest frequency) and single crossovers each at both the regions (I and II) were intermediate in frequency of the parental and double crossover classes.

(ii) In estimating the single crossover frequency at the two regions, for the two loci respectively, the double crossover progeny are added in the number of progeny of single crossovers of both the regions separately.

(iii Sum of the frequencies of the single crossover classes at the two regions excluding the double crossover class, constitute the distance for the loci which are at the two extreme sides.

The above findings can be generalized more clearly, taking 3 loci as A, B and C in linear order and designating the numbers of 4 types of test cross progeny (ignoring the reciprocal classes *i.e.* taking two reciprocal classes as one class) as: N_1 for parental classes, N_2 for recombinants at region I (between A and B gene), N_3 for recombinants at region II (between gene B and C), and N_4 for double crossover classes as under:

Classes	*Phenotypes and Genotypes*	*Types of Progeny*	*No. of Progeny*
1, 2		Parental (most frequent)	N_1
3, 4		Single crossover at region I (A-B loci)	N_2
5, 6		Single crossover at region II (B-C loci)	N_3
7, 8		Double crossover (least frequent)	N_4
Total			N

$$N = N_1 + N_2 + N_3 + N_4$$

= Total number of progenies.

The *map distance* between two loci is calculated as under;

$$\text{A-B loci} = \frac{(N_2 + N_4)}{N}$$

$$\text{B-C loci} = \frac{(N_3 + N_4)}{N}$$

$$\text{A-C loci} = \frac{(N_2 + N_3)}{N}$$

The $\frac{(N_2 + N_3)}{N}$ will give the maximum distance indicating that two loci A and C are located farthest apart at the two extremes and B locus is located in between these two loci.

9.13 INTERFERENCE AND COINCIDENCE

It is fairly characteristic that double crossovers do not occur as often as the single crossover in individual regions and also in some experiments the double crossovers do not appear at all. It may thus be concluded that once crossing over occurs, it reduces the probability of another crossing over in an adjacent region of chromosome. Therefore, the occurrence of crossing over in one part of the chromosome is not independent of its occurrence in other part of the same chromosome. This means that the formation of one chiasma reduces the probability of forming another chiasma in an adjacent region of the same chromosome. This reduction in chiasma formation might be due to physical inability of the chromatids to bend back upon themselves within certain minimum distance. Therefore crossing over in one region decreases the likely hood of crossing over in nearby other region. In other words, the crossing over in one region interferes (inhibits) the second crossing over in the adjacent region of close vicinity. Consequently, fewer than expected double crossover types are observed. This phenomenon of decreased probability of second crossing over in adjacent region of same chromosome due to the occurrence of crossing over at one point is called *interference* (Muller, 1916). Interference is thus the effect of a crossing over in one mathematical term, the *coefficient of coincidence*, which is simply the ratio of observed to the expected double crossovers. Therefore, *Coincidence* = per cent observed D.C.O./per cent expected D.C.O.

The *frequency of double crossovers* (D.C.O.) is obtained by multiplying the frequencies of single crossovers at two regions according to the expectation of the law of probability. Therefore, the *expected double crossovers* = p (crossing over at I region) x p (crossing over at II region). The coincidence is complement of interference and their sum is equal to unity. Thus, *interference* (*I*) = 1- coefficient of coincidence = 1- (observed DCO)/(expected DCO). In general, the interference is more for crossing over to occur over the short distances of loci in the chromosome so that within a certain less distance there is no double crossover (resulting I = 1.0, full interference) and the coincidence is zero. On the contrary, for the farthest apart loci, the interference becomes less and with increasing distance between loci, the interference disappear entirely resulting coincidence equal to unity. The positive interference indicates that the chromosomes show rigidity (stiffness or obstinacy) and do not coil tightly to each other during meiosis.

$$\text{Coincidence} = \frac{\text{Frequency of observed D.C.O.}}{\text{Frequency of expected D.C.O.}}$$

Frequency of expected D.C.O. = (Freq. of C.O. at region I) (Freq. of C.O. at region II)

Frequency of observed D.C.O. = Coincidence × Frequency of expected D.C.O.

Frequency of single C.O. (I) = Map distance (I region) – DCO per cent

Frequency of single C.O. (II) = Map distance (II region) – DCO per cent

Frequency of single C.O. parental type = 100 per cent – (SCO at both regions + DCO)

The parental, single crossover and double crossover are each of two types and hence the frequency obtained of any type of gametes is divided into two parts equally of each type.

The data of four experiments, given under numerical examples, may be analyzed in terms of the interference and coincidence of D.C.O. simultaneously, as under:

Experiment Numbers	*I*	*II*	*III*	*IV*
Gene order	sc ec cv	ec cv ct	y c f	cv ct v
Frequency of S.C.O.: Region I	0.076	0.102	0.339	0.064
Region II	0.097	0.084	0.121	0.132
Double C.O. (Observed)	0.0000	0.0015	0.0258	0.0055
Double C.O. (Expected)	0.0074	0.0086	0.0411	0.0084
Coincidence	0.0000	0.1744	0.6277	0.6548
Interference (1- Coincidence)	1.000	0.8256	0.3723	0.3452
Total no. of progeny	1980	5318	2555	1448

9.14 DISCREPANCY BETWEEN RECOMBINANT FREQUENCY AND GENETIC MAP DISTANCE

The method of chromosome mapping from recombination frequency is better way of mapping genes that are located close together. But the true map distance is not reflected from recombination frequency for the genes located far apart. This can be understood from an example of the experimental findings obtained by Bridges and Olbrycht on mapping of seven sex linked genes on a segment of X chromosome in *Drosophila* from recombination frequencies between each pair of adjacent genes. Seven X –linked genes mapped in *Drosophila* were:

sc (scute bristles), **ec** (echinus eyes), **cv** (crossveinless wings), **ct** (cut wings), **v** (vermilion eyes, **g** (garnet eyes), and **f** (forked bristles).

Bridges and Olbrycht found that **sc** gene was located at one end and **f** was at the other end and the total length of the mapped segment of the X chromosome was found to be 66.8 cM, giving the average number of crossovers in this segment as 0.668. However, the recombination frequency between **sc** and **f** genes was equal to the maximum possible value of 50 percent. Thus, these two loci must be located 50 map units apart but the distance obtained by summing the lengths of the intervening regions on the map was much greater (66.8 cM). This showed that the true genetic distance based on crossovers may be more than the observed recombination frequency. This can be explained on the basis of the occurrence of multiple crossovers between widely located genes and that some of the crossovers may not produce genetically recombinant chromosomes.

The situation that the chromatids with crossing over may not produce genetically recombination chromosome can be understood considering two crossovers between two loci. A single crossover between two chromatids in a tetrad causes recombination of the genes but another crossover between these same two chromatids will bring back the two genes to their original combination. This is because the second crossover between the same two loci will cancel the effect of first crossover by converting the recombinant chromatids back into no recombinants. Therefore, no chromatid will be recombinant, even though two crossovers have occurred and the double crossover between the same chromatid may not contribute to the recombination frequency but it contributes to the average number of exchanges on a chromosome. Similar effect of no recombination will be produced by quadruple crossover. In this way, some of the multiple exchanges produce discrepancy between recombination frequency and genetic map distance.

However, the recombination frequency really estimate the true genetic distance for distances less than 20 cM because the interference suppress multiple exchanges over short distances. The difference or discrepancy between the two estimates of recombination frequency and genetic map distance increases for a distance greater than 20 cM. This discrepancy occurs because of the reason that multiple exchanges are more likely to occur over larger distances and the multiple exchanges do not always produce recombinant chromosomes rather their effect is cancelled. There is linear relationship between these two estimates upto a distance less than 20 cM but the recombination frequency underestimate the map distance for a distance greater than 20 cM.

9.15 CYTOGENETIC MAPPING

The ***cytogenetic mapping*** is a process which was developed to localize genes on the cytological maps of chromosomes. Such a procedure was needed because the recombination mapping is not a way to localize the genes regarding cytological landmarks (bands) on chromosomes. The recombination mapping (genetic maps) uses the frequency of crossing over as a measure of distance and determines only the sequence of genes (relative position of genes on a chromosome). The localization of genes on cytological map requires the knowledge of the phenotypic effects of chromosome rearrangements like deletions and duplications which could be recognized cytologically and hence their occurrence may be correlated with the phenotypic effects of particular region along the length of chromosome. Such a process is called ***cytological mapping*** which associate the phenotypic effects of genes that have already been positioned on a recombination map (genetic map) and used to tie up the map positions of these genes to locations on the cytological map of a chromosome.

The ***necessity*** *of localizing the genes* on the cytological map of chromosome can be understood with an example. Suppose a gene controlling a character is situated at map position 2.5 near one end of a particular chromosome. Now the question is to know that this gene is near to which of the two ends of chromosome and at what distance this gene is from that end in cytological terms. To find the answers of these questions need to know the position of that gene on the cytological map of that chromosome. The large and banded polytene chromosomes of *Drosophila* have provided the extraordinarily detailed cytological maps and hence the geneticists have developed this process of localizing genes (*cytogenetic mapping*) in *Drosophila*.

The ***procedure*** to determine the cytological location of genes has been rested on the *deletions* (deficiency) and *duplications* (additions). Both have their basic principles and have been found useful to apply the process of cytogenetic mapping of localizing the genes of *Drosophila* chromosomes. The procedure is similar to use duplication as well as the deletion. The genes can be localized on maps of the polytene chromosome by combining recessive mutations with cytological deletions and duplications.

The *deletion* (deficiency) is combined with a recessive mutation. The *deletion mapping* has its basic principle that if this deficiency (deletion) does not mask the phenotype of recessive mutation, this indicates that recessive gene must be located within the segment of the chromosome deleted and the wild-type copy of the mutant gene must be lacking within it and this localizes that gene within the boundaries of the deletion. The deletion reveals the phenotype of a recessive mutation located between its endpoints.

Similarly, *duplication* is searched that masks the phenotype of a recessive mutation. Therefore, the *duplication mapping* has its principle that if duplication masks the phenotype of a recessive mutation, the wild-type copy of the mutant gene must be present within it and this localizes that gene within the boundaries of the duplication. The duplication conceals the mutant phenotype and reveals the wild-type phenotype.

9.16 CORRELATION OF PHYSICAL MAP WITH GENETIC AND CYTOLOGICAL MAP

The physical maps of a chromosome can be correlated with the genetic and cytological maps in some of the following ways –

- ☆ The genes that have been cloned by ***In situ*** hybridization can find their position on the cytological map of chromosome,
- ☆ The correlations between the physical and genetic maps can be established by locating clones of genetically mapped genes or RFLPs on the physical map,

- ☆ The physical maps of chromosomes can also be correlated with genetic and cytological maps in several ways:
  - (a) Using PCR to amplify 200 to 500 bp genomic DNA sequences,
  - (b) Using Southern blots to release these sequences to overlapping clones on physical maps, and
  - (c) By *in situ* hybridization to determine their chromosomal locations (cytological map positions).

The genetically and physically mapped markers are called *anchor markers* because they anchor the physical map to the genetic map and vice versa. The short unique anchor sequences are called *sequence-tagged sites* (STSs).

Second approach is to anchor physical maps to RFLP maps (genetic maps) and cytological maps is the use of cDNA sequences (DNA copies of mRNAs), or *expressed-sequence tags* (*ESTs*), as hybridization probes.

The incidence of crossing over between paired chromosomes is used as a procedure to measure the genetic distance and to construct the recombination (genetic) map. The number of crossing over depends on -

- ☆ The length of chromosome, long chromosomes are expected to have more crossovers than short ones, and
- ☆ The region of chromosome because some regions are more prone to recombination than others. This depends on the density of the regions of the chromosome. The terminal regions near the end of chromosome and those around the centromere are more condensed genetically compared to other regions. The crossing over is less likely to occur in these condensed regions due to their greater density.

The recombination mapping reveals the true order of the genes along a chromosome but it does not reveal the actual physical distances between them. The genetic and cytological maps of a chromosome are collinear but the genetic distances are not proportional to cytological distances. There is no direct correlation between physical distances with genetic map distances. This is because some error occurs between the recombination frequencies (genetic map) and molecular distances (physical map). Secondly, no colinearity between genetic and physical distances is the result of the differences in the density of different chromosome regions which affects the frequency of crossing over. In spite of all this, there is reasonable correlation between the genetic and physical maps in euchromatic regions of the chromosomes (1 cM = 1 mb of DNA, on an average).

9.17 USES OF CHROMOSOME MAPPING

- **(1)** The gene mapping in humans contains a broad array of technologies and aims to understand the genome organization and identification of genes.
- **(2)** In farm animals the gene mapping is used to detect genes controlling diseases and quantitative trait loci (QTL) so as to develop more efficient breeding strategies.

(3) The gene mapping has also significant role in the study of evolutionary divergence of mammalian species.

(4) The physical maps are used to prepare clone banks containing catalogued clones covering entire genomes. These clones if required are available on request from clone bank or clone library.

(5) The chromosomal basis of genes was demonstrated by parallelism of actual crossing over between homologous chromosomes (cytological evidence) and genetic crossing over (based on results of crossing of individuals). Thus, the association of genes with chromosome was provided by the fact that there is an interchange of genes by crossing over during meiosis when some material between two homologous chromosomes is interchanged.

(6) The chromosome maps based on linkage and crossing over have already established the validity of the following facts:

- ☆ *Genes are present on the chromosomes,*
- ☆ *Genes are located at specific loci in different chromosomes,*
- ☆ *Genes are arranged in a linear order on chromosomes,*
- ☆ *Specific genes are present in specific chromosomes.*

(7 The available information on genetic maps can be used to predict the results in offspring generation produced from either dihybrid or trihybrid cross. With the help of given gene distance between two loci in a dihybrid cross, the frequency of different types of progeny expected to be produced can be predicted. Similarly, in case of trihybrid cross, the available information on genetic distance between three loci, *viz.* A-B, B-C and A-C, can be used to predict the frequency of different types of progeny expected to be produced *viz.* parental types, single crossover types at two regions and double cross over types.

(*i*) ***Dihybrid cross***: The map distance between two loci can be used to find out the expected results from any type of mating with the help of gametic checker board. In a dihybrid cross, two parental types and two recombinants (crossovers) are produced. Further, each of two parental types is expected to be produced with equal frequencies and same is for the two recombinant types which will also be produced n equal frequencies.

(*See solved example 6.2*)

(*ii*) ***Trihybrid Cross***: In a three point test cross experiment (3 linked loci), 4 classes are produced and each of which is further of 2 types *viz.* two parental types, two crossover type for region I (between A and B locus), two crossover type for region II (between B and C loci), and two double crossover types, each of two types within all the 4 classes will occur with equal frequency. The results of the offspring generation can be predicted, provided map distances, type of mating and coincidence or interference are known. (*See example 5.3*)

NUMERICAL EXAMPLES

9.1. Linkage detection: The following F_2 data on comb shape and leg length in poultry were obtained:

	Comb shape (A locus):		
	Rose comb (A)	Single comb (a)	Total
Length of legs (B locus):			
(B) Short (Creeper)	62	11	73
(b) Normal	12	11	23
Total	74	22	96

Conduct a test for linkage between two genes affecting comb shape and leg length as well as for the two loci segregating according to expected F_2 ratios.

Solution

$$\chi^2_{\text{(A locus)}} = \frac{(C_1 - 3C_2)^2}{3N} = \frac{[(a_1 + a_2)\quad 3(a_3\quad 3a_4)]^2}{3N}$$

$$= \frac{(74 - 3 \times 22)^2}{(3 \times 96)}$$

$$= \frac{64}{288} = 0.222^{NS}$$

$$\chi^2_{\text{(B locus)}} = \frac{(R_1 - 3R_2)^2}{3N} = \frac{[(a_1 + a_3)\quad 3(a_2 + a_4)]^2}{3N}$$

$$= \frac{(73 - 3 \times 23)^2}{(3 \times 96)}$$

$$= \frac{16}{288} = 0.055^{NS}$$

$$\chi^2_{\text{(Linkage)}} = \frac{(a_1\quad 3a_2\quad 3a_3 + 9a_4)^2}{9N}$$

$$= \frac{(62\quad 3 \times 12\quad 3 \times 11 + 9 \times 11)^2}{(9 \times 96)}$$

$$= \frac{(62\quad 36\quad 33 + 99)^2}{864}$$

$$= \frac{8464}{864} = 9.796^{**}$$

$$\chi^2_{\text{(Total)}} = 9.796 + 0.222 + 0.055 = 10.073^{*}$$

Answer: From the chi-square values calculated for segregation of both the loci, it was observed that neither value is significant tested at 1 degree of freedom, proving that the segregation is in agreement with 3:1 ratio for each loci. The chi-square value due to segregation tested at 1 degree of freedom is highly significant, provides an evidence of linkage of two loci. The total chi-square value (10.073) based on 3 degrees of freedom was significant, showed that the joint segregation is not in agreement with 9:3:3:1 ratio.

9.2. The F_1 dihybrid was produced in coupling phase. Find out the expected F_2 results taking the two loci (A and B) located 20 map units apart.

Solution: The recombinants are 20 per cent and hence the frequency of Ab and aB gametes will be 0.10 each and the rest 0.80 will be parental types (0.40 each AB and ab). The F_2 results (frequency of different types of progeny) can be obtained from gametic checker board.

9.3. The test cross on three point cross (Trihybrid) gave the following results: Map distance: A – B =10 units and B – C = 20 units, Interference = 40 per cent.

Find out the frequency of different types of progeny (parental types, SCO at two regions and DCO).

Solution: Coincidence = 1 – interference = 1- 0.40 = 0.60

1. Frequency of expected DCO = (SCO I) (SCO II)
   = 0.1 × 0.2 = 0.02 = 2 per cent

   Frequency of observed DCO = Expected DCO × Coincidence
   = 0.02 × 0.6 = 0.012 = 1.2 per cent

This frequency to be equally divided between two types of double crossovers

2. Frequency of single crossover at region I (SCO I) = 10.0 – 1.2 = 8.8 per cent

   and it will be equally divided between two types of SCO I.
3. Frequency of SCO II = 20.0 – 1.2 = 18.8 per cent

   and it will be equally divided between two types of SCO II.
4. Frequency of parental types = 100 – (SCO I + SCO II + DCO)
   = 100 – (8.8 + 18.8 + 1.2) =71.2 per cent

   and it will be equally divided between two parental types.

9.4. The data given below were recorded on trihybrid crosses on fruit flies in four experiments. The numbers of progenies recorded in these four experiments belonging to different 8 classes have been given below. Find out the frequencies of progenies of different four classes, the crossover percentage, the map distance between loci and the position of 3 genes on the chromosomes.

Classes No.	Class Types	No. of Progenies (Different Expt.)			
		I	II	III	IV
1	Parental	828	2207	725	580
2		810	2125	719	592
3	S.C.O.(I)	62	273	419	45
4		88	265	383	40
5	S.C.O.(II)	103	217	134	89
6		89	223	109	94
7	D.C.O.	0	3	34	3
8		0	5	32	5
Total progenies recorded		1980	5318	2555	1448

Find out the frequency of observed DCO types, if the map distance is 10 and 20 units with 40 per cent interference.

Hint: Find out frequency of expected DCO as $0.10 \times 0.20 = 0.02$ (= 2 per cent);

[Frequency of observed DCO types = Coincidence × frequency of expected DCO.]

9.5. Consider two loci controlling two dominant traits *viz.* an eye abnormality (cataract) and polydactyly (extra finger). These two loci are present 17 cM apart on the same chromosome. Find out the chance that the first child will show both characters from a marriage of a girl who inherited cataract from her father and polydactyly inherited from her mother whereas her husband was normal.

Solution: Both these characters are the result of dominant mutations caused by the alleles C and P. The two genes in the girl will be in repulsion phase because of inheriting one dominant allele from one parent and another from second parent. Therefore, the genotype of the girl will be C + and + P. The girl should produce a recombinant ovum carrying C and P alleles to produce a child having both the traits. The chance of producing such a child can be estimated from the distance between two loci which is 17 cM, equivalent to 17 percent recombination.

As only half of the recombinants will be C P. Therefore, the chance that the child will inherit both the dominant alleles is 17/2 percent = 8.5 percent.

9.6. The full colour (black) in mice is dominant over Himalayan (white with coloured extremities). Another character of hair texture is expressed as frizzy hair coat by recessive allele and normal smooth hair by dominant allele. A number of dihybrid mice were test crossed and the resultant progeny produced were:

14 mice with Himalayan colour smooth hairs

12 mice with black colour frizzy hairs

4 mice with Himalayan colour frizzy hairs

3 mice with black colour smooth hairs

(a) Conduct a test of linkage between two loci and if linkage is present, calculate the crossover percentage. (b) Write down the genotypes of the parents of the dihybrid mice.

Chapter 10

Sex Determination

The sexual reproduction occurs in members of both the kingdoms (plants and animals). There are some aids to sexual reproduction in plants. These include a wide variety of flowers (myriads of flowers), the different attractive colours to attract and enjoy, the scents and perfumes to swoon over, diversity of structures of different parts (inflorescences, flowers, and floral parts having ornamental, social, religious, cultural and aesthetic values, sites of sexual reproduction, and symbols of showing human feelings like love, affection, happiness, mourning, grief, etc) that shows a range of adaptations for sexual reproduction and the production of fruits and seeds.

10.1 SEXUALITY IN ORGANISMS

The two types of gametes (male gamete - *sperm* and female gamete - *ovum*) may be produced either by the same individual or by different individuals. This is called **sexuality**. The sex is the most remarkable and visible phenotype with distinct males and females. Thus, there is ***sexual dimorphism*** (males and females) in animals including man, birds, and some plant species. The sexuality is defined as the condition where the sex cells (Ova and spermatozoa) are produced and the genes of two different individuals are included within the same cell in such a way that recombination and segregation of recombination can occur.

(1) Bisexuality (Bisexual Organisms)

The organisms having both male and female reproductive structures in the same individual are called **bisexual** (individual having both sexes) and this condition is called bisexuality.

The male and female flowers are present in the same flowering plants and such plants are called ***monoecious*** (cucurbits, coconuts). The bisexuality in several fungi and plants is used in terms of **homothallic** and **monoecious**.

The bisexual animals having both male and female reproductive organs in same individual are the earthworms, tapeworm, leech, and sponge and called as the **hermaphrodites**.

(2) Unisexuality (unisexual Organisms)

The individuals (plants/animals) having both types of reproductive organs in different plants/animals are called **unisexual** (individuals having only one sex) and this condition is called unisexuality.

The male and female flowers are present on different plants. Such plants are called called ***dioecious*** (papaya and date palm). The male flower in unisexual flowering plants is called **staminate** (which bears stamens) while the female flower is **pistillate** (which bears pistals). The term unisexuality is used in terms of **heterothallic** and **dioecius.**

Unisexual animal species having two types of reproductive organs in separate individuals is cockroach. *The eukaryotes* (Man, farm animals including poultry, Drosophila and other insects like Grasshoppers, and flies, *etc.*) are unisexual diploids, except some plants which are self fertilized (unisexual) and are polyploids. The ***diploids*** are those in whose cells the chromosomes are present in pairs (*i.e.* two sets of chromosomes or two genomes, symbolized as 2n) whereas the ***polyploids*** are those in whose cells the chromosomes have more than two doses of haploid genome (more than two sets of chromosome or genomes) like triploids (3n), tetraploids (4n), pentaploids (5n), hexaploids (6n), heptaploids (7n), octaploids (8n).

The individuals of two sexes among higher animals are of distinct classes with distinctive features. This means that sexual differences are sharp and indicate clear differences between members of the two sexes of the same species. In many animal and plant species the sexes are readily judged by distinct morphological differences like, size, horns, external genetalia *etc* whereas in others no external morphological differences appeared.

10.2 SEX DETERMINATION MECHANISM

The method/mechanism to explain the primary difference between sexes is called the sex determination. There should have been some definite mechanism of inheritance which determines the fact that one type of individual will be male to produce sperms while the other will be female to produce eggs.

In antiquity, the development of sex was believed to be influenced by the lunar phases, time of day, wind direction at the time of fertilization, sexual desire of male or female parent, fertilization from semen of right or left testicle, and other such environmental factors. The cytologists and geneticists have discovered that the mechanisms of sex determination are different in different species.

The sex is determined by genetic as well as by environmental factors. However, sex determination by environmental factors is in very rare case, *e.g. turtle* species in which temperature has significant role in determining the sex. The incubation of eggs at higher temperature (above 30°C) develop into females while at low temperature the eggs are hatched into males. On the contrary, the genetic factors involving a pair of chromosome called *sex chromosomes* are solely responsible for sexual dimorphism.

10.3 CHROMOSOME THEORY OF SEX DETERMINATION

The mechanism which involves chromosomes in sex determination is called chromosomal mechanism of sex determination. According to this theory, the sex determination was based on numerical inequality in chromosome numbers in two sexes and either of the two sexes will be heterogametic while other will be homogametic. There are two mechanism involved in sex determination based on chromosomal differences between the two opposites sexes. These are XO type and XY type mechanism.

10.3.1 XO Type Mechanism

A German biologist, Henking (1891) made first investigation regarding the inheritance of sex. He observed in a cytological study of the bug (*Pyrrhoeoris*), the different number of chromosomes in the two sexes in which males were with uneven number of chromosomes while the females were with even number. He also traced a particular nuclear body in the spermatogenesis of certain insects which was found to be distributed in 50 per cent of the sperms and that some sperms were different which received this body called as "X body" from the others which did not receive the X body. However, he further could not emphasize the significance of this body. Later on, this X body was identified as a chromosome.

An American cytologist, Mc Clung (1902) based on cytological observations on many species of grasshoppers demonstrated that there are such unpaired chromosomes and postulated that these could be associated with sex determination because the somatic cells in the females carry a different number of chromosome than in the cells of males.

These two workers found that males had 23 chromosomes and the female 24. These existed as pairs of like chromosomes (homologue), thus, 12 pairs in females and 11 pairs plus an unpaired chromosome in the males. Further it was observed that 11 pairs of chromosomes are homologous with the corresponding 11 pairs in the females. These chromosomes which are alike (homologous) in both the sexes are called ***autosomes*** and the remaining one which was paired in female and unpaired in the males was called the ***X chromosome*** by Mc Clung which is now commonly known as ***sex chromosome***. The chromosome which determines the sex of the individual is therefore called the sex chromosome or X chromosome. There is only one pair of sex chromosome involved in the process of determining whether the individual is male or female.

Mc Clung put forth the possible correlation between the sex characteristics and the presence or absence of extra or accessory or X chromosome and postulated that since the sex ratio in every generation is 1:1 the distribution of this X chromosome among the offspring would ensure a 1:1 sex ratio if it is associated with sexuality, because it is present in half of the sperms and absent in other half. The presence of this accessory or sex chromosome was only restricted in males according to Mc Clung and he was unable to follow its presence in females.

Wilson ((1905) and Stevens 1905) found that the X chromosome is present in both the males and females, and its number is two in females but only one in males. Wilson made a notable cytological observation particularly from the genus *Proteuor* (a group of insects) that different numbers of chromosomes were present in the germ cells of the two sexes; all the female gametes had 7 chromosomes whereas some of the male gametes were found to have 6 chromosomes but others from the same individual had 7 chromosomes.

This cytological discovery of sex chromosome put forth by Wilson and Stevens was extended by correns (1907) with plants who found that the pollen of certain plants were sex determining. He pointed out that the eggs were sexually all of one type but the pollens were of two types of equal number. Fertilization of eggs with one kind of pollen produced a male plant whereas other kind of pollen produced a female plant. Thus, females are homogametic and males are heterogametic. This type of sex determination was called the XO method/mechanism of sex determination.

The XO type mechanism has two alternates. One is the XO male type as mentioned above and second is that based on XO female type in which males are homogametic and the females are heterogametic. The XO female mechanism is applicable in the insect *Fumea*. The XO male type mechanism holds true in some other insects (*grasshoppers* and *bug* – squash bug, *Anasa tritis*). In squash bug, the females have 11 pairs of chromosomes and males have 10 pairs plus one odd unpaired chromosome.

According to XO type mechanism, two sexes for their chromosomes are described as –

Sex	*XO Male Type*	*XO Female Type*
Male	n AA + X (heterogametic)	n AA + XX (homogametic)
Female	n AA + XX (homogametic)	n AA + X (heterogametic)
e.g.	Prolinor, grasshopper, Bug (insects)	Fumea

Where, n represents the number of pairs of autosomes.

10.3.2 XY Type Mechanism

Wilson found in milkweed bug (*Lygaeus turcieus*) another chromosome arrangement in the two sexes and it was that the same numbers of chromosomes were present in the cells of both the sexes. The male and female have been found to differ by the presence of a chromosome which is unlike its mate and also unlike any chromosome in the opposite sex. This chromosome was identified as the mate to the X chromosome and it was distinctly smaller and called the Y chromosome. The shape of this Y chromosome is not like chromosome which is being rod like but Y chromosome is hook shaped or bend end of a rod. The rod like shape member (X chromosome) which is alike in both sexes is the sex or X chromosome while the unlike member of this pair in the male is called Y chromosome. This type of sex determination based on equal chromosome numbers in the two sexes but with different kinds of chromosomes (XY type) is called the XY type mechanism of sex determination. Like XO type mechanism, there are also two alternative mechanisms of XY type – one is XY male type and other is XY female type. The chromosome complement of the two sexes can be epresented as –

Sex	*XO Male Type*	*XO Female Type*
Male	n AA + X Y(heterogametic)	n AA + XX or ZZ (homogametic)
Female	n AA + XX (homogametic)	n AA+XY or ZW (heterogametic)
e.g.	Mammals, Amphibia, Drosophila, Coccinia, Rumex, some fishes, Milkweed bug	Birds, moths, some fishes and some insects.

The relative length of X and Y chromosome is different in different species. In Drosophila, Melandrum (flowering plant), Coccinia, the Y chromosome is longer than X chromosome while in man and farm animals, Bryophytes, Angiosperms, the Y chromosome is smaller than X.

Deviation in XY Mechanism

The XY mechanism of sex determination has some deviation in different species. For example, the sex in Drosophila is determined by a genic balance *i.e.* the relative number of X and autosomes as well as by single gene substitution (gene transfer); in man, farm animals, and Coccinia the sex is determined due to the presence or absence of the Y chromosome which carries genes for maleness even in the presence of as many as 3 X chromosome, though this mechanism seems to be changing. The loss of different portions of Y chromosome in Melandrium results in either monoceious, female, or male sterile plants.

Two different strains of fish (*Platypoecilus maculates*) have been reported to behave differently regarding the XY mechanism (Gorden, 1937). One strain (domesticated) is XX in females and XY in males while the other strain of the same species of fish (Mexico) are XX in males and XY in females. In another type of fish (*Xiphophorus*) an individual may become female and male subsequently during its lifetime. Thus, there is a change in sexual mechanism in fishes.

10.4 SEX CHROMOSOMES

In diploid organisms, the chromosomes are in pairs and are of two type *viz.* sex chromosomes and autosomes. There is only one pair of sex chromosome while other pairs are called autosomes. The inequality in chromosome numbers in two sexes has been observed in some animal species like grasshoppers. The female grasshoppers have one more chromosome in comparison to males. This extra chromosome is called the **X chromosome.** The females have two X chromosomes (XX) while males have only one (XO). The meiosis in the two sexes in these species is such that in female two X chromosomes pair, separate, and produce two eggs (gametes) each having only one X chromosome whereas in male the only X chromosome goes into half of the sperms and other half have no X chromosome. Therefore, on fertilization two kinds of zygotes are formed, *viz.* XX which develop into females and XO which develop into males.

On the contrary, same numbers of chromosomes are present in the two sexes of most of other species of plants, animals, humans, *Drosophila,* poultry, *etc.* The presence of a chromosome which makes equal number of chromosomes in two sexes is called the ***Y chromosome.*** This Y chromosome pairs with X chromosome during meiosis. The X and Y chromosomes are called ***sex chromosomes*** whereas other pairs of chromosomes are called ***autosomes.*** The discovery of sex chromosome was made in the early of 20 th century by the cytologists of America during the era of rediscovery of Mendelian principles of heredity. The discovery of sex chromosomes had been of great help in establishing the possible relation between Mendelian factors and chromosome behaviour during meiosis.

Two sex chromosomes are different in two sexes whereas the autosomes are the same. The Y chromosome is much shorter than the X and its centromere is closely located to one end of the chromosome. The genetic material common in X and Y chromosomes is very less. The meiotic cell division also produces two types of gametes in equal proportion in male, *viz.* X bearing and Y bearing while female produce only one type of gamete (X bearing). The Y bearing sperms are lighter, move fast, and have fertilization advantage resulting higher sex ratio at zygotic stage which is diminished during development due to differential viability of two types of zygotes. This eventually results in equal number of two sexes at birth or slightly more number of males than females.

Role of Y Chromosome in Sex Determination in Mammals

According to the chromosome theory of sex determination, the sex is determined by the presence or absence of Y- chromosome. The males of placental animals are developed due to the dominant effect of the Y chromosome. More strong evidence in support of this theory comes from the study of animals having abnormal chromosomes.

The animals without Y chromosome and having a single dose of X chromosome (XO) are females whereas those having a single dose of Y chromosome but two X chromosomes (XXY) are males. The Y chromosome has its dominant effect during early stage of development of foetus when the primordial gonads are developed as testes which then secrete the male hormone, testosterone which stimulates the development of secondary sexual characteristics of maleness. On Y chromosome is a sex determining region which is just near the pseudoautosomal region on the short arm of the Y chromosome. The sex determining region on Y chromosome (**SRY**) has gene (SRY gene) which produces the testis-determining factor (***TDF***). The insertion or deletion of SRY region containg SRY gene that produces TDF determines the sex of the individual. This factor (SRY) was discovered when identified the unusual individuals of inconsistent sex with chromosome constitution of XX which were males and XY which were females.

A small piece of Y chromosome containing SRY gene was found inserted into one of the X chromosome, carried by XX males, and hence these males with XX chromosome complement developed testes. On the other hand, this region of Y chromosome carrying SRY gene was found missing from the Y chromosome of XY females and hence development of testes was prevented in XY female. This clearly showed that this piece of Y chromosome which was found inserted into X chromosome of XX males and that was found missing from Y chromosome of XY females carried a gene responsible for maleness. Therefore, this piece of Y chromosome was required for male development.

The SRY gene in the male determining segment or the testis-determining factor (TDF) on Y chromosome has been identified by molecular analysis. The SRY gene which triggers the development of testis has also been discovered on the Y chromosome in mouse like that present in human. The testosterone hormone secreted by testes binds to receptors in many kinds of cells. This hormone-receptor complex transmits the signals to the nucleus for the way to differentiate the cell. This way the development of male sexual characteristics is initiated. On the contrary, in the absence of the secretion of testosterone hormone the nucleus and hence the cell does not get the signal to differentiate in developing the male characteristics and hence the individual developed is female.

In some cases the XY males fail to make testosterone receptor complex. Such XY individuals lacking this biochemical efficiency are developed as males initially through development of testes and production of testosterone. But there is lacking of transmission of development signal to the target cell. Therefore, such individuals acquire female sexual characteristics due to lack of the formation of hormone-receptor molecule but even fail to develop ovaries and hence remain sterile. This situation is called ***testicular feminization***. Research has indicated that such a syndrome of testicular feminization is the result of a mutation in an X-linked gene, denoted as T*fm* and found responsible to encode the testosterone-receptor protein. Further, it has been found that this mutant allele is transmitted in typical X-linked pattern by the female to the hemizygous offspring (XY) showing such syndrome.

On the contrary, Bridges had shown that Y chromosome has no influence on sex determination in *Drosophila*. In Melandrium plant which is dioceous, the Y chromosome is largest and XY plants are pollen bearing whereas XX plants are egg bearing. However, the sex is determined by a balance between male determining genes in the Y chromosome and the female determining genes in X chromosome and autosomes. The mapping of Y chromosome has shown that 3 distinct parts, besides a part which pair with X chromosome, influence the sex determination (maleness) and male fertility (Washergaard, 1948).

- ☆ The I part of Y chromosome suppresses femaleness and the missing of this part the plant is bisexual,
- ☆ The II part promotes maleness and its missing develops female plant, and
- ☆ The III part controls male fertility and its missing results in male sterility.

In Rumex hastatulus (dioeceous plant) the sex is determined by gene balance with strong male determiners on the Y chromosome (Smith, 1963).

In silkworm Bombyx mori, the Y chromosome determines femaleness (Bacci, 1965).

10.5 GENE THEORY OF SEX DETERMINATION

The gene theory of sex determination indicating that genes play their role in determination of sex, emerged from the study of cytogenetics which had emerged from the fusion of cytology and genetics by the efforts of an American scientist, E. B. Wilson who was cytologist and another American scientist, T. H. Morgan who was geneticist.

The sex is a complex development character and its development is not only affected by chromosomes but also by numerous autosomal genes. It is not the presence or absence of Y or X chromosome which determines the sex in *Drosophila* was demonstrated by Bridges (1925). He showed that female determinants were located in the X chromosome while male determinants were in the autosomes, and that genes for maleness were not present in the Y chromosome od *Drosophila* but were distributed widely among the autosomes, and that all individuals carry genes in certain chromosomes for both the sexes. This is the *gene balance theory* of sex determination proposed by Bridges (1925).

Bridges produced in his experiment the various combinations of X chromosome and autosomes in *Drosophila*. He noticed the failure of paired X chromosome to separate during meiosis (*non-disjunction of X chromosome, i.e. attached X chromosome*) which resulted into female gametes with two X chromosomes as well as devoid of X chromosome. His investigation on non-disjunction demonstrated that upon fertilization some received two X chromosome from mother and Y chromosome from father and the resulting) which resulted into female gametes with two X chromosomes as well as devoid of X chromosome. His investigation on nondisjunction demonstrated that upon fertilization some received two X chromosome from mother and Y chromosome from father and the resulting flies were normal appearing females which were then mated to wild type males (XY). The following results were obtained among progeny generation –

Parents: White eyed female (XX) X Red eyed male (XY)

	Female gametes	X	XX	O
Male gametes	X	XX Red female	XXX Female usually dies	XO Red male (sterile) exception
	Y	XY White male	XXY White female	YO dies

These results indicated that Y chromosome is not involved in sex determination in *Drosophila* but it is essential for male fertility since XO zygote developed into sterile male and XXY zygote as female.

When the XXY females were crossed with the normal male (XY), the following results were obtained –

Parents: XXY (Female) X XY (Male)

	Female gametes	X	XX	XY	Y
Male gametes	X	XX Red female	XXX Female usually dies	XXY Red female exception	XY Red male
	Y	XY White male	XXY White female	XYY White male	YY Dies

Thus, the male determining factors are present on autosomes and female determining on X chromosome and the balance between X chromosomes and autosomes determines the sex. When the number of sets of autosomes was greater, the maleness was expressed. The effect of balance between X chromosomes and autosomes were published by Bridges (1922) in *Drosophila melanogaster*. He found triploid females having every chromosome in triplicate which were fertile and resembled the normal diploid females except for rough eye. The triploid females when mated to normal diploid males produced eight sex types as follows –

Sex	*No. of Sex Chromosome*		*No. of*	*Sex Index Autosomes*	*Remark*
	X	*Y*		*(X:A ratio)*	
Super female	3	–	2	1.5	Sterile
Triploid female	3	–	3	1.0	
Diploid female	2	–	2	1.0	Normal
Diploid XXY female	2	1	2	1.0	Normal
Inter sexes	2	1	3	0.67	Sterile
Inter sexes	2	–	3	0.67	Sterile
Normal male	1	1	2	0.5	
Super males	1	1	3	0.33	Sterile

These results lead to the conclusion that male tendency genes in the autosomes are more effective than those in the X chromosome while the female tendency genes in the X chromosomes are more effective. Thus, the sex is determined by the gene balance which means the preponderance of the male or female tendency genes and the gene balance is controlled by the ratio of X chromosomes to the number of sets of autosomes in the zygote. Equal number of X chromosomes and sets of male determining autosomes produce females but when the number of sets of autosomes was greater than the number of X chromosome, the males are produced. A large overbalance of X chromosome and of autosomes was associated with super females and super males, respectively. When the difference in the proportion was not great, inter sexes were developed. There was a shift of characters from inter sexes (3 A:2 X) in the female direction when added the pieces of X chromosome obtained through breeding this chromosome by X radiation (Dobzhansky and Schultz, 1931) and this shift was greater with the large piece of X chromosome added. This was supported by Pipkin (1940, 1942) who added very short sections of the X chromosome and found that no small section resulted in any more significant shift towards femaleness than did any other. These experiments with the effects of fragments of X chromosome and autosomes indicated that many genes are normally involved in the sex determination in *Drosophila* with small effect individually. The mutated gene has, however, powerful sex modifying action. The transformer gene (tra) when homozygous converts the 2 X: 2 A female individual into male, though sterile.

10.6 GYNANDRISM (SEX MOSAIC)

The different sexes develop in response to genetic differences between them. In the organisms with XY and its analogue WZ sex determining mechanism, the heterogametic sexes produce two types of gametes which determine sex on fertilization. Exceptional individuals have been recorded in various organisms. In these exceptional individuals, some parts of the animal express male characters while other parts express those of females. These individuals have cells of both sexes, differentiating some parts into the male and others as female. This phenomenon is called ***Gynandrism*** *or* ***sexual mosaic*** and the individuals as ***gynanders*** or ***gynandromorphs***. The mosaic organisms are different from hermaphroditic plants which have no sex differential chromosomes and have complete functional sets of reproductive organs of each sex. The *gynanders* do not have two complete reproductive systems but there is a mosaic of parts. The commonest situation in gynanders is a bilateral mosaic, one side being male and other side female. Gynanders are known in insects (Drosophila, moth), crustaceans, birds and some mammals.

The gynandromorphy stands for a combination of male and female (*Gyn* = female and *andro* = male). The different parts of the body are phenotypic either male or female and not a mixture of the two. A gynandromorphy has one half of the body male and other half female as obtained by Morgan and Bridges (1919) and this fly was heterozygous for white eye and miniature wings (Wm/++) which are both sex linked characters. The female portion had both X chromosomes and Wm/++ and the male portion had only one X chromosome with white eyed miniature wings (Wm). Thus, the male portion lacked the X chromosome carrying the two dominant alleles.

Mechanism of Production of Gynanders

The mosaic sex pattern in *Drosophila* is based on an irregularity (abnormality) in chromosome mechanism at the cleavage of the zygote. The gynander arises from zygote that had initially two X chromosomes and therefore should develop into a female fly. On the other, one of the two X chromosomes is lost in some nuclei during cleavage of fertilized egg and consequently the descendent tissues have only one X chromosome and are therefore male. The nuclei which have two X chromosomes differentiated into tissues with two X chromosomes and so those parts being female.

If one cell losses a chromosome at first division after fertilization, one of the first two blastomers gets the normal chromosome complement and the other one losses an X chromosome leading to female genotype into its descendents. But if the chromosome is lost at second division, then ¼ of the resulting fly will have male characteristics. If this happens in later embryonic stage, it then results in a smaller part of male tissue *i.e.* a smaller proportion of the adult body would be the male segment. Therefore, the size of mosaic part is determined by the time of the division of abnormality. The gynanders are produced in every 2000 -3000 flies. When virgin female is not mated until they are 8 – 17 days old, the proportion of gynanders is greatly increased and also greater proportion of gynanders is observed when excess yeast is added to the culture. If a gynander has female sex organ, it is fertile as a female whereas in case if the gynanders are with male sex organs they are invariably sterile because male parts have no Y chromosome. It is a fact that *Drosophila* males lacking Y chromosome are known to be sterile.

The gynanders in ***silkworms*** is not the result of mitotic accident but it appeared as an inherited condition. The experimental evidences indicate that gynanderism is based on single recessive gene in Bomyx moth.

Mosaics for sex chromosome are also known in humans. One case of female athlete was found as XYY/XO mosaic. It was postulated that perhaps the non disjunction of Y chromosome at the first mitotic division might have occurred and produced two cell types: XYY and XO. The XO tissues were presumably enough for the female phenotype.

10.7 HERMAPHRODITISM

It is a condition when an individual is functionally both male and female either at the same time or consecutively. Hermaphroditis is very common among animals and plants but it is very rare in vertebrates. In some species the sex of the individual changes consecutively. The individuals which are male during early part of their reproductive life and females during later part are called ***Protandrous hermaphroditism.*** The reverse of this is called **Protogamous hermaphroditism** (*i.e.* first female and then male). There are some hermaphrodites containing both ovaries and testes (Antheridia in flowering plants). On the other hand, some have combined gonads (***Ovotestes***) as in most snails.

A kind of continuous variation in sexuality *i.e.* a sort of bell curve distribution of sexes (***unbalanced hermaphroditism***) is observed in some animals (Molluscan genera *crepidula* and *Patella.* The unbalanced hermaphrodite species, unisexual forms (*i.e.* individuals that are purely and irreversibly one sex or the other) are found in populations that are otherwise predominantly hermaphroditic. Besides the typical hermaphrodites and the unisexual individuals, other groups of individuals (intermediate) are observed (Bacci, 1965) in *Patella coerulea* and *Crepidula plana.* Most of the individuals in *Patela coerulea* are *protandrous* with male and female phases of about equal duration and rarely unequal male and female individuals also occur. The intermediate individuals between these three types of individuals are observed that have a prolonged male phase and correspondingly short female phase or its reverse. A similar distribution of sexuality is exhibited by *Crepidula plana.*

The sex determination in ***Bonelia*** and in unbalanced hermaphrodites has been postulated to sex polygenes by B**acci (1965).** He assumed that there are four sex-gene loci, each with male and female determining alleles. The genotype with 7 or 8 alleles will produce unisexuality and irreversible sex, if these are male alleles the individual will be male and if female alleles it will then develop as female. The equal distribution of male and female alleles will produce *Protandrous hermaphrodies* of equal male and female duration in *Patella* and *Crepidula* whereas in *Bonellia* such individuals will be unisexual as adults but easily and equally reversible as differentiating larvae.

10.8 ENVIRONMENTAL SEX DETERMINATION

In some lower animals, a single/similar genotype produces both males and females. This depends upon the external environment which gives stimulus and initiates development towards one sex or the other. ***Sea worm*** is example. The sex is related to the ***size of the eggs*** produced by females. Small eggs always produce males but the large ones females.

Another species of ***sea worm***, produce sperms in young age but after getting older the eggs are produced when the ***number of body segments*** increases to more than twenty. However, decreasing the number of body segments of an older female due to any reason, this female reverts to male. Thus, body size is more important than age in controlling the sex.

There is another sea worm (***Bonellia***) whose male is smaller in comparison to the females and live within the reproductive tract of the large female. Genes for both sexes are present in young worm. The free swimming larvae are sexually undifferentiated. Isolated larvae which settle down in sea bottom become females whereas the larvae which attached to the bodies of the adult females are differentiated as males (Baltzer, 1937). Thus, sex differentiation depends on environmental factors related either to ***association or lack of association*** with other members of the species. The newly hatched worms if released in water become attracted to the females if mature females are present in water and they (newly hatched worms) are attached to their body and transformed into males which gradually migrated to the female reproductive tract where they become parasitic on females. Therefore, association of larvae with female body influences the young worms towards maleness while larvae which lead to a free life develop into females.

The developmental sequence of sex has also been observed in the genus ***Crepidula*** (boat-shell snails). The early asexual stage is followed by a male sex and finally transformed into females. The transformation of males into female also depends on the activeness. When the male phase individuals are mated and inactive, the transformation to females is delayed and thus, a mated male remains as such for a long time whereas the unmated males (unable to secure a mate) quickly transformed to female phase. Thus, if the young males get attached to females, they remained males so long as they are attached to females but they start differentiating to become females as soon as they get separated. However, sex is irreversible in the sense that females are unable to change into males. Therefore, snails of the genus *Crepidula* are in intermediate between *Bonellia* and *Ophryotrocha* regarding sex determining mechanism. This phenomenon in which the animal first develops as a male then later is transformed into a female is called ***Protandry*** and the reverse is called ***Protogynous.***

Protandry in ***Osters*** and ***shipworm*** (genus Teredo) has been described by Coe (1933). In Oster the protandry was observed with some individuals as permanent males or females. The protandry is known in ***Tunicates*** and ***Amphibia*** too. If accidentally or experimentally, the testes in a toad are removed, the toad becomes a functional female by enlargement of potential ovaries which are present anterior to the testes in toad. Environmental controlled sex determination in a nematode worm, *Mermis subnigrescens* has also been observed. The eggs of this worm are eaten by grasshoppers along with the foliage and thus the larvae emerge in the intestine of grasshoppers and there itself they complete their development. After full development they come out of the host. The differentiation of sex depends on the number of larvae inside the host. From one to three per host they all develop as females, from 4 to 23 worms per host, the males, females and intersexes are developed. If the number exceeds more than 23, all of them develop as males.

In Equisetum (plant species) the sex is determined by the condition for growth. When the plants are grown under good growth condition the plants develop into female whereas when growth conditions are not very much favourable the plant develops as male.

The development of sex organs in plants may be changed by influence from the environment. Changing the length of day develops the male flowers on female plants and vice versa in dioecious hamp plant.

10.9 HORMONES AND SEXUAL EXPRESSION (SEX REVERSION)

The hormones have the ability to change the sex already determined chromosomally. Fish and Frog fall in this group. The sex determining mechanism in ***Medaka fish*** is the XY based. The XY male young fishes result in their development into fertile females on exposure to female hormone (estrogen). These transformed XY females when mated to XY males also produce YY males and these YY males, like XY males on exposure to estrogen can be changed to females. A cross of YY female with YY males produces only males.

In ***frog,*** the sex determining mechanism is WZ based (Reverse of XY type). Feeding male hormone (androgens) to WZ females results in WW females which can be modified by hormones into males.

Sex reversal through the action of hormones has been observed in ***birds*** (Fowl and Pigeons). When the ovary of female fowl is destroyed, normal egg laying hens underwent complete sex reversa, the male glands developed and finally become functional as a male parent, besides developing male comb, plumage, crowing ability, cock feathering. Crew (1923) reported a classic case of sex reversal which occurred in a mature hen which has already laid fertile eggs. Chickens have two gametes but in females the ovary is developed from left one and the other one remained undifferentiated. In case of destruction of ovary the rudimentary right gonad differentiated into testis.

Removal of gonads of either sex in mammals is followed by the development of secondary sex characters of the opposite sex. The relationship between hormones and secondary sex characters can be shown in ***mammals*** by injecting sex hormones of the opposite sex in normal females or males. It is common experience that hormones imbalances in ***man*** result into maleness in females and femaleness in males. The female characteristics like voice, body built up, and hair pattern on body are expressed in adult human males whose testes are removed before puberty. Injection of male hormone to such males counteracts the female tendencies.

Studies on twins of opposite sex in ***cattle*** have shown that the female calf is usually sterile with many male like traits and is called ***Free-martin***. In this case, the blood of one embryo along with its hormones may enter the blood stream of the other through ***anastomosis*** of blood vessels and the male hormones seem to influence the development of the female embryo in masculinity. Little (1917) demonstrated that placenta of freemartin is fused with that of her male co-twin with consequent mixing of their fetal blood. This leads the gonads of the male to become hormonally functional before the ovaries of the female and the male hormone suppress further ovarian development and induces maleness in a female calf. The sex reversion of the gonads of the freemartin and testosterone secretion by them has been shown by Short *et al.* (1965). They suggested that the sex reversal of her ovaries is attributable not to testosterone from the male but to a substance that causes retention of medullary sex cords. This substance may be derived from the male co-twin or from the gonads of the female herself, because of XX/XY mosaicism in the tissues of both co-twins.

Chapter 11

Sex Controlled Inheritance

The inheritance of some characters is controlled by sex in one or the other way. The expression of these characters is either under the control of genes present on sex chromosomes or under the control of sex hormones. The sex chromosome carry genes which control sexual characters (masculine and feminine characters) as well as other characters not related to sex of the individual. The sex controlled inheritance may be categorized as:

- ✰ Sex influenced characters,
- ✰ Sex limited characters, and
- ✰ Sex linked characters.

11.1 SEX INFLUENCED CHARACTERS

These characters are controlled by such genes whose phenotypic expression in homozygous condition (either dominant or recessive genotype) is similar in two sexes but *the gene expression in heterozygous state is different in two sexes,* in such a way that one allele is dominant in males but it is recessive in females. Thus, the nature of interaction between alleles (expression of heterozygous genotype) depends on the sex of the individual. The allele recessive in males is usually dominant in females. The presence of sex hormone has an influence on gene interaction and hence on the development of the character in the individual. Such genes are present on autosomes, so both the sexes are alike in genetic constitution (same genotypes) and give rise to a sexual dimorphism. These characters are expressed in both the sexes.

In general, secondary sex characters *e.g.* body size, appearance, temperament are the examples. The best known sex influenced characters are the inheritance of horns in sheep, Mohogany colour pattern in Ayreshire cattle and beard in goat. The other characters are white forelock, absence of upper lateral incisor teeth, one type of skin abnormality (ichthyosis), shuttering, baldness, short index finger in human. These characters occur more frequently and more severely among men than women. The inheritance pattern of some of these sex influenced characters is as follows-

(i) Horns in Sheep

Dorset breed of sheep are always horned in both sexes whereas Suffolk, Shropshire and Southdown breeds of sheep never bear horns in either sex. The horn condition is controlled by dominant gene, H. The crossing of these two breeds irrespective of the way the cross was made (reciprocal cross) produces $F_1$with horns if male but without horns (hornless or polled) if female. Thus, the F_2 ratio is 3 horned: 1 polled in males whereas 1 horned: 3 polled among females. This is because the gene for horn is dominant in males but recessive in female. The heterozygous genotype in the two sexes behaved differently in their phenotypic expression by producing horn in males but no horn in female. Further, it was observed that the horns of F_1 heterozygous males are much shorter not only to rams of horned breed but even shorter than the ewes of Dorset breed. This indicated that polled condition is dominant but incompletely. The crosses can be represented as:

Parents Dorset (horned) x Suffolk (polled)

HH ↓ hh

F_1 Hh (Horned if male, Polled if female)

F_2	Genotypes	Sex	HH	Hh	hh
	Phenotypes	Males	Horned	Horned	Polled
		Females	Horned	Polled	Polled

(ii) Coat Colour in Cattle

The coat colour in Ayrshire cattle is also a sex influenced character. The Ayrshire cattle have red and mahogany spotting on a white background. The mahogany is a very deep red, almost maroon and found in Maine-Anjou and Ayrshire cattle. The red colour is observed in Hereford and Shorthorns. The white spotting is almost always associated with red or mahogany colours, though the inheritance of spotting is independent of red or mahogany.

The Ayrshire cattle of both the sexes with MM genotype are mahogany for coat colour while with *mm* genotype are red, but the heterozygote with Mm genotype behaved differently in the two sexes, the males are of mahogany spotting while the females are of red spotting. The gene for mahogany colour is completely dominant in males but completely recessive in females. On the contrary, the gene for red colour is dominant in females but recessive in males. This has been shown below:

Parents	Mahogany	x	Red		
	(MM)	↓	(mm)		
F_1		Mm (Mahogany if male, Red if female)			
F_2	Genotypes	Sex	MM	Mm	mm
	Phenotypes	Males	Mahogany	Mahogany	Red
		Females	Mahogany	Red	Red

(iii) Baldness in Men

The pattern baldness in men is a familiar example of sex influenced character. The baldness may be genetic or environmental. It may occur due to some disease, thyroid defects or radiation and also it is found to be an inherited character. The condition of getting hair thinner progressively on the top of head until little or none is left is due to a single mutant gene, B. This gene for pattern baldness (B) express differently in two sexes. It exhibits dominance in men but acts recessive in women. Therefore, the pattern baldness is developed in men when the gene is in either the homozygous (BB) or heterozygous (Bb) condition but in women it will develop only when homozygous (BB). Thus, the individuals of both sexes with genotype BB are bald and with genotype bb are non-bald (normal hair) whereas the heterozygous men (Bb) are bald but heterozygous women are normal (non-bald). Therefore, the expression of heterozygous genotype is different in the two sexes, depending on ***internal biological environment*** (presence of male sex hormone). The testosterone, the male hormone probably triggers the expression of the allele. Women produce this hormone in much less quantity not enough to trigger the expression of the allele and hence they have less risk to develop baldness. This shows that biological factor (environment – hormone) may control the gene expression. The cross will be as:

Parents	Bald	x	Non bald		
	(BB)	↓	(bb)		
F_1		Bb (Bald if male, Non bald if female)			
F_2	Genotypes	Sex	BB	Bb	bb
	Phenotypes	Males	Bald	Bald	Non-bald
		Females	Bald	Non-bald	Non-bald

The expression of the gene as a character is related to the concentration of male hormone when the expression of the heterozygous class is altered by the cellular environment or biological environment (hormone concentration). The gender of person is the relevant biological facor. This means that the gene B gets its effect in association with male hormone.

This is supported by the evidence that the women after developing a tumour in the adrenal cortex became bald, developed a beard condition and also a deep voice because adrenal cortex normally produces a small amount of male sex hormone, bur after surgical removal of tumour the hairs on head appear, beard condition disappear and female voice resumed. Likewise, under male hormone therapy, the women suffer thinning of the hair on the head and growth of hair on the upper lip appears. The normal baldness in women with genotype BB may be due to small amount of male sex hormone present in the blood stream of women and this amount is sufficient to cause baldness in BB women but insufficient to cause baldness in Bb women.

(iv) Index Finger in Men

The gene for short finger (S) is dominant over long (s) in men but the dominance of gene is changed in women. The expression of the character (finger size) is such that:

SS genotype = Short index finger in men and women,

Ss genotype = Short index finger in men but long finger in women,

ss genotype = long index finger in both men and women

(v) White Forelock in Men

The gene W producing white forelock acts as dominant in males but recessive in females.

WW genotype = white forelock in men and women

Ww genotype = white forelock in men but normal in women

ww genotype = normal forelock in men and women

11.2 SEX LIMITED INHERITANCE

Some characters are an extreme type of sex-influenced characters. However, *these characters are expressed only in one sex* in contrast to sex influenced characters and hence called as sex limited characters. The genes controlling these characters are present on autosomes and hence both the sexes are alike in genetic constitution (same genotype) but their phenotypic expression is different in two sexes, being limited to only one of the two sexes, depending on the presence or absence of one of the sex-hormones. These characters give rise to a sexual dimorphism. These genes control the expression of primary and secondary sexual characters and their action is clearly related to the sex hormone.

The genes, which express themselves in the presence of certain sex hormones, are considered to be sex-limited. For example, the genes for *beard, size and shape of the penis* are present in both the sexes but the genes are expressed only in males. Likewise, the genes for *breast development* in human beings and *udder development* in farm animals are present in both the sexes but their expression is limited in females only. *Milk production in mammals* and the *egg production in birds etc.* fit beautifully in this category as the expression is limited to females of the species in spite of the fact that milk production and egg production genes are carried on chromosomes of bulls and cocks also. The expression of these characters is dependent on the development of certain anatomical structure which provides the particular product (semen, milk, egg). Men have *beard* but women normally do not, though some abnormalities in hormone secretion may cause appearance of beard in women and breast development in men.

The other *secondary sex characters* include not only physical traits (penis, breast, udder, ovary) but differential response of the nervous system depend upon gene whose expression is sex limited.

(i) Creamy Puff Plumage Colour in Fowl

Morejohn (1953) had demonstrated that the adult plumage of red jungle fowl, the ancestor of domestic chicken, showed sex limited pattern of inheritance for plumage colour. The adult females of recessive genotype (ss) develop a *creamy buff plumage*, whereas the males of ss genotype develop the normal plumage (wild type) indistinguishable from that of the males which have SS or Ss genotype. The *creamy buff plumage* is limited to only in females. The female sex hormone is necessary for creamy puff plumage gene to express.

Genotypes	Sex	SS	Ss	ss
Phenotypes	Males	Wild	Wild	Wild
	Females	Wild	Wild	Creamy buff plumage

(ii) Plumage Type (Cock Feathering) in Fowl

The *cock feathering* is sex limited character controlled by single pair of autosomal genes. The plumage type (feathering) of the two sexes in most breeds of poultry is strikingly different. The feathering pattern is hormone dependent. The cock feathering is being a showy plumage represents larger comb and wattles and long, pointed curved, fringed feathers on neck, tail (sickle feathers), is expressed only in males and produced by recessive allele h. The *hen feathering* (short and round feathers without a fringe) is expressed in both the sexes and produced by dominant gene H. Thus, the males are of two types (hen feathered and cock feathered) but all females are hen feathered. The hen feathering gene (H) is dominant over cock feathering gene (h). Therefore, hen feathering genotypes can be HH or Hh. The chicks of the genotypes HH and Hh of either sex are hen feathered, whereas the homozygous recessive (hh) are hen feathered if females but cock feathered if males. The *cock feathering is produced by homozygous recessive genotype (hh) limited to the male sex* and also requires the presence of male hormone. Thus, the male hormone is apparently necessary for the cock feathering gene to express. This indicated that the poultry breeds having different plumage in the two sexes (Hamberg, Campines) are homozygous recessive (hh) while other breeds (Sebright) having hen feathering in both sexes are homozygous dominant (HH). The hybrids of these two types of birds will express their feathering pattern according to the genotype and sex (presence or absence of male sex hormone). In these crosses, all the females are hen-feathered irrespective of the genotype but the males are hen-feathered if carry H gene and cock-feathered if carry hh genotype. *In other words*, the gene for hen feathering (H) is dominant over cock feathering gene (h) in the presence of any sex hormone and thus the allele H causes hen feathering. The cock feathering is limited only in males and thus the recessive gene (h) in homozygous condition (hh) produces cock feathering in the presence of male sex hormone but produces hen feathering in the presence of female sex hormone.

Genotypes	Sex	HH	Hh	hh
Phenotypes	Males	Hen feathering	Hen feathering	Cock feathering
	Females	Hen feathering	Hen feathering	Hen feathering

The expression of the gene H and h depends on sex hormone. The experimental evidences indicated that removal of testes of male with hen feathering or the ovary in female results in the production of cock feathering (Donn, 1929). Thus cock feathering occurs even in the presence of H gene and in the absence of sex hormone either due to removal of gonads or destruction by disease. This indicated that the hen feathering gene H appears to be dominant over cock feathering in the presence of either sex hormone. The cock feathering is produced by the genotype hh only in males or in ovariectomised females. The allele h thus does not prevent cock feathering but it cannot express itself in the presence of sex hormone. The hh genotype leads to cock feathering in castrated chickens of either sex, and if the castrated chickens are treated with male hormone the cock feathering is developed while treatment with female sex hormone develop the hen feathering. This indicates that feathering pattern is hormone dependent.

(iii) Colour Pattern in Butterfly

The white colour in butterfly is a sex limited character, expressed only in females (Gerould, 1911). The males are yellow but females are of two types – yellow and white. The white colour appeared in the female only and depends on a dominant gene (W) so that the females of the genotype WW, Ww are white and of ww are yellow, but the males of all the 3 genotypes are yellow. Thus, males are always yellow. The *white colour is a sex limited character* which depends upon the genotype (WW, Ww) and also requires the presence of female sex hormone. The mating of yellow male (WW) with yellow female (ww) produces yellow F_1 male but white F_1 females, and the F_2 ratio with all yellow males but 3 white: 1 yellow female as:

Genotypes		WW	Ww	ww
Phenotypes	Males	Yellow	Yellow	Yellow
	Females	White	White	Yellow

11.3 SIMILARITIES AND DIFFERENCES IN SEX INFLUENCED AND SEX LIMITED CHARACTERS

The similarity lies in that the genes for both kinds of characters are present on the autosomes and hence the genetic constitution (genotype) is same for both the sexes. The difference between two types of inheritance is that the dominance of gene is sex dependent for sex influenced traits in a way that the expression of gene in heterozygous genotype is determined by the sex hormone. On the contrary, in case of sex-limited inheritance, the gene dominant in the male is also dominant in female. The effect of sex hormone is different in two types of inheritance, in a way that sex hormone determines the gene interaction (dominance or recessive alleles) for sex influenced inheritance while the sex hormone, in case of sex limited inheritance, determine expression of the trait (*i.e.* whether the trait will or will not be expressed). Thus, the expression of any genotype for the sex limited trait is determined by the sex hormone.

11.4 SEX-LINKED CHARACTERS

The *genes present on the sex chromosome* (X chromosome in mammals and Drosophila or Z chromosome in birds and moth) are said to be *sex-linked genes*. The inheritance of these genes is called as the *sex-linked inheritance*. The characters controlled by the sex-linked genes are called as *sex linked-characters*. Morgan and his associates gave the concept of sex-linked inheritance, working on the inheritance pattern of eye colour in Drosophila, concluding their experimental findings that gene for eye colour is located on the X-chromosome and hence sex linked.

11.4.1 Inheritance Pattern of Sex-Linked Characters

The genes present on the X chromosome in mammals are represented twice in females (XX) but once in males (XY). Therefore, recessive characters of this type are expected to express ***more often in males than in females.*** This is because that the recessive character can express itself in a female if the recessive gene is present on both the X chromosomes (double dose of gene is required) while the character in males can be expressed with single dose of gene. A female parent transmits its genes to both of her male as well as female offspring but the male parent transmits its genes only to his female progeny and not to his male offspring because the Y chromosome, which has no gene, is transmitted to male progeny by male parent.

These characters are expressed in both the sexes but the expression of the character depends on the sex of the parent in which the character was introduced in to the cross.

In case of the characters controlled by autosomes, the sex of the parent has no effect on the appearance of the character in the progeny. As a consequence, the reciprocal crosses for autosomal genes give similar results but *the results of reciprocal crosses are different for sex linked traits*. This means that a given character brought in by the male or female parent produces different results for sex linked characters. This is because the two members of sex chromosomes are not homologous either morphologically or genetically and so there is no crossing over between sex chromosomes (X and Y).

11.4.2 Complete vs Incomplete Sex-linked Genes

The linkage of genes may be complete or incomplete, depending upon the presence of genes on the homologous part or non-homologous part of X and Y chromosomes. Some part of X and Y chromosome are identical (homologous) having homologous genes and called as homologous region whereas other portion of X and Y chromosomes are non-homologous.

The synapsis and crossing over takes place between homologous parts of the two chromosomes (X and Y) and therefore, genes present on homologous parts of the two chromosomes do not always inherit along with other genes of their respective chromosomes. Such genes are called as *partially sex linked*. In contrast to this, the genes located on non-homologous parts of X chromosome and inherit together due to no crossing over between non-homologous parts are called *completely sex-linked genes*. The genes for haulandric inheritance are completely sex-linked because of their presence on differential parts of chromosome having no homologous genes. Thus, the Y-linked genes inherit along Y chromosome and hence expressed only in males. Therefore, the Y linked (haulandric) genes and the sex-linked (X-linked) genes present on non-homologous part (of X chromosome) are known as *sex-linked genes* and their inheritance is called as *sex linkage.*

Characteristics of sex linked recessive and dominant characters:

The sex linked genes show dominance-recessive relationship and the co-dominance among the alleles affecting a character. The dominance of alleles changes the inheritance pattern of the sex-linked characters.

11.4.3 Ways of Expression of a Sex Linked Recessive Gene (Character)

(i) The incidence of ***sex linked recessive trait*** is *more in males* (q) than in females (q^2). The proportion of male recessive to female recessive is 1:q if the recessive gene is more. The red-green colour blindness in humans is due to sex linked recessive gene. When the sex linked recessive gene is very rare (low frequency), its frequency in females (q^2) will be too low as there will be hardly any homozygous recessive female at all and the recessive gene of the female will remain hidden in the heterozygous condition. The hemophilia is a sex linked recessive trait and it is extremely rare in women for two reasons- one is the low frequency of the gene and second is that homozygous females are not viable.

(ii) The sex linked recessive traits express themselves showing the *crisscross inheritance* (To *skip a generation*). The process of skipping of generation is called as *crisscross inheritance or skip- generation inheritance.* The skip generation inheritance occurs when the female is homozygous. But when the female is carrier (heterozygous) the recessive trait appears in father as well as in sons.

(iii) The females do not express the trait unless it was expressed in the paternal parent.

A ***dominant sex linked gene*** and hence sex linked dominant character expresses in the following ways:

(i) The carrier female will express the trait. The *female dominant are always more numerous* than male dominants. Thus the dominant trait is mostly present in females than in males. This is in the contrary to the sex link recessive characters that the women have twice as many chances as men of receiving the gene for the reason of having two X chromosomes.

(ii) There is *no skipping of generation* for sex linked dominant traits. It is expressed in all female progeny of a male which express the trait. The ocular albinism in man is controlled by partially dominant gene.

(iii) If the female parent does not express the trait, it is not expressed in male progeny from the mother.

11.4.4 Sex-linked Inheritance in different Species

The examples of sex-linked genes in various species of animals with their details have been given as under:

(1) Sex Linkage in Drosophila

Morgan (1910) first time noted that reciprocal crosses in Drosophila produced different results in F_1 and F_2 progeny. He found that white eye was recessive to red eye. He made the *first cross* by crossing the red eye female (wild type - dominant) to white eye (recessive) male and observed that all the F_1 individuals of both sexes were red eyed. But F_2 data did not fit a 3:1 ratio of red: white eyed. Interestingly all the F_2 white eyed flies were males whereas among the F_2 red eyed progeny both the males and females were observed. There was a deficiency of recessive white eyed males among F_2 due to their low survivability. All the F_2 females were red eyed with no white eye whereas the F_2 males were red as well as white in a 1:1 ratio.

The *reciprocal cross* made by changing the sex of parents exhibiting the character (*i.e.* red males were crossed with white females) gave quite different result. Among the F_1 progeny, all the females were red eyed and all the males were white eyed. When these F_1 were crossed among themselves (*inter se* mating of F_1), the F_2 progeny had red and white eyed individuals in about equal numbers in both the sexes. Thus, the results of reciprocal for F_1 as well as for F_2 generation were different to the first cross. The results of two crosses have been shown digrametically as:

	I. Original cross	II. Reciprocal cross
Parents	X^+X^+ x X^wY	X^wX^w x X^+Y
	Red female ↓ white male	White female ↓ Red male
F_1	X^+X^w : X^+Y	X^+X^w : X^wY
	Red female red male	Red female white male
F_2	X^+X^+ : X^+X^w : X^+Y : X^wY	X^+X^w : X^wX^w : X^wY : X^+Y
	Red females, red male, white male	red female, white female, white male, red male
	2459, 1011, 782	¼, ¼, ¼, ¼
	3470	

Morgan postulated that Y chromosome is inert and therefore the genes on the single chromosome of a male are expressed even if they are recessive. On the other hand, female have two X chromosome and hence the females express the recessive trait only when homozygous for recessive gene. The conclusions drawn were:

(i) The white gene (w) is present on the X chromosome (Sex linked character) and Y chromosome had no allele, hence white gene will be transmitted from the male parent to only females of F_1 and the males will receive the Y chromosome,

(ii) The white eyed females had gene for white eye on both its chromosome (X^wX^w),

(iii) The white eyed males receive X chromosome with *w* gene from mother and Y chromosome (no gene) from father, producing white eye in all the males,

(iv) The female progeny received one X chromosome with w gene from mother and the other X chromosome with dominant W^+ gene from father,

(v) One X chromosome having red allele will come from the red female parent. Thus, the F_1 female will be heterozygous. This heterozygous female will transmit X chromosome to F_2 males which will result 50 per cent of F_2 males as white eye.

These results clearly indicated the linkage of genes expressing two colours (presence of two colour genes on X chromosome). Moreover, the sex linked genes are transmitted from father to grandson through the daughters and never directly through sons. Thus, the *crisscross* pattern of inheritance (from male parent to F_1 females and then to the F_2 males) of recessive X linked gene was evident. Morgan called this phenomenon as sex linkage. The sex linkage is due to genes located on X chromosome and the character (eye colour) controlled by sex linked genes has no association with sex of the individual.

In *Drosophila, some other sex linked characters* controlled by sex-linked genes (completely) have also been reported. The followings are the examples:

Dominant gene (B) producing bar eye (narrow reduced eye);

Recessive gene (v) producing vermillion eye colour;

Recessive gene (ec) producing echinus (rough eye);

Recessive gene (y) producing yellow body colour;

Recessive gene (sc) producing scute bristles (abscences of some bristles);

Recessive gene (f) producing forked bristles;

Incomplete recessive gene (bb) producing bobbed bristles (short);

Recessive gene (cv) producing crossveinless wings;

Recessive gene (ct) producing cut wings margin and

Recessive gene (m) producing miniature wings

(2) Sex Linkage in Humans

About 120 inherited characters are controlled by sex linked genes. Some of them are *red- green colour blindness, hemophilia (bleeder's disease), agammaglobulinemia, deafness, white forelock, toothlessness, oscillation of the eye ball, optic atrophy, near sightedness (myopia), defective iris, muscular dystrophy (pseudohypertrophic), double eye lashes (distichiasis), etc.* The inheritance pattern is similar to that for white eye colour in Drosophila.

(i) Hemophilia in Humans-Blood Clotting Disorder

The best known and earliest example of sex-linked character in men is the *hemophilia* known as bleeding disease or bleeder's disease, reported only in males in the royal family of Spain. This disease occurs in those humans who lack to produce a blood clotting factor and hence it is characterized by continuous blooding from the cuts, bruises, and wounds, if not treated. The hemophilic condition stops the blood to clot on exposing to the air. It has been seen that a small cut or injury cause continuous bleeding which may lead to death due to loss of blood as a result of excessive bleeding. Such persons are called ***hemophiliacs.*** The hemophiliacs need treatment when they are injured, by transfusion with clotting factor. The hemophilia is a fatal disease and the hemophiliacs die in infancy before the age of 20. However, this disease is curable effectively with an inexpensive treatment and consequently the hemophiliacs may live healthy long life.

This is completely *sex linked recessive* character in human. This is a mutant allele. The disease occurs more only in men. This is due to the reason that the hemophilic males are ubable to produce children because of their death before reproductive age. The hemophilic people in the population are nearly 0.01 percent which means that hardly one person in 10,000 is suffered with this disease and taking the same frequency of homozygous females will be around 0.0001 percent which is negligible which means that one in one crore women will be homozygous. The chances of homozygous girl to be born are very rare and further a girl with severe bleeding die before adolescence.

The hemophilia is under the control of a sex-linked recessive allele present on X chromosome and hence the single dose of the allele causes this ailment. On the other hand, a woman requires two genes to cause the problem. A person who has normal gene for the sex linked recessive trait cannot transmit the disease (defect) caused by sex linked recessive gene. Thus, a man whose blood clots normally cannot transmit the allele for hemophilia to his children, irrespective of high incidence of the disease in his family. The reason is that a man has only one X chromosome on which the allele for hemophilia may be located and therefore a normal man (whose blood clots normally) will not have gene for hemophilia. If the recessive allele is present on the X chromosome of a man, then he will bleed, even with small injury. The hemophilic girls surviving to marriageable age can produce normal daughters, though they will be carrier for the hemophilic gene. But theses carrier daughters on marriage with normal man transmit the hemophilic gene to half of their sons which are grand-sons of the hemophilic man. But a carrier daughter on marriage to a hemophilic man can produce a hemophilic girl.

(ii) Colour Blindness in Human-Vision Disorder

The colour blindness in human is another example of completely *sex linked recessive* character. It is characterized as the inability of a person to distinguish between some colours. There are three light absorbing proteins in the specialized cells of retina in the eyes. The colour perception is mediated by these three proteins, synthesized by three genes. One of the three proteins absorbs *blue light*, other absorb *green light*, and another third protein absorb red light. There are thus three colour receptors, controlled by three genes. Out of these three receptor genes, two receptors (genes) have similar structure. This may probably be because the genes controlling these two receptors have been evolved from same ancestral colour-receptor gene and located on sex chromosomes.

On the contrary, third receptor-gene which encodes blue light is located on an autosome. An abnormality in any of the colour recepting proteins causes colour blindness. The red-green colour blindness is caused by any defect in any of the two color receptor proteins controlled by two genes present on sex chromosome.

Among various types of colour blindness, the ***red-green colour blindness*** is most common described by Horner (1876). It is caused by sex linked recessive allele which fails to produce colour sensitive cells in the retina of eye and hence the eyes results in colour blindness. This disorder involves faulty perception of red and green light which is controlled by sex linked gene. One gene encodes the receptor for green light and the second gene encodes the receptor for red light.

The condition of colour blindness is more common in men than women. About 5- 10 per cent human males and less than 1 per cent females have red-green colour blindless. This suggests that this character is controlled by recessive mutant allele. This is because two dose of recessive gene are required for expression of recessive character (colour blindness) in females while only one dose of recessive gene is required to express the recessive character in males. Men are not carrier because they have only one X chromosome in their genome. Colour blind woman always have colour blind father, and if this woman marry with colour blid man, will always produce colour blind sons as well as colour blind daughters only. Normal woman whose father is colour blind produce sons having both colour visions in equal ratio.

The *inheritance of colour blindness* (genotypes and phenotypes of parents and the progeny) can be studied from all possible marriages among the couples of different visions. There will be 6 possible combinations of marriages among women of three vision types (normal XX; carrier XX^c; colour blind $X^c X^c$) and men of two vision types (normal XY; colour blind X^cY). The progeny (sons and daughters) from marriage of persons with similar vision types (normal x normal and colour blind x colour blind) will have vision of the parental types. Now, the remaining couples can marry in 4 possible combinations. These 4 possible marriage combinations will produce the sons and daughters with genotypes and the vision types as shown below:

Parents	$XX \times X^cY$	$X^c X^c \times XY$	$XX^c \times XY$	$XX^c \times X^cY$
	↓	↓	↓	↓
Sons	XY	X^cY	XY X^cY	XY X^cY
Daughters	XX^c	X^cX	XX X^cX	XX^c X^cX^c

(iii) Some Incompletely Sex Linked Genes

In man are present on that portion of the X chromosome which is homologue with a portion of Y chromosome. These are the genes causing total *colour blindness, Xeroderma pigmentation, progressive degeneration of retina and nephritis* (*kidney disease*). These genes segregate like autosomal genes but in association with sex of individual and represent in the X and Y chromosome as allelic pairs. Therefore, the incompletely sex linked characters do not show crisscross inheritance.

(iv) The Sex Linked Dominant Character

In man is the *defective enamel of teeth*. It occurs more frequently in women compared to men because the women have two X chromosomes but men have only one X chromosome.

(v) Sex-Linked Lethal in Man

The gene causing *muscular dystrophy* is recessive sex-linked lethal gene. This is the condition when the muscles wear up in early age, leading to death in early age.

(3) Sex Linkage in Birds

The female is heterogametic (having one X chromosome) in birds (fowl, pigeon, duck), moths, butterflies whereas the males are homogametic (having two X chromosomes, XX), in contrast to mammals and Drosophila.

(i) ***Barred Feathers in Poultry*** (white bars on top of head, feathers are banded with bars of black on white background), is a colour pattern characteristic of Plymouth Rock breed of fowl and is a *sex linked dominant* colour pattern over black or red unbarred plumage. This forms the best example. The barred is normal and dominant (B) over black (b). The crossing of barred with black male produces only barred males and black females in F_1 generation. The *inter se mating* produces barred and black individuals in equal ratio among males as well as among females. The *reciprocal cross* of black female with barred male produced all the F_1 progeny as barred (males as well as females). In F_2 generation, barred and black individuals were found in a ratio of 1:1 among females but all F_2 males were barred.

(ii) ***Slow and rapid feathering in domestic chicken*** is another example. Early feathering (rapid feathering) is observed in Mediterranean breeds (Leghorn, Minorcha, Andulasian, Ancona) whereas the Asiatic (Brahma, Cochin), English and (Australorp, Cornix, Sussex), American (Plymouth Rock, RIR, New Hampshire) are slow feathering (feathers grow at slow rate). The difference is more apparent from 8-10 days after hatching. The slow feather chicks have no tail feathers and only very small wing feathers whereas a rapid feathering chick has tail feathers of about one inch long and wing feathers extended to the tail. The slow normal feathering (K gene) or late feathering is dominant over rapid feathering (k gene) or early feathering, the recessive gene causes an increase in feathering rate. The rapid feathering is thus a recessive sex-linked trait. The fast feathering gene (k gene) is correlated with better growth rate and egg production.

(iii) ***Silver coloured plumage in chickens*** is produced by dominant gene (S) whereas recessive gene (s) produces gold coloured plumage.

(iv) **Dark shank colour** is recessive to non-dark skin and shank colour.

(4) Sex Linked Characters in other Species of Animals

Hemophilia in dogs is a sex linked recessive trait. The hemophilia is a genetic disease, caused by a deficiency of some factor that influences blood clotting reaction. The mating of normal males (AY) to carrier female (Aa) can only produce hemophilic pups. From this mating, only half of the pups produced (aY) will be hemophilic and other half will be normal (AY). On the other hand, all the females produced from this mating will be either AA or Aa and hence will be normal phenotypically.

***Tortoiseshell* or *calico pattern in cats*:** The sex-linked locus controlling coat colour in cat has been reported. This locus controls the production of the black and yellow (orange) pigment in the coat of the cats. This is due to a pair of co-dominant alleles (B, Y) present on X chromosome. The black coat colour is due to the allele represented by B in homozygous state (BB) whereas the yellow (or orange) colour is due to the allele Y in homozygous condition (YY). The two alleles are co-dominant and hence produce another colour in heterozygous state (BY), called as tortoise pattern which is due to the presence of both black and yellow hairs, as the roan colour pattern occurs in cattle due to the presence of red and white hairs. As the locus is sex-linked, only the females are heterozygous having both the alleles (B and Y) and hence produce the tortoiseshell colour pattern. The males are hemizygous and hence cannot produce tortoiseshell or calico pattern. The females on the other hand, have black (BB), tortoise (BY) and yellow (YY) coat colours.

The X chromosome in cats and mice carries a gene for pigmentation of the fur. The *tortoiseshell* coat colour in cat is a patchy phenotype produced by two alleles present in heterozygous individuals - one allele produces black pigment (dark patches) and other produces orange pigment (light patches). Thus, the tortoiseshell coat colour in females shows two different phenotypes (phenotypic mosaicism) due to *genetic mosaics* having two types of cell lineage by females.

The tortoiseshell coat colour in cat is an example of *inactivation of–linked genes* in female mammals. The maternally inherited X-chromosome is inactivated in roughly half of the cells while the paternally inherited X chromosome is inactivated in other half of the cells.

Wing colour in moth: Sex linkage is also observed in ***moth***, similar to sex linkage in fowl. Normal dark *wing colour* (large black spots on wings) in currant moth (*Abraxas grossulariata*) is dominant (L allele) over lacti colour (l, allele), a pale milky coloured variety having small black spots. The breeding results on these two wing colours of currant moth (*Abraxas*) were reported by British biologist Doncaster, L. and Rayno, G. H. (1906) from crossing between lacticolour females with grossulariata males (large black spots). They found that this is a sex linked character. The females are heterogametic (ZW) while the males are homogametic (ZZ). Thus, the females are hemizygous for a recessive allele (l) located on Z chromosome and the males are homozygous for a dominant allele on this sex chromosome.

About 20 sex linked genes have been reported in mouse.

11.5 CONTRIBUTION OF SEX LINKAGE

The *sex-linked inheritance* has made it clear that homogametic sex receives equal inheritance from both the parents for sex linked genes but the hemizygous sex receives only from homozygous parent. Thus the two parents for sex linked genes do not contribute equally to their offspring and hence the reciprocal crosses yield different results. The female progeny receives equal inheritance from both the parents for sex linked characters but the male progeny receives only from their mother.

The sex linked recessive traits *skip a generation* remaining unexpressed in the F_1 generation. The genes are transmitted from a parent of one sex to the progeny of other sex in subsequent generation. A male transmit sex linked traits to his grand sons through his daughters and not through his sons and likewise the female parent transmit the sex linked character to her grand-daughter through her sons and not through her daughters. This *crisscross inheritance* has the importance in establishing the relationship between gene and the sex chromosome, and to study the transmission of the sex linked disorders casing the disease.

11.6 USE OF KNOWLEDGE OF SEX LINKAGE

The knowledge of sex linkage is helpful to predict about the children of affected individuals which is evident from hemophilia in men. The principle of sex linkage in poultry has been practically used to determine the sex of the baby chicks. Sexing is done on the basis of marker genes for colour pattern such as barred feathers and this type of sexing is called *auto sexing*. There is another marker gene which is used for auto sexing without involving different colour in poultry. The growth of feathers is influenced by this gene. When male homozygous for the slow feathering gene are crossed with females having normal allele for rapid feathering, the females to be produced from this cross will be slow feathering because they receive marker gene (K) from their father and can be distinguished from the heterozygous males (Kk) within few hours of hatching because males will show rapid feathering.

11.7 Y-CHROMOSOME HEREDITY

Though Y- chromosome is genetically inactive or inert, but some genes have been reported to be located on Y chromosome and such genes are called as haulandric genes. The word haulandric is derived from two words *viz. haul* means whole and *andro* means male. This is because of their presence only in males. In Drosophila, one gene, b, has been found on both X and Y chromosomes. The homologous recessive genotype (bb) in either sex produced shorter and slender bristles (bobbed). The traits controlled by the Y linked genes have a very simple pattern of inheritance. All the male offspring express the trait of the father whereas none of the female progeny expresses the trait. The inheritance controlled by Y linked genes is called *haulandric inheritance* and it is sex limited.

Morgan (1942) mentioned at least 5 gene loci which have alleles on X and Y chromosomes in human. A dense growth of long hair on the outer rim of ears in man (hairy pinna) is one of the characters transmitted from fathers to all of their sons and to none of their daughters (Dronamraju, 1965). The gene controlling the *hairy pinna* (*hypertrichosis of ears*) seems to be present on non-homologous part of the Y chromosome. This gene has high penetrance but not 100 per cent for an occasion it may skip a generation. The same phenotypic effect like Y linked gene has another gene which is autosomal. Therefore, it requires nearly complete pedigree for positive identification.

Another example of haulandric inheritance is a type of *ichthyosis* (*scaly skin*) called as porcupine man. However, there are some evidences of doubt on its being Y linked (Penrose and Stern, 1958).

Very little was known about the genetic make up of Y chromosome before Human Genome Project. It has now been observed about 397 genes on human Y chromosome during Human Genome Project. However, all of them are not functional. On the contrary more than 1000 genes have been identifies on human X - chromosome. A number of genes on Y chromosomes have been found to be required for male fertility.

11.8 PSEUDO-AUTOSOMAL GENES

The terminal regions of both X and Y chromosomes are common and hence some genes are present on both X and Y chromosomes. Such genes are transmitted like the inheritance pattern of autosomes rather than a distinct X or Y linked pattern of inheritance. Therefore, these genes are called ***pseudoautosomal genes.*** The regions of sex chromosomes containing these genes allow pairing them (sex chromosomes).

NUMERICAL EXERCISES

11.1 The coat colour pattern in Ayrshire breed of cattle is a sex influenced character. A cow with pure mahogany coat colour was mated with a bull with red coat. Find out the genotypes and phenotypes for F_1 and F_2 animals.

11.2 Baldness in human is a sex influenced trait. A normal man is married with a normal girl for this character. They produced one son and one daughter. The baldness appeared in their son at the age of 30. What were the genotypes of the parents?

11.3 A shepherd has a horned ram in the flock of hornless ewes. He is interested to develop a polled flock. He succeeds in his goal. What were the genotypes of male and females of parental generation?

11.4 Cock feathering in poultry is a sex limited character recessive to hen feathering. Give the genotypes and phenotypes of all the progeny of two sexes produced from heterozygous mating.

11.5 What will be the genotypes of the parents of colour blind boy who had his colour blind sister and normal brother? [Hint: XX^{c} and X^{c} Y].

11.6 Hemophilia in man is caused due to recessive sex-linked gene. List out the genotypes and phenotypes of different sons and daughters born from (i) the marriage of carrier women with a normal man and (ii) if a carrier girl marry with a man suffered with the disease (hemophilia).

11.7 Three sons and two daughters were born to a couple. One of their sons was found hemophilic. What is the chance of their other children to develop this ailment?.

[Hint: Since one of the two sons develops the disease, so father should be normal and the mother seems to be carrier].

11.8 A normal girl having a colour blind brother marries with a normal boy. Predict the chance of developing colour blindness in her son.

[Hint: The girl may be normal or carrier].

11.9 Barred feather pattern is dominant sex linked character over black. What will be the genotypes and phenotypes of the progeny of two sexes produced by mating of two birds differing in feather pattern?

Part 2

Molecular Genetics

Chapter 12

Microbial Genetics: Bacteria and Viruses

The bacteria are a large group of typically unicellular microscopic organisms widely distributed everywhere. The synonymous terms with bacteria are the microbes and germs. The word germ implies especially to any of the pathogenic or disease producing bacteria whereas the microbe is a French word means microscopic organisms or microorganism, being usually applied to the pathogenic forms.

12.1 PLACE OF BACTERIA IN PLANT KINGDOM

The bacteria display the characteristics of both plants and animals. However, these are classified with the plants. The plants are dvided into following 5 divisions -

- ☆ Protophyta (primary plants) which includes 3 classes *viz.*
    1. Schizophyceae (blue- green algae),
    2. Schizomycetes (***bacteria*** which lacks photosynthetic pigments) divided in 10 orders,
    3. Microtatobiotes which have 2 orders *viz.* Rickettsiales and ***virales***,
- ☆ Thallophyta (Thallus plants) which have 3 subdivision -
    1. Algae: containing chlorophyll green, brown, and red algae,
    2. *Fungi* (Yeasts and moulds) having 5 classes *viz.* Myxomycetetes (slim moulds), phycomycetes (moulds), ascomycetes (some mould and all yeasts), basidiomycetes (moulds), and fungi imperfecti (moulds), and
    3. Lichens - composite organism having of mould living symbiotically with an alga,

- ☆ Bryophyta divided into 2 classes *viz.* hepaticae (Liverworts), and Musci (Mosses),
- ☆ Pteridohpyta (flowerless plants like *ferns* which includes 7 classes, and
- ☆ Spermatophyte (seed plants) which includes 2 subdivisions of
  1. Gymnospermae (cone bearing plants, nacked seed plants *viz.* pines, himlocks, and
  2. Angiosperms (Flowering plants) which has following two classes - (a) Dicotyledoneae and (b) Monocotyledoneae.

Classification of Organisms on the Basis of Nutrition/Feed Habits

1. ***Autotrophs*** – those organisms that synthesize their food from inorganic raw material, *e.g.* plants, and
2 ***Heterotrophs*** – those organisms which feed on high energy organic molecules, *e.g. animals and protozoans.* The heterotrophs are of the following 4 types –
   - ***(i)*** *Parasitic* – which generally consume liquid food derived from the body of the host, *e.g.* Tape worm, Ascaris and Leech
   - ***(ii)*** *Symbiotic* – which live in association with other animals by obtaining food material from each other *e.g.* Bacteria (E. Coli present in human gut, consume food materials from the intestine and in turn provide vitamins to human body)
   - ***(iii)*** *Saprophytic* – which survive on dead organic matter by digesting them outside the body *e.g.* housefly, spider
   - ***(iv)*** *Holozoic* – which consume whole or part of a plant/animal food in liquid or solid form *e.g. animals*. Such animals can be classified into following 3 groups –
     - *(a)* *Herbivorous* – which consume plant material *e.g.* cows, rabbit
     - *(b)* *Carnivorous* – which consume flesh or animal meat *e.g. Lion, Tiger*
     - *(c)* *Omnivorous* – which consume both plants and animals *e.g.* Cockroach, crow, rat and man.

The ***heterotrophs*** have some special categories depending on the type/form of food they consume. Such heterotrophs may be classified as –

- ☆ Insectivorous (frog, lizard, ant-eaters) which feed on insects,
- ☆ Larvivorous (Gambusia fish) which feed on mosquito larvae,
- ☆ Corpophagous (rabbit, pig) which feed on faecal matter,
- ☆ Cannibals – which feed on the members of the same species,
- ☆ Detritivores (Earthworm) which feed directly on decaying organic matter,
- ☆ Osmotrophs (Tape worm) which absorb pre-digested food material through skin by osmosis,
- ☆ Sanguivores (Leech, louse, bedbug, female mosquito, vampire bat) which feed on blood of vertebrates,

- ☆ Frugivores (birds, monkey, bat) which feed on fruits,
- ☆ Grainivores (birds) which feed on grains.

12.2 IMPORTANCE OF BACTERIA

The bacteria are generally considered as the disease causing organisms. Only few bacterial species are harmful to man and great majority are not only harmless but also absolutely necessary for the existence of life to the extent that life cannot exist without bacteria.

(i) The bacteria (***Soil organism***) are very important in *agriculture*. The plants cannot grow in the absence of soil organisms. The soil bacteria by invading the roots of certain plants convert the free nitrogen of the air into organic compounds (nitrogen fixation) which are utilized by plants (symbiotic relation). The bacteria also convert sulfur and phosphorus into soluble inorganic salts for absorption by plant roots. The bacteria also erode rock.

(ii) Bacteria are necessary for the ***disposal of sewage*** containing human excreta and municipal waste water (with large amount of organic matter and microbes). The sewage is treated in sewage treatment plants (STPs) to make it less polluting first through filtration and sedimentation to remove large and small particles (known as sludge) and the supernatant forming the effluent and then secondly by biological treatment by pumping the air in the tank and allowing the growth of useful aerobic microbes. These microbes consume the major part of organic matter in the effluent. Other kinds of bacteria digest the bacteria and fungi in the sludge and a mixture of gases (biogas) like methane, CO_2, and hydrogen sulphide are produced which can be used as a source of energy due to its inflammability. The microbes thus convert the insoluble proteins, fats, and carbohydrates (cellulose) into soluble, odorless compounds.

(iii) ***Souring of milk*** for making *dahi* (production of curd from milk) is the result of bacterial action. A small amount of curd called starter is added to the fresh milk as inoculums or starter culture which contain millions of ***lactic acid bacteria*** (*lactobacillus and others*). These bacteria grow in milk and multiply at suitable temperature, produce acid that coagulates and partially digest proteins, and converts milk to curd. This also improves its nutritional quality by increasing vitamin B_{12}. *Dahi* is also subsequently used to make the butter and ghee. The bacteria also improve the aroma and flavor of the butter. The lactic acid bacteria in human stomach have a beneficial role in checking disease causing microbes. The microbes are also used to prepare cheese which is an oldest food item.

(iv) The ***industrial fermentation*** by acting on carbohydrates is the important role of bacteria in addition to yeast and moulds. Organic acids (Lactic acid, citric acid, acetic acid, butyric acid, and propionic acid; alcohols (butyl alcohol), acetone; and enzymes are produced by microbes. Acetic acid is produced by a bacterium (*Acetobactor aceti*), butyric acid by another bacterium *clostridium butylicum*, and lactic acid by *lactobacillus* bacterium.

Ethyl alcohol is formed by yeasts while glutamic acid and citric acid are produced by moulds (fungus). Ethanol is produced by yeast (Baker's).

The enzyme ***Streptokinase*** (used as blood clot removers from blood vessels of heart patients) is produced by a bacterium *Streptococcus*.

Cyclosporin, a bioactive molecule produced by a fungus (*trichoderma polysporum*) is used as an immunosuppressive agent in organ-transplant patient. ***Statins*** produced by yeast (*Monascus purpureus*) is used as blood-cholesterol lowering agent by inhibiting the enzyme which synthesizes the cholesterol.

The moistened and kneaded flour (called ***dough***) fermented by bacteria has puffed-up appearance due to production of CO_2 gas and is used to make food items like *dosa* and *idli*. The dough is fermented using baker's yeast (*Saccharomyces cerevisiae*) and used to make *bread*.

The microbes are used to ferment and preparing a number of traditional drinks and foods, to ferment fish, soyabean and bamboo shoots to make foods. The microbes are also used to make fermented ***beverages***. These beverages are wine and beer which are produced without distillation whereas whiskey, brandy malted cereals and fruit juices and to produce ethanol.

Microbes are used to produce ***antibiotics*** which are chemical substances and used to kill or retard the growth of disease- causing microbes. The *anti* is a *Greek* word means *'against'* and *bio* means life. Thus, in context of microbes it means against life while in case of humans and animals the antibiotics are 'pro life' rather than against life. This is most important discovery of last century for the welfare of the human society. The *Penicillin* was the first antibiotic produced as a chance discovery by Alexander Fleming while working with *Staphylococci* bacteria and he observed the growth of a mould (in unwashed culture plate) around which *Staphylococci* could not grow. This was due to a chemical that was found to be produced by the mould *Penicillium notatum* and hence this chemical was named as *penicillin* which checked the growth of *Staphylococci* bacteria and hence acted as antibiotic. Fleming and others (Chain E. and Flory H. who established the full potentiality of penicillin as an effective antibiotic) were awarded Noble Prize in 1945. Later on other antibiotics were also purified from other microbes which are effective in treating diseases like plague, diphtheria (*gal ghotu*), whooping cough (*Kali Khansi*), and leprosy (*kusht rog*).

(v) The microbes are also used as ***biocontrol agents*** in controlling the plant diseases and pests in place of chemicals (insecticides and pesticides) which are toxic affecting human beings and animals as well as polluting the environment and the soil (by use of weedicides).

The aphids and mosquitoes are get rid of by the beetles (ladybird with red and black markings) and Dragonflies, respectively. Another example to control butterfly caterpillars is bacteria *bacillus thuringiensis* (Bt) which is available in sachets as dried spores and can be sprayed after mixing in water on brassicas and fruit trees.

The bacteria Bt toxin genes has been introduced into plants by genetic engineering by which the plants become resistant to insect pests, The Bt-cotton is an example.

The fungus *Trichoderma* species present in root ecosystem are effective agent to control several plant pathogens. Baculoviruses are pathogens to attack on insects and have no negative impact on plants and animals. These are species-specific and thus do not harm the beneficial insects.

(vi) The use of ***biofertilizers*** is the need of the day to reduce pollution by reducing the overuse of chemical fertilizers. The fertilizers are organisms (bacteria, fungi and cynobacteria) that enrich the soil quality. The symbiotic association of *Rhizobium* produces nodules on the roots of leguminous plants and fixe atmospheric nitrogen into organic forms used by plants as nutrient. The nitrogen content of the soil are also enriched by other bacteria like *Azospirillum* and *Azotobacter*.

(vii) The microbes are good source of good protein as ***single cell protein*** (SCP). The ***mushroom*** is a good source of protein, is eaten by the people accepting it as food, and its culture is growing on large scale turning it into an industry. Another microbe is *Spirulina* which can be grown easily on waste material like waste water containing starch produced from potato processing plant, molasses, straw, animal manure and these microbes can be produced on large scale to serve as food rich in protein, fat, carbohydrates, minerals and vitamins. Still another microorganism *Methylophilus methylotropus*, has quick growth and high rate of biomass production, and hence expected to produce protein in large quantity.

12.3 IMPORTANCE OF BACTERIA IN GENETIC STUDIES

Bacteria: The Suitable Material for Genetic Studies

The bacteria and viruses have made significant contributions to the science of genetics. The followings are the advantages to conduct genetic research on bacteria and viruses compared to that on *Drosophila*

- ☆ The bacteria have a short generation interval, some bacteria divide about once every half an hour and hence about 30 generations are produced within 15 hours period(quick reproduction), producing about a billion progeny cells.
- ☆ Secondly, the sexuality in bacteria, short generation interval, less cost involved in producing large population in a small place (10^{10} bacteria in a small culture tube) with less investment, *etc.* made the bacteria as the suitable materials for genetic studies. Thus, the experiments which may not be conducted on large animals can be carried out on bacteria easily with lesser cost and man power.

- Thirdly, the bacteria and viruses have simple structures and physiology and hence more suited for conducting experiment to study fundamental biological processes.
- Finally, it is easy to detect genetic variability in these organisms. These are able to mutate which make easy to analyse complex phenomena. This has made advances in the field of basic genetics.

The bacteria have proved useful and meritorious organism for conducting genetic experimentation and have been made several landmark discoveries to probe the chemical nature of genes and their products, like identification of DNA and RNA as the genetic material, protein synthesis, genetic code and gene regulation studies, fetching Noble prize. The studies on bacteria and viruses have founded the molecular biology.

12.4 ADVANTAGES OF USING BACTERIA IN GENETIC STUDIES

These microorganisms are unicellular having only one set of chromosomes and hence like that of the haploid gamete of the diploid organism. Thus, there is no phenomenon of dominance among alleles because only one allele is present in individual. This makes the study simple due to the fact that each gene will be expressed in phenotype. The study of mutation on these microorganisms is simple and easy because a large population can be grown in small field (petri dish or tube) and the use of selective media can isolate a mutant easily in a million individuals. The microorganisms like virus provide best opportunity to study the gene structure and function at molecular level.

12.5 DISADVANTAGES OF USING BACTERIA IN GENETIC STUDIES

- The first is the relative dearth (scarcity) of regular recombination events. Mostly the mode of reproduction in microorganisms is asexual (vegetative) by amitosis, which is a direct nuclear division, though some sexual reproduction is also known to occur.
- Secondly, the morphological variations in microorganisms are lacking.
- The small body size is also a limiting factor to study the gross phenotypic characteristics of an individual.
- Further, the genetically different clones may respond differently to the nutrients, drugs, pathogens *etc.* in the culture medium. The wild type and mutant strains grow on different culture medium *viz. mutant strains* (auxotrophic) requires supplementation whereas *wild type* grow on minimal medium (prototrophic) containing the basic growth requirements (glucose, sodium citrate, magnesium sulfate and ammonium sulfate required for growth).
- Fifth point is that they are though haploid but most of them are multinucleate. The presence of more nuclei makes delay the expression

of the traits. Due to their small size, the variation may become clear after several recombination events have occurred and hence the population dynamics may be a source of confusion for genetic analysis. Lastly, they also do not have easily visible chromosomes compared to the organism of higher order.

Earlier it was believed that bacteria and virus reproduce asexually and hence these were not considered as suitable materials for conducting genetic studies. Asexual progeny of a single bacterium are genetically identical except mutants and these progenies (produced asexually) are referred to as a clone or colony when grown on a medium like agar plate.

Later on, the work of American scientists Lederberg, J. and Tatum, E.L. (1946) have demonstrated that sexuality exist in bacteria. This discovery proved very important to include bacteria in genetic studies and hence this opened a new area of research in genetics.

12.6 BACTERIAL CELL: PROKARYOTIC CELL

The bacteria are single-celled plant with small cells, sometimes ultramicroscopic, being frequently motile and reproduce normally by transverse or binary fission. Most of the common species belong to the order Eubacterales which is the largest order.

These cells are motile (by means of peritrichous flagella) or non-motile, and not acid-fast. The flagella used for locomotion protrude from an intracellular "basal granule" through the plasma membrane and cell wall. The flagellum is composed of three parts (filament, hook, and basal body).

They are living forms found everywhere in abiotic (air, water, earth) and biotic (animals and plants) ecological habitats of earth. Thus, the respiration may be aerobic or anaerobic. The bacteria are autotrophic or heterotrophic (saprotrophic and parasitic to plants and animals), for their nourishment.

There are ***two types of bacteria*** *viz.* Gran positive and gram negative. These two types are distinguished by a stain (Gram stain, developed by C. Gram in 1884). The gram positive are stained, by the Gram stain and their cell wall contains polysaccharides and mucopeptides (*Pneumococcus, Streptococcus, Bacillus, Clostridium, Mycobacterium,* and *Streptomyces*). The gram negative bacteria are not stained by Gram stain. The cell wall of these bacteria contains additionally an outer layer of lipids, complex with protein and polysaccharides (*Escherichia, Pseudomonas, Salmonella, Vibrio, Rhizobium, Haemophilus,* and *Helicobacter*). However, the cell wall of both the types of bacteria contains murein which can be dissolved by lysozyme.

12.7 BACTERIAL GENETIC: GENETIC MATERIAL OF BACTERIA

The genetic material of bacteria is the DNA mostly present in the main chromosome as well as in the variable number of mini chromosomes, called plasmids and episomes.

12.7.1 Structure of Prokaryotic main Chromosome

The genetic information in bacteria is stored in a single main chromosome carrying a few thousand genes. The DNA molecule is the genetic material of all bacteria. Some RNA is present. The prokaryotic chromosomes (bacterial chromosome) are devoid of nuclear membrane and called as ***nucleoid*** rather than nucleus. There is also no protein and RNA around the DNA molecule like present in eukaryotes.

The hereditary material (DNA) is one large circular chromosome (100 µ long) made up of a circular molecule of double strand DNA and called as bacterial chromosome or nucleoid. The DNA occurs in the ribosome-free cytoplasmic regions of the bacterial cell.

The bacterial chromosome has no protein around the DNA molecule as in case of eukaryotes. The DNA molecule is super coiled which is due to nucleoid proteins and RNA. The length of the circular DNA molecule of the chromosome of bacterium, *Escherichia coli* is about 1500 µm or about 1.5 mm with a diameter of only 1 – 2 µm. The DNA is tightly coiled up in nucleiod in such a way that most of the cytoplasmic particles are excluded but without surrounding the nucleoid by a membrane.

The structure of the functional state of *E.coli* chromosome is that it is 350 µm (circular, unfolded chromosome), 30 µm (folded chromosome of about 40-50 loops), 2 µm (super coiled folded chromosome).The large DNA molecule in the folded genome of circular chromosome of *Escherichia coli* has about 50 or more (about 100) highly twisted or super-coiled loops (domains). Each of these loops is independently negatively super-coiled.

The DNA of *E. coli* has about 4 million nucleotide pairs and molecular weight of 2.8×10^9. The single molecule of DNA of *E.coli* has 3500 to 4000 genes. The DNA is tightly coiled up in nucleiod in such a way that most of the cytoplasmic particles are excluded but without surrounding the nucleoid by a membrane.

The DNA molecule is having highly condensed configuration (super coiled or folded) called as ***folded genome*** which is due to nucleoid proteins and RNA. The DNA is tightly coiled up in nucleiod in such a way that most of the cytoplasmic particles are excluded but without surrounding the nucleoid by a membrane. The chromosome of E. *coli* are seen in a highly condensed state comparable in size to the nucleoid *in vivo,* when isolated in the absence of ionic detergent (so that the bacterial cell does not lyse) and kept in high concentration of cations like polyamines (which is basic or positively charged protein) or in 1M salt, to neutralize the negatively charged phosphate group of DNA. The bacterial chromosome functions in the condensed state. The DNA and RNA are both present in folded genome. These two components can be partially relaxed (cleaved) by treating with enzyme DNase or RNase.

12.7.2 Plasmids and Episomes - Mini-chromosomes

Each bacterial cell besides one large circular chromosome also contains much smaller circular duplex (1 to 20 in number) DNA molecules. These are the variable number of "mini-chromosomes" found in bacterial cell and called as *plasmids* and *episomes*.

(i) Plasmids

These are ***extra-chromosomal*** DNA molecules which are replicating autonomously (self-replicating genetic elements). The plasmids are small, circular, double-stranded DNA molecules. The plasmids are similar to viral DNA in size and replicates in fixed numbers along with the bacterial chromosome. The functions of plasmids vary to the extent that they are incorporated into the host cell chromosome and called ***episomes***, to sometimes their transfer from one bacterial cell to another during conjugation.

The *plasmids* in *E. coli* are of the following three types -

- ***F factors***: These are the fertility (F) factors responsible for transfer of genetic material which have been discussed under conjugation,
- ***R factor***: These are the resistant (R) plasmids which carry genes that make host cells resistant to antibiotics and other antibacterial drugs, and
- ***Col plasmids*** (or colicinogenic factors): They encode proteins (*colicines*) that kill other bacteria (sensitive *E. coli* cells). These are numerous and distinct.

The plasmids may be conjugative or non-conjugative depending upon their ability to provide host cells to conjugate. All the F^+ plasmids, many R plasmids and some Col plasmids are conjugative. Many of the R plasmids due to their conjugative nature are important fot rapidly spreading the antibiotic and drug resistant genes through populations of pathogenic bacteria and this has made a serious medical problem.

(ii) Episomes

F. Jacob and E. Wollman (1958) recognized the unique properties of *F factor* and some other genetic elements which were called as ***episomes.*** The episomes are similar to plasmids and can replicate either autonomously or as part (integrated component) of the main bacterial chromosome. These episomes are not essential to the host. However, the plasmids and episomes are not synonyms. The episomes are those plasmids which can get associated temporarily with nucleoid. Thus, many of the plasmids are not episomes because they do not exist in integrate state. Likewise, many lysogenic phage chromosomes (such as phage lambda genome) are episomes but are not the plastids.

The short DNA sequences of about 800 to 1400 nucleotide pairs long called as *insertion sequences* (*IS* elements) are present in episomes and bacterial chromosomes. These IS elements provide episomes the ability to insert themselves into chromosomes and also to mediate recombination between nonhomologous genetic elements (episomes and chromosomes). The F factor in *E. coli* is an evidence of integration of episomes due to IS elements.

12.8 *E.COLI* – MOST INTENSIVELY STUDIED BACTERIUM

The *Escherichia coli* (*E.coli*) is a bacillus bacterium, a common colon bacterium, and non-pathogenic intestinal parasite of man and other mammals. It has been very much useful to gain our knowledge of molecular genetics, for its rapid proliferation rate and easy to culture. The *E. coli* has been named after its discoverer's name (T. Escherich) and its habitat (presence in human intestine).

The *E. coli* has one major chromosome in circular form. The gentle lysis can loosen the tight DNA meshwork of its nucleiods and its enormous circular duplex molecule has been identified among the liberated DNA in many favourable preparations. Its molecular weight is 2.6 x 10^9 daltons and 1100 *u* length. The E. coli cell, besides having a major chromosome often contain one or more minor chromosomes, which are called as ***plasmids*** and contain 0.5 to 2 per cent of the DNA of the cell. The plasmids exist distinctly from main chromosome and also replicate independently of the major chromosome. Thus more than one genetic element is transmitted from parent to offspring in E. coli. This bacterium though reproduce asexually, but still there are a number of sources by which there is genetic exchange from one bacterial cell to the other *i.e.* DNA from one bacterial cell can undergo genetic exchange with the DNA from another bacterial cell. E.coli synthesizes all necessary vitamins and amino acids required for growth (auxotroph strain). However, there are also some strains of E.coli which may not grow on minimal medium and need addition of some particular vitamin or amino acid which they may not synthesize (prototroph strain).

Each bacterium divides and grows exponentially. The bacteria may grow in liquid as well as in semisolid medium containing agar. They require aeration to grow in liquid medium. As a result of bacterial growth a visible colony of each bacterium is produced on the surface of the medium. It is to see that each bacterial species has its specific colour and morphology. The mutation results into another strain and hence the colour or morphology or both clolour and morphology of colony may be changed. The numbers of bacteria used to grow the colonies are used to estimate the number of bacteria that were initially present in the suspension put on the agar plate. Not only this but also the mutation may change the growth rate as well as the morphology of the bacterium. The mutants with slow growth rate produce small colonies called petite.

The ***wild-type E. coli*** have the following characteristics -

- ☆ *Energy source of bacteria:* They use any sugar in the medium as a source of energy,
- ☆ *Synthesis process:* They can synthesize the essential metabolites (purines, pyrimidines, amino acids, vitamins, *etc.*) and do not require in the growing media an energy source and some inorganic salts.
- ☆ *Prototroph bacteria:* Such bacteria of wild-type that can grow on minimal medium are known as ***prototrops,***
- ☆ *Susceptible bacteria:* The antibiotics like ampicillin, tetracycline, *etc.* were invented to kill bacteria.

12.9 MUTATION IN BACTERIA

The mutation (genetic change) occurs in wild-type *E. coli*. The ***mutant types E. coli*** have the following characteristics:

- *Energy sources for mutants:* Some mutants cannot utilize the milk sugar (lactose) like wild-types but they require another medium containing lactose, some other mutants are unable to use galactose, some other mutations are those that are unable to grow on arabinose.
- *Mutant bacteria nomenclature:* The mutant types of bacteria are described using three-letter abbreviations. In describing the phenotype of bacteria, the first letter is kept of upper case while for genotypes all the letters are of lower case. For example, the wild-type *E. coli* is able to use lactose as an energy source and hence its phenotype is written as Lac + and genotype as lac^{+}. On the contrary, the phenotype of the mutant type of *E. coli* that is unable to use lactose as energy source is written as Lac^{-} and genotype as lac^{-} or simply *lac.*
- *Lack of synthetic process in mutants:* The mutant bacteria cannot grow on minimal medium and need addition of metabolites (auxiliary nutrients) in their medium for their growth because they cannot synthesize the auxiliary nutrients.
- *Auxotroph mutants:* These mutant type bacteria that require additional metabolites for their growth are known as ***auxotrophs.*** The example is of the requirement of the amino acid *tryptophan.* Wild-type *E. coli* can synthesize this amino acid but the mutant cannot. Therefore, *E. coli* that are prototrophs are designated as Trp^{+} phenotypically and trp^{+} genotypically. The mutant type that are tryptophan autotrophs are written phenotypically as Trp^{-} and genotypically as trp^{-}.
- *Resistant mutants:* The genetic change in gene (mutation) occurred. This change makes the bacteria resistant to the antibiotics. The bacteria with this mutant allele can grow on media containing antibiotics. The mutant allele which is resistant to the drugs acts dominant selectable marker.

12.10 GENETIC EXCHANGE MECHANISM IN BACTERIA

In diploid organisms of higher order, there are a number of mechanisms by which the genetic variations are produced *viz.* genes in pairs, multiple alleles, number of gene loci, gene action, mutation and chromosomal aberration, genetic recombination (segregation and crossing over), sex controlled genes and extra chromosomal variation, *etc.* In case of bacteria, the genetic recombination is important.

The most bacteria reproduce asexually which is accomplished by *amitosis* and often called as *binary fission.* The mutant cell can be detected by use of selective media in a colony of millions of bacteria grown in liquid media and then distributed over an agar plate. The mutant strain of bacteria resistant to streptomycin (antibiotic) can be detected in a way that all cells without mutation will be sensitive to antibiotic and hence will not grow but the antibiotic resistant mutant will form a colony. The spontaneous mutations occur in bacteria.

Gene Transfer in Bacteria

The gene transfer in bacteria is unidirectional. The genes are transferred from donor cell to a recipient cell and this gene transfer is not in a reverse way from recipient to donor cell, whereas in case of eukaryotes there is reciprocal exchange of genes during meiosis and hence bidirectional. In case of bacteria, a fragment of one chromosome from the donor cell is combined with a complete chromosome in a recipient cell instead of the gene exchange between two complete chromosomes, as in case of eukaryotes.

Genetic Recombination Mechanisms in Bacteria

The bacteria do not reproduce sexually but the genetic recombination in bacteria is very important in their evolution like the recombination events of crossing over and independent assortment as an integral part of sexual reproduction in eukaryotes. The work conducted on *E. coli* concluded that bacteria exhibit sexual differentiation behaving like the male and female gametes of higher orders.

Some mechanisms for exchanging the genetic information have been evolved which enable to produce the recombinant combinations of genes in bacteria. This is the *genetic recombination* which means bringing together of genetic material of two bacterial cells. In this process, the genetic material of one bacterial cell goes to other bacterial cell. There are three different mechanisms (*transformation, transduction,* and *conjugation*) through which the bacteria exchange the genetic material from one bacterium to another. These mechanisms are called ***para-sexual*** processes, akin to sexual reproduction and occur as one of the following ways:

12.10.1 Transformation – Uptake of Free DNA by Bacteria

- to make a change. It is recombination of naked DNA molecule from one bacterial strain to another to produce new phenotype.

The *genetic transformation* is the genetic change of an organism brought about by the incorporation of foreign DNA into cells. The genetic material of one bacterial cell moves into another bacterial cell by some unknown mechanism. This is called transformation as it converts one type of bacterium into another type like non-capsulated to capsulated form.

The phenomenon of bacterial transformation was discovered by Griffith (1928) in *Diplococcus pneumonia.* Thus, it is also called as ***Griffith effect.*** This refers to the genetic change in the properties of one bacterium mediated by soluble DNA from another bacterium. The avirulent type bacteria (type II R - with no polysaccharide capsule around the bacterial cell producing small and rough colony) are transformed into virulent type III S (with a capsule and producing large and smooth colony). The *transformation* occurs when the living bacterial cells take up the fragments of DNA released by dead cells (naked DNA or free DNA molecule). The dead cells are donor cells and the living bacterium cell is the recipient cell.

The transformation of avirulent form into virulent form was shown by Griffth (1928) by conducting experiments on *Streptococcus pneumonia* (Pneumococci). These pneumococci had genetic variability showing different phenotype. He injected virulent heat-killed Type III S pneumococci (thus these were avirulent due to heat treatment) plus avirulent live Type II R pneumococci into mice. The result was that the mice were died of pneumonia and live type III S cells with Type III polysaccharide capsules recovered. Thus virulence was observed. But when mice were injected with heat killed Type III S pneumococci alone, the result was no death of mice. These results have indicated that the transformation of avirulent Type II R cells to virulent Type III S cells was not due to the mutation but it was due to the transformation (conversion) of some dead Type III S cells (heat killed) from living Type II R cells (avirulent) into Type III S cells (virulent).

The result of these two experiments can be shown as under:

(a) Mice injected with virulent but heat killed Type III S (avirulent) + avirulent live Type II R

Result = mice died with recovery of live Type III S cells containing capsule

= virulence was observed

= Avirulent living Type II R cells were transformed to virulent Type III S because of the presence of dead Type III S cells genetic material (DNA).

(b) Mice injected with heat killed (avirulent) Type III S alone

Result = no death of mice because of no alternate of transformation of dead Type III cells (avirulent) to virulent form.

This process of transformation does not require cell contact and secondly, the process is sensitive to deoxyribonuclease (DNase), an enzyme that degrades DNA. Thus, the living cells have additional DNA showing additional characteristics (Griffith, 1928). This provides new combination of genes and produce new phenotype.

12.10.2 Conjugation – Contact of Donor Cell to a Recipient Cell

Requires cell contact.

It is the unidirectional transfer of DNA from F^+ bacterial cell to F^- bacterial cell through cytoplasmic bridge.

The transformation does not occur in *E.coli* under natural conditions. The gene transfer between *E. coli* cells is by another mechanism called as *conjugation* which means to unite two bacterial cells sexually. The conjugation in *E. coli* is one way transfer of genetic material from a donor (male cell) to a recipient (female cell). The DNA is transferred through a specialized intercellular conjugation channel formed between donor and recipient cells. It thus requires cell contact, though it is not sensitive to DNase to degrade the DNA.

This is the unidirectional transfer of DNA from donor bacterium having sex pilli and F factor (F^+ bacterial cell) to recipient bacterium lacking both sex pilli and F factor (F^- bacterial cell). This type of bacterial recombination was first demonstrated by J. Lederberg and E. Tatum (1946) in *E. coli.* In the process of conjugation, two bacterial cells come in contact physically and the genetic material (DNA) of one bacterial cell moves to another cell through conjugation tube formed by sex pilli.

The experiment was conducted on two mutant strains of E.coli which were biochemically or nutritionally deficient unable to grow on minimal medium because both the strains had one or more mutation in nutritional genes that control synthesis of certain growth substances. One strain (A) was deficient in vitamin biotin (B-) and amino acid methionine (M-) and hence unable to synthesize them but able to synthesize the amino acid threonine (T+) and leucine (L+) and vitamin B_1 (B_{1+}). The other strain (B) was able to synthesize vitamin biotin (B+) and amino acid methionine (M+) but unable to synthesize amino acids (Thereonine, T-; leucine, L-) and vitamin B_1 (B_1-). The genotypes of the two strains can be written as under:

Strain A: $B^- M^- T^+ L^+ B_1^+$

Strain B: $B^+ M^+ T^- L^- B_1^-$

The + and – sign indicates the presence or absence of particular gene responsible for synthesizing or not synthesizing the particular vitamin or amino acid.

Both the strains were cultured on complete medium having glucose, yeast extract and peptone. The suspensions of the washed cells after one or two generations were placed on minimal medium. It was found that most of the cells failed to grow (multiply) and only a few cells had grown. It was thus postulated that these cells which grew were waild type with all the genes dominant ($B^+ M^+ T^+ L^+ B_1^+$) and were formed due to recombination of genes from the two mutant strains.

Under *conjugation,* the F^+ means male factor (donor strain possessing sex factor or fertility factor, or f factor) containing genes for maleness. The F^+ strain transfers their genetic material to F^- bacterial cell and change them to F^+. The F^- represents the female strain or recipient without f-factor. The sex factor is composed of DNA containing about 100 genes, is autonomous and self replicating, the replication being rapid than the bacterial chromosome. Usually one f-factor is present per male bacterial cell and F^+ male cells can be changed to F^- female cell by losing f-factor. The conjugation is like uniting sexually and it occurs between f+ and F- strains in which the F factor from F^+ donor is transferred to F^- recipient cell producing all the daughter bacterial cells as F^+. The F factors that contain chromosomal genes (F^+ factors) are transferred to F^- cells by sexduction. The transfer of F^+ factors to recipient cell (F^-) is called sexduction.

The integration of F^+ factor is mediated by short DNA sequences which are present in multiple copies in both F factor and the bacterial chromosome. Thus F^+ factors integrate in bacterial chromosome at many different sites and such a bacterial cell that carries an integrated F factors is called an **Hfr cell** (high frequency recombination).

The conjugation is used for genetic mapping in bacterial species and it is valuable in genetic research.

12.10.3 Transduction – Exchange of DNA from One Bacterium to another through Virus (Bacteriophage)

The phenomenon of transduction is another mode of gene transfer in bacteria and this was discovered by Zinder and Lederberg (1952) in *Salmonella typhimurium*. The *transduction* is also the unidirectional genetic exchange in bacteria. This is a process of genetic recombination (transfer of genetic material of one bacterial cell to other bacterial cell) in bacteria which is mediated by *bacteriophage*. The bacterial DNA is injected by a phage into a bacterium, but it does not replicate. It neither require cell contact nor sensitive to DNase for degradation of DNA.

Two auxotrophic strains of *Salmonella typhimurium* requiring amino acid supplements in their growing medium were selected by Lederberg and Zinder (1952). One strain needed phenylalanine, tryptophan, and tyrosine while other strain needed methionine and histidine to grow. They grew both the strains together and observed rare prototrophs. Secondly, the prototroph bacteria were also produced on growing the strains in medium containing DNase. The appearance of the prototroph strain proved that there was gene exchange. This gene exchange did not require cell contact and hence ruled out the mechanism of conjugation and the insensitivity to DNase ruled out the transformation of gene exchange mechanism. It was observed later on that one strain was infected with a virus (bacteriophage P 22) through which the genes were carried from one strain (donor) to another strain (recipient). Therefore, the recombination occurred between the bacterial DNA (carried by the virus) and the DNA of the recipient cell.

The transduction occurs by carrying the fragments of DNA from one bacterial cell (donor cell) to other cell (recipient cell) through bacterial virus (*bacteriophage*). The bacteriophage attacking the bacteria injects its DNA into bacterial cell. The bacterial DNA breaks down and the viral DNA replicates within the bacterium. The lysis of bacterial cell liberates the phages carrying bacterial DNA. The phage carrying bacterial DNA infects other bacterial cells. The viral DNA, which is the donor of genetic information, is incorporated into bacterial DNA (recipient bacterium) and thus provides new combination of genes.

In this process of transduction, the bacteriophage transports the bacterial gene from one cell to another and hence called ***transduction***. The phage particles that contain bacterial DNA are called *transducting particles* which may be generalized transducting particles (containing only the bacterial DNA) and specialized transducting particles (containing both bacterial and phage DNA). The P22 in *Salmonella* and P1 in *E. coli* are the generalized transducting phages whereas the bacterophage lambda is the specialized transducting phage that carries only the *gal* and *bio* genes from one *E. coli* cell to another. The *gal* genes stands for the gene that is required for the utilization of galactose as an energy source while the *bio* stands for the gene essential for the synthesis of biotin.

There is also the simultaneous transduction of two different genetic markers to a single recipient cell. This is called ***co-transductions***. The frequency of co-transduction of any two markers is inversely related to the distance between them on chromosome.

12.11 DISTINCTION AMONG THREE PARA-SEXUAL PROCESSES

In view of the above findings, the three parasexual processes can be distinguished on the two criteria *viz.*

- ✰ Whether the process requires the cell contact (donor and recipient cell), and
- ✰ Whether the process is sensitive to DNase that degrades the DNA.

Only the process conjugation requires cell contact and the transformation is the only process that is sensitive to DNase which degrades the DNA.

It is easy to test these two criteria. The cell contact between donor and recipient cell is tested by growing bacteria of different genotypes in opposite arms of U – tube. The U – tube is separated by a glass filter that prevents contact between two different genotypes of bacteria. The glass filter contains pores so as the DNA molecules and viruses pass through this filter but the bacteria cannot pass through. The occurrence of gene transfers between the bacteria in opposite arms of U – tube rule out the possibility of conjugation because the conjugation requires direct contact between donor and recipient cells.

Transformation: Uptake of free DNA by bacteria.

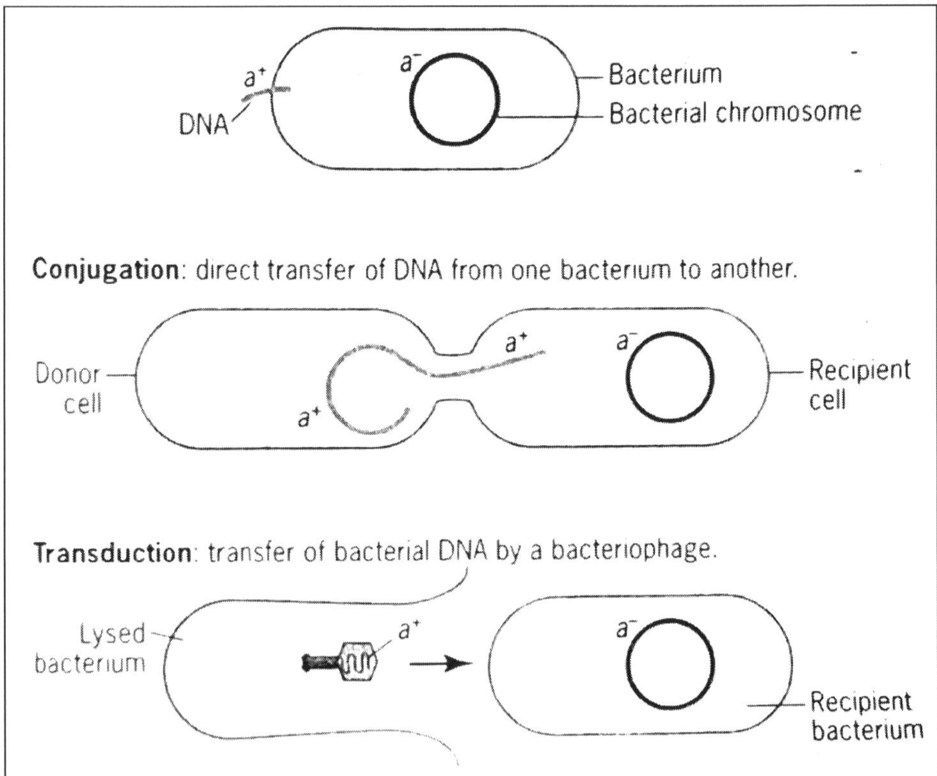

Figure 12.1: Comparision of Three Processes of Genetic Recombination.

The test of sensitivity to DNase is carried out by adding the enzyme DNase to the growing medium of bacteria. If there is no transfer of genes, the process indicates the degradation of DNA and hence ***transformatio***n. There is no gene left for transfer because the DNA of donor cell is degraded by DNase.

In other two processes of conjugation and transduction the degradation of DNA of donor cell is protected. This protection is provided by the protein coats of bacteriophage during transduction whereas the bacterial cell walls and membranes protect the donor DNA from DNase during conjugation.

The process involves ***transduction*** if there is occurrence of gene transfer in the presence of DNase and in the absence of cell contact.

The ***conjugation*** is indicated when the gene transfer occurs in the presence of DNase (means no degradation of DNA of donor cell) while in contact of recipient cell. Thus during conjugation there is cell contact but there is no degradation of DNA of donor cell by DNase.

Transformation: Uptake of free DNA

The three parasexual mechanisms of gene exchange in bacteria based on above two criteria may be shown in a tabular form as under:

		I. Criterion *(Cell contact)*:	
II. Criterion		Yes (required)	No (not required)
Sensitive to DNase (degradation of donor DNA)	Yes	- - -	***Transformation*** *(degradation)*
	No	***Conjugation*** *(Unite sexually) Or cell fusion*	***Transduction*** *(Transport through virus)*

The gene exchange does not occur by all the above mentioned three parasexual processes in all the bacterial species, except probably the transduction. The occurrence of transformation and conjugation depends on the evolution of genes and metabolic machinery in the bacterial species. The transformation does not occur in *E. coli* under natural conditions because this species of bacteria (*E. coli*) does not contain the genes that synthesize proteins required to take up free DNA (requirement of transformation). The gene transfer in *E. coli* occurs through conjugation and transduction.

Cyanobacteria

At present there are 24 cynobacteria for which a total genome sequences are available. The marine environment contains 15 of these cyanobacteria. Several studies have demonstrated how these sequences could be used very successfully to infer important ecological and physiological characteristics of marine cyanobacteria.

However, there are many more genome projects currently in progress. Thus, the growing body of genome information can also be tapped in a more general way to address global problems by applying a comparative approach. Some new and exciting examples of progress in this field are the identification of genes for regulatory RNAs, insights into the evolutionary origin of photosynthesis, or estimation of the contribution of horizontal gene transfer to the genomes that have been analyzed.

12.12 ENZYMES OF BACTERIA

The ***enzyme*** is a protein that accelerates a specific chemical reaction in a living system. Such enzyme which accelerates a reaction is called as a ***catalyst.*** Thus, the protein which acts as a catalyst is known as enzyme. The catalyst is an agent that accelerates a chemical reaction without itself being used up or destroyed. Therefore, a catalyst (enzyme) may be recovered practically unchanged (active condition) at the end of the reaction. The ***catalysis*** may be defined as the acceleration of a chemical reaction produced by the presence of a catalyst. An enzyme acts by catalysis which means that an enzyme increases the velocity of a chemical reaction without itself being permanently changed.

An ***enzyme or ferment*** is a thermolabile organic catalyst elaborated by a living cell and capable of functioning independently of the cell. Every living cell may be considered a gross catalyst. It converts nutrients to waste products and obtains energy.

The photosynthetic reaction occurring in green plants utilizes solar energy, 6 CO_2 and 6 H_2O to produce carbohydrates ($C_6H_{12}O_6$) and oxygen (6 O_2). The reverse to this reaction occurs in animals, plants, and microorganisms.

The enzymes possess the properties of proteins. The enzymes are classified according to their action. The general names have been given for groups of enzymes *viz.* proteases, oxidases, nucleases, esterases, and dehydrogenases. It is customary to name the enzyme after the substance acted upon adding the suffix – ase with some exceptions like rennin, pepsin, and trypsin. The lysozyme is an enzyme present in nasal mucus and lyses many bacteria. It is also present in egg white.

12.13 VIRUSES

The *virus* was discovered in 1899 by Beijrnick, M.W. The virus has been taken from Latin word, venom or poisonous fluid. The viruses demarket a line between the living and the nonliving. These are the non-living, inert, and acellular particles outside the host cell. They are regarded as a living chemical, lacking their own enzyme systems, depend on host cell for all metabolic activities, multiply only inside the living cells, and are obligatory intracellular parasites. In classifying the organisms the viruses have been placed in the order virales of class *microtatobiotes* of the division *Protophyta* of ***plant kingdom.***

The viruses are considered as living on the basis of the criteria that they reproduce and transmit their genes to progeny viruses. They utilize energy provided by host cells and respond to environmental and cellular signals like other living organisms. On the other hand, they are considered non-living because they are obligate parasites, can reproduce only in appropriate host cells, and have no free life.

The biologists consider the viruses as individual cells. However, at the same time, the *viruses* have been considered as an exception to the cell theory. The THV (Tobacco mosaic virus) can be taken as an example. This virus can be crystallized and stored for years, and it does not show any property of living systems, *viz.* reproduction, growth and development, utilization of energy, and response to environmental stimuli. However, TMV exhibit the properties of living systems when a liquid suspension containing TMV comes in contact of living system (tobacco leaves). The virus in suspension infects the cells, reproduce, utilize energy, and respond to cellular signals.

The viruses are smallest organism consisting of nucleic acid (DNA or RNA) as central core and protein coat called capsid. They exist as the replicating nucleic acid molecules devoid of capsid inside the host cell. The viruses can be crystallized like inorganic or organic compounds.

There are also some other organisms which do not fit in cell theory. For example, the living substance in Paramecium (protozoa), Rhizopus (fungus) and Vaucheria (alga) is enclosed in a wall and there is no organization like that of the cell.

The *virus* is a unicellular (single unit of body), ultramicroscopic and infectious particle (pathogenic agent). The viruses are capable of passing filters to which the bacteria cannot, typically of small size of < 0.1 μ in diameter except for a few pox viruses. They are transmitted by infection and replicated only within the specific cells (host cell). Thus, the viruses are etiological agents of diseases. They cause a number of diseases in man, animals and plants, besides bacterial virus known as *bacteriophage* which parasitizes the bacterial cell. The viruses have parasitic mode of existence (living). They are obligate parasites that can only reproduce after infecting living host cells.

The virus following infection causes cell ***lysis*** which is the bursting of a cell by the destruction of the cell wall. A virus (phage) that destroys the host (bacteria) cell is called ***virulent phage***. On the contrary, a phage (virus) that invades but may not destroy (lyse) the host (bacterial cell) is called ***temperate phage.*** However, subsequently it may enter the lytic cycle. The bacteria harbouring temperate bacteriophages are called ***lysogenic bacteria.*** The genome of a temperate bacteriophage intergrated into the chromosome of a lysogenic bacterium and replicated along with the host chromosome is called ***prophage*** or ***provirus*** (viral chromosome that has integrated into a host genome).

According to the parasitic mode of existence, the viruses have been given the names after the host cell to which they parasitize *viz.*

- ☆ Plant viruses (parasitizing the plant cell),
- ☆ Animal viruses,
- ☆ Fungal viruses,
- ☆ Bacterial viruses, called as *Bacteriphage* (parasitizing bacteria), and
- ☆ *Cynophages* (parasite to blue green algae).

The virus is an ideal research tool for genetic analysis. The viruses have two major advantages over the cellular and multicellular organisms. The first is their structural simplicity, having only a single chromosome with a relatively small number of genes compared to more complicated eukaryotic systems. The second is their short life cycle of about 20 minutes to a few hours.

The experiments conducted on viruses have given evidence that genetic information is stored in DNA and RNA. The viruses have also been used in experiments to elucidate the mechanisms of DNA replication, transcription, and translation.

12.14 VIRAL CHROMOSOME

The viruses are the simplest forms of life, have only one type of nucleic acid either DNA or RNA, called as ***viral chromosome***, and enclosed in a coat of protein molecule (capsid). The viral chromosome may be single stranded or double stranded.

The nucleic acid of virus and bacteriophage occurs as a single molecule of DNA or RNA (single set of genes in a single chromosome – monoploid, like bacteria) which is either linear or circular formed by 1000 to 250,000 nucleotides. The viral chromosome may be single-stranded or double stranded.

However, the viruses have no plasma membrane, cytoplasm and nucleus as well as no energy yielding and no synthetic enzyme system, and their metabolic activities depend on host cell. Therefore, viruses cannot live a free mode of life but lead a ***parasitic mode of existence,*** as intra-cellular parasites of specific host (animals, plants and bacteria) and cause damage to the cellular structure of the host. The viruses can multiply only in the living cells of the host.

There are only 4 genes in the RNA of smallest virus (bacteriophage MS2) consisting 3569 nucleotides. There are some other smallest DNA viruses having 9 to 11 genes. The chromosome of another bacteriophage (X 174) contains DNA molecule having 11 genes with 5386 nucleotides. The largest DNA viruses (bacteriophage T2, pox virus of animals) contain about 150 genes, and the phage T4 have about 200 genes. The DNA molecules of viruses are organized into negatively super-coiled loops.

The size and structure of the genomes of some viruses are as under:

Type and Name	*Molecular Weight ($x\ 10^{-6}$ daltons)*	*Approx. No. of Genes*
Linear single stranded RNA:		
(i) Potato spindle tuber virus	0.025 – 0.11	< 1
(ii) Polio virus	2.6	4
(iii) Influenza virus	3.6	12
(iv) Mouse leukemia virus	11.2	37
Linear double stranded DNA:		
(v) Reovirus	15	25
(vi) Adinivirus type 12	21	38
(vii) Herpes simplex	96	160

Type and Name	*Molecular Weight (x 10^{-6} daltons)*	*Approx. No. of Genes*
Circular single stranded DNA:		
(viii) x 174 coliphage	1.7	6
Circular double-stranded DNA:		
(ix) Polyoma virus	3.0	5
(x) SV 40 virus	3.2	6

12.15 BACTERIOPHAGES

The viruses also infect bacteria and such viruses are called ***bacteriophages*** (Greek word meaning "to eat bacteria"). Felix D'Herelle (1917) used the term bacteriophage. Bacteriophages have played and continue to play a key role in bacterial genetics and molecular biology. The *bacteriophages* had been the best experimental materials for molecular genetics, such as discovery of DNA as the carrier of genetic information, discovery of genetic code and protein synthesis mechanism. Delbruck, Lauria, Hershey (1940) discovered genetic recombination in phages.

Historically, they were used to define gene structure and gene regulation. Also the first genome to be sequenced was of a bacteriophage. However, bacteriophage research did not lead the genomics revolution, which is clearly dominated by bacterial genomics. Only very recently has the study of bacteriophage genomes become prominent, thereby enabling researchers to understand the mechanisms underlying phage evolution. Bacteriophage genome sequences can be obtained through direct sequencing of isolated bacteriophages, but can also be derived as part of microbial genomes. Analysis of bacterial genomes has shown that a substantial amount of microbial DNA consists of prophage sequences and prophage-like elements. A detailed database mining of these sequences offers insights into the role of prophages in shaping the bacterial genome.

The bacteriophages are of two types based on their lifestyle in the infected cells *viz.* virulent and temperate. The most important bacteriophages played the roles to elucidate genetic concepts had been bacteriophage T4 (phage T4) and bacteriophage lambda. Both these viruses infect the *E. coli* (colon bacillus) and hence called coliphage. Phage T4 is a virulent page, produces progeny using the metabolic machinery of host cell, and kills the host during this process. The bacteriophage lambda is a temperate phage that infects also to the *E. coli.* The bacteriophage lambda either kills the host cell or integrates in the host genome and replicated along with the host cell's genome in each cell division.

(i) Bacteriophage T4

It is a lytic phage (virulent phage) virus that infect *E. coli*, reproduces (replicates) and lyses (kills) the host cell. This is a large virus having a double-stranded DNA molecule which is packed in a proteinaceous head. Thus, the DNA is present inside head. It is about 168,800 bp long containing about 150 characterized genes with many more uncharacterized. The page DNA is injected into the bacterium through central hollow core of phage.

The phage is mainly divided into head and tail. Whereas the head of phage contains its DNA, the tail of the virus has many components to help the phage to infect the *E. coli.* These components include the *central hollow core* that forms a channel for entry of phage DNA into the bacterial cell, *tail sheath* to function as small muscle and pushing the tail core through the bacterial cell wall, 6 *tail fibers* to help in locating receptors on host cell, and *tail pins* on the base plate to attach firmly to the receptors.

The phage DNA within 2 minutes of infecting the host cell stops all the functions of bacterial genes (transcription, translation, and replication) and takes over the control of the metabolic machinery of the host. The host DNA is degraded by the enzyme nucleases encoded by the phage genes and the replication of phage DNA is initiated by some phage proteins and produces about 300 progeny in each infected cell. After about 17 minutes of infection, the assembly of progeny phage begins and starts accumulating in the host cell. An enzyme *lysozyme* encoded by the phage about 25 minutes of infection degrades the bacterial cell wall for its rupture and about 300 progeny phage from each infected cell are released.

It is very interesting that the phage DNA is synthesized by the degraded products that are produced through the degradation of host DNA by nucleases encoded by T4 phage. But at the same time, the enzyme nuclease does not degrade the viral DNA. This is because the base cytosine of T4 phage DNA contains an additional CH_2OH group attach to one of the atom of cytosine molecule and converting the cytosine into 5-bromo-hydroxymethylcytosine (MHC) as well as the derivatives of glucose molecules are also attached to the MHC. The phage DNA is protected from being degraded by nucleases due to this modification.

(ii) Bacteriophage Lambda (λ)

The bacteriophage lambda (λ) was discovered by Andre Lwoff who shared the 1965 Noble Prize in Physiology or Medicine. This virus is smaller than phage T4. Bacteriophage lambda contains a single linear molecule of DNA only 17.5 μm long. The phage lambda chromosome has three forms *viz.* linear chromosome, hydrogen-bonded circular form, and covalently closed circular form.

The phage lambda chromosome is unusual to have a single-stranded region, 12 nucleotides long, at the 5′ end of each complementary strand. The 12 nucleotides single stranded cohesive ends of linear phage lambda chromosome are:

3′ G..................CCCCGCCGCTGGA 5′

5′ GGGCGGCGACCTC..................G 3′

These single stranded ends, called *cohesive* or *sticky ends* are complementary to each other. The cohesive ends being complementary, base pair to form a hydrogen-bonded circular structure.

Its genome has a double stranded molecule of 48,502 bp long containing about 50 genes. The DNA molecule is linear packaged in the lambda head. But this lambda DNA gets converted into circular form of DNA after injecting into a host cell (*E. coli*). This conversion from the hydrogen-bonded circular form to the covalently closed circular form occurs prior to replicating in the host cell and the conversion is catalyzed by DNA *ligase* that seals single-strand breaks in DNA double helices.

One of the features of lambda chromosome is its differentiation into regions containing high concentrations of adenine and thymine (AT-rich regions) and also the regions containing large amounts of guanine and cytosine (GC-rich regions). There are very few segments with high AT content. These AT clusters had been used as physical markers by Maria Schnos and Ross Inman (1960s).

This virus as the circular lambda chromosome after entering into host cell adapts either of the two pathway *viz.* as a lytic pathway to reproduce and lyse the host cell by encoding the enzyme like the bacteriophage T4 or it may enter a lysogenic pathway by inserting into the bacterial chromosome where it is replicated along with host chromosome. The lambda chromosome is called a prophage in its integrated state and its lytic genes are kept turned off to continue this state. This means that the genes of the prophage are not expressed and hence do not encode the products required in lytic pathway *viz.* the enzymes (involved in the replication of phage DNA), structural proteins (involved in phage morphogenesis), and lysozyme (involved in catalyzing the cell lysis).

It is interesting that the lambda prophage after every 10^5 cell divisions is spontaneously excised from the host chromosome by two enzymes (integrase and excisase) and entered the lytic pathway. Thus, the prophage is said in a *lysogenic* state capable to cause lysis.

Chapter 13

Structure of Genetic Material: Nucleic Acids (DNA and RNA)

The classical genetics has shown the transmission of genetic information by genes and their pattern of inheritance providing the *chromosomal theory of heredity* but could not provide information about the molecular structure of genes. The study of *molecular structure of genetic material and its functions* to carry out the phenotypic expression of characters is called the ***molecular genetics.***

The foundation of the molecular genetics dates back to the discovery of nucleic acids by Miescher in 1868, almost with or soon after the theory of evolution based on natural selection and theory of pangenesis proposed by Charles Darwin in 1859 and Mendelian discovery in 1866 formulating the *laws of heredity* and a base to the classical genetics. The molecular genetics is rooted in the discovery of Johann Friedrich Miescher (1844-1895), a young Swiss medical student who discovered (1868) in the human pus cells, the acidic substance to which he called ***"nuclein"***, now called ***nucleic acid.***

However, this acidic substance, nuclein (nucleic acid) could get importance only after the documentation of the presence of polynucleotide chains of the nucleic acid in 1940s (Levene, 1869-1940). The role of nucleic acid in storing and transmitting genetic information was discovered by Avery *et al.* (1944) and the double helical structure of DNA was discovered by Watson and Crick (1953).

13.1 EVIDENCE OF GENETIC MATERIAL (NUCLEIC ACIDS)

The chromosomes, known as hereditary vehicles, are chemically composed mainly of large organic molecules (macromolecules) called as ***nucleoproteins*** which are composed of nucleic acids (DNA and RNA) and proteins, although other chemical constituents are present. The large DNA units in association with proteins can be stained with dyes and visualized in the light microscope as chromosomes.

Earlier, it was thought that one of the two component parts of nucleoproteins (protein + nucleic acid) should be the genetic material. Thus, there had been controversy about the proteins or the nucleic acids as the genetic material. The genetic information in all the living systems (organisms) is stored in DNA, except the RNA virus. The DNA is usually double-stranded while RNA is usually single-stranded. The double-stranded DNA molecule is formed by pairing adenine base with thymine and guanine with cytosine. The RNA contains the base uracil in place of thymine.

The information in favour of nucleic acids as the the genetic materials comes from the indirect evidences as well as from the experiments conducted.

13.1.1 Indirect Evidences from Comparisons

Some of the indirect evidences in favour of the nucleic acids, particularly the DNA as the genetic material compared to RNA and proteins, though these do not prove, are as under:

- ☆ The DNA in most of the amount is present in the chromosomes whereas the RNA and proteins are also present in abundant amount in the cytoplasm,
- ☆ All the cells of an organism have the same molecular composition of DNA but it does not hold true for RNA and proteins whose composition is highly variable among cell types. Further, the composition of DNA is same in all the organisms of a species but different in the other species,
- ☆ The amount of DNA present in the cell has positive and precise correlation with the number of sets of chromosomes per cell. There is corresponding increase in the amount of DNA of the cells of polyploids,
- ☆ The somatic cells of diploid organisms contain twice the amount of DNA than haploid cells (gamete) of the species concerned. The gametes (haploid reproductive cells) contain half the amount of DNA present in the mother cells or somatic cells. The fertilization (Union of male and female gamete – zygote formation) makes the amount of DNA double in zygote equal to the amount of DNA present in somatic cells, and
- ☆ The DNA is more stable compared to RNA and protein, and this stable property of genetic material is essential to store and transmit the information generation by generation. The integrity of DNA is maintained during cell metabolism except during mutation. The mutagenic agents change the chemical structure of DNA.

13.1.2 Direct Evidences from Experiments

The experiments have clearly established that the genetic material (having genetic information) is present in nucleic acids and not in proteins. The nucleic acid is of two type *viz. Deoxyribonucleic acid* (*DNA*) and the *Ribonucleic acid* (*RNA*) as per details in next section, 13.2. The DNA is the genetic material in eukaryotes and prokaryotes whereas the genetic material is RNA in some viruses. Molecular biologists conducted experiments on bacteria, bacteriophage and virus to get proof of genetic material.

(1) DNA is Genetic Material Based on Bacterial Recombination

The experiments conducted by various groups of scientists (molecular biologists) had provided direct evidence of DNA in its favour as the genetic material. Three groups of scientists had conducted experiments on bacteria in 1928, 1931, and 1944 by repeating the earlier experiment. The details of these experiments are as under -

Bacterial transformation, bacterial recombination, transduction and bacteriophage infection have provided direct evidence that DNA is the genetic material.

I. Bacterial Transformation

The results of three groups of molecular biologists in favour of DNA as the genetic material are given here as under -

(*i*) ***F. Griffith* (1928)**, bacteriologist in England, conducted an experiment on mice. He injected in mice a mixture of the following two strains of bacteria, pneumococcus (pneumonia causing bacteria):

- ☆ One strain was S-III which was *pathogenic* (**virulent**) when alive but lost the infectivity due to their heat killing.
- ☆ Second strain was R-II which was *non-pathogenic* (***avirulent***) and alive.

Many mice developed pneumonia and died, and type S – III cells were found in the dead body of mice. This showed that heat killed virulent bacteria (S-III) has caused transformation of non-pathogenic bacteria (R-II) into pathogenic (virulent) bacteria. This phenomenon of transferring the character (virulence) of the virulent but heat killed strain (S-III) into another strain (non-virulent, R-II) by using a DNA extract of virulent strain (S-III) was called as *bacterial transformation* or *Griffith effect*. However, Griffith could not explain the cause of bacterial transformation.

(*ii*) ***Richard, S. and Martin, D.* (1931)** did this same experiment *in vitro*. They found that the transformation did not occur by a living host and hence mice were not responsible for the phenomenon of transformation.

(*iii*) ***Oswald Avery, Colin MacLeod, and Maclyn McCarty* (1944)** later on, repeated the Griffith's experiment. They concluded that DNA is the transforming substance which could bring about transformation of avirulent bacteria (Type II R cells in pneumococci) into virulent form (Type III S cells). Thus, it was established that DNA is the genetic material.

However, it required the use of enzyme that could degrade DNA, RNA, and protein. Therefore, highly purified DNA from virulent form (Type III S cells) was treated with 3 enzymes that degrade (hydrolyze) the DNA (DNase), RNA (RNase) and protein (proteases). It was observed that it was only the DNase treatment that affected transforming activity of the DNA preparation and eliminated all transforming activity. The results of six sets of experiment conducted by Avery and coworkers can be illustrated as under:

	Type of Cells (Avirulent)		*DNA Source (Virulent but made avirulent)*	*Serum*	*Enzyme that Degrades*	*Colony Developed*
1.	Type II R cells		—	—	—	II R colonies
2.	—		DNA from heat killed III S cells	—	—	No colony
3.	"	+	"	+ Serum that Precipitates II R cells from mixture	—	III S colonies
4.	"	+	"	+ "	+ Protease	"
5.	"	+	"	+ "	+ RNase	"
6.	"	+	"	+ "	+ DNase	No colonies

The above results showed that the DNA that carries the genetic information specifying the synthesis of Type III capsule is inserted physically into the chromosome of Type II R recipient cell.

***Test of determining the presence of genetic information in a mixture* of DNA and protein**: The enzymes have the biological specificity to provide a powerful test. The enzyme deoxyribonuclease (DNase) degrades DNA to mononucleotides while the enzyme protease degrades proteins to smaller components. If the mixture of DNA and protein lost the genetic information treated with DNase it indicates that the DNA stores the genetic information or if the genetic information is lost on treating the mixture with protease it shows that the genetic information is present in protein.

II. Evidence from Bacterial Conjugation

Laderberg and Tatum (1946) discovered the genetic recombination in bacteria (called conjugation) from two different strains of *E. coli*. On the basis of the findings of their results they have shown that conjugation (genetic recombination in bacteria) resulted in the transfer of DNA (genetic material) from one bacterium to another bacterium mutant strain. Their experiment was based on two mutant strain of *E. coli bacterium*- mutant strain A and mutant strain B with their genetic compodition as Met, Bio, Thr, Leu, Thi.

Both the strains coud not grow in a minimal culture medium. The strain A was used as male strain which could not manufacture vitamin *methionine and biotin* and can grow in a culture medium having these vitamins besides sugar and starch. The strain B was used as female strain or recipient which could not manufacture *threonine, leucine and thionine* and can grow after supplementing the culture medium with these vitamins. However, growing of the mixture of two strains in the same minimal culture medium has shown that a number of colonies were produced. This was the evidence that the portion of donor DNA containing information to manufacture *threonine, leucine and thionine* were transferred and incorporated in the recipient genotype during conjugation.

III. Evidence from Bacterial Transduction

This is the transfer of small part of DNA by means of a phage from one bacterial cell to another. The phage formed within the bacterial cell occasionally encloses a DNA part of bacterial chromosome and may infect another bacterium. In this process of infection the phage releases its own DNA and liberates the DNA fragment of previous host bacteria. The process of crossing over between the segments of two bacterial chromosomes incorporates th genes from previous host. This indicated that the genes (DNA fragments) are made up of DNA because only DNA is transferred.

(2) UV Light as Evidence of the DNA as Genetic Material

The UV light is absorbed by nucleic acid very strongly with in maximum absorption occurring at a wavelength of 260 milli microns. The UV light is also a mutagen at this wavelength of 260 millimicrons. There was found a close correlation between action spectrum for the production of mutation and the absorption spectrum for nucleic acid. This showed that genes are composed of nucleic acids, because the mutation is the result of nucleic acid to absorb energy which is effective in causing mutation (change of the nucleic acid molecules).

(3) Gene Synthesis

The chemical synthesis of one gene of yeast containing 77 nucleotides by H. Khurana and synthesis of more complex gene in rabbit containing 650 nucleotides by the biochemical scientists of Harward University of America have undoubtedly proved that genes are made up of DNA molecules.

(4) Biochemical Evidences in Favour of DNA as Genetic Material

The biochemical study on approximate DNA content per cell in various organisms indicated that the amount od DNA per cell appeara to be proportion to the complexity of cell structure and the amount of genetic information contained in the cells. This has been indicated on the information given below:

Species	*DNA Amount (pg per cell)*	*No. of Nucleotide Pairs (Millions)*
T4 bacteriophage	0.00024	0.7
Bacteria	0.002 to 0.06	2
Fungi	0.02 to 0.17	20
Sponge	0.1	100
Molluscs	1.2	1000
Birds	2	2000
Fishes	2	2800
Reptiles	5	4500
Amphibia	7	6500
Mammals	6	5500

(5) Nitrogen Bases in DNA

A quantitative study of 4 nitrogen bases in hybridization of DNA specimens isolated from different organisms by Chargaff, E. (1949- 1953) concluded that

- ✰ The base composition of DNA show species differences,
- ✰ The base composition is same in different tissues of the same species,
- ✰ The base composition of DNA of a species does not change with change in environment like age, nutritional state and so by other environmental factors, and
- ✰ The base composition of closely related species has similar composition while widely different species are expected to have different base composition.
- ✰ The base pairing is such that A + T and G = C. Thus purines are equal to pyrimidine residues (A + G = C + T), and

(6) DNA is Genetic Material in Bacteriophage

Another experiment on bacteriophage infection (infection of bacteria by bacteriophage) was carried out by Alfred Harshey (1969 Noble Prize winner) and Martha Chase (1952). This also indicated that DNA is the genetic material of certain bacterial virus (bacteriophage T2). On this finding it was accepted that DNA is the genetic material.

The viruses are acellular parasites that can only reproduce in host cells depending on the metabolic machinery (ribosome, *etc.*) of the host. The bacteriophage T2 (infects *E. coli*) has DNA and protein in equal amount of 50 percent each. It is known that DNA contains phosphorus but it does not contain sulphur. On the contrary, the proteins have sulphur but no phosphorus. This difference in chemical composition of the two components was the base of their experiment. Secondly, they showed that DNA of the virus particle is able to enter the cell while most of the protein of the virus is adsorbed to the outside of the cell. This showed that the genetic information required for viral reproduction lies in DNA.

The basic idea of Harshey and Chase experiment was to see whether it was the radioactive protein or the radioactive DNA remain outside the host cell after mixing. This could be proved from the presence of particular radioactivity of the infected phage cells.

They conducted two experiments involving the following steps in each of the two experiment:

(i) Labelling of phage DNA or protein with radioactive isotopes: In one experiment, they labelled the phage DNA in a medium having the radioactive isotope of phosphorus ^{32}P rather than normal isotope ^{31}P. In the second experiment, they labelled the phage protein coats in a medium having radioactive sulphur, ^{35}S rather than having normal isotope ^{32}S.

(ii) Mixing of *E. coli* cell with phage particle: The T2 phage particles labelled with ^{35}S as well as those labelled with ^{32}P were mixed with *E. coli* cells,

(iii) Time of infection: Allowed a time of about 10 minutes to phage particle to infect bacteria in both the sets of experiment.

(iv) Use of shearing forces: The phage infected cells of both the experiments were then subjected to shearing forces in a Waring blender.

(v) Separate bacteria from phage by centrifugation: Low speed centrifugation was used to separate the sheared off phage coats from infected cells in both the sets. The cells got sediment but the page particles remained suspended.

Observations

(a) It was observed that most of the radioactivity of the phage infected cells (labelled with ^{35}S) was removed on shearing from the cells without affecting phage production and hence protein was removed.

(b) On the contrary, when T2 phage particles that were labelled with ^{32}P and subjected to mixing with *E. coli* and shearing, essentially all of the radioactivity was found inside the cells and hence the DNA was not removed by shearing.

Results

This showed that DNA of the virus entered the host cell but the protein coat remained outside the cell. This was because the progeny viruses were produced inside the cell and moreover the progeny particles were shown to have some of the ^{32}P but not the ^{35}S of parental phage.

Conclusion

These results indicated that the genetic information (directing the synthesis of both the DNA molecules and the protein coats of the progeny viruses) must be present in the parental DNA.

The DNA differs from protein in its chemical structure. This difference helps to label these macromolecules with a radioactive isotope. The DNA contains phosphorus with a common isotoe ^{31}P, has no sulfur, and it can be labelled by growing cells on medium containing the radioactive isotope of phosphorus^{32}P. On the contrary, the proteins contain sulfur with common isotope ^{32}S, have little or no phosphorus, and these can be labelled by growing cells on medium containing the radioactive isotope of sulfur, ^{35}S.

(7) RNA is Genetic Material in some Viruses

Many of the plant viruses contain RNA and proteins but no DNA. However, these RNA viruses contain their genetic information in nucleic acid and not in the proteins, like all other organisms but in these cases the nucleic acid that store genetic information is the RNA instead of DNA.

The experiment called as reconstitution experiment to establish that RNA is the genetic material in such viruses was conducted by Heinz Fraenkel-Conret and coworker Stanley (1957) in California on *tobacco mosaic virus* (TMV), which is a small virus contains only single molecule of RNA encapsulated in a protein coat and it does not contain the DNA. The chemical composition of protein coats of different strains of TMV differs.

Fraenkel-Conrat and coworkers conducted infectivity test of RNA and proteins of TMV. They treated two strains of TMV with chemicals that dissociated the protein coats of the viruses from the RNA molecules and hence separated the proteins from the RNA. They conducted the reconstitution experiment by mixing protein from one strain and RNA of other strain. This resulted into the reconstitution of complete infective viruses having the proteins and RNA molecules of separate (different) strains. Now infecting the tobacco leaves with these reconstituted viruses, the progeny viruses were found genetic and phenotypic identical to the strain from which the RNA was taken.

This infectivity test of both RNA and protein fractions of TMV had shown that RNA alone and not the protein fraction of TMV was a cause of infection. This gave the evidence that RNA also carry genetic information in some viruses. Thus, the *nucleic acids* actually constitute the *genetic material.* However, *DNA* is always the *genetic material* and RNA is non-genetic in most of the cases except where DNA is absent (virus).

13.2 MOLECULAR STRUCTURE OF GENETIC MATERIAL: THE NUCLEIC ACIDS

There are three most important facets of understanding the nature of life:

- ☆ DNA structure,
- ☆ The form in which the genetic information are stored in DNA, and
- ☆ Mechanism of the structure of DNA to facilitate the accurate transmission of genetic information from generation to generation.

(1) Discovery of Nuclein or Nucleic Acid

The answer of the above facets started coming with the notable work of a young Swiss medical student, Johann Friedrich Miescher, to discover an acidic substance which he isolated from pus cells adhered to the bandages used to dress human wounds. He separated the pus cells and debris, and treated the cells with the proteolytic enzyme ***pepsin***. The pepsin was isolated from the stomach of pigs. The substance obtained from pus cells after pepsin treatment was found acidic in nature.

- ☆ J. F. Miescher (1868) observed that the acidic substance obtained from pus cells was a unique substance to which he called as ***nuclein.*** The nuclein was unusual to have large amounts of both nitrogen and phosphorus which were known at the time to coexist only in certain types of fat. The Miescher's work could get publish after 2 years later of its submission because the Editor was skeptical of the results and hence repeated himself the experiment. This *nuclein* of Miescher was later named as ***nucleic acid.***
- ☆ Kossell and Neumann in 1894 identified three of the bases in DNA
- ☆ Hammersten in 1900 showed the presence of pentose sugar in DNA.
- ☆ Levens (1929) demonstrated that this sugar was 2′-deoxyribose.
- ☆ Caspersson (1934) showed that the DNA is a macromolecule and gave the tetranucleotide theory of its structure.
- ☆ Levene (1869-1940) separated the nucleic acid from protein. He found that the nucleic acid is macromolecule composed of repeating subunits (thousands of smaller units) called ***nucleotides***.

The nucleotides, in addition to be present in DNA, are also found in nucleoplasm and cytoplasm but with the difference in the form of phosphate. The phosphate present in DNA is in monophosphate form whereas that present in nucleoplasm and cytoplasm is in its triphosphate form. The triphosphate form is essential because during DNA replication, the DNA polymerase enzyme can act only on triphosphate of deoxyribonucleotides (DNA).

- ☆ The key component of the acidic material in Miescher's nuclein (nucleic acid) was found the polynucleotide chains, documented in 1940s,
- ☆ The role of nucleic acids in storing and transmitting the genetic information could not be established until 1944 (Avery *et al.*, 1944). They discovered that the transforming principle is DNA, the first indication of DNA as the genetic material,
- ☆ Chargaff (1950) published the results showing a consistency of the base ratios in DNA from different sources,
- ☆ Hershey and Chase (1952) showed that DNA is the phage gene,
- ☆ Franklin (1952) indicated that DNA is a helix based on the X-ray differentiation pictures, and
- ☆ The double-helix structure of the nucleic acid (DNA) was discovered in 1953 (Watson and Crick, 1953).

(2) Types of Nucleic Acids

The ***nucleic acids*** are complex molecules, bigger than proteins, containing carbon, oxygen, hydrogen, nitrogen and large amount of phosphorus but no sulfur in contrast to proteins. The nucleic acid is found to associate with various proteins in combinations called ***nucleoproteins*** (Nucleic acid + Proteins). The nucleic acid is a macromolecule composed of phosphoric acid, pentose sugar, and organic bases.

There are two types of nucleic acids. They (two nucleic acids) differ in their location in the cell, in chemical structure, and in function. The two nucleic acids are named depending upon the type of sugar present *viz.* ribose and deoxyribose (lacking one oxygen atom). These are accordingly called as:

- ☆ ***Ribonucleic acid* (RNA):** In RNA, the sugar is pentose *ribose* which has hydroxyl (OH) group on the 2-carbon. The RNA is commonly found in cytoplasm as well as nucleus and hence through cells. The RNA in viruses forms the genetic material
- ☆ ***Deoxyribonucleic acid* (DNA):** In DNA, the sugar is *deoxyribose* (contains the sugar 2′- deoxyribose with only hydrogen on the 2-carbon). The DNA is found mainly in chromosomes (the nucleus) and some in cytoplasmic organelles (mitochondria and chloroplasts). The DNA is not present in chromosomes in some cases (plant virus) in which RNA is genetic material. The DNA in eukaryotic cells is long double-stranded spirally coiled, in virus there is a single molecule of DNA (single strand) which is enclosed in protein coat whereas in bacteria, mitochondria and plastids of eukaryotic cells it is circular lying naked in the cytoplasm. Sinsheimer (1959) found a single strand DNA in a small bacteriophage 174 which attack *E. coli* and this DNA contains 5500 nucleotides without helical configuration and without equivalence of molar ratio of bases (A and T or G and C). This was circular DNA and single strand.

(3) Components of Nucleic Acids

The nucleic acids are polymers of nucleotides (***polynucleotides*** – a linear sequence of joined nucleotides in DNA or RNA) or say that the nucleic acids are formed by the *polymerization of nucleotides*. All nucleotides have a common structure. Each of the ***nucleotide,*** which forms the nucleic acids (DNA and RNA, the polynucleotides), is a *monomer* (single chemical unit) and composed of three subunits:

- ☆ a *phosphate* group (phosphoric acid),
- ☆ a *five-carbon sugar* (pentose), and
- ☆ *a base* (heterocyclic nitrogen-containing compound).

(i) The ***phosphate group*** of each nucleotide is linked by a phosphoester bond to a pentose sugar (a five-carbon sugar molecule) at its number 5 carbon position, forming sugar-phosphate backbone of DNA strand. There is chemical connection between the sugars of one nucleotide to the phosphate of next nucleotide. The sugar and phosphate groups are the constant components of all nucleotides in a nucleic acid.

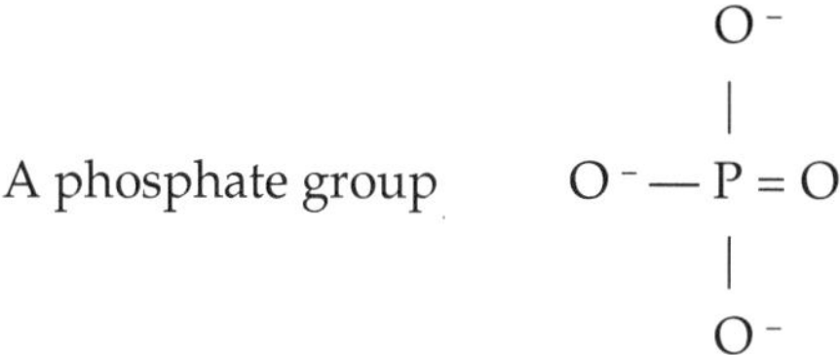

(ii) The ***sugar*** of nucleotide is a 5- carbons sugar (pentose sugar). There are two types of sugars in nucleic acids which are named as *ribose* and *deoxyribose.* In case the sugar is lacking one oxygen atom, it is called as deoxyribose. Both these sugars are not ordinarily found at the same time in any particular nucleic acid.

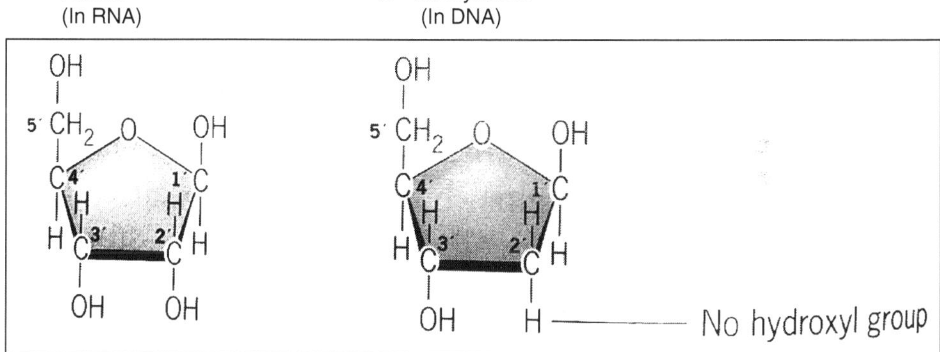

Figure 13.1: Structure of a Five-Carbon Sugar Molecule (Pentose).

Each sugar molecule is covalently linked to one of 4 possible bases (**A**denine, **G**uanine, **C**ytosine and **T**hymine).

(iii) A ***nitrogen base*** (heterocyclic nitrogen-containing compound) of nucleotide is present in association with each sugar at its number 1 carbon position. The nitrogen containing group is more variable having either one or two carbon-nitrogen rings and function as a base called as nitrogen base (hydrogen-ion acceptor) whereas the phosphate group has its acidic nature.

There are found 4 different nitrogen bases (two purines and two pyrimidines) in polynucleotides of DNA and RNA. These four different nitrogen bases are as:

- *Pyrimidines:* They have one carbon-nitrogen (C-N) ring. These are *cytosine* (C) and *thymine* (T) present in DNA; and *cytosine* (C) and *Uracil* (U) present in RNA. Thus, uracil (U) is present only in RNA in place of thymine present in DNA;
- *Purines:* They have two C-N rings (a pair of fused rings). These are *adenine* (A) and *guanine* (G), present in both DNA and RNA.

The bases present in nucleic acids are heterocyclic compounds with the rings containing nitrogen and carbon. The acidic character of nucleotides is due to the presence of phosphate, which dissociates at the pH found inside cells, freeing hydrogen ions and leaving the phosphate negatively charged. These charges attract proteins and hence most nucleic acids in cells are associated with proteins. In nucleic acids and nucleotides, the 1′ carbon atom of the sugar (ribose or deoxyribose) is attached to the nitrogen at position 9 of a purine (N_9) or at position 1 of a pyrimidine (N_1).

The structural chemical formulae of cyclic nitrogen-containing compounds (two purines and three pyrimidines) present in nucleic acids are as given below:

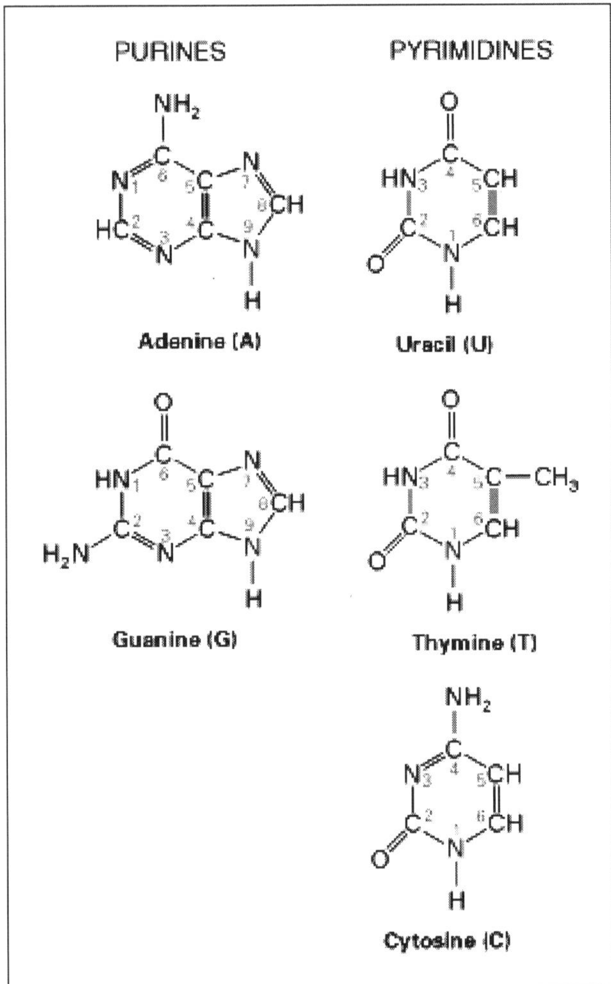

Figure 13.2: Structural Formulae of Purines and Pyrimidine.

The RNA has also four nitrogen bases which are also the same two purines (adenine and guanine) and also two pyrimidines (cytosine and uracil) but one is different from that present in DNA (uracil, in place of thymine). The base pairs often called *Watson-Crick base pairs.*

The organisms contain small concentrations of nucleosides (combinations of a base and a sugar without a phosphate) in their cells and extracellular fluids.

Nucleotides are nucleosides that have one, two, or three phosphate groups esterified at the 5′ hydroxyl. The *nucleotide*

- ✰ *Monophosphate* has a single esterified phosphate,
- ✰ *Diphosphate* contains a pyrophosphate group, and
- ✰ *Triphosphate* has a third phosphate.

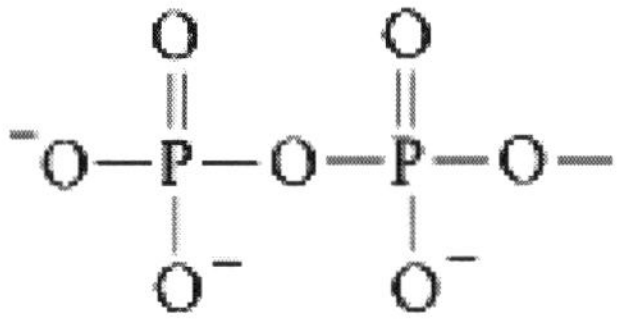

$$^{-}O-\underset{O^{-}}{\overset{O}{\overset{\|}{\underset{|}{P}}}}-O-\underset{O^{-}}{\overset{O}{\overset{\|}{\underset{|}{P}}}}-O-$$

The nucleoside triphosphates are used in the synthesis of nucleic acids. In addition, these compounds also serve many other functions in the cell: ATP, for example, is the most widely used energy carrier in the cell, and GTP plays crucial roles in intracellular signaling and acts as an energy reservoir, particularly in protein synthesis.

(4) Types of Nucleotides

The DNA contains four deoxyribonucleotides whereas the RNA contains four ribonuleotides and these are named according to the nitrogen base attached.

The term ***nucleoside*** is used for a combination of a nitrogen base and a sugar without the phosphate group. The nitrogenous base is linked to C-1 of deoxyribose in a nucleotide though N-glycoside bond. The nucleotide is formed of one molecule of deoxyribose, one molecule of the four nitrogenous bases, and one molecule of phosphoric acid. The four nitrogen bases, nucleosides (Nitrogen base + sugar) and ***nucleotides*** (Nitrogen base + sugar + phosphate group) of DNA molecule are as under:

Nitrogen Base	*Deoxyribonucleoside (Nitrogen Base + Sugar) = Nucleosides*	*Deoxyribonucleotide (Nucleoside + Phosphate) = Nucleotides*
Purines (Two C-N rings):		
Adenine (A)	Adenosine or Deoxyadenosine	Deoxyadenylic acid
Guanine (G)	Guanosine or Deoxyguanosine	Deoxyguanylic acid
Pyrimidine (One C-N ring):		
Cytosine (C)	Cytidine or Deoxycytidine	Deoxycytidylic acid
Thymine (T)	Thymidine or Deoxythymidine	Deoxythymidylic acid

The nucleotides in polynucleotide chains of the DNA molecule are joined by phosphodiester linkage. The nucleotides have a top (5′) to bottom (3′) chemical polarity because each phosphodiester linkage joins the 5′ carbon of 2′-deoxiribose in one nucleotide to the 3′ carbon of 2′-deoxyribose in the adjacent nucleotide. Thus, the chain has a 5′ carbon (5′ P) terminus at the top and a 3′ carbon (3′-OH) terminus at the bottom.

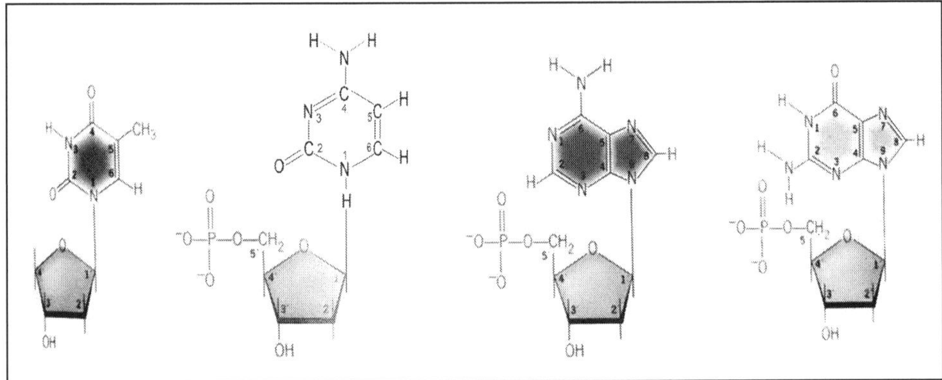

Figure 13.3: Four Types of Nucleotides.

(5) Polymerization of Nucleotides

The primary structure of nucleic acids is constituted by the linear sequence of nucleotides linked by phosphodiester bonds. This structure so formed is called the poly-nucleotides which can twist and fold into three-dimensional conformations stabilized by non-covalent bonds. In this respect, the nucleic acids are similar to polypeptides.

Both the nucleic acids are *linear* and *unbranched* polymers (multiple chemical units) of nucleotides, called polynucleotides. The polymer means many parts (*poly* means many and *mer* means parts). The thousands of nucleotides are joined together in long chains in forming the polynucleotides (DNA and RNA). Thus, each of the nucleic acid (DNA and RNA) is a long chain polymer of nucleotides (polynucleotide) or that the nucleic acids are formed by the *polymerization of nucleotides*. Each of the two nucleic acids contains four different nucleotides among which two are purines and two are pyrimidine nucleotides. Each nucleotide consists of a heterocyclic base linked to a five-carbon sugar (deoxyribose or ribose) which in turn is linked to a phosphate group. Both the nucleic acids have great chemical similarities.

Cellular RNAs range in length from less than one hundred to many thousands of nucleotides. Cellular DNA molecules can be as long as several hundred million nucleotides.

Each nucleotide contains a special nitrogen base, the sugar (deoxyribose) and phosphoric acid, as mentioned above and shown below:

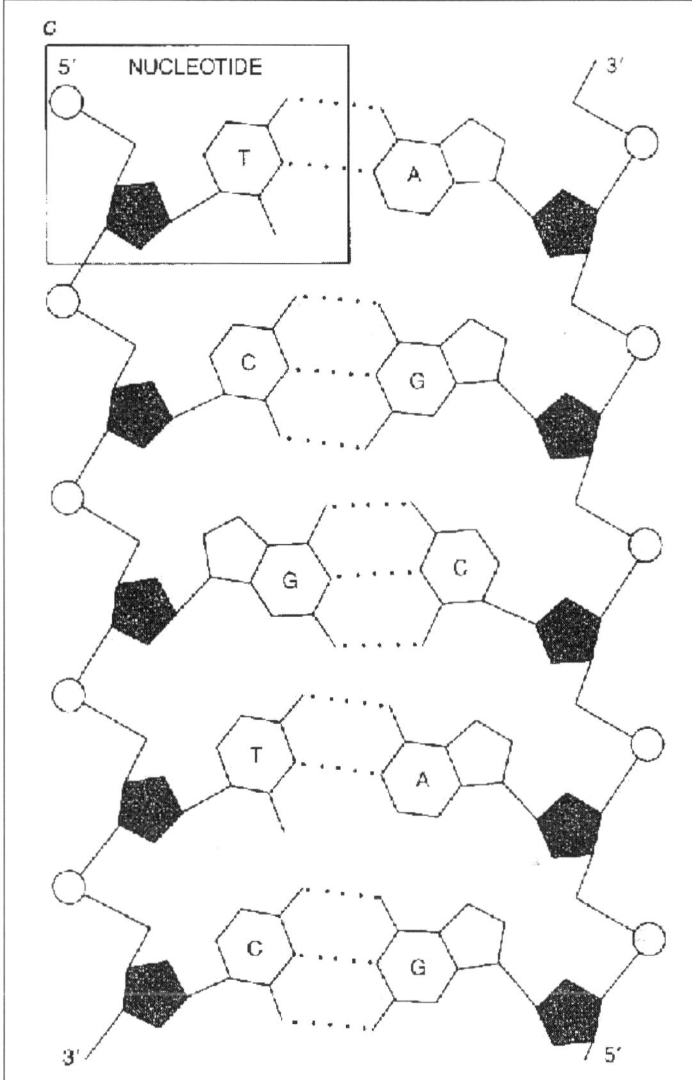

Figure 13.4: Polymerization of Nucleotides.

Phosphodiester Bond

The nucleotides in a polynucleotide chain of each strand of DNA are linked together by a chemical connection between the sugar (deoxyribose) of one nucleotide and the phosphoric acid molecule of the next. This chemical connection of linking together two nucleotides in a polynucleotide chain is called the *phosphodiester bond*.

When nucleotides polymerize to form nucleic acids, the hydroxyl group (OH) attached to the 3′ carbon of a sugar of one nucleotide forms an ester bond to the phosphate of another nucleotide, eliminating a molecule of water:

$$\begin{array}{c} (\text{Base})_1 \\ | \\ (\text{Sugar})\text{—OH} \end{array} + \text{HO—}\overset{\overset{\displaystyle O}{\|}}{\underset{\underset{\displaystyle O^-}{|}}{P}}\text{—O—}\begin{array}{c} (\text{Base})_2 \\ | \\ (\text{Sugar}) \end{array} \longrightarrow$$

$$\begin{array}{c} (\text{Base})_1 \\ | \\ (\text{Sugar})\text{—O—} \end{array}\overset{\overset{\displaystyle O}{\|}}{\underset{\underset{\displaystyle O^-}{|}}{P}}\text{—O—}\begin{array}{c} (\text{Base})_2 \\ | \\ (\text{Sugar}) \end{array} + H_2O$$

This condensation reaction is similar to that in which a peptide bond is formed between two amino acids. Thus, a single nucleic acid strand is a phosphate-pentose polymer (polyester) with purine and pyrimidine bases as side groups. The two adjacent nucleotides in a polynucleotide are linked by phosphodiester bonds.

Chemical Orientation

Like a polypeptide, entire strand of nucleic acid has an end-to-end chemical orientation. The *5′ end* has a free hydroxyl or phosphate group on the 5′ carbon of its terminal sugar while the *3′ end* has a free hydroxyl group on the 3′ carbon of its terminal sugar. The polynucleotide sequences are conventionally written and read in the 5′ → 3′ direction (from left to right). This is due to the reasons that there is directionality (5′ to 3′) of an end-to-end chemical orientation of nucleic acid strand and that the synthesis proceeds 5′ to 3′. For example, the sequence AUG is written to be (5′) AUG (3′). The 5′ → 3′ directionality of a nucleic acid strand is an extremely important property of the molecule.

13.3 DEOXYRIBONUCLEIC ACID (DNA)

The cells of all living organisms except plant virus contain the DNA. But the RNA is present in plant viruses as the genetic material in place of DNA.

There is single molecule of DNA in bacteriophages and viruses in which it remains coiled and enclosed in the protein coat, while the DNA is circular and lies naked in the cytoplasm in bacteria, mitochondria and plastids of eukaryotic cells. On the other, the DNA occurs in the form of long spirally coiled and unbranched threads like structure in the nuclei of eukaryotic cells. The DNA molecule is divided into chromosomes in eukaryotes, the number of DNA molecules is equal to the number of chromosomes per cell, DNA is found in combination with proteins in the form of nucleoproteins which is called as the chromatin material (or chromatin network), and is enclosed in the nucleus.

Chemically, the DNA is composed of three units *viz.*

- ✰ *Sugar molecule* (pentose sugar- deoxyribose or 2′-deoxyribose),
- ✰ *Nitrogen bases* (Nitrogen containing organic ring compounds that are 4 in number) and *phosphoric acid*. Of the 4 nitrogen bases, two are single ring nitrogen organic compounds called pyrimidines (cytosine, thymine) and other two are double nitrogen ring organic compounds called purines

(adenine and guanine). The structural formulae of pyrimidines and purines nitrogen bases have been given above (Figure 13.2).

- *Phosphorus group.*

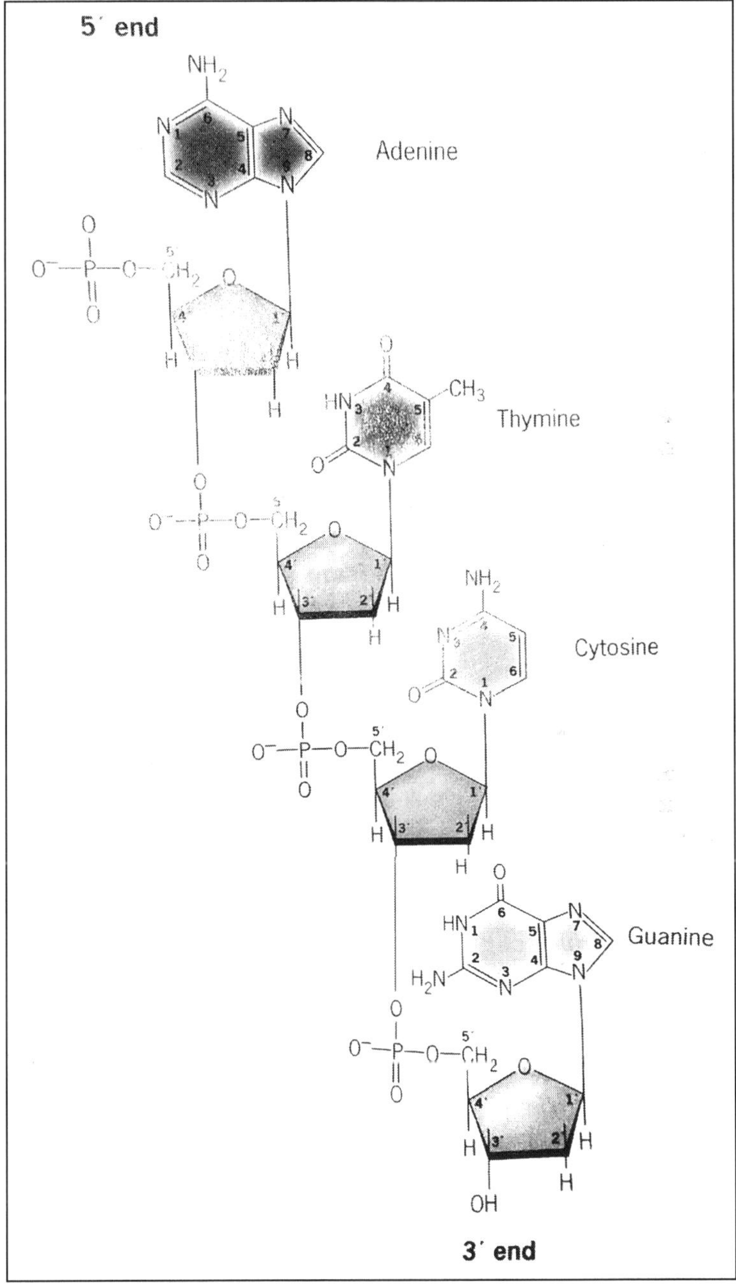

Figure 13.5: Polynucleotide Chain of DNA with 2'-deoxyribose Joined by Phosphodister Linkages showing 5' to 3' Chemical Polarity.

Molecular Ratio of Nitrogen Bases in DNA

Chargaff described three fundamental features of DNA known as *Chargaff's base ratio*. These are as under:

- ☆ ***The purines and pyrimidine*** components occur in equal amounts in a DNA molecule irrespective of its source,
- ☆ The A = T and C = G
- ☆ The base ratio A = T/G = C may vary in the DNA of different groups of animals but constant for a species. This information is therefore useful to identify the DNA from a particular source.

Chemical data of Erwin Chargaff et al: They analyzed the composition of DNA of many different organisms. They found that there exists -

(i) A fix interrelationship of thymine and adenine as well as cytosine and guanine in DNA. The concentration of thymine was always equal to the concentration of adenine whereas the concentration of cytosine was always equal to the concentration of guanine. According to the base pairing principles, the ratios of (A + T: G + C) is 1.53 in humans, 1.51 in D. *melanogaster, 1.80 in S.* cerevisiae, and 1.04 in Zea mays.

(ii) Equal concentration of pyrimidine (C + T) and purine (A + G). The molar ratios of purines (A + G) to pyrimidine (T + C) in human DNA and *Drosophila melanogaster* is 1. 01 while in *Saccharamyces cerevisiae* and Zea mays (Corn) is 1.00. This ratio in *E. coli is 1.04.* Among *viruses,* the ratio is *0.99* in *bacteriophage lambda, 1.03* in *bacteriophage T2,* and is *1.06* in *Herpes simplex.*

- ☆ *X-ray diffraction data of Wilkins and coworkers*: The X – ray diffraction patterns can be recorded on X-ray – sensitive film on the same principle just as the patterns of light are recorded with a camera on light-sensitive film. On focusing the X - rays through fibers of purified molecules, the rays are deflected by the atoms of the molecules in specific patterns, called diffraction patterns, which provide information about the organization of the components of the molecules. The X – ray diffraction data on DNA structure was provided by Maurice Wilkins, Rosalind Franklin, Francis Crick and James Watson.
- ☆ Inferences from careful model building.

Structure of DNA

The DNA molecule, called the ***"thread of life"***, is present in the chromosome resides in the nucleus of the cell, extends the length of the chromosome, more or less in its center. In spite of the isolation of DNA constituents quite early in 1930s that DNA is long chain polymer it remained unknown about the knowledge of the arrangement of its different constituents so as to carry out their cytological and genetical activities. The DNA is a macromolecule formed by linking of several thousand nucleotides and hence polymer of nucleotides. The nucleotides are thus monomers and building block of DNA. The phosphate molecule in a nucleotide is attached to 5- carbon atom of deoxyribose molecule through a phosphodiester linkage.

Watson and Crick (1953) proposed the *"double helical"* structure of DNA on the basis of the followings:

Francis Crick and James Watson (1953) proposed that DNA molecule in eukaryotic cells is a long two-stranded structure of polynucleotide chains running in opposite directions. Watson, Crick, and Wilkins shared the 1962 Noble Prize for their pioneer work on double-helix model of DNA. In this respect, Franklin had been unfortunate not to share Noble Prize due to death in 1958 at the age of only 37.

Double Helical Structure

The natural DNA (***B*** DNA) contains two polynucleotide strands which are complementary and wind together through space to form a structure often described as a **double helix.** Each of the two strands of DNA contains thousands of units of *nucleotides.* Thus, each strand of DNA is called a polymer of nucleotides (*polynucleotide*), because these are composed of many repeated units of *nucleotides.*

The double helix structure is characterized by twisting the two strands of DNA (coiled like a rope) to form a regular right-handed double helix (spiral-like structure, in which two polynucleotide chains are coiled about one another in a spiral way). Such a twisted structure like a rope is ***called helix***. The double helix has the nitrogen bases on the inside and the sugar-phosphate backbones on the outside. Base pairing (A:T and G:C) and hydrophobic interactions between adjacent bases in the same strand stabilize this native structure.

There are following 7 important features of DNA double helix:

(i) The double helix has 2 chains of polynucleotide,

(ii) The two chains (known as strands) are antiparallel,

(iii) Each of the two chain has a backbone of sugar-phosphate while the nitrogenous bases are inside the helix being stacked on top of each other like a pile of saucers,

(iv) The nitrogen bases of two antiparallel strands are linked through hydrogen bonds which are two between A and T but three between G and C. These hydrogen bonds are attractive forces between two strands of DNA to hold together the structure,

(v) The two strands or chains of polynucleotides are complementary. The sequence of nitrogenous bases in one strand determines the sequence of nitrogenous bases in the other strand. This is called complementary base pairing,

(vi) The each turn of helix contain 10 base pairs with spacing between adjacent base pairs as 10 A° and the helix is 20 A° in diameter, and

(vii) There are two groves in double helix which are major and minor groove.

- ☆ ***Sugar-phosphate backbone:*** Each DNA strand has a *sugar-phosphate backbone* which is made up of sugar molecules (deoxy-ribose) linked together by phosphate groups. Each of the two chains of sugar-phosphate backbones is on the outside of the double helix, with the bases oriented into the interior. In each nucleotide, the nitrogenous base is linked to a sugar which is linked to a phosphoric acid molecule. The adjoining bases in each DNA strand stack on top of one another in parallel planes.

  The backbone of polynucleotides is highly charged (1 unit negative charge for each phosphate group; 2 negative charges per base-pair). The two strands of DNA show strong repulsion and fall apart in the absence of salt in the surrounding medium. Therefore, counter-ions are essential for the double-helical structure. Counter-ions shield the charges on the sugar-phosphate backbone. They may also contribute to an *attractive interaction* from fluctuating counter-ions around the backbone.

- ☆ ***Opposite chemical polarity:*** The orientation of the *sugar-phosphate backbones* of the two complementary strands (double helix) is anti-parallel; that is, the $5' \rightarrow 3'$ directions of two strands are in opposite direction. The $3'$ - OH of deoxyribose present in one strand and the $5'$ – phosphate residue of other strand are located at the same end of the double helix. Thus, the

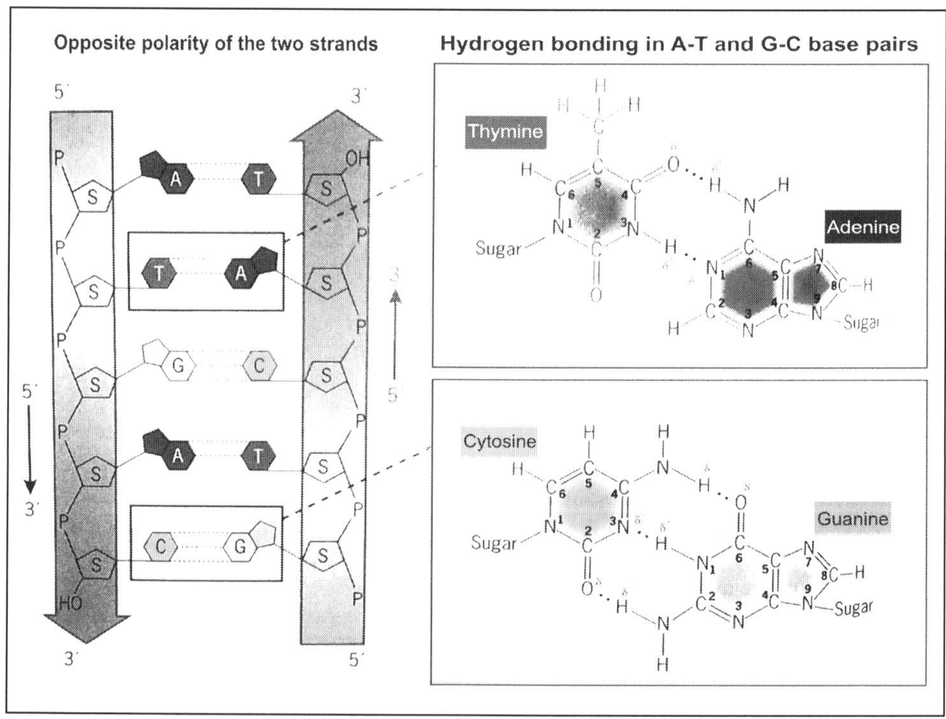

Figure 13.6: DNA Double Helix Showing Opposite Chemical Polarity and Hydrogen Bonding.

two strands of a double helix of DNA have *opposite chemical polarity*. More clearly, unidirectionally along a DNA double helix, the phosphodiester bonds in one strand go from a 5′ carbon of one nucleotide to a 3′ carbon of the adjacent nucleotide, whereas in the complementary strand go from a 3′ carbon to a 5′ carbon. This opposite polarity of the complementary strands of a DNA double helix has its very important part to play in DNA replication, transcription, and recombination.

☆ ***Phosphodiester linkage:*** The 3′ C of a sugar molecule is connected through a phosphate group to the 5′ C of the next sugar. This linkage is also called *3′-5′ phosphodiester linkage*. All DNA strands are read from the 5′ to the 3′ end where the 5′ end terminates in a phosphate group and the 3′ end terminates in a sugar molecule.

☆ ***Complementary of two DNA strands:*** The two strands are called as *complementary* because the base pairs are complementary to each other for their pairing. The sequence of bases in one polynucleotide should determine the sequence of bases in the other polynucleotide of double helix. The complementary of the two strands of the double helix is very important property, because this makes DNA uniquely suited to store and transmit genetic information from generation to generation as a result of DNA replication and equal division in daughter cells.

The two complementary strands of DNA are coiled in a manner so as to be separated from one another only by uncoiling allowing their ends to revolve freely. The coiling is helical (spiral) structure like a circular stair case maintaining same diameter and same width of the steps with a connecting railing on either side. The railing (backbone) of each strand (side) is composed of the phosphate-sugar linkage which are continuously repeated without change.

This *base-pair complementary* is a consequence of the size, shape, and chemical composition of the bases. The presence of thousands of such hydrogen bonds in a DNA molecule contributes greatly to the stability of the double helix. *Hydrophobic* (association of nonpolar groups with each other when present in aqueous solutions due to their insolubility in water) and *van der Waals* interactions (weak interactions between atoms placed in close proximity) between the stacked adjacent base pairs also contribute to the stability of the DNA structure.

☆ ***Base pairing principle and hydrogen bonding:*** The geometry of the double-helical structure is maintained by pairing a larger purine (A or G) with a smaller pyrimidine (C or T). This is the *base pairing principle* which indicates that all base pairs consist of one purine and one pyrimidine.

The nature of *hydrogen bonding* is such that adenine and thymine are attracted to each other and there is a chemical bonding between them by two hydrogen bonds (A to G) and likewise is the attraction between cytosine and guanine and the chemical bonding by three hydrogen bonds (G to C), without any exception. The hydrogen bonding is neither possible between C and A bases nor between T and G in their common structural states. The bases of double stranded DNA has a quantitative relationship in which A = T and G = C, or A + G = C + T, or A + G/C + T = 1.0. However, it is not necessary that A + T equal G + C.

The three hydrogen bonds make the G-C interaction stronger (by about 30 per cent) than A-T interaction. The A-T rich regions of DNA are more prone to thermal fluctuations. The base pairs in DNA are stacked between the two polynucleotide chains perpendicular to the axis of the molecule like the steps of a spiral staircase.

The relatively weak connections of hydrogen bonds between two nitrogen bases of two strands (called base pair or complementary base pair) hold together the two polynucleotide chains in a double helix (two strands of DNA molecule of polypeptide chain). The ***hydrogen bonds*** are weak interactions between electro-negative atoms and hydrogen atoms (electro-positive) that are linked to other electro-negative atoms.

The base pairing of purines with pyrimidines results to a constant diameter of 20°A of the DNA molecule. This is because the two pyrimidines (single C-N ring) require lesser space whereas the two purines (two C-N rings) require more space to pair. The distance between two base pairs (one step) in the nucleotide chain is 3.4°A (0.34 nm apart) along the axis of the molecule with each turn of about 34°A long and hence there are 10 base pairs in each turn (360°) of double helix.

The base-pairing is as shown as under Figure 13.7.

Now, the DNA structure can be shown as under Figure 13.8.

There is stability of DNA double helices. This is due to large number of hydrogen bonds between base pairs and also due to the hydrophobic (water-insoluble) bonding (or stacking forces) between adjacent base pairs. The DNA molecules present in the aqueous protoplasm of living cells have considerable stability. This is the result of insolubility in water the hydrophobic core of stacked base pairs.

Reversible DNA Strand Separation

The X-ray diffraction pictures suggest that a DNA molecule is not a rigid and static structure. In reality, it is under constant thermal fluctuations, which result in local twisting, stretching, bending, and unwinding of the double-strands. Certain sequences also lead to permanent bends or kinks in the direction of the helix. These local (sequence-specific) fluctuations are essential for the recognition of specific binding sites along the DNA molecule where proteins involved in replication, transcription, regulation of gene expression, or DNA-damage repair can bind.

The DNA strands of the double helix must separate at least temporarily during DNA replication and copying of DNA to RNA. During DNA synthesis two new strands are formed (one copied from each of the original strands) resulting in two double helices identical with the original one. The RNA is released and the two DNA strands re-associate with each other after completion of the synthesis of RNA from DNA template.

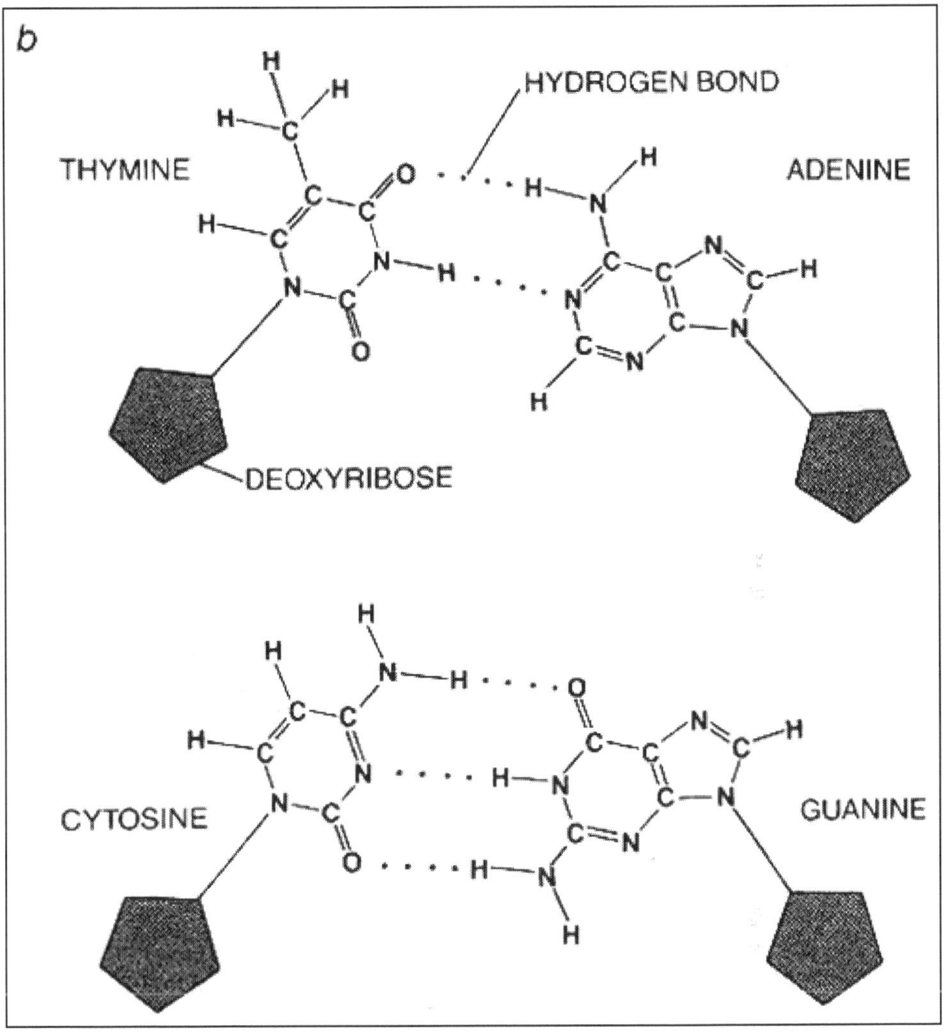

b

HYDROGEN BOND

THYMINE

ADENINE

DEOXYRIBOSE

CYTOSINE

GUANINE

Figure 13.7: Base Pairing and Hydrogen Bonding.

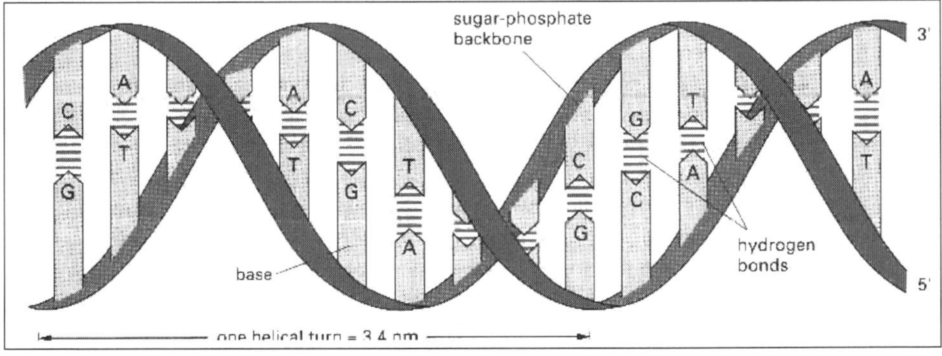

Figure 13.8: Double Helicle Structure of DNA.

Biological Significance of DNA Double Helix

Watson and Crick model of DNA has its biological significance as:

(I) *Self duplication*: The structure is most convenient to duplicate easily the molecule with particular sequence of base pairs. This is because each strand can construct its complementary strand by acting as a template and the sequence of nitrogenous bases in one strand determine the sequence of other strand,

(II) *Transmission of information*: Such a structure explains the transmitting information for the synthesis of protein. The genetic information are coded in the sequence of nitrogenous bases and hence the same sequence coded in some other molecule (mRNA) can be carried out to the site of protein synthesis. Moreover, a new strand of mRNA is coded or produced by either of the two strand of DNA molecule and this mRNA controls the proper alignment of amino acids in the polypeptide chain so formed, and

(III) *DNA repairs*: Under the influence of a number of factors like bending, shear forces and change in pH, the DNA is easily damaged and hence relatively fragile. The base sequences of DNA are changed by chemical agents and by radiations. However, the DNA preserve its integrity after several millions of replications, is a most stable structure, and most suited for preservation of the coded information for longer time. The reasons are that the base sequence in the strands is complementary and the coded information is stored in duplicate. A correct sequence of bases in a strand help in correcting the error that are likely to occur in the other strand (complementary) to send correct message.

Forms of DNA

The DNA exists in 6 different forms – A, B, C, D, E, and Z.

The most common DNA structure in solution is the B-DNA. Under conditions of applied force or twists in the DNA, or under low hydration conditions, it can adopt several helical conformations, referred to as the A-DNA, Z-DNA, B-DNA. The ***helix*** is a structure with a spiral shape. The A-form crystallizes under low hydration conditions and is not normally found for DNA in the cell. It is, however, the structure adopted by double-stranded regions in RNA as well as the transient double-helix between DNA and RNA during transcription. Both A- and B-DNA are right-handed helices whereas Z-DNA is a left-handed helix and is commonly found in regions of DNA that have an alternating purine-pyrimidine (*e.g.* 5′-CGCGCGCG-3′ or 5′-CGCGCATGC-3′) sequences.

- ✰ The DNA structure described above is its conformation under physiological conditions of aqueous solutions with low concentrations of salts. This DNA structure is called ***B-DNA*** and it is natural DNA. The DNA molecules mostly exist in the B conformation in aqueous protoplasm of living cells. However, considerable conformational flexibility exists in the structure of DNA molecules in accordance to the environment depending on the nature of the molecules to which it interacts. The two polynucleotide strands of natural DNA form right handed helix because the geometry of the sugar-phosphate backbone is more compatible for right-handed helix, long and thin double helix, helix diameter of 23.7 A°. The helix makes a complete turn every 3.4 nm (rise/base pair 3.4 A°); thus there are about 10 pairs per turn. The helix pitch is of 34 A° and tilts of bases -1 deg. The X-ray diffraction pattern of DNA indicates that the stacked bases are regularly spaced 0.34 nm apart along the helix axis. This is referred to as the *B form* of DNA, the normal form present in most DNA stretches in cells.

- ☆ The DNA present in high concentrations of salts or in a partially dehydrated state is called as ***A – DNA*** which is also right handed like B – DNA. In very low humidity, the crystallographic structure of B DNA is changed to the *A form*. The *A-DNA* differ from B-DNA in that it is shorter and thicker double helix, having a diameter of 2.3 nm (1 nm = 10^{-9} meter) or 25.5 A, rise/base pair 2.3 A. The A form is more compact than the B form, resulting 11 bp/helical turn, helix pitch of 25 A and tilt of bases 20 deg. This A – DNA molecule never exist *in vivo*. But this A-DNA conformation is important. This is because DNA-RNA hetero-duplex (DNA strand base-paired with a complementary RNA strand) or RNA-RNA duplexes exist in a very similar structure *in vivo*.
- ☆ Another form of DNA also exists. These are some short DNA molecules composed of alternating purine-pyrimidine nucleotides (especially Gs and Cs) adopt an alternative left-handed configuration instead of the normal right-handed helix.
- ☆ The Z-DNA is GC-rich left handed. Such a form is called ***Z-DNA*** after the zigzag path of the structure of sugar-phosphate backbone when viewed from the side. It is longer and thinner double helix, having a diameter of 18.4 A, rise/base pair 3.8 A, with 12 bp/helical turn, helix pitch of 47 A and tilt of bases -9 deg. It is entirely possible that both A-form and Z-form stretches of DNA exist in cells.
- ☆ The C-DNA and E-DNA are right handed with slight different configuration but seen under special environmental circumstances and hence do not occur *in vivo*.

Many DNA Molecules are Circular

All prokaryotic genomic DNAs and many viral DNAs are circular molecules. Circular DNA molecules also occur in mitochondria, which are present in almost all eukaryotic cells, and in chloroplasts present in plants and some unicellular eukaryotes.

Functions of DNA

Deoxyribonucleic acid (DNA) is the genetic material which carries information to specify the amino acid sequences of proteins. It is transcribed into several types of ribonucleic acid (RNA) including messenger RNA (mRNA), transfer RNA (tRNA), and ribosomal RNA (rRNA), which function in protein synthesis.

Denaturation of DNA

The unwinding and separation of DNA strands, referred to as denaturation, or "melting," can be induced experimentally. For example, if a solution of DNA is heated, the thermal energy increases molecular motion, eventually breaking the hydrogen bonds and other forces that stabilize the double helix, and the strands separate. This melting of DNA changes its absorption of ultraviolet (UV) light (in the 260-nm range), which is routinely used to measure DNA concentration because of the high absorbance of UV light by nucleic acid bases. Native double-stranded DNA absorbs about one-half as much light at 260 nm as does the equivalent amount of single-stranded DNA. Thus, as DNA denatures, its absorption of UV light increases. Near the denaturation temperature, a small increase in temperature causes an abrupt, near simultaneous, loss of the multiple, weak, cooperative interactions holding the two strands together, so that denaturation rapidly occurs throughout the entire length of the DNA. The *melting temperature,* T_m, at which the strands of DNA will separate, depends on several factors. Molecules that contain a greater proportion of G·C pairs require higher temperatures to denature because the three hydrogen bonds in G·C pairs make them more stable than A·T pairs with two hydrogen bonds. Indeed, the percentage of G·C base pairs in a DNA sample can be estimated from its T_m. In addition to heat, solutions of low ion concentration destabilize the double helix, causing it to melt at lower temperatures. DNA is also denatured by exposure to other agents that destabilize hydrogen bonds, such as alkaline solutions and concentrated solutions of formamide or urea:

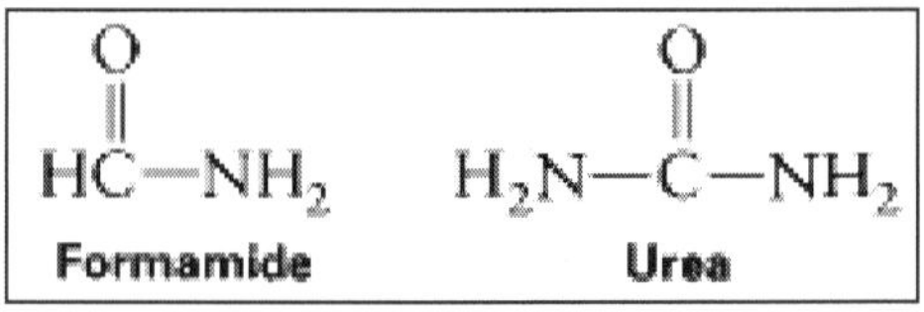

$HC(=O)—NH_2$	$H_2N—C(=O)—NH_2$
Formamide	**Urea**

The single-stranded DNA molecules that result from denaturation form random coils without a regular structure.

Renaturation

Lowering the temperature or increasing the ion concentration causes the two complementary strands to reassociate into a perfect double helix. This is called renaturation. The extent of such *renaturation* is dependent on time, the DNA concentration, and the ionic content of the solution. Two DNA strands not related in sequence will remain as random coils and will not renature and, most important, will not greatly inhibit complementary DNA partner strands from finding each other.

Denaturation and renaturation of DNA are the basis of nucleic acid hybridization, a powerful technique used to study the relatedness of two DNA samples and to detect and isolate specific DNA molecules in a mixture containing numerous different DNA sequences.

Heteroduplex DNA

It is the hybrid DNA formed by recombination. This DNA contains mismatched base pair or heterogous base sequence and also known as heterozygous DNA. The heteroduplex segregate by DNA replication. This DNA may replicate and produce two daughter homoduplexes. On the other, one strand of heteroduplex is removed and replaced by a new matching segment producing homologous DNA.

In vitro Synthesis of DNA

Kornberg, A. and coworkers (1967) synthesized DNA molecule in a test tube with the help of enzyme DNA polymerase from *E. coli*. They added in the test tube four different types of deoxyribonucleotides in the form of triphosphate, polymerase enzyme, magnesium ions and some amount of DNA. They found that DNA was synthesized about 20 times more than the amount of initial DNA added in the tube. The enzyme has the function to hook together the nucleotide units freely available in the tube into a DNA strand. The nucleotides are added to the hydroxyl group at number 3 carbon atom of deoxyribose sugar at one end of the chain. There is spontaneous bounding of nitrogenous base of the newly added triphosphate to the complementary base of the primer strand by hydrogen bond. Between 3′-OH group of newly added nucleotide and 5′ –OH group of the next arriving nucleotide is formed a phosphodiester bond. Thus, new and complementary nucleotides are added to the 5′ 3′ strand from 5′ and towards the 3′ end.

13.4 RNA STRUCTURE AND ITS TYPES

The RNA is found in cytoplasm and in nucleolus. The RNA occurs freely in cytoplasm as well as in the ribosomes. The RNA stores and transmits the genetic information in some viruses which do not have the DNA. The RNA is more frequently a single-stranded molecule of polynucleotides that form well-defined secondary and tertiary structures but some RNAs are double stranded. The polynucleotides are arranged in a linear sequence connected together by 3′-5′ phosphodiester bonds. RNA molecules are also polynucleotides with a sugar-phosphate backbone and four kinds of bases.

Some RNAs, called *ribozymes,* have catalytic activity.

The picture shows an ATP molecule (adenosine tri-phosphate) about to be incorporated into an RNA chain with the release of a di-phosphate.

RNA molecules do not have a regular helical structure like DNA. Instead, they can form complicated 3-dimensional structures where the strands can loop back and form **intra-strand** base-pairs from self-complementary regions along the chain. The RNA in reality is a molecule derived from DNA molecule by transcription that may carry information (mRNA), provide subcellular structure (rRNA), transport amino acids (tRNA), or facilitate the biochemical modification of itself or other RNA molecules.

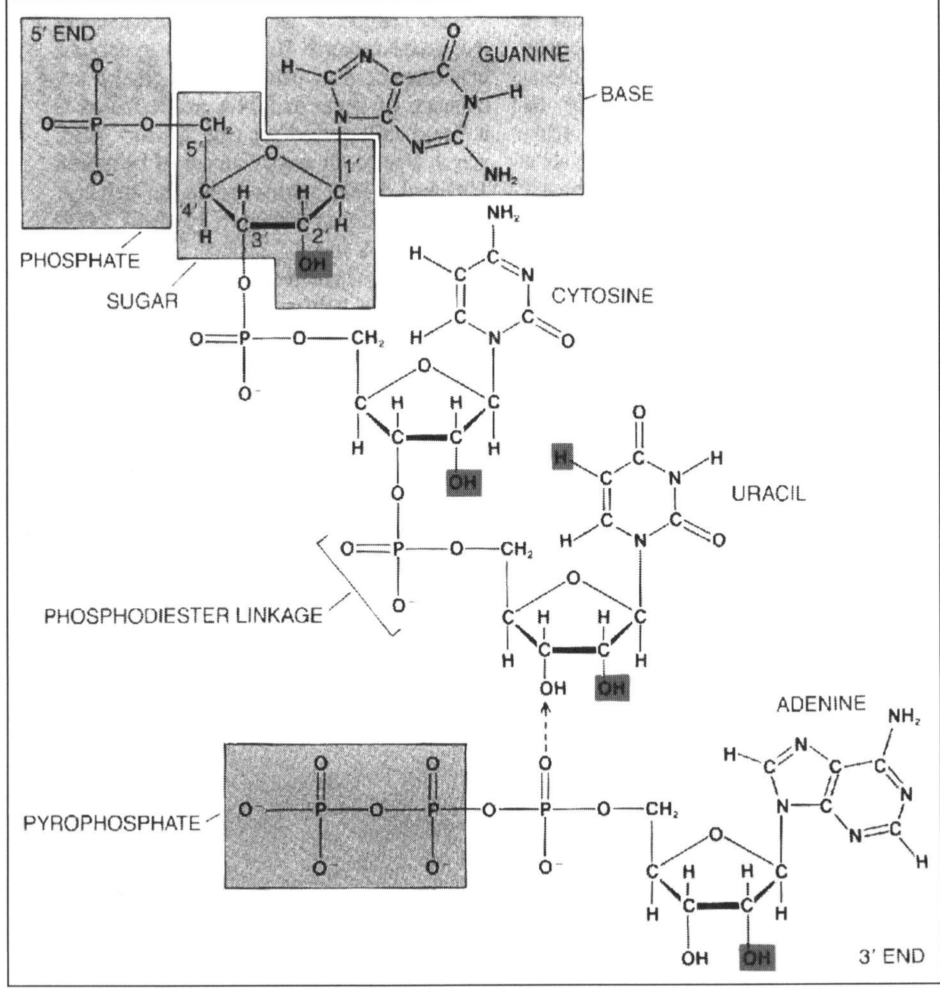

Figure 13.9: Structure of RNA.

Types of RNA

The RNA is of different types specially depending on performing different functions in protein synthesis.

(1) Genetic RNA

The RNA is also the genetic material in most of the plant viruses and some animal viruses in which DNA is not present. The experiment conducted by H. Fraenkel in California on tobacco mosaic virus (TMV) showed that RNA is the genetic material. The RNA may be double stranded or single strand. The base pairing rules in double stranded RNA are same to that of DNA. The different genetic RNAs are as under:

Types of Genetic RNA	*Type of Viruses*	*Name of Viruses*
Single stranded	Plant virus	TMV
" "	Animal viruses	Influenza virus
" "	"	Poliomyelitis
" "	Bacteriophages	MS2
" "	"	F2
" "	"	r17
Double stranded	Plant virus	Wound tumour
" "	Animal virus	Reo virus

(2) Non-genetic RNA

In case of eukaryotes in which the DNA is the genetic material, there are 3 major forms of RNA molecules which are non-genetic. These three forms are the messenger RNA (mRNA), ribosomal RNA (rRNA) and transfer RNA (tRNA) or soluble RNA (sRNA). The DNA is transcribed into all these types of ribonucleic acid (RNA) and all these forms function in protein synthesis.

Each kind of RNA molecule differs among them, each is transcribed from different genes and each has a unique function in the cells but all the three forms are likely to be produced in the nucleus by transcription of the DNA. The rRNA and tRNA live longer than mRNA. This is because after a short time, RNA hydrolyzing enzyme (*RNases*) cause the mRNA to break down after protein synthesis takes place.

Both prokaryotic and eukaryotic organisms contain all the above 3 types of RNAs. In addition to the above 3 major RNA molecules, 2 other types of RNAs are found in eukaryotes. These are the *small nuclear RNAs* **(snRNAs) and** *the micro RNAs* **(*miRNA*)** found only in eukaryotic organisms.

(a) Messenger RNA (mRNAs)

The mRNA is synthesized in the nucleus as a complementary strand to one of the two strands of the DNA. This synthesized mRNA carries the genetic information from the chromosomal DNA to the cytoplasm for protein synthesis. Thus, this RNA is called messenger RNA because it sends the message. The mRNA acts as a template for protein synthesis and has the same sequence of bases (read from the 5′ to the 3′ end) as the DNA strand that has the gene sequence. An mRNA can range from ~300 nucleotides to ~7000 nucleotides, depending on the size and the number of proteins that they are coding for.

mRNA synthesis: One of the two DNA strand is used for the synthesis of mRNA. The synthesis takes place from 5′ end towards 3′ end. The RNA polymerase catalyzes RNA synthesis by attaching to the initiator site or promoter end of structural gene or DNA cistron. This process of mRNA synthesis is called ***transcription***.

The mRNA constitutes about 10 per cent of the total RNA present in the cell. The developing mRNA molecule is anti- parallel and its nucleotides are complementary to those of the DNA template strand. The mRNA diffuses out of the nucleus into the cytoplasm after synthesis and deposited on some ribosomes. The mRNA is of short duration in prokaryotes. Its lifespan is of about 2 minutes in bacteria. However, in eukaryotes, the mRNA remains for more times, say from a number of hours to even for days.

The mRNA contains the same information as coded in that part of DNA. The main function of mRNA is to carry the genetic information from DNA to the ribosomes in the cytoplasm where the information is expressed for protein synthesis. Thus, the mRNAs are intermediaries to carry genetic information from DNA to the ribosomes where proteins are synthesized. The linear sequence of triplet codons in an mRNA molecule specifies the linear sequence of amino acids in the polypeptides produced during translation of that mRNA. The RNA after its synthesis immediately diffuses out of the nucleus into the cytoplasm through nuclear pores and deposited on some ribosomes in cytoplasm. The synthesis of mRNA from DNA is called as ***transcription.***

The specificity for a particular amino acid sequence is determined by mRNA. The transcription of eukaryotic DNA to produce mRNA begins with the synthesis of long precursor molecule by RNA polymerase II from the template strand of DNA. This enzyme functions by catalyzing formation of 5′ end towards 3′ phosphodiester of RNA "backbone" by "reading" the DNA template in the 3′ to 5′ direction. The mRNA chain growth is rapid from 15 to 100 nucleotides per second *in vitro.*

The immediate product of transcription in eukaryotes is a molecule of many more ribonucleotides that comprising the ultimate functional mRNA. This primary transcript in eukaryotes is generally referred to as heterogeneous nuclear RNA (hn RNA). The molecules of hnRNA range from 500 to 50,000 nucleotides long. They are very rapidly processed in to much smaller molecules. Some estimates predict that as little as 10 per cent of most original transcript eventually reaches the cytoplasm as mRNA. Following its transcription in eukaryotes, hnRNA is processed into functional mRNA in 3 steps.

Types of mRNA

The mRNA of different organisms may be alike in gross base content but differ in their arrangement. The molecules of mRNA are ***heterogeneous*** for their different sizes of different mol. Wt. The size and number of cistrons and the size of the protein molecule are two factors to decide the heterogeneity. Based on the presence of the number of cistrons there two types of mRNA *viz.* ***monocistronic mRNA*** which contains the codons of a single cistron to code for one complete molecule of protein and ***polycistronic mRNA*** molecule which contains the codons for more than one cistrons that may lie close together and synthesizes more than one protein chains, *e.g.* the mRNA molecule for controlling the metabolism of histidine codes for the synthesis of 10 specific enzymes.

Informosomes

According to Spirin, these are some ribonucleoprotein complexes in eukaryotes formed by the association of mRNA with protein in a ratio of 1:4 and remain free in the cytoplasm with no attachment to the polyribosomes. These complexes are stable for several days due to the presence of protein sheath around mRNA. The informosomes occur in the form of particles of 80S or less. These are used by the cell in protein synthesis only in case of delay in translation. The informosomes control the protein synthesis in early stage of cleavage when there is no rRNA and the genetic apparatus starts functioning only late during organogenesis in embryonic cells.

(b) Ribosomal RNA (rRNAs)

This is the RNA molecule that is structural components of ribosomes. It is bulk of the cellular RNA up to about 80 per cent of the total RNA of the cell and occurs in ribosomes that are nucleoprotein molecules. The rRNA is formed inside the nucleus. The rRNA inside the ribosomes of eukaryotic cells occurs in the form of particles of three different dimensions of 28S, 18S, and 5S.

There is large subunit (60S subunit) of ribosome to have 28S and 5S while the small subunit (50S subunit) of ribosome contain 18S molecule. In prokaryotic cells there are only 23S and 16S rRNA. The base contents of rRNA are different to those of mRNA and tRNA. The rRNA is relatively rich in cytosine and guanine. The molar ratio of guanine, cytosine, adenine and uracil in rRNA of *E. coli* is 36:23:21:19. The 5S RNA is transcribed from genes present outside the NOR and thus has an extra-nucleolar origin.

The structures of ribosomal RNA can get very complicated because of the large number of ways in which hairpins and loops can be formed.

Synthesis of rRNA

The DNA associated with the nucleolus is responsible for coding rRNA and known as nucleolar organizer. About 10-210 cistrons are involved with the rRNA synthesis in bacteria whereas the number is 210-2100 tightly clustered rDNA cistrons in higher organisms. The nucleolar DNA as a single unit of 45S synthesizes two types of rRNA of 28S and 18S. There is methylation of 45S RNA and complexed with protein inside the nucleolus. This 45S RNA is finally cleaved into 32S and 18S segments. Small subunits of ribosome are formed by association of 18S RNA with basic proteins. The 32S segment finally changes to 28S RNA and forms the large subunit of ribosome after getting associated with proteins. Now these units come out of into the cytoplasm.

Function of rRNA

The rRNAs are molecules to provide part of the structure and function of ribosomes and also represent an important part of the machinery required for the polypeptide synthesis. Thus, the rRNAs are structural and catalytic components of the ribosomes (an intricate machine) to translate nucleotide sequences of mRNAs into amino acid sequences of polypeptides. The set of polypeptides synthesis is the ribose which is a small peptide that averaged about 175×225 A°, composed of protein and rRNA.

The ribosomes that function in polypeptide synthesis occur in linear groups connected by mRNA and such groups of ribosomes are called ***polysomes***.

(c) Transfer RNAs (tRNAs)

The tRNA comprises about 10 - 15 per cent of the total RNA present in a cell at any one time. It is also called as soluble RNA (sRNA) or sometimes as adapter RNA. The tRNA is a small RNA molecule of about 80 nucleotides long, in the range ~70-90 nucleotides. They have a molecular weight of ~25,000 and have sedimentation constant ~ 4 Svedberg (S) units. The polypeptide chain of tRNA is bent in the middle and folded back on itself giving clover leaf model and some of the bases of two arms coiled over one another.

The 3′ end of the chain ends in CCA base sequence which represents the site for the attachment of activated amino acid. tRNA mole is present in both active and inactive forms. The inactive form of tRNA does not contain the CCA sequence at 3′ end of the chain. The active tRNA molecule can be activated by the addition of this nucleotide sequence under the control og the enzyme cytidine triphospate and ATP.

Each tRNA molecule in addition to the usual bases of RNA also contains many unusual bases like pseudouridine, inosinic acid, methylguanine, methyl aminopurins, *etc.* However, these additional bases do not affect the pairing of tRNA with mRNA.

Function of tRNA

This molecule (tRNA) serves as adapter molecule mediating the interaction between amino acids and the ***codons*** in mRNA during translation. This means that tRNA bring amino acids to the ribosomes (site of protein synthesis) and provide codon-recognition specificity during translation. Thus, these are the RNAs that transport amino acids to the ribosomes where the amino acids are assembled into protein. The tRNA picks up a specific activated amino acid from the cytoplasm, carries it to the site of protein synthesis (ribosome) and attaches itself on ribosome according to the sequence specified by mRNA. The tRNA transmits its amino acid to the newly polypeptide chain under formation.

Transfer RNA (tRNA), one for each triplet codon that codes for a specific amino-acid. The tRNA molecules are covalently attached to the corresponding amino-acid at one end, and at the other end they have a triplet sequence (called the *anti-codon*) that is complementary to the triplet codon on the mRNA.

The tRNA functions as an adaptor molecule of three bases known as *anticodon*. The ***anticodons*** are the nucleotide triplets in the tRNA molecule that are complementary to the three bases (nucleotide triplets) of mRNA. The anticodon (definite sequence of 3 nitrogeneous bases) which recognizes the codon of mRNA is contained in the bent of the polynucleotide chain of each tRNA molecule. There is at least one tRNA that is specific for each of the 20 amino acids. There are more than one tRNA molecules for each amino acid. Thus, the tRNA is a family of about 60 small sized RNA which can recognize the codons of mRNA,have high affinity for 21 activated amino acids, combine with them to carry them to the ribosome (site of protein synthesis).

The tRNA molecule has following 4 different special sites:

1. *Amino acid attachment site* – which occurs at the 3′ end of tRNA chain and has OH group combines with specific amino acid in the presence of ATp forming amino-acyl tRNA,
2. *Recognition site* – which contains a specific base sequence to indicate the attachment of correct amino acid to the tRNA molecule,
3. *Anticodon or codon recognition site* – which has 3 unpaired bases with complementary sequence with a codon in mRNA so as to determine the pairing of tRNA with the specific codon of mRNA, and
4. *Ribosome recognition site* – which help in the attachment of tRNA to the ribosome.

The covalent attachment between the *t*RNA and its corresponding amino-acid is achieved by yet another adaptor molecule (this time a protein molecule called aminoacyl-tRNA synthetase) of which there are at least 20 varieties, one for each kind of amino-acid. The synthetases recognize the detailed shape and properties of a specific amino-acid and the detailed shape of the acceptor stem in the folded tRNA molecule and catalyze the covalent attachment between the amino-acid and its corresponding tRNA.

During protein synthesis, codon on the mRNA attracts the proper tRNA by specific interaction between codons of mRNA and antcodons of tRNA. The amino acid phenyalanine is coded by UUU, the anticodon on one type of tRNA to accept phenylalanine is AAA. The tRNA is transcribed from several particular sites on template DNA.

tRNA Synthesis

The tRNA synthesis involves about 40 to 80 genes or cistron in bacteria scattered on the chromosome and 55 in *Drosophila*. There are particular regions of the DNA to synthesize tRNA molecules. The complementary in base composition and sequence to its particular cistron in the DNA is shown in the beginning by each tRNA molecule but the nitrogenous bases at certain specific points are changed through enzyme action after the complete tRNA molecule is transcribed from DNA.

RNA Synthesis In vitro

Weiss and coworkers (1960) isolated another RNA polymerase which could work in the presence of DNA as a template for RNA *in vitro* synthesis.

Grunbergmango and Ochada (1965) isolated an enzyme RNA polymerase which can link different nucleotides into a long RNA chain or it can also break the chain in small sections. The RNS synthesis can occur in the presence of this enzyme even in the absence of primer, in any proportion of nucleotides even in the presence of only one kind of nucleotides. Thus, the RNA chain may be formed with a single repeating base.

Synthesis of RNA requires nucleotide diphospate for adenosine (ADP), uridine (UDP), guanine (GDP), and cytosine (CDP). However, all these 4 substrates may not be necessarily present at the same time.

(d) Small Nuclear RNAs (snRNAs)

These are small RNA molecules that are located in the nucleus of eukaryotic cells. Most of them are the structural components of *spliceosomes,* nuclear organelles that excise introns from pre-mRNAs (nuclear gene transcripts).

The RNA-protein complexes that are components of spliceosomes are called ***small nuclear ribonucleoproteins* (*snRNPs*).**

(e) Micro RNAs (miRNA)

The micro RNAs (miRNAs) or short interfering RNAs (siRNAs) are short double-stranded RNA molecules (21 to 28 base pairs long). They mediate the phenomenon of RNA interference (RNAi). The RNAi is a phenomenon in which double-stranded RNA prevents the expression of a gene homologous to at least part of the RNA. There are a number of sources from which these small RNA molecules that induce RNAi (RNA interference) are produced -

- ☆ The *transcripts of microRNA genes* (genes denoted by *mir*) produce the RNAi. Hundreds of the genes for miRNAs (*mir* genes) are present in the genomes of different eukaryotes. Few of these genes were identified through analysis of mutations that changed the regulation of other genes. These genes have little or no protein-coding potential but they have a peculiar structure, and each gene has a short stretch of nucleotides repeated in opposite orientation around a short intervening segment of DNA.
- ☆ The transcription of some elements in the genome like *transposones* and *transgenes* may also stimulate/produce the RNAi (siRNAs). Some RNA viruses also produce RNAi. The RNAi derived from these sources (transposons, transgenes, and RNA viruses) are targeted for repression or degradation. This application of RNAi has an important function of protecting the organisms against viral infection and from transposition.
- ☆ The transcription of the double-stranded RNA prepared *in vitro* from cloned genes or gene segments can also induce RNAi. The double-stranded RNA molecules derived from the transcripts of such clones can be introduced into cultured cells or may be injected into living organisms. Now, the double-stranded RNA entering into the cells takes part in RNAi pathway. This double-stranded RNA after diced into siRNA molecules is incorporated into RNA-protein complexes and targeted to mRNAs of complementary sequences. The targeted mRNAa are generally degraded. Therefore, a particular type of double-stranded RNA can be used to treat the cells or organisms for an effect of striking out (empty) or knocking down (strike down) the expression of the gene that corresponds to that RNA. This approach can be used to study the effect of attenuating the expression of particular genes, particularly in those organisms in which genetic analysis is difficult, slow or impossible. This way the function of genes may be analyzed by using the RNAi as a *research tool,* in the cells and complete organism of many eukaryotes.

The short interfering RNAs and micro RNAs of 21 to 28 bp long are produced from longer double-stranded precursors (RNA molecules) by the enzymatic action of proteins that are double-stranded RNA specific endonucleases. These endonucleases are called ***dicer enzymes*** because they "dice" large RNA into small pieces. Thus, the siRNAs and miRNAs are produced by dicer activity and they base-pair throughout their lengths except at their 3′ ends with two nucleotides remaining unpaired. Different eukaryotes produce different dicer enzymes. These enzymes act in cytoplasm in *C. elegans* and *Drosophila* but probably act in the nucleus in *Arabidopsis.*

The small RNA molecules have their important role to play in both plants and animals. They either cause the cleavage and subsequent degradation of mRNA or prevent the mRNA to translate them into polypeptide.

All the above 5 types of RNAs are produced by transcription. The mRNAs is translated and specify polypeptides whereas the final products of other 4 types of RNA genes are RNA molecules. These 4 types of RNA molecules are not translated.

The functions of 5 types are RNAs in the cells having both the DNA as well as the RNA, are as follows:

(i) mRNA acts as an intermediary in protein synthesis to carry the information from DNA to the cytoplasm and ribosomes where the proteins are synthesized,

(ii) rRNA molecules are essential components of the ribosomes,

(iii) tRNAs carry amino acids to the ribosomes and function in codon recognition during the synthesis of polypeptides,

(iv) snRNAs are major components of spiceosomes, and

(v) miRNAs play key roles in regulating gene expression.

13.5 DIFFERENCES AND SIMILARITIES BETWEEN DNA AND RNA

The two nucleic acids have the following main differences and similarities:

- ✰ The DNA is a double-stranded molecule having two intertwined polynucleotide chains (strands) but some DNAs are single-stranded. RNA molecules are mostly single-stranded (single polynucleotide chain or strand) but in some viruses, the RNA is double-stranded. Although the primary structures of DNA and RNA are generally similar, but their conformations are quite different. This structural difference (single and double-stranded) is critical to the different functions of the two types of nucleic acids.
- ✰ Both DNA and RNA are long, unbranched polymers of nucleotides. Each nucleotide in both the nucleic acids consists of a heterocyclic base linked via a five-carbon sugar (deoxyribose or ribose) to a phosphate group.
- ✰ The RNA contains the sugar ribose in place of deoxyribose contained in DNA. Thus the nucleotides in RNA are called *ribonucleotides* whereas in DNA the nucleotides are the *deoxyribonucleotides.* The sugar in RNA has

an –OH at the 2′ C position highlighted in red in the figure below (DNA sugars have –H at that position)

- DNA and RNA each contain four bases, out of which 3 are common in both DNA and RNA. The purines adenine (A) and guanine (G) and the pyrimidine cytosine (C) are present in both DNA and RNA. The pyrimidine thymine (T) present in DNA molecule is replaced by the pyrimidine uracil (U) in RNA molecule. However, some DNAs contain uracil, and some RNAs contain thymine. T has a methyl ($-CH_3$) group instead of the H atom shown in red in U.
- The standard base pairs are G:C and A:T in DNA; and G:C and A:U in RNA (Watson-Crick). The bases in nucleic acids interact via hydrogen bonds. Base pairing stabilizes the native three-dimensional structures of DNA and RNA.
- The purines are equal to pyrimidine in DNA (A + G = C + T) but purines are not necessarily equal to pyrimidine in RNA.

13.6 GENE CONCEPT

After the discovery of Mendel's law of inheritance, the gene concept came into existence and known as part of chromosome. **The *gene has become a part of DNA molecule,*** after the discovery of the components of chromosome.

On an average, a gene (sometimes called a *cistron*) probably contains about 600 consecutive nucleotide base pairs but this number vary from gene to gene. Thus, the gene is a structural part of a chromosome. Hundreds and possibly thousands of genes are present in each chromosome and each gene has a fix or especial position called a *locus*. Each gene has at least two alternate forms called as *allelomorphs* which have contrasting or different effects on the trait.

This model of DNA structure has helped to explain that how the changes in heredity (mutation) may occur. The error in base pairing may happen occasionally due to some reason (environmental effects, *viz.* radiation *etc.*) and this may result the substitution of different nucleotide during replication in place of the nucleotide usually present at that position. Thus, all descendant molecules will have the new sequence of nucleotides in the DNA.

The different concepts of gene have been given in different ways as:

(*i*) ***Mendelian factor*** – Mendel on the basis of his experimental results used the term factor or determinants to the hereditary entity for which the term gene was introduced by Johannsen (1909).

(*ii*) ***Concept of gene*** was introduced by Sutton and elaborated by Morgan, Bridges, and Muller. The *classical concept of gene* is given as the hereditary or genetic unit based on some essential features which are the followings:

- A gene is a unit of physical or physiological function (character), located at a definite position in a specific chromosome (locus, plural loci). There are some situations like chromosome aberration that bring change in relative position. The genes on the chromosome are numerous (about 50,000 genes are known on 23 pairs of human chromosomes) and they produces a specific phenotypic action or expression (character).

- ☆ There is a single linear order arrangement of genes on chromosomes looking like beads on a string. A gene occurs in its various structural forms called mutants or alleles which arise as a result of cgange in the original gene called mutation and the phenomenon as the allelomorphisms. Thus, a gene is a unit of change by mutation. Some genes have only two alternate forms while others have many structural forms called as multiple alleles. The alternative structure of gene (mutants) shows the existence of gene. These alleles have their functional nature or relationship as dominant and recessive.
- ☆ The genes have the ability for self duplicate (DNA replication) exactly in two copies very accurately. The gene is a unit of structure which cannot be divided by crossing over and hence a unit of segregation or transmission.
- ☆ The genes exert their action or express by producing enzymes (proteins) and each gene synthesize a particular protein by a two stage process of gene transcription and translation.

(iii) ***Molecular structure (concept) of gene*** is given in relation to the parallel behavior of DNA with chromosomes. Molecular studies (structure and function of DNA in protein synthesis) had shown that chemically, a gene is a part of DNA as one or a sequence of nucleotides. The three nucleotides in a sequence produce one amino acids which are assembled to form peptide (two amino acids) and polypeptides chains forming the part of protein. The molecular structure of gene can be given in the following terms (Benzer, S.):

- ☆ *CISTRON:* The cistron is a part of DNA containing a number of nucleotides which can synthesize a single polypeptide chain of an enzyme. It is the unit of physiological function and in real a gene. It is synonymous with the gene function. A polypeptide chain is formed of a number of amino acids and each amino acid molecule contains 3 nucleotides. Therefore, the haemoglobin for its globin protein fraction would need two cistron, one each for α and β chains.
- ☆ *MUTON:* The muton is the smallest unit of DNA which may undergo a change resulting mutation and produce a phenotypic effect. The mutation occurs as a result of change in any nucleotide. There are thus many positions or sites within a cistron as per the number of nucleotides where the mutation can occur. In this way, the muton may thus be a single nucleotide or some part of nucleotide, as the smallest unit of mutation to occur and hence to qualify the term gene. This is because any change in a nucleotide (base pair of triplet) modifies the message carried by the codon.

- ☆ *RECON:* It is the smallest unit of DNA capable of crossing over and hence recombination between two adjacent nucleotides. The crossing over may take place anywhere in DNA. A recon may be as small as one nucleotide pair in DNA.
- ☆ *REPLICON:* It is the unit of replication. It is a segment of DNA which is under the control of one origin of replication and two termini. In this context entire prokaryotic chromosome is usually one replicon whereas each of the eukaryotic chromosomes contains multiple replicons distributed throughout the chromosome at an interval of about 30,000 to 300,000 bp.
- ☆ *OPERON:* The combination of operator gene and sequence of structural gene acting together as a unit is called *operon*. Thus, it is composed of several genes.
- ☆ *COMPLON:* Two or more polypeptide chains which complements to each other through their active groups. This unit of complementation is called complon and used to replace cistron.

(iv) ***Modern concept of gene*** in terms of its essential features is that-

"The genes are part of DNA, located on chromosomes, at a specific position (*locus*), *arranged in linear order like the beads on a string, and transmitted from parents to the offspring. A gene may occur in many alternate forms* (*multiple alleles*) *due to mutation and hence a gene is capable of mutation. The genes duplicate themselves very accurately through DNA replication, express themselves by producing enzymes* (*proteins*) *through genetic code and finally determine the various characteristics of organisms".*

SPLIT GENES: Some genes are called as split genes that are splitted into several distinct units separated by regions of non-coding DNA. These intervene.ing non-coding sequences are called as ***introns*** whereas those having biological information are called as ***exons***. These split genes are also called as ***discontinuous genes***, or the ***mosaic genes***. A gene may have no introns or many introns.

The eukaryotes and their viruses have introns but the prokaryotes and their viruses are lacking in introns. Archaebacteria have these introns while the mitochondris do not have introns. The number of introns may not be present in a single gene or it may have as many as 52 as found in mammalian α- collagen gene.

Gene splicing *– reunion of introns*: The exons from different discontinuous genes can form new combinations of biological information by their shuffling as the shuffling may produce new functional proteins according to ***Gilber hypothesis***.

The coding strand of the gene on its transcription produces its faithful copy. The primary transcript may therefore have introns if these are already present in the gene. It is therefore essential the removal of introns and exon regions of the transcript should be reattached to each other before translation. Such a process of reattachment of exons is called gene splicing.

Identification of introns: The comparison of the nucleotide sequence of a gene with the nucleotide or amino acid sequence of the gene product can easily indentify the introns. Moreover, the introns detection is also possible by a method that depends on the ability of gene in base pair to its RNA transcript. Absence of introns will produce continuous copy of DNA producing an uninterrupted heteroduplex. Presence of one or more introns produces a series of loops within the heteroduplex.

Chapter 14

Mutation: General Aspects

The history of mutation dates back to the appearance of a lamb with exceptionally short legs during 1791 in a flock of sheep maintained by Seth Wright. He developed a flock of sheep having short legs considering the economic significance of short leg sheep. This newly developed flock of sheep was named as ***Ancon breed*** of sheep. The short leg character was found later on a recessive trait developed in homozygous recessive condition.

Morgan, T.H. (1910) reported white eyed *Drosophila* males among red eyed males. He along with his colleagues started work on this aspect on *Drosophila.* A number of mutations were discovered in *Drosophila* and in other organisms including bacteria, plants, and animals.

However, Hugo De Vries during early of twentieth century was the first to coin the term mutation to a sudden and permanent change in the genome observed phenotypically in the evening primrose, *oenothera lamarckiana.*

The mutation in general is used to cover all genetic changes including changes in gene (gene mutation) and changes in chromosome (chromosome mutation). However, the *gene mutation* is the chemical change in gene at specific site which is called as point mutation or mutation. A definite mechanism is involved in bringing this change in a gene at particular site. The *chromosome mutation* is the change in either structure of the chromosome (inversions, translocations, deletions, duplications of nucleotide sequence) or in the number of chromosomes (heteroploidy). However, the term mutation is restricted to a change at a particular locus (called point mutation or gene mutation) and thus differs from chromosome aberration. Therefore, the mutation is a change at gene level rather than at chromosome level.

14.1 DEFINITION AND CONCEPT OF MUTATION

The nucleotide is the basic and structural unit of genetic material, the DNA (gene – the DNA segment) as well as of RNA. The DNA is transmitted from generation to generation through sexual reproduction and also from one cell to another through cell division which requires DNA duplication (replication). The DNA (genetic material) stores the genetic information which is encoded in the sequences of nucleotide pairs, duplicates the genetic information (DNA duplication or replication), and transmits the information from parents to the offspring to produce the different characteristics of all the living beings. The accurate replication of DNA depends on proofreading activities of DNA polymerases which catalyze DNA synthesis. However, the DNA replication is not perfect but some mistakes do occur in the replication of DNA. This DNA with mistake in replication is transmitted causing the heritable changes in the phenotype of the individual.

The heritable changes in the DNA are called ***mutations***. Therefore, the mutation is the heritable change in the genetic material of an organism other than recombination of genes or a process of occurrence of the genetic change. Mutation is a sudden and spontaneous heritable change produced by a change in the base pair of nucleotide of the DNA segment (gene) so that a new allele produced is different from the original gene in its base sequence and has an effect on the expression of a particular character.

The change in genetic material at DNA level occurs during its replication due to incorrect incorporation of nucleotides into replicating DNA and this change is capable to change or disrupt the information encoded in gene. The gene with this change in its nucleotide sequence is called *mutant gene* which causes different phenotype in an organism. The organism showing the changed phenotype due to having received the mutant allele is called *mutant*. The change in polypeptide β- globulin chain of haemoglobin is the best known example of gene mutation.

The mutant allele has an effect different to that of the normal allele and produces an alternate phenotype of the trait. For example, in *Drosophila melanogaster*, the normal colour of the eyes is red. A white eyed male fly appeared in the normal population of red eyes. It was later on found that white eye colour is recessive to the normal red eye colour. The appearance of white eye due to recessive allele was referred to as the gene mutation. Thus, mutation provides new genetic material on which selection can operate.

A gene can change into another form which may either exist in the population or it may be a new allele that does not exist in the population. The different allelic forms of one or the other gene (A, a) arise only as a result of mutation. It is taken that one of the two alleles at a locus arises by mutation from the other.

14.2 TYPES OF MUTATIONS

The mutation may be classified in a number of ways depending upon the cell type of the body in which mutation occurs, nature or origin of cause (known or unknown causes), size of the part of chromosome affected by mutation (single nucleotide to entire gene or chromosome), different phenotypic effect, recurrence of mutation (once or repeatedly), direction of change (forward or reverse mutation) and change in nucleotide content or in location of gene (basis of mutation).

(i) Somatic and Germinal Mutations: Cell Types of Body in which Mutation Occur

The mutation may occur in any cell and any age. The mutation can be somatic and gametic (germinal). When the mutation occurs in somatic cells (body cells that are not reproductive cells or non-germ line cells) it is called as somatic mutations but if the mutation occurs in germ cells or sex cells, it is called as gametic or germinal mutation.

The somatic mutations are not heritable and remain limited to the organism in which they occur. Thus, somatic mutations are not genetically important. However, the *Delicious apple* (discovered in 1881by Jessie Hiatt, an Iowa farmer) and the *Novel orange* have resulted from mutations that occurred in somatic tissues. The cells carrying the mutant gene give rise to more of its own kind, eventually producing an entire branch on its respective tree which had the characteristics of the mutant type gene. The fruit trees with these mutations were somatic mosaics and the vegetative propagation is possible in these fruit species. The progeny from grafts and buds have perpetuated the original mutation. Somatic mutations also occur in animals. The occurrence of hair spot in red portion of the coat of Hereford cattle is an example of somatic cell mutation.

The *gametic* or *germ cell mutations* occur in germ-line cells, at any stage in the reproductive cycle of the organism, and produce permanent heritable change. The stage of the occurrence of mutation is important in the spread of mutant allele. The mutation if occurring in primordial germ-line cell of the testis or ovary, the mutant allele will be received by several gametes with increased potential for perpetuation but if the mutation occurs in a gamete, it will be received only by a single progeny. Further, the effect of mutant allele is observed immediately on the phenotype if the mutant allele is dominant over its wild allele. Therefore, the stage in the reproductive cycle for the occurrence of mutation and the dominance of a mutant allele are important factors.

These mutations create genetic variations, producing numerous varieties of plants and animals, colours in farm animals. Seth Wright (1791) first observed in his flock of sheep a peculiar male lamb with short legs and this was found to be due to a dominant germinal mutation. The owner of this male lamb (Wright) used this for breeding ewes and succeeded to develop a line of short-legged sheep (Ancon breed). The other examples of germ cell mutations in animals have been mentioned elsewhere in this book dealing with multiple alleles and other topics.

(ii) Spontaneous and Induced Mutations: Origin or Cause of Mutation

The mutation may occur spontaneously without a known cause or agent present in the environment. These are called as *background mutations or* ***spontaneous mutations.***

The spontaneous mutations are rare and arise randomly in nature without any readily apparent cause. Even gene has its own characteristic mutational behavior.

Some genes undergo mutation more frequently than others in the same organism. Highly mutable genes frequently occur in somatic tissues and occasionally in germ cells, are unstable and also influenced by other factors in the genetic component.

The spontaneous mutation may result of natural radiations (gamma rays and cosmic rays produced from radium and other radioactive substances), natural gases, sudden change in temperature and metabolic activities as a result of formation of certain chemical compounds. The mutation rate is increased with the increase in age of animals and plants. The plants grown from old seeds (5-6 years) have more mutations than grown from fresh seeds. The exposure to extreme temperature also produces mutation. The spontaneous mutation rates are relatively low, with most occurring one in a million or more.

Secondly, the mutations can be induced artificially (Hermann J. Muller, 1927) and hence called as ***induced mutation***. The mutations are induced by exposure of organisms to physical, like ionizing radiations (X rays, gamma rays, and cosmic rays) as well as nonionizing radiation (Ultraviolet light) and chemicals agents, called mutagenic agents that cause changes in DNA.

The spontaneous and induced mutations can be compared in terms of their frequency (rate), source and nature of origin, and use. The spontaneous mutations occur rarely, due to unknown natural causes, and as a result of natural electromagnetic energy, *e.g.* natural radiation, sudden change in temperature, *etc.* while the rate of induced mutation is more, produced artificially, and as a result of treating the organism with radiations and chemical mutagens. However, both the spontaneous as well as induced mutations form the basis of improvement in plants and animals.

The details of induced mutations along with mutagenic agents have been discussed further in subsequent pages of this chapter.

(iii) Point and Gross Mutation: Size of Mutation

A very small part of DNA *viz.* single nucleotide or nucleotide pair may be involved and called as *point mutation*. The mutation may involve more than one nucleotide pair, *gross mutation*, to the entire chromosome or set of chromosome, chromosomal aberration.

(iv) Single and Recurrent Mutations: Recurrence of Mutation

The newly arisen mutant allele may be due to a single mutational event and called as *single mutant allele* or the mutational event recurred regularly called as *recurrent mutation*.

A newly mutant allele may increase or decrease in its frequency or may be lost from population by chance elimination or fixed in the population. The fate of a new single mutation depends on the population size, selective advantage and the distribution of progenies in families in which the mutant gene is arises.

The recurrent mutation results to an increase in frequency in a large population and cannot be lost by sampling process but they are established in the population. The frequency of this mutant gene depends on mutation rate per generation which varies for different loci but seems to be reasonably constant for a particular locus under constant environmental conditions.

(v) Forward and Back or Reverse Mutation: Direction of Mutation – A Reversible Process

The wild-type gene is changed by mutation resulting in abnormal phenotype. This is called the *forward mutation.* Likewise, the abnormal phenotype is changed into wild type due to the reason that the mutant allele mutate back to the original form (wild type). This is called as *reverse or back mutation.* The rate of forward and reverse mutation is different. However, sometimes the mutation causes two different but normal phenotypes, *e.g.* brown and blue eye colour in human. The frequency of the individuals in a large population decides that which allele is wild or mutant. The allele with least frequency is considered as mutant.

(vi) Random and Non-adaptive Process

The environment factor (stress – temperature, use of antibiotics does not causes genetic changes but it simply selects the pre-existing change (mutation – mutant phenotype) having better adapted phenotype to the changed (new) environment. Thus, the mutation is a randomly occurring and a non-adaptive process. The examples are that the rats may not be affected by the anticoagulant (rodent poison), many cockroach are insensitive to chlordane (poison to control the cockroach), high level of resistance of houseflies to many insecticides and pesticides, the pathogenic microorganisms becoming resistant to antibiotics.

The mutations are occurring to produce resistance to the pesticides and antibiotics. The sensitive microorganisms are killed but the mutants are multiplied to produce new resistant strains. Thus, mutation and natural selection give rise to evolution by producing new mutant strains and their survival to the new environment. The environmental stress simply preserves pre-existing mutations. The environmental stress (antibiotic) simply select rare, randomly occurring mutants pre-existing in the population subjected to environmental stress.

Joshua and Lederberg, E. (1952) developed a new technique (*replica plating*) to know whether the resistant organisms are present prior to exposure to new environment (antibiotic treatment) or resistant strain was developed (induced) in the presence of new environment (antibiotic). This technique was able to demonstrate the presence of antibiotic-resistant mutants in the culture prior to exposure to the antibiotic.

(vii) Knockout Mutation

A mutation that impairs or abolishes gene expression or the function of a gene product is called ***knockout mutation*** or ***loss-of-function mutation***.

A mutant allele that completely abolishes gene expression is called an ***amorphic*** or ***null mutation.*** Such mutant form of a gene that either produces no product or a nonfunctional product is called ***null allele***. Such genes do not encode functional products because they have sustained one or more lesions like frame shifting or nonsense mutations. Such alleles are called ***pseudoalleles*** - the duplicated genes.

A *pseudogene* is an inactive but stable component of a genome resembling a gene, apparently derived from active genes by mutation.

However, ***pseudoautosomal gene*** is different from *pseudogene*. The pseudoautosomal gene is that which is located on both the X and Y chromosomes.

The gene mutations with no effect on phenotype or small effect are called ***isoalleles***. These are different forms of a gene that produce the same phenotype or very similar phenotype. These are detected by special techniques.

The mutations that are both structurally and functionally allelic and hence the mutations arising at the same site in the same gene are called ***homoalleles.*** The genes that have evolved from a common ancestral gene are called ***homologous genes***. The chromosomes having the same array of genes are called ***homologous chromosomes.*** The chromosomes that occur in pairs, similar in size and shape, and one each coming from two parents (male amd female) are also called *homologous*.

A mutant allele that has less expression than a wild-type allele but does not completely but partially abolish expression is called ***hypomorphic***. The ***suppressor mutation*** is that which partially or completely cancels the phenotypic effect of another mutation. An organism that can grow in the presence of a second genetic factor (suppressor) but not in the absence of this factor is called ***suppressor-sensitive mutant.***

The mutation that changes a codon specifying an amino acid to a chain-termination codon (triplets) within genes is known as ***nonsense mutation.*** The nonsense mutations produce completely nonfunctional polypeptide fragments. On the contrary, the ***missense mutation*** changes a codon (triplet) specifying an amino acid to a codon specifying a different amino acid. The gene with missense mutation encodes a complete polypeptide but with an amino acid substitution in the polypeptide gene product. The mutations are ***suppressor mutations*** which are nucleotide substitutions and suppressed the effect of other mutations.

A DNA sequence that helps to 'reduce' or 'shut off' the expression of a nearby gene is called ***silencer.*** A variant in DNA that does not alter the amino acid sequence of a protein is called ***silent polymorphism.*** This occurs due to degeneracy of genetic codes.

(viii) Insertion Mutation

A mutation caused by the insertion of foreign DNA such as a transposable element or the T-DNA of the Ti plasmid of *Agrobacterium tumefaciens.*

(ix) Mutator Genes

The genes which increase the mutation rate are called ***mutable genes*** or ***mutator genes.*** The mutable or mutator genes have their effect on other genes to make them mutate with higher and lower frequency. The effect of mutator genes may either be limited to one locus (specific mutators) or have simultaneous effects on many loci (non-specific mutations). The mutator genes are mainly the structural genes, produce mutant phenotype, and widely present in both animals and plants. The example of mutator gene is the gene ***Dt*** which influences another gene a_1 for green colour in plants to mutate it to A_1 causing variegated leaves and seeds having purple streaks or dots (Rhoades, 1938) in maize. The mutator genes have also been reported in *Drosophila* (Demerec, 1937) and *E. coli* (Goldstein, 1955).

On the other hand, there are also some ***mutation suppressor genes*** which may decrease the mutation rate. The mutation suppressor is called when a mutation occurs at a locus different from the locus of already mutated locus and reverses the mutational effects of already mutated gene. Likewise the *photo-reactivation* and *dark-reactivation* also cause reverse mutation. The thymine dimmers produced by UV rays induce mutation that is reverted by specific enzymes in the presence of light waves as a result of cleavage of dimmers and to restore their original forms. The reverse mutation may also occur in the absence of light (dark-reactivation) by some enzymes (endonuclease that make a cut in dimer, exonuclease, DNA polymerase, and some unknown enzyme).

14.3 PHENOTYPIC EFFECTS OF MUTATIONS

The analysis of the properties of mutations has proved useful not only to identify the genes but to know more about them. The mutations bring change in phenotype of character (colour and shape of body parts like eyes). The mutations vary in their effects which shows that each individual carries many different kinds of genes and that each gene can mutate in different ways resulting different effects. The mutated alleles may produce slightly modified phenotype or clearly identified phenotype in homozygous or in heterozygous combination with other alleles.

(i) Mechanism of Producing Phenotype by a Gene

It is well known from the variation produced by gene mutation that there are many different genes in an organism and that these genes have also their multiple allelic forms. The different genes are responsible to produce the different characters of an organism (plant height, seed coat colour, eye colour, *etc.*) and different alleles of a gene produce different forms of any character (tall versus dwarf plant height, yellow versus green seeds, red versus white eye colour in *Drosophila*).

It has become clear that most of the genes specify a product that produces and influences the phenotype of a character. These products are known as gene products which are the *polypeptides* as discovered by Beadle George and Tatum Edward. There is a relationship between genes and polypeptides. Each gene synthesizes a particular polypeptide which in turn influences the phenotype of a character.

The polypeptides are the linear chains of amino acids and are thus macromolecules. There are formed thousands of different polypeptides in each organism. Each of the polypeptide has a sequence of specific amino acids. These amino acids are the building blocks of each polypeptide chain. Two or more polypeptides are combined and form a protein. Thus, the amino acids are the constituents of polypeptides and the polypeptides are the constituents of proteins.

The proteins have to perform different functions of the cell(s) depending on the type of protein formed, *viz.*

☆ Some proteins are the structural components of the cells,

- ☆ Some proteins are catalysts in biochemical reactions known as *enzymes*, and
- ☆ Some other proteins are involved in transporting the substances within and between cells.

Each gene specifies a specific polypeptide made up of amino acids (See chapter 16 - Mechanism of gene expression). Each polypeptide forms its product called the gene product. Thus, the *genes function* by producing *polypeptides*. The mutation brings a change in polypeptide and its product (gene product). As a result, the polypeptide product is either not formed or it is different from that produced by wild-type allele and hence its role is changed. The mutations therefore, either eliminating the formation of polypeptide or bringing a change in the polypeptide (section 14.2 – molecular pathway/mechanism of mutation) has an effect on the character by changing its phenotype.

(ii) Variable Effects of Mutations on Phenotype – Lethal, Semi-lethal and Detrimental

The mutations may change the various aspects of morphology of the individual as a whole or of any body part. Such mutations are called ***visible mutations*** *or visible change, e.g.* red eye gene in *Drosophila* is mutated and produced white eye. These mutations may be dominant or recessive and can alter any character of the organism.

The mutations limiting the reproduction are called ***sterile mutations***. The sterile mutations affect the reproduction to different extent *viz.* some of them impair the reproduction slightly while others prevent the reproduction completely.

A mutation is called ***neutral mutation*** that changes the nucleotide sequence of a gene but it has no effect on the fitness of the individual. The ***neutral theory*** *of molecular evolution* is the one that explains the evolution of DNA and protein sequences by neutral mutation rate, random genetic drift, and purifying selection which eliminates fitness depressing mutation and hence has little or no effect on fitness.

The production of ***null alleles*** by mutation in growth affecting genes has their effect on the vital functions (viability) of organism to different extent. This is because *null mutations* produce no gene product or totally nonfunctional gene products. Thus, such mutations interfering with necessary vital functions are called ***lethal mutations***. These mutations cause the death of the individuals homozygous for mutation. They are classified as ***lethal*** which kill all individuals before adult age; ***semi- lethal*** which kill most of the individuals (say up to 90 per cent); and ***sub-vital*** (*detrimental*) which have relatively greater viability.

The visible as well as lethal effects of mutants are used to measure the mutation rate. Some treatment is given to a sample of organisms. The rate of mutation in treated and control groups is compared. If the differences are more, it indicates that the treatment produced mutation. The lethal effect is detected by the entire absence of an expected genotype/phenotypic class of progeny. However, the *semi-lethal* kill only a fraction of the embryos, but the semi-lethal are rare as compared to lethal.

The lethal alleles may be dominant or recessive. The dominant lethal kill the individuals before or soon after birth. It is difficult to study the dominant lethal genetically unless death occurs only after the reproductive stage. But the genetic studies of recessive lethal can be conducted because they are inherited from generation to generation in heterozygous individuals. If a recessive lethal is sex linked, it then survives as a heterozygote only in the sex having two X chromosomes and is inherited whereas the sex having only one X chromosome carrying lethal dies. This results the sex ratio in crosses with heterozygous female instead of being 1:1 as 1 M: 2F.

(iii) Conditional Lethal Mutations

These are another category of mutations. These mutations are lethal under one set of environmental conditions like nutrition and temperature, called the *restrictive conditions* but these are viable in another environment, called the *permissive condition.* These environmental conditions resulting in *conditional lethal mutations* and in complete loss of gene-product activity allows to identify and study the mutations in essential genes. The mutants carrying the conditional lethal are propagated under the permissive environmental conditions. The function of gene products may be inferred from the consequences of their absence under the restrictive conditions. The conditional lethal phenotypes can be categorized as:

Auxotrophic Mutants

Mutation affecting the nutritional properties of the organism may be considered conditional lethal when the mutant fails to survive long on minimal medium but survive on appropriately supplemented medium. The auxotrophs are the mutants which cannot synthesize the essential metabolites (amino acid, purine, pyrimidine, vitamin, etc) which are synthesized by the wild-type organisms of the same species known as *prototrophic.* Thus, the auxotrophs need the supply of the metabolites in the medium (permissive condition) for their growth and reproduction, and they (auxotrophs) cannot grow in restrictive condition (minimal medium - in the absence of essential metabolite).

Temperature-Sensitive Mutants

Temperature sensitive lethal mutations form another category of conditional lethal. These are mutations that make essential genes inactive at high temperature but not at low temperature. The mutant organisms grow at specific temperature but not at other temperature. Most of them are heat-sensitive while some are cold-sensitive. The increased heat or cold labile nature of the mutant gene product gives rise to the temperature sensitivity. For example, an enzyme which is active at low temperature but it is partially or completely inactive at high temperatures. It is only the synthesis of gene product which is sensitive to temperature and after being synthesized it is equally stable to the wild-gene product.

Suppressor-sensitive Mutants

These mutants require the presence of a second genetic factor (called suppressor) for their viability otherwise they are not viable. The presence of suppressor gene makes ineffective the effect of mutation of a gene by compensating or correcting the defect caused by the mutation.

Example: The expression of *Himalayan* allele of the coat colour gene in mammals like rabbits and mice is *temperature-sensitive*. The Himalayan *albino rabbits* have black colour on feet, ears, nose, and tail but the remaining body is white. If the rabbits are shifted to cold place after cutting of white hairs (from white parts), the black hairs appear instead of white hairs. This is the case when recessive mutation results in a partial loss of gene function. The *Himalayan* allele specifies a polypeptide which functions only in the body parts with reduced temperature. The rabbits homozygous for the *Himalayan* allele have pigmented (black) hair on their extremities, *viz.* tail, legs, ears, and tip of nose but not on the rest of the body which have white coat colour. The reason being that the polypeptide specified by this allele is functional only in the body parts which have low temperature but the polypeptide in the rest of the body is not functional due to their exposure to high temperature.

Another example of temperature-sensitive allele is the *shibire* mutation. The word shibire means "paralysis" in Japanese. The temperature for normal viability and fertility of *Drosophila* flies is 25°C but these are extremely sensitive to a sudden shock. The temperature of shibire culture raised to 29°C becomes lethal to the flies. This is because the mutant gene produces a totally non-functional protein at higher temperature of 29°C.

14.4 MUTATION RATE

Each gene has a potential to mutate. The mutation rate varies roughly from 10^{-7} to 10^{-4} for a locus. However, some genes mutate with higher frequency than others while others with lower frequency. There are some genes which may increase or decrease the mutation rate.

There are some genetic and non-genetic (environmental) factors that influence the mutation rate. The mutation rate is increased by -

- ☆ Certain *genes* (called mutator genes) and by some transposable genetic elements (transposons),
- ☆ Some *viruses* also influence the mutability of host's genes as reported by Sprague (1963) in maize and Baumiliar (1967) in *Drosophila melanogaster*, and by
- ☆ Some *environmental factors* like radiation, temperature, chemicals, called as mutagens.

The ***occurrence of mutations*** have been observed in many organisms of animal species like, *Drosophila* (eye colour, body colour), mice and other rodents (coat colour like black, white, brown), rabbits (body colour), guinea pigs, sheep, and man (hair colour, eye colour, skin pigmentation).

14.5 DETECTION OF MUTATION

Muller, H.J. (1927) was the first to discover that X rays induced mutations in *Drosophila*. This discovery proved to be a very important field in Genetics in helping the genetic analysis to study the effects of missing gene products. Muller, H. J.

noticed that X ray treated sperm of *Drosophila* had increased frequency of X-linked recessive lethal and it was the first study of induction of mutation by external factor for which he received in 1946 the Noble Prize in Physiology or Medicine. Muller developed a technique which was very simple and accurate to identify lethal mutations on the X chromosome of *Drosophila.*

(i) ClB Method: Detection of Sex-linked Lethal

The technique devised by Muller to detect linkage is known as ClB method or triple gene method. This technique detect the sex-linked lethal. The three genes involved/present on X chromosome of *Drosophila* are as:

C = ***Crossover suppressor gene*** which governs the long inversion of X chromosome. This suppresses the recombination (crossing over) between the *ClB* chromosome and normal X chromosome. The inversion though does not interfere of crossing over but it causes to abort the progeny carrying recombinant chromosome (produced by crossing over between two chromosomes) due to duplications and deficiencies

l = ***Lethal recessive gene*** on X chromosome. The homozygous female and hemizygous male carrying this X-linked lethal gene die and

B = ***Bar eye gene,*** producing eyes with reduced size known as bar eyes (small/ narrow eyes like a bar) in *Drosophila.* This gene is partially dominant and hence female heterozygous for the ClB chromosome can be easily identified and used as genotype marker for this chromosome.

The flies having these 3 genes on X-chromosome are known as ClB females whose other X-chromosome is normal. The recessive lethal ((*l*) and the bar-eye gene (B) are present within the inverted segment of the ClB chromosome.

This technique involves the treating of male *Drosophila* with X rays or mutagenic agent to test its ability to induce mutation. The treated males with mutagenic agent (X-ray) are mated to ClB females. The F_1 daughters carrying ClB chromosome from mother and treated X-chromosome from father are then mated with normal male. The two crosses made have been shown below:

Cross I:

Parents	ClB female			Irradiated male
	$X^{ClB}X^{+}$	x ↓		$X^{m}Y$
F_1	$X^{ClB}X^{m}$ $X^{+}X^{m}$		$X^{ClB}Y$	$X^{+}Y$

Cross II:

	$X^{ClB}X^{+}$	x ↓	$X^{+}Y$ (wild type male)	
F_2	$X^{ClB}X^{+}$ $X^{m}X^{+}$		$X^{ClB}Y$ (Dies)	$X^{m}Y$ (Dies if lethal mutation is induced)

Figure 14.1: Muller's CLB Method of Detecting Induced Mutation in X Chromosome of Drosophila.

The sex ratio among F_2 progenies gives an indication of mutation. If only females are produced in the F_2 generation, it indicates that lethal mutations have been induced by X-ray treatment. But the production of both females and males among F_2 generation indicates that no lethal mutation was induced. This is because ClB chromosome received from mother is lethal for males ($X^{ClB}Y$). In other males ($X^{m}Y$) the X-ray treated chromosome is inherited and if this chromosome has lethal mutants, then these types of males ($X^{m}Y$) also die.

The ClB method of detecting mutation has its limitation. The limitation is that the inversion of the X chromosome in the ClB females does not completely act as crossover suppressor. This results in misleading of the results.

(ii) Attached-X Method – Detection of Sex-linked Visible Mutations

In *Drosophila* some females carry attached X and also the Y chromosome (XXY – female). The normal males (XY) are treated with X-rays and mated to attached X females.

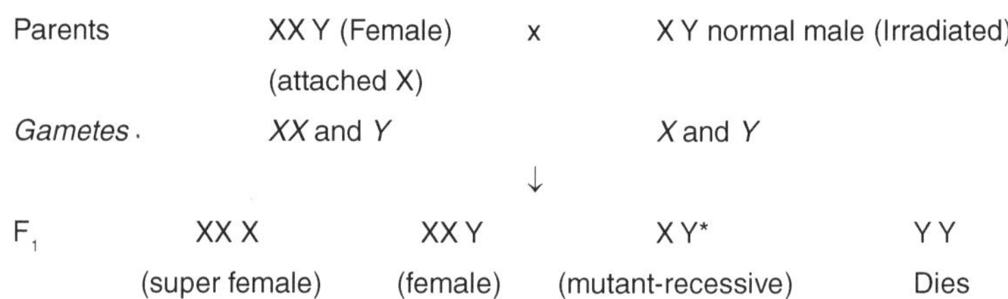

Figure 14.2: Attached X-Method of Detecting Sex Linked Visible Mutation.

The XX chromosomes in females (among parents and also among $F_{1'S}$) indicate the attached X chromosome. The XY* males among $F_{1'S}$ express visible recessive mutation or they die if lethal. This male (X Y*) receives X chromosome from their father which was treated with X rays.

(iii) Balanced Lethal System

Detection of Autosomal Mutation: The balanced lethal system is the one wherein the heterozygote is at advantage (*i.e.* survival of heterozygote and death of homozygote). Lethal mutations in different genes on the same pair of chromosomes that remain in repulsion because of close linkage or crossover suppression are called *balanced lethal*. The balanced lethal stock used to detect the autosomal mutations is the ***curly-Lobe-Plum*** (Cy L Pm) in *Drosophila*. The detection of mutation in autosomes is more difficult compared to that used for detecting mutation in sex chromosome. The complication arises due to the reason that it requires to introduce the same mutation in both the autosomes of a pair. In a closed population, only the trans-heterozygote ($a\,b^+/a^+b$) for the lethal mutations survive.

The balanced lethal stock carries recessive alleles on each of two homologous chromosomes while their normal alleles are present on its homologue. As a result the heterozygous individuals survive but homozygous recessives do not survive and hence lethal. A stock of *Drosophila* carrying dominant alleles for the curly wing (Cy) and lobed eyes (L) present on one chromosome whereas the dominant gene for plum eye or brownish eye (Pm) on its homologue is used to detect visible mutation. Thus, the *Drosophila* stock crossed among itself was heterozygous Cy + L/ + Pm + and the phenotype was curly wings, lobed eye with brownish (plum) eye colour. The crossing of these heterozygous individuals (Cy + L/ + Pm +) among themselves produces heterozygous progenies always. This has been shown below:

Cy + L/+ Pm + X Cy + L/+ Pm +

↓

Cy + L/Cy + L: Cy + L/+ Pm +: ***+ Pm +/+ Pm +***

(Cyrly lobe plum)

Dies Survive Dies

Figure 14.3: Balanced Lethal System in *Drosophila* Flies.

The Cy + L/ + Pm + are trans-heterozygote showing curly lobe plum characters. These trans-heterozygote fies survive because both chromosomes of these flies carry different recessive lethal genes. All the three loci in homozygous condition are lethal and hence the homozygous genotypes for all the three lethal alleles do not survive.

(iv) Complementation Test of Mutation

Edward Lewis (1940s) working on *Drosophila* (fruit flies) developed a test, called as *complementation test* or *trans- test* which defines ***functional allelism.*** This test of functional allelism is used to identify whether two mutations producing the same or similar phenotypes are in the same gene or in two different genes. The ***complementation test*** is the introduction of two recessive mutations into the same cell to determine whether two mutations are alleles of the same gene, *i.e.* whether the two mutations affect the same genetic function.

The complementation is the result of the functionality of the gene product specified by chromosomes carrying two different mutations when they are present in the same cell. The complementation or its lacking is assessed by the phenotype (wild type or mutant) of each *trans-* heterozygote (repulsion phase or trans-configuration). *Trans-* heterozygote is that contains two mutations arranged in the *trans*-configuration, *e.g.* a b^+/a^+b.

The *trans*-heterozygote is produced by crossing homozygous for each of the mutations of interest in case of diploid organisms. In viruses, these are produced by simultaneously infecting host cells with two different mutants. The *trans*-heterozygote irrespective of their production provides the same information on trans-or complementation test.

(i) When the *trans*-heterozygote has the *wild-type phenotype*, two mutations will then be in two different units of function (two different genes, the mutations are non-allelic). In this situation, the two mutations are said to complement each other (show complementation) and are located in different genes. Such heterozygote will have functional products of both genes and hence will have the wild-type phenotype.

(ii) When the *trans*-heterozygote has the *mutant phenotype* of the organism homozygous for either one of the two mutations, the two mutations will then be in the same unit of function (same gene, the mutations are allelic). In this situation, the two mutations (being present in a *trans*-heterozygote) do not complement each other and are both in the same gene. Both chromosomes will have defective copies of that gene (non-functional products of the gene) and will have a mutant phenotype.

On the contrary is the ***structural allelism*** which is the occurrence of two or more different mutations at the same site on a chromosome and is determined by the recombination test. Two mutations that do not recombine are structurally allelic; the mutations either occur at the same site or overlap a common site. The recombination involves the actual breakage of chromosomes and reunion of parts to produce wild-type and double-mutant chromosomes. The complementation does not depend on recombination of two chromosomes.

The mutations that are both structurally and functionally allelic are called ***homo-alleles***. These are mutations at the same site in the same gene. They do not complement or recombine with each other. The mutant homo-alleles have defects at the same site or overlapping a common site in the same gene.

The mutations that are functionally allelic but structurally non-allelic are called ***hetero-alleles***. These are mutations at different sites in the same gene. The hetero-alleles recombine with each other but do not complement one another.

14.6 METABOLIC PATHWAY OF MUTATION

The effects of the recessive and deleterious mutations are explained on the basis of the genetic control of metabolism through the sequences of chemical reactions wherein each step is catalyzed by a specific enzyme encoded by one or more genes. The recessive mutations cause the metabolic blocks and produce the abnormal phenotype. The effects of mutations on human metabolism have been studied in terms of metabolic pathway. The best known examples are the metabolism of aromatic amino acids *phenylalanine* and *tyrosine* that are essential amino acids, required for protein synthesis, do not synthesize in humans like that in microorganism, and hence must be supplied through diet (dietary proteins). This is because the blocks in the metabolic pathway have been observed.

(*i*) ***Mutations block the metabolic pathway***: Five different inherited disorders (autosomal recessive traits) are caused by mutations in genes that control steps in a single metabolic pathway of phenylalanine-tyrosine metabolism. These disorders are *alkaptonuria* (first studied inherited disorder), *phenylketouria* (PKU), *tyrosinosis, tyrosinemia*, and *albinism* (See chapter 20 – Biochemical genetics).

(*ii*) ***Recessive and deleterious effects of mutations- reasons***: *Active and inactive forms of an enzyme*: Geneticists have observed that most of the mutations are recessive and deleterious. This can be explained considering the genetic control of metabolism through the sequences of chemical reactions wherein each step is catalyzed by a specific enzyme encoded by one or more genes. The metabolic pathways are frequently blocked by the action of mutant alleles. It is known that mutation results into the change in base-pair sequences of gene which in turn cause change in the amino acid sequences in polypeptide. Ultimately, this results in change of normal and functional gene products into nonfunctional products (inactive enzyme). It will make it clear that why most of the mutations are recessive taking that wild type allele (normal allele) encodes an active or functional enzyme whereas the mutant allele encodes less active or totally inactive or nonfunctional enzyme. Therefore, after mutation, the cell will contain two alleles that are different in structure (amino acid sequence) and function (active verses inactive gene products). The cell will have thus active and inactive forms of an enzyme and the active form will catalyze the reaction and will produce the gene product whereas the inactive form of allele (mutant allele) being nonfunctional will produce inactive product. Therefore, the allele will be dominant that specifies the active product (wild allele) and the allele will be recessive that specifies the inactive product (mutant allele).

In view of the above, it can be said that there is a loss of gene function due to mutation. This means that the gene does not specify a polypeptide or specifies a nonfunctional or less functional polypeptide. Thus, the different mutations in the same gene produce different alleles (a, a^+, a′, a^h, etc) and these different alleles will produce different polypeptides having different sequences of amino acids which produce different polypeptide products (gene products). This is called as *loss of function* alleles.

(iii ***Most mutations are recessive but others are dominant - reasons:*** *Loss or gain-in-gene function:* The dominant and recessive nature of mutation could be explained after it was discovered by Beadle and Tatum that the genes specify polypeptides. There are striking differences in the expression of dominant and recessive mutations. The dominant mutations have their phenotypic effect in heterozygous as well as in homozygous states whereas the recessive mutations have their phenotypic effects only in homozygous state.

The *recessive mutations* are said to have a *loss-of-gene function* which occurs either when the gene fails to specify a polypeptide or specify a nonfunctional polypeptide or impairs (abolishes) gene expression (or the function of a gene product). Thus, the recessive mutation has no effect in the presence of wild-type allele (heterozygous state) whereas the wild-type allele produces the functional polypeptide and hence the phenotype that will be produced by a heterozygous genotype will be the same as that produced by the wild-type homozygote. The wild-type allele produces enough amount of the enzyme to synthesize normal amount of the gene product (say pigment production for colour development). On the contrary, the recessive mutation being a loss-of-function allele produces no enzyme or gene product. The recessive mutations may have complete loss or partial loss-of-gene function (polypeptide activity).

Complete loss-of-gene function can be explained by citing the example of eye colour in *Drosophila.* A brown pigment in normal amount is synthesized by an enzyme (polypeptide) produced by a wild-type allele. Thus, the wild-type allele produces a polypeptide that functions as an enzyme to synthesize brown pigment in the eyes. This pigment is deposited in the eyes of *Drosophila* and produces dark red eyes. The mutation in this wild-type allele (for dark red eye colour) produces a recessive loss-of-function allele, called *cinnabar mutation.* The flies homozygous for this *cinnabar* gene do not produce the enzyme responsible to synthesize the brown pigment in their eyes. Consequently, the phenotype of flies homozygous with *cinnabar* mutants is bright red which is the colour of the mineral cinnabar, because these flies lack the brown pigment.

Partial loss-of-gene function can be explained by an example of the *Himalayan allele* of the coat colour gene in rabbits and cats. This allele specifies a polypeptide that functions under reduced temperature. The homozygous state of this allele (*himalayan*) specifies a polypeptide which is functional to produce pigmented hairs in the extremities of the body parts (tail, ears, legs, and tip of the nose) which are exposed to low temperature.

Dominant mutations, like recessive mutations, may also have a loss-of-gene function or interference with its function. Such gene mutations are called the *dominant mutations.* This occurs when the amount of gene product controls the phenotype. The wild-type allele in this case is not likely to produce its product in sufficient amount for full and normal function. Consequently, the mutation lowers down the amount of gene product necessary for the wild phenotype. Secondly, the dominant mutation actually interfere the function of wild-type allele. The dominant mutation specifies polypeptide that inhibits, antagonize, or interfere the activity of the wild-type polypeptide. The mutations of this type are called *dominant-negative mutations.* The example of such mutation is the *T* allele affecting tail length in mice. The wild-type allele of the T gene is essential for life of mice. The mutation in heterozygous condition shortens the tail while in homozygous state these are lethal. The dominant-negative T alleles cause the shortening of the length of polypeptides than the wild-type T allele and the short polypeptide in heterozygous condition interferes the function of the wild-type polypeptide which results in completely tailless mouse.

The *gain-of-function mutation* also occurs when the heterozygote with mutant allele shows the mutant phenotype. This is due to the fact that the mutant allele increases the function of the gene product because the mutation specifies a novel polypeptide. Alternately, as a result of mutation, the wild-type polypeptide is produced irrespective of its requirement at that location and time. Such mutations are called *gain-of-function mutation.* The example of such mutation (dominant gain-of-mutation) is the *Antennapedia* which causes in heterozygous state to develop the legs instead of antennae on the head of *Drosophila.* This is because the polypeptide product of mutant gene (*Antennapedia*) is produced in the head where it is not usually produced. Therefore, the mutant gene product has expanded the place of function.

14.7 MOLECULAR BASIS OF MUTATION

The hereditary specialty depends on the sequential arrangement of the nucleotides of DNA molecule (polynucleotide chain) in chromosomes and maintained by DNA replication. The nucleotide sequence determines the amino acid sequence and produces a specific protein which in turn influences the expression of a gene in term of the production of a phenotype of a particular character. Some copy error in nucleotide may occur during replication of DNA and this copy error leads to a change in DNA structure, resulting in a new gene (DNA). This is because the change in nucleotide (mutation) changes the ***genetic code*** (nucleotide triplet) which forms an amino acid, the building stone of protein. The amino acids are formed according to the sequence of nucleotides in DNA. This means that the nucleotide sequence in DNA determines the amino acid sequence as per nucleotide triplet. A change in the sequence of nucleotide results in the change of amino acid sequence which in turn produce a different protein and consequently a new phenotype is produced.

Different Types of Mutations on Molecular Basis

The type of change in arrangement of nucleotides (base pairs in DNA molecule – polypeptide chain) determines the type of mutation. The different types of changes in the arrangement of nucleotides are the *substitution mutation* caused by substitution of bases; *frame shift mutation* caused by the deletion (loss) and duplication (addition) of bases causing the frame shifting of codons, and *transposition of bases* from one position to another.

1. Substitution Mutation – Base Pair Substitution

These mutations involve the *substitution* of a base with another base. For example, the *substitution* of 3rd nucleotide of 2nd triplet (T) with G will form new arrangement of nucleotide triplets as –

Origional chain: TAG CAT TAG CAT TAG CAT TAG CAT ... ... and so on

Mutated chain: TAG CAG TTA GCA TTA GCA TTA GCA T. ... ... and so on

These are spontaneous and point mutations. The substitution mutation involves the substitution of one nucleotide (nitrogen base in a triplet codon) for another in DNA. These are base pair replacements (substitutions), change the codons which code for different amino acids resulting into the formation of different protein and causing the changed phenotype. The substitution mutation is of two type depending on the type of base pair to be substituted *viz. transition and transversion.*

(i) Transition Mutation

This involves the replacement of a purine in a polypeptide chain with other purine (substitution within purine bases), or replacement of a pyrimidine with other pyrimidine (substitution within pyrimidine bases) in a strand of DNA.

The transitional substitution mutations occur through the followings -

- ☆ Tautomerization (shifting of hydrogen atom),
- ☆ Ionization (loss of Hydrogen atom),
- ☆ Deamination of nitrogen bases (replacing amino group $-NH_2$ by hydroxyl group –OH), and
- ☆ Base analogue (incorporation of unnatural bases).

See ***annexure 14.1*** for mechanism of transition mutation.

(ii) Transversions

Freese, E (1959) proposed the occurrence of transversion. It is the base-pair substitution involving the replacement of a purine with a pyrimidine and vice versa (substitution between purine and pyrimidine bases). The transversion mutations occur through ***depurination*** (removal of a purine from DNA strand – leaving a gap at that point) caused by alkylating agents. This gap is filled at the time of replication by insertion of any of the four bases in the complementary strand.

For every base pair there are three possible substitutions – one transition and two transversions. Therefore, a total of 12 different base substitutions can occur in DNA comprising 4 different transitions and 8 different transversions as:

Transition mutations	Transversions
A to G; G to A;	A to C; C to A;
C to T; and T to A	C to G; G to C;
	G to T; T to G;
	T to A; and A to T

Example: The transversion results in conversion of normal Hb A into abnormal Hb S responsible for producing *sickle cell anemia.*

2. Frame Shift Mutations

This involves the additions and deletions of one or a few base pairs within the coding regions of genes. These are called frame shift mutations because these mutations alter the reading frame of an mRNA. This includes the insertion (addition) or deletion of one or more base pairs (nucleotides) between any two base pairs of a gene and this changes the reading frame of that portion of the gene. The shift in reading frame changes all of the codons in the mRNA and all of the amino acids in the polypeptide specified by base-pair triplets.

The deletion or addition of a single base pair has been found to be caused by acridine dyes. The acridine dyes become intercalated between two adjacent purines. A nitrogenous base is either inserted in the gap of there is a loss of a base at the time of DNA replication. The removal of ethylated bases also causes the deletion and hence results in the frame-shift mutations.

The *frame shift mutations* leading to loss of some portion of a gene (deletion of one or more base pairs) are called *deletion mutation.* The changes in base-pairs that may lead to addition of one or more extra nucleotide in a gene are called as *insertion mutation.*

***(i) Deletion Mutation (Deletion of a base)*:** The *deletion* of the 1st nucleotide (T) in 3rd triplet (TAG) will produce the new arrangement of nucleotide triplets (Code) as under:

Original chain: TAG CAT TAG CAT TAG CAT TAG CAT … … … and so on

Changed chain: TAG CAT AGC ATT AGC ATT AGC AT. … … … and so on

(ii) *Insertion mutation* (*Addition* of a base): The *addition* or *duplication* or *insertion* of 2nd nucleotide (A) in 1st triplet (TAG) will produce the following rearrangement of nucleotide triplets (Code) –

Original chain: TAG CAT TAG CAT TAG CAT TAG CAT ... ... and so on

Mutated chain: TAA GCA TAG CAT TAG CAT TAG CAT ... ... and so on

3. Transposition

It means the change in position of a base. For example, when the 2nd nucleotide of 2nd triplet (A) changes its position in between 3rd and 4th triplet, it is called *transposition*. This change will produce new arrangement of nucleotide triplets as –

Original chain: TAG CAT TAG CAT TAG CAT TAG CAT ... ... and so on

Mutated chain: TAG CTT AGA CAT TAG CAT TAG CAT ... ... and so on

The induced base during replication is either one of the 3 natural occurring bases (Code) or it is different which is analogous to them (base analogue). This changes the genetic code and hence the amino acid which result into production of different protein.

See ***annexure 14.2*** for mechanism of transposition.

14.8 MUTATION IN HUMAN β-GLOBIN CHAIN

The change in DNA structure is due to a change in nucleotide sequence (codon) in different ways (deletion, insertion of one or a few base pairs or substitution of one base pair for another, as mentioned above). This change in nucleotide sequence results in a different amino acid in a particular protein, *e.g.* in sickle cell anemia (Hb S).

The haemoglobin is the complex protein that carries oxygen from the lungs to other tissues. This haemoglobin contains 4 polypeptides – 2 identical α-globin chains and 2 identical β-globin chains, and an iron containing heme group. Each α chain (polypeptide) consists of a specific sequence of 141 amino acids whereas each β chain is 146 amino acids long.

Ingram, V. and colleagues (1957) showed that the sixth amino acid of the β-globin chains of sickle-cell haemoglobin was valine instead of glutamic acid found at this position in normal haemoglobin of adult human. A codon changes from GAA (glutamic acid) to GUA (valine) and thus valine is incorporated instead of a glutamic acid residue, resulting in production of another protein (abnormal protein, Hb S) and another phenotypic expression of the character (anemia, known as sickle-cell anemia). The RBCs of anemic person are changed to sickle shape, thin and elongated instead of round shape and haemoglobin is half of the normal level, as per repeated blood test observations made by James Herrick, a Chicago physician and Ernest Irons, a medical intern (1910). All the symptoms of sickle-cell anemia are the result of the single amino acid change in a single polypeptide chain (β) of haemoglobin. Many different variants of adult haemoglobin with amino acid changes are known in human population. Several of these variants have severe phenotypic effects. The variants were initially detected by their movement in an electric field due to charge differences (altered electrophoretic bahaviour). These variants have helped to know the effects of mutation on the structures and functions of gene products as well as the phenotypes of the mutants. Over 100 Hb variants with amino acid changes in the β chain are known. Mostly the differences have been observed from the normal β chain of Hb A by a single amino acid substitution and some by two amino acids. α polypeptide has also been identified to have numerous variants.

Illustration of Mutation in Human Haemoglobin

A single change in a single base pair (nucleotide) may results in a change of gene product, *e.g.* production of abnormal human haemoglobin S, in place of Hb A and Hb B at its beta chain. There are about 140 amino acid residues in each of alpha and beta chain of normal haemoglobin A. The sequence of amino acids in the beta chain of Hb A is:

Position: 1 2 3 4 5 6 7 8

Amino acid: Valine-histidine-leucin-theorine-proline-glutamic acid-glutamic acid-lysine *etc.*

The triplet codes for three amino acids *viz.* glutamic acid, valine and lysine are:

Glutamic acid	Valine	Lysine
GAA		*AAA*
GAG	GUU	AAG
	GUC	
	GUA	
	GUG	

The glutamic acid at 6th position of beta chain of Hb A is replaced by valine and abnormal haemoglobin (Hb S) is produced but when the glutamic acid at 6th position of Hb A is replaced by lysine, it also produces another type of abnormal haemoglobin called as haemoglobin C which is lethal.

The replacement of first A base (adenine) of glutamic acid (GAA) by U changes the codon as GUA and translates into valine. Likewise, the G base (guanine) in codon for glutamic acid (GAA) is replaced by A (adenine base) and produces the codon as AAA which codes for lysine. Thus, a change in the single nitrogen base (nucleotide, A to U or G to A) of the gene Hb A produces the change in amino acid (glutamic acid, GAA into valine, GUA and the glutamic acid, GAA into lysine, AAA) of the chain and hence the gene product (protein, haemoglobin) is changed which has phenotypic effect other than the original gene product.

The mutations are random, permanent and rare. This means that most genes are stable. The mutation rate is 1×10^{-5} to 1×10^{-6} which means that one gamete in 1000, 000 to one million contain a mutation at a locus. However, the mutation rate varies from one strain to others, from one individual to another and from one locus to another in the same strain. There are some genes whose effect is only to increase the mutation rate of other genes (loci) and such genes are called "*mutator genes*". For example, in corn a dominant gene (Dt) on 9th chromosome is a mutator gene which mutates the colourless gene (a) present on 3rd chromosome into coloured gene responsible for producing dots in maize grain.

The mutations are recessive, lethal or semi-lethal and may occur simultaneously at two or more loci. The mutations, being deleterious to the organism, are at low frequencies in the population. This is because the individuals showing mutant trait are less adapted and hence the natural selection acts against mutations keeping their frequencies less than expected. The action of natural selection against mutant types is indicated by the observed deviations from expected ratios of phenotypes.

14.9 SIGNIFICANCE OF MUTATION

The mutation is said to be a necessary evil. This statement can be supported from the fact that the mutations are important in causing genetic variation for selection to work and for evolution to occur but on the other hand, the mutations are harmful. However, the mutations due to their low rate play a relatively minor role as a factor to disturb the genetic equilibrium.

(1) Mutation is Necessary

The mutations are of biological importance as they lead to the *biological evolution.* In the absence of mutation the new genetic variation will not arise, the members of a species will remain alike and the new species would have not come up without mutation. The mutation is the ultimate source of the genetic variations and hence it is the essential first step to provide the raw materials for *evolution.*

Mutation, the change in genetic material (mutational property of the gene) is thus the *evolutionary function* of DNA. The presence and occurrence of alleles producing different phenotypes of a character is the evidence of this property of genes. Thus, the functional differences arise due to this mutational property of the gene. All the genes without mutation would have existed in only one form.

Moreover, the mutations are essential for *biological existence* which depends on change and not by maintaining the *status quo* under the changed environmental conditions. The organism would cease to exist or would have remained in very simple form in the changing environment. The absence of mutation would eliminate the genetic variability which is essentially required for adaptation of any species in a changing environment. Thus, in the absence of mutation the possibility of evolution through natural selection favouring hereditary alternative forms is eliminated.

There is a reference in Holy Bible about a man of great stature born to the giant having polydactyly (6 fingers) on each hand and foot. This character is dominant originating from a mutation affecting finger numbers. In cattle mutation occurred in gene controlling horn (p) and the gene mutated to its allele producing *polled condition* (P, without horn). The polled trait is dominant over horn. Short leg sheep of *Ancon breed* is also the result of mutation in gene controlling normal leg size. Likewise, *different colours in farm animals* have been originated as a result of mutation in gene for original colour.

The induced mutations are more useful in plants. A number of useful mutations particularly for high yield of crop have been produced in:

- ✰ *Wheat* (branched ears, high protein and lysine content, lodging resistance, high yielding varieties),
- ✰ *Rice* (high yielding variety developed by mutation after gamma radiation, mutation for increased protein and lysine content, development of short duration variety),
- ✰ *Barley* (high yield and other useful mutations), and
- ✰ *Peppermint, cotton, caster* plant (short duration variety named *Aruna*), *legumes* (*French bean, Pea, Lentil*), *mustard, ornamental* plants, *fruit trees, etc.*

As a result of several mutations in the same gene, various alternative forms of a gene (multiple alleles) occur in the population and produce different phenotypic effects. It is generally agreed that more than two alternate forms of a gene (multiple alleles) are present in the population for a number of loci. These multiple alleles are created by mutation. The creation of a new allele causes change in the existing genetic structure of the population by increasing the number of genotypes.

The *mutation* is the sole, primary and ultimate source of genetic variation of a population, and provides the raw material while genetic recombination, selection and migration are of the secondary level of genetic variation.

The genetic *recombination* mechanism produces new combinations of genetic variation caused by mutation. The role of secondary level factors to give rise to genetic differences starts only if there are allelic differences at a number of gene loci which arise due to mutation. This is because without the existence of mutational variability at individual locus there is nothing different to recombine.

The *selection* (natural or artificial) preserves the new mutants as well as the combinations which produce organisms that are the best adapted to environments in which they live. The mutation leads to genetic differences and for selection and evolution. The occurrence of mutation consistently in every generation over a long period of time gradually changes the gene frequency in a population. All the local populations of a species would have been identical without mutation.

Likewise, *migration* is only effective to create genetic differences in a population only when there is genetic variability between migrants and native population. Thus, the mutant conditions have allowed the present evolutionary stage. The allele in a population is either got fixed or lost irrespective of the size of population, though the rate of fixation and loss of allele from a large population is very small. The allele once lost can be regained through mutation. Thus mutation provides a means of genetic variability and plays a special role as the *spoiler of genetic fixation.*

(2) Powerful Tool for Dissection of Biological Processes

The *conditional lethal mutations* are useful and powerful tools in genetic studies to investigate and dissect into the individual steps of many biological processes from development to photosynthesis. The mutation eliminates the activity of a single polypeptide and helps to break down the processes into individual steps which make easy to isolate and characterize the gene products. The mutation studies have dissected successfully many biological processes. Robert Edgar and coworkers had worked out the process of complete pathway of morphogenesis for *bacteriophage T4* which involves the products of about 50 genes wherein each gene encodes a structural protein or an enzyme to catalyze one or more steps in this process of morphogenesis. They established the complete pathway of phage T4 morphogenesis by isolating the mutant strains of the virus (bacteriophage T4) with temperature-sensitive and suppressor-sensitive conditional lethal mutations in each of the 50 genes, and by use of electron microscopy and biochemical techniques to analyze the structures that accumulated when these mutant strains are grown under restrictive conditions. Other examples of dissecting the biological pathways by mutational studies are the pathways of nitrogen fixation in bacteria and the photosynthetic electron transport chains in plants. The behavior and learning studies on *Drosophila* and the process of differentiation and development in higher plants and animals are under progress through mutational dissection. The mutation can be used to dissect any biological process because every gene can mutate to a nonfunctional state.

The action of the conditional lethal mutations can be understood by a simple biosynthetic pathway wherein gene A produces an enzyme (A) which acts on a precursor X and converts it into intermediate product Y which in turn is quickly converted to a product Z by the action of another enzyme (B) produced by another gene B. Therefore, the intermediate Y is present in small quantity unable to isolate and characterize. Now, consider two situations. In the first situation, suppose there is mutation in gene B. This mutation will either produce no enzyme B or it may produce an inactive form of enzyme B. As a result the intermediate Y will not be converted into the product Z and hence there will be accumulation of Y intermediate in higher concentration. This will allow the isolation and characterization of Y. Second situation is that the gene A is mutated. The mutation in gene A will help to identify the precursor X. This can be shown as under:

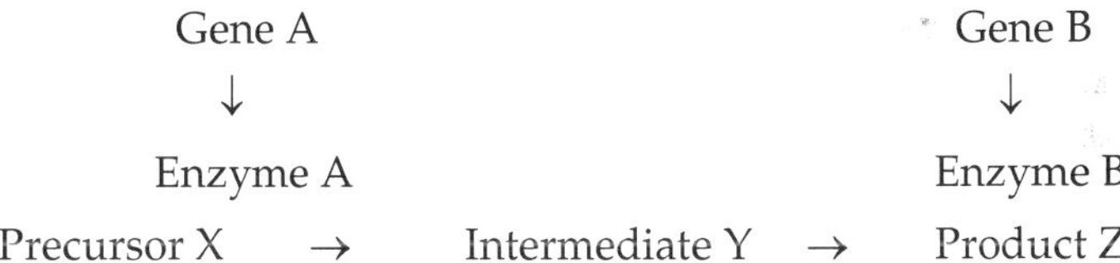

(3) Mutation is Harmful

The mutation exerts an adverse effect on the genetic structure of population. The mutation induced changes (mutant alleles) are mostly unfavourable because most of the mutant alleles are harmful and deleterious. The change caused by mutation depends on its degree of harmfulness and the rate at which the mutant alleles arise (mutation rate). The mutant alleles can do harm to the extent that they cause death of the individual and these mutant alleles are called as *lethal* or *semi-lethal genes.* The process of mutation and reduced viability brings down the frequency of the gene under mutation.

Higher mutation rate are harmful and dangerous for the existence of any species due to the fact that most of the mutant forms of alleles are deleterious. Therefore, if there would have been too much mutation, the species could have not continued to exist because of accumulation of so many deleterious effects of mutant alleles.

Thus, the level of mutation must be less. The direction of mutation is random and unpredictable for which the mutations are usually deleterious.

However, the mutations are rare and hence their direct effect on gene frequencies is very small. It requires many generations to bring a change in gene frequencies due to mutation. The mutation rates are not constant for any locus being influenced by temperature, radiation hazards, chemical treatments *etc.* The mutation rates also vary between loci and also between races or species. The mutation rates have been indicated ranging between one gamete in one lakh gametes to one gamete in hundred million gametes (10^{-5} to 10^{-8}) contain a mutation at a locus. Thus, mutation alone can produce only very slow changes in gene frequency and hence they are not important. However, the effect of mutation which is seemingly minute become important and may play a substantial role in the process. Mutation at separate locus is slow but each locus is capable of mutation and hence a number of mutations are expected in every gamete each generation because the entire genome contains thousands of loci. A number of loci determine the general functions (viability, fertility, disease resistance, vigour *etc.*) and hence the mutations at these loci may accumulate resulting in the total genetic variation to affect these functions to a greater extent than individual locus mutants.

EXERCISES - SOLVED

14.1 The following is a trinucleotide-pair sequence of β chain of Hb A gene and specifies the glutamic acid at 6th position.

5′-GAG-3′

3′-CTC-5′

In case of the change of the second base pair of this triplet from A:T to T:A, the DNA sequence will become as –

5′-GTG-3′

3′-CAC-5′

This bas-pair change will encode which amino acid.

Answer: Codon 5′- GAG-3′ is for glutamic acid. Thus, the bottom strand of DNA (3′-CTC-5′) is the template strand. The transcription of β chain of Hb A gene produces mRNA sequence 5′-GAG-3′ which is a glutamic acid codon whereas the transcription of the changed DNA sequence produces the mRNA sequence 5′-GUG′3′ which is a valine codon. Thus, the base-pair change in DNA will produce amino acid valine.

14.2 The following is given a short nucleotide sequence of a wild-type gene –

5′-ATG TCC GCA TGG GGA -3′

3′-TAC AGG CGT ACC CCT -5′

This gene transcribes the mRNA nucleotide sequence 5′ –AUG UCC GCA UGG GGA -3′ and translation of this mRNA produces the amino acid sequence:

Methionine-serine-alanine-tryptophan-glycine

Now, there occurs a single nucleotide-pair substitution at position 7 in the above gene changing G:C to A:T. Determine the effect of this change (mutation) on the polypeptide that will be produced by the mutant gene.

Answer: Since there has been a change in nucleotide sequence of gene due to mutation of base-pair substitution, the resultant nucleotide sequence in mRNA produced after transcription of the mutant gene will be –

5′-AUG UCC ACA UGG GGA-3′

And this mRNA will be translated into amino acids sequence as –

Methionine-serine-threonine-tryptophan-glycine

Therefore, the mutation has changed the third amino acid of the mutant polypeptide as threonine in place of alanine and has resulted in a single amino acid substitution in the polypeptide encoded by the gene.

14.3 Consider the gene segment of exercise 14.2 above and a change of a single nucleotide-pair substitution from G:C to A:T at position 12. Determine the effect of this mutation on the polypeptide that will be produced by this gene.

Answer: Transcription of the DNA segment will produce the mRNA sequence as -

5′- AUG UCC GCA UGA GGA-3′

In this case the change is in the fourth codon which was for tryptophan (UGG) but after the change the codon produced is the *termination* codon (UGA). This will result the mutant polypeptide to be prematurely terminated at this position.

14.4 Again consider the gene segment referred in exercise 14.2. This time consider a single base-pair insertion between nucleotide airs 6 and 7 in the gene segment. Now, determine the effect of this mutational change on the polypeptide produced by the gene.

Answer: Mutant gene segment will transcribe the mRNA nucleotide sequence as -

5′-AUG UCC AGC AUG GGGG-3′

Altered mRNA will translate/produce the following polypeptide with the amino acids as –

Methionine-serine-serine-methionine-glycine.

Thus, this mutational change has changed the reading frame of mRNA (which is the trinucleotides read as codons), resulting the changes of all of the amino acids specified by codons downstream from the site of insertion (mutation). This will produce ultimately the abnormal protein.

Chapter 15

Induction of Mutation

The mutations can be induced by exposure of organisms to some physical and chemical factors. These may be radiations, chemicals, transposable genetic elements (transposons), and repeated trinucleotides. These factors cause changes in DNA (mutation). The factors causing mutation are called the *mutagenic agents* or *mutagens* and the mutation caused by these factors is known as *induced mutation.*

The mutagenic agents either radiation or chemicals do not have selective mutagenic effects. But all mutagenic agents produce all kinds of mutations. Thus, their effects are random. The various mutagenic agents are as under:

- ✰ Radiations (ionizing and non-ionizing),
- ✰ Chemicals,
- ✰ Transposons (transposable genetic elements), and
- ✰ Expanded trinucleotide repeats.

15.1 RADIATION INDUCED MUTATIONS

The radiation is a physical phenomenon in which energy travels through space. The sun is the source of spectrum of radiation such as radio waves, infra red, UV, X-ray, gamma, and cosmic rays.

The radiations include ionizing radiation (X-rays, gamma rays, and cosmic rays) and non-ionizing radiation (Ultraviolet light) depending on the part of the electromagnetic spectrum (shown below) with wavelengths shorter and of higher energy than visible light, as shown below:

Energy Level	*Electromagnetic Spectrum*	*Wavelength*	*Rays/Light*
Highest	Ionizing radiation	10^{-5} nm	Cosmic rays
"	"	10^{-3} nm	Gamma rays
"	"	1 nm	X rays
Medium (greater)	Non ionizing radiation	254 nm	U.V. radiation
—	Visible light	380 nm	Blue light
—	"	—	Green
—	"	—	Yellow
—	"	750 nm	Red
—	Infrared	10^{3} nm to 10^{6} nm	—
—	Microwaves	10^{6} nm to 10^{9} nm	—
Lowest	Radio-waves	10^{9}nm to 10^{3}m [1 m = 10^{9}nm]	—

(i) Ionizing Radiations

These are the portion of the electromagnetic spectrum that produces the positive and negative charges (ion pairs) in molecules. These radiations cause ionization and are of high energy with shorter wavelength than visible light. They penetrate the living tissues for substantial distances and hence used in medical diagnosis. There is release of electrons on striking the high energy rays with atoms and the positively charged *free radicals* or *ions* are produced. The ions then strike with other molecules causing release of additional electrons. Thus, a *cone of ions* is formed along the track of each high energy ray on passing through living tissues. This is the process of *ionization* which is induced by machine - produced *X - rays, protons, and electrons,* and also by α, β, *and gamma rays* and other fasr moving particles released by radioactive substances (isotopes) like the ^{32}P, ^{35}S, and the uranium-238 used in nuclear reactors.

The radioactive isotopes give off sub atomic particles such as protons, neutrons, electrons, and helium nucleic acid called α particle in the process of decomposition from an unstable state to a more stable condition. The ionization process results in breakage of the sugar-phosphate strand of DNA. The ionizing radiation thus induces mutation and breaks in chromosomes more during the cell division in the blood forming cells in the bone marrow and reproductive cells. The embryos are particularly sensitive to radiation damage. The free ions produced/released combine with oxygen and produce highly reactive chemicals which affect the genes and chromosomes. They produce changes in chemical valence through the ejection of electrons. The atomic and hydrogen bombs are now familiar and terrible source of ionizing radiations.

The atom which is electrically neutral is made up of a positively charged atomic nucleus (consisting protons and neutrons) surrounded by negatively charged electrons. The proton carries a positive charge while the neutrons are uncharged particles. The electron is the lightest particle of these atomic particles. During the process of radiation (diffusion of light rays) the electrons are ejected from outer shell of the atom and the unstable nucleus gives out energy and attains a more stable state. The atom becomes positively charged on the loss of balancing negatively charged electrons from the atom. The charged atom is said to be ionized and called *ions.* The atom after being ionized (ion) becomes chemically reactive and reacts with another atom of the molecule. This results into a change. When this changed molecule is a gene, it causes mutation.

Among the ionizing radiation, the X -rays are more commonly used these days due to the reasons that facilities are available in most of the research labs, its use is simple, easy, and cheap than other radiations to treat any part of plant and seeds, and its amount can be measured and controlled easily. The *X - rays* are electromagnetic radiation with shorter wavelength and higher energy than visible light. The X - rays have many effects on living tissues and hence the mutations induced by X - rays give little information about molecular mechanism of producing mutation.

Muller (1927) was the first to demonstrate that X rays can induce mutation in flies. In the next year (1928), Stadler, L. J. demonstrated that X rays can increase the rate of mutations in barley and maize. The X-rays have another pathway to induce mutation. They break water into neutral H and OH free radicals. The H can combine with dissolved O_2 of water and form an unusual compound HO_2 whereas another H can combine with HO_2 and form H_2O_2. The two OH produced by X-rays acting on water may combine to form H_2O_2. Thus, the X-rays break the water and produces H_2O_2 (*hydrogen peroxide*) which is highly mutagenic.

The mutation rate is independent of the wavelength of the X – rays used. The wavelength of X – rays varies from 1°A to 10 °A (°A = Angstrom unit which is equal to hundred millionth of a cm). However, the dosage of X-rays influences the mutation rate. The weak X-rays (low intensity of irradiation) used for long period produce the same dose of irradiation in *roentgen* units and hence same effect as the strong X-rays (high intensity of irradiation) over a short period. Further, the effectiveness of radiation to induce mutation depends upon the stages of gamete formation. *Drosophila* sperms are more sensitive to radiation. The frequency of breaks in chromosomes induced by radiation is greatly reduced by active metabolism and protein synthesis. The ionizing radiations (X-rays) are very efficient agent to produce breaks in chromosome which in turn produce all types of chromosomal rearrangements (inversion, translocation, deletions, and duplications) through at least two breaks in chromosomes.

The *ionizing radiations* including X - rays are quantified in ***roentgen*** (*r*) units under a standard set of conditions. The roentgen is a measure of the number of ionizations per unit volume. A quantity of ionizing radiation producing 2.083×10^9 ion pairs in one cc of air at 0 °C and a pressure of 760 mm of mercury is equal to one unit. The dose of irradiation is important as it influences directly proportionally the frequency of induced point mutations. In *Drosophila,* it has been observed that the acute and chronic irradiations are equally effective. The chronic irradiation means low levels of irradiation for longer time while acute irradiation means the same total dose of irradiation given at high intensity for shorter time.

Any form of radiation which produces ions is expected to produce mutation. Radium is found in a kind of rock and gives off three forms of radiation (alpha, beta, and gamma radiation). The cosmic rays are more penetrating than X-rays and gamma rays but they are extremely dilute. The cosmic rays – the radiation which enters the earth's atmosphere from outer space – from rocks and soil in the form of radioisotopes and radio active compounds reach to the plants and then transferred to animals, are natural source of genetic changes.

Manmade Radiations

The followings have become the manmade radiations:

- ✰ Use of X-rays in diagnostic use;
- ✰ Atomic power plants (to meet increasing demand for energy) produce nuclear wastes in the form of spent fuel rods of uranium, plutonium, radioactive iodine;
- ✰ Wastes from production of nuclear weapons (plutonium) produce radioactive strontium and caeseim which are carcinogenic;
- ✰ Use of nuclear weapons (hydrogen and atomic bombs); and
- ✰ The nuclear wastes which also include contaminated dust, debris, clothing, sweeping, gloves, and shoes, etc defile the atmosphere when damped into disposal tank and pollute the drinking water through seepage into soil.

Therapeutic Use of X-rays

The X-rays usually have more damaging effect on dividing cells than the resting cells. This principle is used in treating cancer cells with X-rays. Thus, they have therapeutic use. The little exposure to X-rays is less harmful if not repeated often. This is because the genetic effect of X-rays is cumulative and so repeated use of X-rays in small dose is equal one large dose.

Use of Radiation in Genetics

It becomes possible to know the nature of mutation more effectively on its occurrence at will. Secondly, the breaks producing effects of X-rays make it possible to cut and dissect a chromosome and to test the properties of various parts. Muller has studied the properties of heterochromatin. Muller and co-workers studied that the spindle fiber attachment points and chromosome ends have distinctive structures. The study of X – chromosome by breaking it into fragments showed the effect of each part on sex and it was observed that there is more than one gene for sex in X – chromosome of *Drosophila.* It was also known by breaking of chromosome by X-rays that the broken ends are sticky and tends to unite with one another with perfect healing. This leads to chromosomal rearrangements which are produced by X-rays to be helpful in the construction of cytological maps. All these discoveries have brought a new science called the ***radiation genetics***.

The *damage due to radiation* depends on a number of factors like stage of development of an organism, its age, sex and type.

- ✰ The embryos and growing parts (tastes, ovaries, lymph glands, and bone marrow) are more prone to radiation because they have actively dividing cells, and are less protected and less resistant to radiations.
- ✰ In *Drosophila* the males are more affected by radiations than females.
- ✰ Higher plants are more resistant to radiation damage than animals.
- ✰ The onion is more resistant than corn plants.
- ✰ The seeds are more resistant than seedlings.

The damage caused by radiation is decreased by some reducing agents and other chemical agents such as alcohol, sulfhydral compounds, *etc.* However, the complete effect of radiation is not neutralized and also they cannot prevent death due to large dose of radiation.

(ii) Non-ionizing Radiation

These are the portion of the electromagnetic spectrum that does not lead to the production of positive and negative charges (ion pairs) in molecules. The radiation of shorter wavelength having greater energy and cause injury to the surface tissues only and increases the mutation rate. They raise the energy level of atoms which make the atoms less stable. These *do not cause ionization.* The *ultraviolet ray* (light) and visible light are the examples. These rays have low energy compared to ionizing radiations. This low energy is not sufficient to cause ionizations. The UV light is a radiation like visible light but of shorter wavelength not visible to human eyes. They penetrate only the surface layer (epidermal layer) of cells in higher plants and animals and hence penetrate tissue only slightly.

The smallest divisible amount called *photon* of UV light has enough energy to dislodge an electron from atoms. Some of the electrons are raised to higher level and this state is known as *excitation.* The effect of an UV photon is limited to one atom and thus localized. This is because the UV photon does not give much speed to the electron and hence it does not cause much secondary ionization. Thus, its effect is less drastic than complete ejection of electrons. However, it causes an increase in the chemical reactivity on the part of the affected molecule. The UV light may make the atom in an unstable state by knocking an electron from one shell of the atom to another farther out and an atom in unstable state is chemically reactive. It is known to be "sensitized". However, the unstable condition of atom is only for a small fraction of a second during which the atom enter into chemical reaction to a more extent than usual.

The UV rays penetrate tissues only very slightly than X-rays. Thus, they have very weak penetrating power. The most effective wavelength for inducing mutation is about 2600 °A with a range of 1800 to 3100 °A. The UV penetrates only the most superficial layers of the skin and therefore in man it causes no mutation in germ cells. The UV light in comparison to X-rays produces very few chromosome breakages and if produced, they are healed immediately without causing any rearrangement.

However, the UV radiation is effective mutagen for unicellular organisms. The UV radiation is easily absorbed by the organic molecules like bases in DNA and then they enter a more reactive or excited state. The purines and pyrimidine absorb the UV and mediate UV-induced mutation process. The DNA absorbs the maximum UV at a wavelength of 254 nm at which the maximum mutagenicity also occurs. These rays loss their energy to the atoms and raise the electrons in the outer orbits to higher energy levels, known as *excitation*. The molecules become chemically more reactive when they have atoms in either ionic forms or excited states than when containing atoms in their normal stable states.

Most of the mutagenicity of ionizing radiation and UV light is due to the increased reactivity of atoms present in DNA molecules.

The UV alterations of DNA are more evident during replication, indicating that error occurs during base incorporation. The nucleic acid specifically absorbs UV. This means that the wavelengths of the UV region are especially highly absorbed by nucleic acid. At this wavelength the proteins absorb little energy. Thus, the UV acts directly on DNA.

The pyrimidines are more sensitive to UV than purines. The pyrimidine (Thymine and cytosine) absorb UV light and produce two major products (pyrimidine hydrates and pyrimidine dimmers). There is hydrolysis of cytosine to a hydrate form (cytosine + H_2O, *i.e.* addition of H_2O -hydrolysis) which results in mis-pairing of a base (cytosine) pair during replication. The cross-linking of thymine molecules forms thymine dimmers (two thymine molecules) which block DNA replication. The UV generates pyrimidine dimmers which mean the bonding between pyrimidine bases on the same strand, *i.e.* covalent linking of two pyrimidine bases (cytosine and thymine). Thus, the pairing property of the DNA is affected. Therefore, dimmers affect the structure and function of DNA and inhibit separation of DNA strands during replication. The most changes are found to be cytosine to thymine transition. The UV causes addition of water (H_2O) in pyrimidine which weakens the H bonding besides being causing the formation of pyrimidine dimmers.

The *heat* also speeds up the mutation rate because it speeds up chemical reaction. Muller found that heat produces mutation but to a lesser amount than X-rays.

However, the white light has little or no photo-reactivating effect if provided after treating with X-rays. This gives an indication that the manner of action to produce mutation by X-rays and UV light is different.

Mutagenic Effects of Radiations

The penetration and ionizing power of rays determine the harmful effect of radiations. The α and β rays do not penetrate beyond the human skin and hence cannot affect body cells. The gamma and X –rays struck at high speed with the molecules of the cells and eject electrons from the outer shells of atoms which become positively charged ions. Moreover, the ejected electrons move at high speed and knock other electrons free from their respective atom. The free electrons attach to other atoms which become negative charged ions. These ions reach a stable state after neutralizing their charge under chemical reactions. However, the mutagenic effects of ionizing radiations are produced during the chemical reactions.

The ionizing radiations have two fold effects of producing the breaks in chromosomes and by producing abnormal mitosis in the irradiated cells. The chromosome breaks seems to involve the sugar-phosphate backbone of the polynucleotide chains and lead to loss of chromosomes or chromosome segments, deficiencies, duplications, translocations or inversions. Thus, abnormal chromosomes regarding their structure and number in the daughter cells cause abnormal functioning of the cell or resulting in cell death. The radiation also causes various types of cancers particularly the blood cancer or leukemia.

On the contrary to the effect of ionizing radiations, the non ionizing radiations like UV light have much less penetration power than X rays due to their longer wavelength and to carry much low energy. The UV rays are absorbed in the skin remaining unaffected the gonads, though they may be effective on lower organisms (microorganisms, pollen grains of plants or gametes of animals).

The nucleic acids absorb the UV rays causing the change in their bond characteristics. These changed bases are known as ***photoproducts***. Comparatively, the pyrimidine are more prone to these changes by forming covalent bonds and hence the ***dimmers***. The most easily formed dimer is of thymine and the dimer formation interferes with proper base pairing of thymine. The tymine may pairs with guanine rather than adenine resulting in the substitution of A:T to CUG. In a similar way, the cytosine thimer become deaminated to uracil dimmers and produce G:C to A:T transition mutation.

More chromosomal aberrations are produced by stronger treatments than weaker ones. The short but intense treatments produce more abnormalities in chromosomes compared to long but slow treatments with same number of r-units of radiations. Moreover, continuous treatment with acute doses of radiations produce more changes in chromosomes.

15.2 CHEMICALLY INDUCED MUTATIONS

There are some chemical substances which increase the mutability of genes. This important discovery was made by C. Auerbach during II world War to show that certain chemicals can also induce mutations. She tried a number of chemicals. The chemical mutagens are unlimited, the most powerful are –

- Mustard gas and related compounds,
- Ethyl urethane,
- Formaldehyde,
- Organic peroxides,
- Ferrous and magnesium salts,
- LSD (Lysergic acid dimethylamide) in large doses becomes carcinogenic and teratogenic. The use of sleeping pills made of thalidomide by pregnant woman results in the birth of deformed new born with no arms or with flippers.
- The drugs, pesticides and chemical preservatives and colouring agents added to the foods are threat to human due to their mutagenic nature.

The chemical mutagens can be put in two groups:

(*i*) Chemicals which are mutagenic to replicating and non-replicating DNA. The chemicals in this group are the

- ☆ ***Nitrous acid*** and
- ☆ ***Alkylating agents*** like nitrogen mustard, sulphur mustard (mustard gas), and sulfonate compounds (diethyl sulfonate, ethyl ethane sulfonate, ethyl methane sulfonate).

(*ii*) Chemicals which are effective to induce mutations only during DNA synthesis/replication. The chemicals in this group are the

- ☆ ***Base analogous*** (like 5-bromouracil, 2-aminopurine, 5-flurouracil) and
- ☆ ***Acridine dyes*** (proflavin, acridine orange and related compounds).

Most of the chemicals except mustard gas and peroxides have little effect and effective only in certain organisms, at certain stages in mitosis or certain stages of development and in one sex only. For example, the *formaldehyde* causes mutation in male *Drosophila* but not in female.

A chemical mutagen requires the penetration of nuclear wall in a resting nucleus. Some organisms destroy chemicals in their cytoplasm before it is penetrated in the nucleus. The chemical property of a chemical mutagen is not a criterion to judge about its mutagenic activity. The chemicals which are chemically similar may or may not produce mutation, *e.g.* Mustard gas.

(a) ***NITROUS ACID*** (HNO_2) is a direct acting mutagen. It acts on either replicating or non-replicating DNA. It results into point mutation by causing oxidative deamination (removal of amino group by hydroxyl group) in A, C, and G bases. The nitrous acid changes the base structure directly by converting the *amino groups* to *keto groups* which results in hydrogen-bonding potential of the changed bases. This change results into mispairing and hence base-pair substitution mutations occurs.

(b ***ALKYLATING AGENTS*** are the chemicals that transfer alkyl (methyl, ethyl, and so on) groups to the bases in DNA. They induce all types of mutations (transitions, transversions, frame shifts, and chromosomal aberrations). They react chemically with intact DNA and modify its structure. However, the alkylating agents have less specific mutagenic effects than others (nitrous acid, base analogs, or acridines).

The alkylating agents donate alkyl groups to other molecules and have multiple effects on DNA. These agents reacting with DNA add the ethyl or methyl groups to the bases. This results in mispairing of the affected base or its loss entirely, creating a gap. The most affected base is the guanine. These agents produce mutations as under:

- ☆ Addition of methyl or ethyl groups to G causing it to behave as a base analogous of A and thereby producing errors,
- ☆ Loss of alkylated G base (depurination) producing gaps in the DNA chain which may interfere with DNA replication or cause a shortened

nucleotide sequence. In ***depurination,*** the chemicals alkylate the purine in the nitrogen at the 7 position in the guanine and adenine and finally cause its separation from DNA strand, and

- ☆ Cross-linkage between the strands of the same or different DNA molecule causing the loss or excision of nucleotides and introduce chromosome breaks.

The sulfonate compounds (EMS, EES) result into transversion. They cause G to behave like base analogous to A. This produces G:C to T:A. The EMS causes ethylation of the bases in DNA at the 7-N and the 6-O positions. On producing 7-ethylguanine it base-pairs with T and results into G:C to AT transitions.

(c) *BASE ANALOGS* mutagens: See ***annexure 14.1***

(d) *HYDROXYLATING AGENT:* The hydroxylamine (NH_2OH) is a mutagen having its effect only G:C to A:T transition. The hydroxylamine makes complexe with cytosine. This cytosine pairs with adenine rather than with guanine. The amino group of cytosine (C) at carbon 6 position is hydroxylated by treating the DNA with hydroxylamine. This means the amino group of cytosine is changed to hydroxyl group. This results the hydroxylaminocytosine complex to base pair with A and produces G:C to A:T transition (figure 14.7 above).

The use of this mutagen (hydroxylamine) has its significant role to classify transition mutations, whether a particular mutation was an A:T to G:C or a G:C to A:T transition. The hydroxylamine cannot revert back those mutations with an A:T base pair at the mutant site whereas it can revert the mutation with a G:C base pair at the mutant site.

(e) *ACRIDINE DYES* includes *proflavin, acridine orange* and related compounds. These mutagens produce frameshift mutation. The positively charges acridines become sandwiched between the stacked pairs in DNA and hence changes the conformation of the double helix with slight bends or kinks in DNA. The replication of such DNA of intercalated or sandwiched acridines results into additions and deletions of single base pair. This alters the reading frame for the portion of the gene distal to the mutation. The acridine-induced mutation produces non-functional gene products.

Manmade Chemical Hazards or Environmental Mutagens

Besides the chemical or physical mutagenic agents, there are some chemicals to which human population is exposed. These include air and water pollutants, food additives and preservatives, and agricultural chemicals (used in crop production). In addition many potentially mutagenic compounds may be carcinogenic capable of inducing cancer like benopyrene which is a hydrocarbon in cooking meat, alfatoxin β1 which is a fungal toxin produced on seeds of crop plants (pea nut and corn) and several chemical components of hair dyes. Many carcinogens are also mutagens. About 70 per cent of the carcinogens tested have also been shown to be mutagens.

The genetic changes in bacteria, fungi, higher animals and plants are caused by some chemicals such as formaldehyde, phenol, permagnate, peroxides and even caffine and theobromine. The acrdine dyes used in certain antimalarial and anticancerous drugs, and food colours causes damage to chromosomes. The caffine and theobromine are stimulating agents of coffee, tea, and cocoa also induce mutation in *E. Coli,* and chromosomal changes in onion root tip cells, *Drosophila,* gonads and human lymphocytes.

The chemicals used for the production of antibodies (immune-suppressants) and cyclamates act as mutagens and carcinogenic agents. The sodium nitrate used as food preservative also act as mutagenic as it is converted into nitrous acid in stomach. These are thus manmade chemical hazards. Likewise, the insecticides, pesticides and herbicides (like DDT) remain in soil for many years and are dangerous to animals and human beings. Thus, there is a constant threat of exposure to a number of chemical hazards to man and animals. The other health hazards come from chemical industries (Bhopal Gas tragedy, 1984). The methyl isocyanate (MIC) also called cyanate methane is the killer gas which was involved in Bhopal tragedy. The phosgene or carbonyl chloride is another toxic gas which was used in World War II. Its brief exposure is fatal and is used in the manufacture of dyestuff, coal tar and urea, and sometimes in pharmaceuticals and metallurgical industries. The blood capillaries are affected by these gases in a way that water leaks out of the capillaries and causes oedema which slow down or stopped the normal body functions, *e.g.* pulmonary oedema affects respiration and cause death.

Mutagenicity of Chemicals – Ames Test

The mutagens also induce *cancers* and called *carcinogens.* All types of cancers have their common feature that the malignant cells continue to divide, even after the normal cells have stopped to divide. However, the cell division like other biological process is genetically controlled. The cell division is regulated by the products encoded by the specific genes in response to intra- as well as inter-cellular and environmental signals. Mutation of these genes that regulate cell division to become non-functional results the cell division to be uncontrolled. Therefore, it is advisable not to be exposed to the mutagenic and carcinogenic agents. This emphasizes that before a new chemical is started to be used for some purpose, its mutagenicity should be tested.

The rodents particularly the new born mice are traditionally used to test the carcinogenicity of a chemical by feeding or injecting the substance under test and examining the animals for tumours. Similar way the mutagenicity test is carried out. However, such test for mutagenicity has limitation. The limitation is due to low-frequency of mutation. Thus, the test requires to maintain a large population of mice and hence expensive and insensitive as it cannot detect the low levels of mutagenicity.

A rapid, inexpensive, and sensitive technique was developed by Ames Bruce and his colleagues for testing the mutagenicity of chemicals. They developed auxotrophic strains (a mutant microorganism which cannot grow on a minimal medium and needs the addition of some amino acid or vitamin) of the bacteria

Salmonella typhimurium having various types of mutations (transitions, transversions, and frame shifts) in genes required for the biosynthesis of histitine amino acid.

They kept a number of mutant bacteria (auxotrophs) on histidine lacking medium (*prototroph* - an organism that can grow on a minimal medium) and monitored the reversion of the auxotrophic mutants to prototrophy by scoring the number of colonies produced by prototrophic revertants. They compared the frequency of reversion in its presence with the spontaneous reversion frequency to measure the mutagenicity by using a set of tester strains carrying different types of mutations, taking different strain for different mutation types. They observed more than 90 percent correlation between the mutagenicity and the carcinogenicity of the substances tested.

15.3 TRANSPOSABLE GENETIC ELEMENTS INDUCING MUTATIONS

There are some DNA sequences that can move (transpose) from one location to another in a chromosome (DNA molecule) and even to a different chromosome or inactive sequences. Such sequences are called ***Transposons* (*transposable genetic elements*).**

The movement of DNA sequences from one position to another is a process or phenomenon called ***transposition.*** An enzyme that catalyzes the movement of a DNA sequence to a different site in a DNA molecule is called ***transposase.*** The insertion of transposon into or near a gene for marking that gene with a known DNA sequence is called ***transposon tagging.***

When these transposons are inserted in a gene, they make the gene non-functional, thus resulting in mutation. For example, the first mutation (w') causing *white eyes* in *Drosophila* and *wrinkled* allele in garden pea reported by Mendel have been the results of insertion of transposons.

This phenomenon of transposition was first discovered in maize and found responsible to give rise the colourful patterns on maize ears (strips and spots found on maize kernels). The mutation caused by insertion of transposons in *Drosophila, E. coli,* maize, and other organisms are known.

The transposons are the most prevalent repeated DNA sequences, structurally and functionally diverse, and have been identified in many organisms including bacteria, fungi, protists, plants, and animals. The transposons constitute appreciable fraction of the genome accounting for about 85 percent of DNA in maize, and nearly 44 percent of human genome.

Significance of Transposons

The transposable elements have their genetic significance in causing breaks in chromosomes and mutating genes, genetic transformation, shaping the structure of chromosomes (genome organization), and to play role in evolution of chromosome structure.

(i) *Mutagenic effect of transposons:* The transposons have the mutagenic potential to disrupt genes and are said to be nature's intrinsic mutagens as they mutate genes and break chromosomes on moving through the genome. Thus, these genetic elements produce the spontaneous mutations and hence used in genetic research to induce mutation. The first mutation discovered by T. H. Morgan in *Drosophila* was in the allele of the *white* gene which was resulted by a transposon insertion. The production of dysgenic hybrid in *Drosophila* transposes the P elements in the germ-line cells of hybrid offspring of P x M strains.

The spontaneous mutations or mutagenesis with transposons have an advantage. The gene mutated by insertion of transposable element can be *tagged* with a known DNA sequence. This is used to isolate the gene from a large heterogenous mixture of DNA with the help of a probe derived from cloned transposon. Therefore, this procedure of mutagenesis by *transposon tagging* has become a routine genetic practice.

(ii) *Transposons used as vectors in genetic transformation:* There is peculiar characteristic of some bacterial transposons, like composite transposons as well as the Tn3 transposons, to carry genes producing their product unrelated to transposition. This means the transposons are used as vectors to move DNA within and between genomes. This has made possible the use of transposons to transfer genes of different kinds between organisms. Thus, an organism can be transformed with the DNA of another organism. Gerald Rubin and Allan Spradling tested this idea of carrying a cloned gene by a transposon into an organism, for which they selected one of the many genes controlling eye colour in *Drosophila.* They were successful to genetically transform mutant flies (brown eyes) with DNA from wild-type flies (red eyes). The technique developed by them is now used by geneticists to transform the organism (*Drosophila*) with cloned DNA.

(iii) *Change in chromosome organization* (*deletion* and *addition*)*:* The centric heterochromatin region and the heterochromatin near the euchromatin of each chromosome arm are rich in transposons sequences. Interestingly, the mutations have occurred in many of these transposons to the extent that they cannot be mobilized and have become dead, and therefore the heterochromatin is composed of the degenerate transposable elements.

Some of the transposons seem to have played their role in the evolution of chromosome structure, and some in the formation of chromosome rearrangements. The mechanism involved is crossing over between homologous transposons located at different positions in a chromosome. The crossing over between two neighbouring transposons can contract a region of the genome by deleting the region between them or can expand the region of the genome by duplicating the chromosome segment. The deletion of the chromosome segment between two transposons results by crossing over between them present in the same orientation. The crossing over that occurs between transposons located in different chromosomes and oriented in the same direction results in two structurally changed chromatids – one lacking the DNA segment between the two transposons and another having an extra copy of that segment.

15.4 REPEATED TRINUCLEOTIDE INDUCED MUTATIONS

The repeated sequences of 1 to 6 nucleotide pairs are called as *simple tandem repeats*. These repeats are present in human genome throughout. The tandem repeats with three nucleotide pairs are called ***trinucleotide repeats***. The trinucleotide repeats have been found to cause some inherited diseases in humans.

The ***fragile X syndrome*** is the second most common form of an inherited mental retardation in humans. This disorder is caused by expanded CGG trinucleotide repeats on X chromosome. The occurrence of this disorder is about 1 among 4000 males and 1 among 7000 females. The people with this syndrome also exhibit facial and behaviour abnormalities. This abnormality is caused by a dominant X-linked mutation with incomplete penetrance since about 20 percent of hemizygous males and about 30 percent of heterozygous females do not show this disorder. The number of copies in mutant X chromosome contains up to 1000 copies of the tandem CGG repeat while the normal X chromosome contains from 6 to about 5o copies of the CGG repeat.

Several inherited ***neurological diseases*** like Huntington disease, myotonic dystrophy, Kennedy disease, dentatorubral pallidoluysian atrophy, spinocerebellar ataxia, and Machado-Joseph are caused by CAG and CTG trinucleotide repeats. The copy numbers of these repeats has direct relation with severity of the disease. However, the expanded trinucleotides causing these disorders are unstable in somatic cells and between generations.

15.5 CANCER: DISEASE OF CELL DIVISION

The different phases of cell division and the entry of a cell into different phases of cell cycle are under genetic control through the regulation of a mechanism (***checkpoint*** – *chapter 9*) that stops progression in the cell cycle until DNA synthesis is completed or damaged DNA is repaired. The checkpoints are regulatory mechanisms that are responsible for control and regulation of cell growth and differentiation.

The cancer is a genetic disease though environmental factors (physical, chemical and biological) are involved in many cancers. The cancer results from mutations in genes whose protein products are involved in the **regulation of cell cycle (growth and division).** Therefore, the mutation causes the biochemical processes to lead the unregulated proliferation of cells. The most peculiar characteristic of cancerous cells is that their growth is unregulated which results the cells to divide unstopped. These unstopped divided cells form tumour by piling up on top of each other.

See ***annexure 15.1*** for more details about cancer

15.6 DNA REPAIR MECHANISMS

The multiple DNA repair mechanisms have been evolved in different organisms to repair a specific type of damage in DNA. There are five well known mechanisms to repair DNA defects in *E. coli*. These mechanisms are light-dependent repair (photo-reactivation), excision repair (base excision repair and nucleotide excision repair), mismatch repair, post-replication repair, and error-prone repair. The mammals have all the five but photo-reactivation mechanism. The UV light has very weak penetrating power and causes injury to the surface tissues only. The mammals are multi-cellular and hence their cells do not have access to light.

(1) ***Photo-reactivation*** (*light-dependent repair*): Exposing the DNA to UV light produces the thymine dimmers by covalent cross-linkage between adjacent thymine molecules. The white light prevents the lethal action of UV light. This is a light-dependent DNA repair process and it is called ***photo-reactivation***. Thus, the *photo-reactivation* means the action of white light to prevent the damaging effect of UV light. The enzyme ***DNA photolyase*** present in bacteria is activated by light, recognizes and binds to thymine dimmers in DNA, and cleaves the covalent cross-links by using the energy from visible light within the blue region of the spectrum. The bacteria treated with UV light are reactivated by the effect of white light and thus, they escape death and grow colonies. The white light neutralizes the lethal effect of UV light and prevents to some extent the genetic damage caused by UV light. Likewise, *photolyase* enzyme also splits the cytosine dimmers and cytosine-thymine dimmers.

(2) **Excision repair mechanism**: This DNA repair process involves the removal of the damaged segment of DNA by means of synthesizing of a new strand using the complementary strand of DNA as template. This repair mechanism involves three enzymes, *viz.* the *endonuclease* recognizes, binds to, and excises the damaged base in DNA; the *DNA polymerase* makes use of undamaged complementary strand of DNA as a template to fill in the gaps; and the *DNA ligase* seals the break left by DNA polymerase.

The excision repair may be:

- ✰ For the repair of abnormal or chemically modified bases in DNA (base excision repair). This removes the abnormal bases, or
- ✰ For the repair of larger lesions (defects) like thymine dimmers (nucleotide excision repair) from DNA.

(3 ***Mismatch repair mechanism:*** Sometimes there is mismatching of base-pairing among the normal four bases in DNA. The DNA repair process to correct base pairs that are not properly hydrogen-bonded is called the *mismatch repair.* There is a mechanism by which the 3′ to 5′ exonuclease activity of DNA polymerases proofreads DNA strands during their synthesis and removes any mismatched nucleotide at the 3′ termini of growing stands (See DNA replication).

(4) ***Post-replication repair mechanism***: This DNA repair mechanism also involves mismatch repair. This is a recombination-dependent mechanism for repairing of damaged DNA. This mechanism provides a backup to the proofreading during DNA synthesis by correcting mismatched nucleotides which could not be corrected by replicative proofreading. This mechanism identifies the template strand having the original nucleotide sequence and distinguishes it from the nascent strand having mismatched bases (the error). The pattern of methylation in nascent DNA strand is made use of distinction between original and nascent DNA strands

in *E. coli.* The methylation of DNA sequence occurs subsequent to its synthesis. A time interval thus occurs during which the template strand is methylated and the nascent strand is un-methylated. This difference in methylation state is used by the mismatch repair mechanism to excise the mismatched nucleotide in the nascent strand and to replace it with the correct nucleotide by use of the methylated parental strand of DNA as template.

(5) ***Error-prone repair mechanism:*** The *E. coli* cell damaged by mutagenic agent (UV light) adapts some drastic steps for the survival. This is called the ***SOS response*** during which a whole battery of proteins is synthesized involving DNA repair, recombination, and replication. Two regulatory proteins control SOS response. The DNA polymerase V initiates the replication across damaged segments of template strands but this cannot accurately replicate the nucleotide sequences in the damaged region. This mechanism removes gaps in the nascent strands opposite damaged nucleotides in the template strands but with increased frequency of replication errors.

15.7 DEFECTS IN DNA REPAIR: INHERITED DISEASES (HUMAN)

The defects in DNA repair pathways have resulted into many inherited disorders in human beings. The inherited disorders result from the failure to repair DNA damaged by physical and chemical agents. These disorders have the life-threatening consequences due to defects in DNA repair enzymes. The known inherited human diseases due to the defects in DNA repair pathways are given below:

Inherited Disorders	*Ch. Nos.*	*Major Symptoms*
1. Ataxia-telangiectasia	11	Radiation sensitive, neuro-degradation, cancer prone.
2. Bloom syndrome	15	Chromosome instability, mental retardation, cancer prone.
3. Cockayne syndrome	5, 10	UV sensitive, neurological disorders, premature aging.
4. Fanconi anemia	(8 genes on 5 chromosomes)	Chromosome instability, cancer prone.
5. Nonpolyposis colon cancer (Lynch syndrome)	2, 3, 7 (5 genes)	High risk of familial colon cancer.
6. Nijmegan syndrome	8	Chromosome instability, microcephaly, cancer prone.
7. Rothmund –Thomson	8	Chromosome instability, mental retardation, cancer syndrome prone.

Inherited Disorders	*Ch. Nos.*	*Major Symptoms*
8. Trichothiodystrophy	2, 6, 9	UV sensitive, neurological disorder, mental retardation.
9. Werner syndrome	8	Chromosome instability, neuro-degeneration, cancer prone.
10. Xeroderma pigmentation	2, 3, 6, 9, 11, 13, 16, 19	UV sensitive, early onset skin cancer, neurological disorders.

Chapter 16

DNA Replication

Development of new cell, organism and strain has a genetic base that the body cell within it has its intrinsic power to have the genetic material (gene, DNA, chromosomes, and genome) with enormous genetic variability. The gene is a part of DNA which makes up the chromosome by combining with proteins, collectively called nucleoprotein and perform its functions to produce its phenotypic effect by specifying the amino acid sequences of specific protein.

The gene is a portion of DNA molecule and acts mainly by producing the enzymes. These enzymes are proteins formed of polypeptide chain of amino acids and involved in different steps of metabolism. The type of protein produced is determined by the arrangement of amino acids (sequence of amino acids in a polypeptide chain) and determined by the genes.

The genes perform the following three major functions:

- ☆ The gene are self-replicating (*duplication of chromatin, or replication of DNA*),
- ☆ Gene mutation due to error in DNA replication, and
- ☆ The genes synthesize the *proteins* through a two stage process *viz.* production of messenger RNA molecules (mRNA), called *transcription* and protein synthesis with the help of the ribosomes, called the *translation.*

Before the process of protein synthesis is described, it is essential to know about the constituents of proteins (amino acids), the arrangement of different amino acids in sequential order to form different proteins, and the linear arrangement of nucleotide bases in DNA to determine the sequence of amino acids in RNA (genetic code).

The two functions of genes *viz.* duplication of DNA molecule and protein synthesis have been explained here:

16.1 IMPORTANCE AND BASIS OF DNA REPLICATION

It is well known that the chromosomes are duplicated during cell division (both mitosis and meiosis). Each chromosome synthesizes a new chromosome identical to itself. This is known as DNA replication.

Replication of genetic material is the *genotypic function.* The ability of double-stranded DNA molecule to replicate has made possible the transmission of genetic material from one cell or organism to another. The base to the process of DNA replication has been provided by the followings -

- ✰ The complementary nature of the DNA strands and its double-stranded molecular structure,
- ✰ The base pairing principle (pairing of A with T, and of C with G), and
- ✰ Holding together the specific base pairs in the double strands of DNA by relatively weak hydrogen bonds.

16.2 MAIN FEATURES (NATURE) OF DNA REPLICATION

The DNA replication has the following four characteristics –

- ✰ The DNA replication is ***semi-conservative,***
- ✰ It is initiated at unique origins,
- ✰ It usually proceeds bi-directionally from each origin of replication, and
- ✰ Polarity in DNA replication.

(1) Semi-conservative Nature of DNA Replication

This is a mechanism of the DNA replication in which the parental strands are conserved (remain intact) and serve as templates for the synthesis of new complementary strand. This means that each daughter DNA molecule synthesized is a hybrid, conserving one parental polynucleotide chain and the other strand is the newly synthesized strand. Watson and Crick after proposing the double-helix structure of DNA with its complementary base-pairing, also thought that this base-pairing characteristic may provide the basis of simple mechanism of DNA replication, and hence postulated a possible mechanism of replication of DNA.

Proposed Mechanism of Replication

Watson and Crick proposed the semi-conservative DNA replication wherein each of the parental strands of the double helix is conserved and served as a template for the synthesis of a new complementary strand.

The first step in duplication process (DNA synthesis) is the untwisting (uncoiling or straightening) of the double-stranded DNA molecule and the two strands are separated into single strands. The replication occurs by separation of the two DNA strands. The separate strands serve as template for the synthesis of new partner strands. Two new DNA strands are assembled by the stepwise incorporation of nucleotides opposite to the nucleotides of the template strand following the base pairing rule of uniting A with T and C with G. Thus, the base-pairing principle dictates the sequence of bases (nucleotides) in the newly synthesized strand on the basis of sequence of nucleotides in the template strand. Thus, each of the original single-strand guides the manufacture of its new complementary strand by attracting the appropriate nucleotides according to base pairing principle. In this way the two identical DNA duplicates are formed from original DNA duplex. These two newly produced double-stranded DNA molecules are exactly the same to the original double-stranded DNA molecule, except few copy errors (gene mutations). Such a mechanism of DNA duplication is called ***semi-conservative.***

Experimental Evidences

J. Herbert Taylor, Philips Woods, and Walter Hughes (1957) conducted experiment on root-tip cells of broad bean (*Vicia faba*) and demonstrated that the eukaryotic chromosomes have semi-conservative replication. They labelled the chromosomes by growing root tips for less than one cell generation of 8 hours in a medium containing radioactive ^{3}H-thymidine. The technique of autoradiography was used by them to examine the distribution of radioactivity in the chromosomes of cells. They removed the root tips from radioactive medium, washed them, and transferred to nonradioactive medium containing the alkaloid colchicines at metaphase. The colchicine binds to microtubules and prevents the formation of functional spindle fibers so as the daughter chromosomes do not undergo their normal anaphase separation resulting the doubling of the number of chromosomes per nucleus per cell cycle. This helped to determine the number of DNA duplications, each cell had undergone after incorporating the radioactive thymidine. They observed that both chromatids of each pair were radioactive at the first metaphase of colchicines but only one of the chromatids of each pair was found radioactive at the second metaphase of colchicines. Such results were in accordance to the expectation of the semi-conservative nature of DNA duplication.

Matthew Meselson and Franklin Stahl (1958) and John Cairns (1962) also demonstrated that the chromosomes of *E. coli* replicate semi-conservatively. The experiments on eukaryotic chromosome replication had been subsequently carried out by other workers. The results of all such experiments had indicated the semi-conservative nature of DNA replication.

(2) Unique Origins of DNA Replication

The site of initiation of DNA replication in the circular chromosome of *E. coli* was reported *by* J. Cairns (1962) but could not decide the exact site of initiation whether it was a unique site or it occurred at randomly. It has now been known that there is unique and single origin of replication per chromosome to control the replication of the entire chromosome in bacteria and viruses whereas in case of large chromosomes of eukaryotes there are multiple origins that occur at specific sites and control collectively the replication of the giant DNA molecule in each chromosome.

The site or nucleotide sequence on a chromosome or DNA molecule at which replication is initiated is called the ***origin of replication.*** The replication of *replicon* (a unit of DNA) is controlled by each origin of replication. Therefore, the numbers of replicon are many in eukaryotic chromosomes while there is only a single replicon in prokaryotic chromosome.

The single origin of replication in *E. coli* chromosome is 245 nucleotide pairs in length containing two different conserved repeat sequences. One of the sequences is of 13 bp long:

G A T C T N T T N T T T T

This sequence is present as 3 tandem repeats which are rich in A:T base pairs. These AT-rich base pairs are held together by only two hydrogen bonds for which the two strands of AT-rich regions of DNA are separated more easily with the input of less energy. Thus, a localized region of complementary strand separation is formed at the origin of replication during the initiation of DNA replication and it is called the ***replication bubble.*** The formation of replication bubble is an essential and first step in the replication of all double-stranded DNAs. The second conserved component of sequence is the 9-bp long sequence:

T T A T N C A N A

This sequence is repeated 4 times, interspersed with other sequences, and these 4 sequences act as binding sites for a protein which has its role in formation of the replication bubble.

The eukaryotic chromosomes to have the multiple origins of replication also appear to be specific DNA sequences. The baker's yeast (*Saccharomyces cerevisiae*) which is a fungus and eukaryote has been characterized for its segments of chromosomal DNA that allow a fragment of circularized DNA to replicate as an independent unit like an extra-chromosomal self-replicating unit. As these sequences are autonomously replicating and hence called ARS (autonomously replicating sequences) elements. The frequencies of ARS elements in this yeast genome are equal to the number of origins of replication and some of them may function as origins. These ARS elements are of about 50 bp long including a core 11-bp AT-rich sequence:

A T T T A T Pu T T T A

T A A A T A Py A A A T

and additional imperfect copies of this sequence.

However, the scientists could not get success to identify the origins of replication in multi-cellular eukaryotes in spite of the facts that replication is initiated at specific sequences *in vivo* and that the DNA sequence of the entire genome is available. The reasons of failure in indentifying the origin of replication could be assigned to the initiation of replication at random or multiple sites and also involving relatively long DNA sequences.

(3) Bi-directional DNA Replication

John Cairns (1963) was the first to determine the gross structure of replicating bacterial chromosome by growing *E. coli* cells in medium containing ^{3}H-thymidine with the help of the technique of autoradiography. This autoradiography showed that the chromosomes are circular, winding of the two complementary parental strands and their semi-conservative replication occur simultaneously or coupled closely. The replication of *E. coli* chromosome occurs bi-directionally from the unique origin of replication. The Y-shaped structure known as ***replication fork*** is seen by autoradiography and the two replication forks move in opposite direction sequentially around the circular chromosome. The bi-directional replication occurs during cell division.

Distinction between Uni- and Bi-directional Replication

The cells growing in ^{3}H-thymidine medium for a short period of time and then transferred to nonradioactive medium for further growth (pulse-chase experiment), uni – and bi-directional replication predict different labelling patters, distinguished by autoradiography. In unidirectional replication there is origin with single fork, and a single tail of decreasing silver grain density appears at only one end of each fork by autoradiographs. In bidirectional replication, the origin has two forks and the audiographs show two tails of decreasing silver grain density. Bidirectional replication produces tails of decreasing grain density at each growing point at both ends of an autoradiographic track.

The experiment conducted on bacteriophage lambda (small virus that infects *E. coli*) demonstrated that DNA replication is bi-directional. The AT-rich and GC-rich clusters of phage lambda were used as physical markers using the technique of denaturation mapping by Maria Schnos and Ross Inman (1960s) and demonstrated that lambda chromosome replication is initiated at a unique origin and proceeds bi-directionally. The ***denaturation*** is a process of separation of two DNA strands on exposing the DNA molecules to high temperature (100 ° C) or high pH (11.4). Such a treatment or condition breaks the double-helix configuration resulting by holding the complementary strands together by the hydrogen and hydrophobic bonds.

The replication of chromosomal DNA in eukaryotes and other organisms with chromosomes that replicate as linear structures is also bi-directional. However, the bi-directional replication of DNA is not universal as in case of coliphage P2 the chromosome replicates from a unique origin uni-directionally.

(4) Polarity in DNA Synthesis

Two strands of a DNA double helix have opposite chemical polarity wherein one strand has 5′ to 3′ polarity and the other has 3′ to 5′ polarity when both are read in the same direction. This is because it is customary to write sequences starting with the 5′ –terminus on the left and ending with the 3′ –terminus on the right. All DNA synthesis occurs in the 5′ to 3′ direction. This means that the synthesis occurs by adding of nucleotides to the 3′ –OH end (terminus) of the primer strand. Therefore, new strand of DNA is formed on RNA primers in 5′ – 3′ direction from 3′ – 5′ template DNA by the addition of deoxyribonucleotides to the 3′ –OH end of primer RNA. The sequence of the new DNA chain synthesized with strand 1 as template is read 5′ to 3′ from the left to the right on the computer printout. The addition is by DNA polymerase III in the presence of ATP. All DNA polymerase have an absolute requirement for a free 3′-OH (hydroxyl) on the end of the primary strand that will be extended by DNA polymerization reaction.

The RNA primer is the primer strands of RNA which are synthesized by DNA directed RNA polymerase. The DNA synthesis proceeds simultaneously on both the strands as small segments of 1000 – 2000 nucleotides. The enzyme polynucleotide ligase helps to join them and in completing the formation of polynucleotide chain. The enzyme RNA polymerase initiates the replication of DNA or RNA strand and recognizes 5′ end of DNA strand. The unzipping (uncoiling) of original DNA strand and synthesis of fresh DNA strands go simultaneously.

The addition of a 2′, 3′ –dideoxyribonucleoside monophosphate to the 3′ end of a primer strand blocks its extension.

16.3 ENZYMES INVOLVED IN DNA REPLICATION

A number of proteins and enzymes are required in DNA replication and these form a DNA replicase system or ***replisome.*** An enzyme that catalyzes the formation of DNA or RNA is called ***polymerase.*** The enzymes are of the following types which are involved in DNA replication:

(i) DNA Polymerases

The ***DNA polymerase*** enzyme is responsible for the synthesis of DNA and this enzyme can only catalyze the synthesis in the 5′ to 3′ direction. These enzymes participating in the process of DNA replication are of 3 types. These are DNA polymerase I, II, and III.

(a) The *DNA polymerase I* was discovered by Kornberg and colleagues (1955) who were awarded 1959 Noble Prize. The DNA polymerase I studied in *E. coli* is spherical formed by a single polynucleotide chain of about 1000 amino acids. It has a diameter of about 6.5 nm and a molecular weight of 190,000.

It is a multi-functional enzyme participating in DNA repair by catalyzing the addition of mononucleotide units to the free 3′- hydroxyl end of DNA chain @ about 1000 nucleotides per minute, catalyzes 3′-5′ exonuclease activity and removes nucleotides of primer RNA at 3′ end, and also catalyzes 2′-3′ exonuclease activity. The DNA polymerase I in *E. coli* excises (removes) the RNA primers during chromosome replication.

The ***enzyme primase*** catalyzes the synthesis of RNA primers in the semi-conservative replication in prokaryotes.

The DNA polymerase I have three distinct enzyme activities to play:

- ✰ *Polymerase activity* of covalent extension of a DNA primer strand in the 5′ to 3′ direction,
- ✰ 5′ to 3′ *exonuclease activity of DNA polymerase I* catalyses the removal of RNA primers to cut back DNA strands starting at 5′ termini in semi-conservative replication in prokaryotes, and

☆ 3′ to 5′ *exonuclease activity* to cleave off nucleotides from the 3′ termini of DNA strand.

(b) The *DNA polymerase II* is effective on DNA-duplex with gaps only but cannot replicate long strands. Not much more is known about this enzyme.

(c) The *polymerase III enzyme* is main and most active enzyme in DNA replication. This enzyme is true replicase in *E. coli* and it does not remove the DNA primers. The enzyme polymerase III catalyzes the semi-conservative replication of the chromosome in *E. coli*. It catalyzes the addition of deoxyribonucleotids to RNA primers. This enzyme elongates the DNA in 5′ to 3′ direction by adding new units to the 3′ end of primer strand and thus cannot initiates replication.

It was discovered by Kornberg, T. and Gefter, M.L. (1972) as a large complex molecule with a molecular weight of about 550,000 formed by a number of subunits (α, β, γ, δ, ε, θ). The subunit β (also called co-polymerase III) recognizes and binds to the primer strand of parental DNA and it is released after binding of polymerase III to the correct initiation point.

Requirement of DNA polymerases: The DNA polymerases catalyze the covalent extension at the 3′ termini of growing polynucleotide chain and hence called processive enzymes. There is an absolute requirement of all known DNA polymerase that there should be a free 3′- OH on the end of the DNA strand being extended/ synthesized and an appropriate DNA template (specifying the complementary new strand) for its activity and no DNA polymerase can initiate the synthesis of a new strand of DNA without this requirement. Thus, all the DNA polymerases require preexisting DNA with its two essential components (***primer*** DNA and ***template*** DNA). The synthesis of DNA chains cannot be initiated *de novo* but all known DNA polymerases absolutely require for a free 3′ –OH on a preexisting polynucleotide chain.

This means that DNA polymerases can only extend/grow either DNA or RNA chains containing a free 3′-OH. This is because the mechanism of extension involves a nucleophilic attack by the 3′-OH on the interior phosphorus of the deoxyribonucleoside triphosphate precursor with elimination of pyrophosphate. The strand with the 3′-OH is the primer strand which is extended during synthesis. The *primer DNA* strand provides a terminus with a free 3′-OH to which nucleotides are added during DNA synthesis. The **primer** is a short nucleotide sequence with a reactive 3′ –OH that can initiate DNA synthesis along a template. Therefore, all the DNA polymerases require a primer strand with a free 3′-OH and this strand is covalently extended by the addition of nucleotides. All the DNA polymerases catalyze the formation of a phosphodiester bridge between 3′ –OH at the end of the primer DNA chain and the 5′-phosphate of the incoming deoxyribonucleotide.

Also all the DNA polymerases require a *template strand* which determines the base sequence of newly synthesized strand. Thus, the *template DNA* provides the nucleotide sequence that specifies the complementary sequence of the growing DNA chain. The template strand in transcription is the DNA strand that is copied to produce a complementary strand of RNA. The base sequence of DNA template strand dictates the synthesis of a complementary nucleotide base sequence in the newly synthesized strand by the base pairing rule. Thus, the new strand will be complementary to the template strand as shown below:

(Template strand)

3′ G T C A T C   G T C A A G C 5′

5′ C A G T A G OH → P

(Primer strand)

The DNA polymerase III in *E. coli* has many subunits (multimeric enzyme) having a molecular mass of about 900,000 daltons (mass of a hydrogen atom) in its complete form and the minimal core with catalytic activity *in vitro* has 3 subunits (α, ε, and θ) which are gene products.

There are at least 5 DNA polymerases in *E. coli viz.* DNA *polymerase I to V*. The first 2 polymerases (I and II) are DNA repair enzymes. The DNA polymerase III is composed of many different subunits. Like the DNA polymerase I, it has 5′ to 3′ polymerase and 3′ to 5′ exonuclease activities, though its 5′ to 3′ exonuclease that is active only on single-stranded DNA. The 5′ to 3′ polymerase activity of DNA polymerase III catalyzes the covalent extension of DNA chains at the 3′-OH termini of primer strands in the semi-conservative replication of DNA in prokaryotes. The DNA polymerases IV and V along with polymerase II have been recognized to be involved in the replication of damaged DNA.

There have been identified at least 15 different polymerases in eukaryotic organisms. These different polymerases have been named as α, β, γ, δ, ε, κ, ζ, η, θ, κ, λ, μ, σ, φ, and Rev I. These different DNA polymerases have different roles to play in DNA replication. Two or more of them (α, δ and or ε) are involved in semi-conservative replication of nuclear DNA. Polymerase δ and or ε catalyze the continuous synthesis of leading strand while polymerase α functions as a primase in the discontinuous synthesis of the lagging strand, and polymerase γ catalyzes the replication of mitochondrial DNA (organellar chromosome). The remaining enzymes are said to be involved in DNA repair pathways or in metabolic functions.

The 3′ to 5′ exonuclease activity present in most prokaryotic DNA polymerase is said to be lacking in some of the eukaryotic DNA polymerases. However, all of the DNA polymerase either prokaryotic or eukaryotic catalyzes the same basic reaction of a nucleophilic attack by the free 3′-OH at the primer strand terminus on the nucleotidyl phosphorus of the nucleoside triphosphate precursor. Therefore, the absolute requirement of all the DNA polymerases is the free 3′-hydroxyl group on a preexisting primer strand. It is well known that none of the DNA polymerase can initiate new DNA chain *de novo*, and all DNA synthesis occurs in the 5′ to 3′ direction.

The shape of polymerase is such that the incoming nucleoside triphosphate, the template, and the primer terminus are tightly grasped and provides a simple mechanism for the template-directed selection of incoming nucleotides during DNA synthesis. There is high fidelity of DNA synthesis due to the crystal structure of the complex formed by a monomeric DNA polymerase, a nucleoside triphosphate precursor, and a template primer DNA.

(ii) DNA Helicases

The enzymes ***helicases*** catalyzes the unwinding process of double helix during replication of DNA molecules. In *E. coli,* the major replicative DNA helicase is the product of the *dna**B*** gene. This enzyme derived energy from ATP to unwind the DNA molecules.

(iii) DNA Ligase or Polynucleotide Ligase

As the name indicates, this enzyme joins the ends of two fragments of DNA chain. This process of joining the two fragments by this enzyme is by catalyzing the synthesis of a phosphodiester bond between a 3′-OH group at the one end of one chain and 5′-phosphate group at the end of other chain. The DNA ligase isolated from *E. coli* has a single polypeptide chain with a molecular weight of about 17,000. There are multiple copies (200 to 400 copies) of this enzyme in each cell of *E. coli.*

Besides joining the segments of DNA during DNA replication, and also in the process of recombination during meiosis and in transduction or genetic transformation, the enzyme DNA ligase also links the ends of linear DNA duplexes to make circles, and repairs the single-strand phosphodiester linkage (nicks).

(iv) DNA Topoisomerases

These are enzymes that catalyze the introduction or removal of supercoils from DNA. These enzymes induce transient breaks in DNA and are of the following two types -

(a) The first is the ***DNA topoisomerase I*** which produces temporary single-strand breaks or nicks in DNA. It plays its role in activities to remove supercoils from DNA one at a time. The transient single-strand break provides an axis of rotation to allow the DNA segment on opposite sides of the break to spin independently with the phosphodiester bond in the intact strand to serve as a swivel (turning on a pivot). These enzymes are energy efficient and conserve the energy of the cleaved phosphodiester linkages in the form of storing in covalent linkages between themselves and the phosphate groups at the cleavage sites for use in resealing the breaks.

(b) The second is the ***DNA topoisomerase II*** and termed as ***DNA gyrase*** in *E. coli.* The topoisomerase II induces transient double-strand breaks in DNA. The important role played by this enzyme is to remove positive supercoils and introduce negative supercoils in DNA two at a time by ATP requiring mechanism. These enzymes perform this process by cutting both strands of DNA, holding on to the ends at the cleavage site through covalent bonds, passing the intact double helix through the cut, and resealing the break. This enzyme can separate interlocking circular molecules of DNA.

In *E. coli,* the enzyme topoisomerase II (DNA gyrase) has been best characterized. It is tetramer of two α subunits and two β subunits. α subunit is specified by a *gyrA* gene (nalidixic acid) while the β subunit is encoded by the *gyrB* gene (coumermycin). The nalidixic acid and coumermycin are antibiotics that inhibit the activity of DNA gyrase and DNA synthesis by binding to α and β subunits, respectively of DNA gyrase whose activity is needed for DNA replication in *E. coli.*

The chromosomal DNA is negatively supercoiled in bacteria (*E. coli*) and introduced by DNA gyrase with ATP energy. The ***DNA gyrase*** activity of forming the negative supercoils in progeny DNA molecules also provides help in solving the unwinding problem. The separation of strand is favoured due to reduction in superhelical tension during unwinding, the negative supercoiling behind the fork may result the unwinding. This shows that DNA gyrase activity is required for DNA replication in bacteria or the gyrase may remove forming the positive supercoils ahead of the replication fork.

16.4 SIMILARITIES AND DIFFERENCES IN DNA REPLICATION OF PROKARYOTES AND EUKARYOTIC CHROMOSOMES

Mostly the information on DNA replication have come from studies on *E. coli* and its viruses compared to less information on eukaryotes for their DNA replication. However, based on the studies made on DNA replication it has been said that most of the aspects of DNA replication are almost similar in prokaryotes and eukaryotes.

The continuous and discontinuous mechanisms exist for replication of leading and lagging strands, respectively for both prokaryotes as well as in eukaryotes. However, the RNA primers and Okazaki fragments are shorter in eukaryotes compared to prokaryotes. The eukaryotic chromosomes besides being longer in size also differ in structure than of the prokaryotic chromosomes. The longer size of eukaryotic chromosomes requires multiple origin of replication.

(i) There is nonstop DNA replication throughout the cell cycle in bacteria. On the contrary, the DNA replication in eukaryotes is restricted to a period during cell cycle known as the synthetic phase (S phase) which is in between the G_1 phase (after completion of mitosis) and G_2 phase (preparation for mitosis) followed by M phase (mitosis). The G stands for gap. The DNA replication occurs once and only once during each cell division in eukaryotes. Thus, the uniqueness in DNA replication in eukaryotes is that DNA synthesis takes place within a small period of the cell cycle instead of continuously as in case of prokaryotes.

(ii) The eukaryotic chromosomes contain multiple origins of replication because of the giant size of their DNA molecules for which long time would require to replicate with a single origin. The prokaryotic chromosomes have a single origin of replication.

(iii) The eukaryotic organisms utilize two or more different polymerases instead of using two catalytic complexes of one DNA polymerase to replicate the leading and lagging strands, but the prokaryotes utilize two catalytic complexes containing the same DNA polymerase to replicate the leading and lagging strands.

(iv) The eukaryotic chromosomes have linear DNA molecules and the DNA is packaged in nucleosomes (histone- containing structure). Thus, the eukaryotes require the partial disassembly of nucleosomes as the replisome move along the parental DNA and then assembly after the replisome is passed to nucleosome.

(v) The prokaryotic chromosomes are circular and hence no ends but eukaryotic chromosomes are linear having unique termini (telomeres) that are replicated by a unique RNA-containing enzyme (called telomerase) and the termini are added to replicating DNA molecules.

(vi) The replication rates are slower in eukaryotes than in prokaryotes and depends on the rate of growth of replication bubble.

16.5 WATSON AND CRICK (1953) MODEL OF REPLICATION

The DNA replication is more complicated than thought earlier and put forth by Watson and Crick (1953) proposing the semi-conservative mechanism of replication.

(i) Unwinding of Two Parental DNA Strand

The first requirement of semi-conservative replication of DNA molecule is the unwinding (separation) of two strands of a parental DNA. Therefore, the two strands should be separated during the synthesis of new complementary strands. The separation requires the untwisting of two DNA strands turn by turn and hence requires unwinding mechanism. The DNA molecule must be rotated 360° once for each 10 bp that are required for one turn (gyre). The *E. coli* chromosome contains about 4×10^6 nucleotide pairs and replicates as a single bidirectional replicon in about 40 minutes. The DNA replicates 30,000 nucleotides in one minute in *E. coli.* A replicating DNA molecule to meet this replication requirement must spin 3000 revolutions per minute for unwinding of the parental DNA strand.

The DNA replication or duplication requires unwinding mechanism of two strands so as the two strands are separated for synthesis new complementary strands of a parental DNA molecule (nascent chain of DNA). The separation requires their untwisting turn by turn. The process of unwinding requires ***three different proteins***, namely the DNA helicase, single-strand DNA binding protein coats, and DNA gyrase.

(*a*) The enzymes **DNA helicases** unwinds the DNA double-helix. These helicases are the gene product and are the major replicative DNA enzyme in *E. coli.* The DNA helicases unwind the DNA molecules using the energy derived from ATP.

(*b*) *DNA binding proteins:* The DNA strands after being unwound by DNA helicases are kept in an extended, single-stranded form for replication. A coating of single-strand DNA-binding protein (SSBP) maintains the DNA strand unwound. The SSb protein is encoded by the *ssb* gene in *E. coli.* The binding is cooperative as the binding of the first SSB monomer stimulates the binding of additional monomers at contiguous sites on the DNA chain. The entire single-stranded region of DNA is rapidly coated with SSB protein due to the cooperative activity of SSB protein binding. The SSB protein coating is essential not to allow the formation of intra-strand hairpin structures on the complementary strand by hydrogen bonding between short segments of complementary or partially complementary nucleotide sequences. The activity of DNA polymerases is impeded by these hairpin structures.

(c) ***DNA gyrase*** catalyzes the formation of negative supercoiling in *E. coli* DNA. This negative supercoiling behind the replication fork drives the unwinding process.

The *E. coli* chromosome has a circular DNA molecule and the unwinding of the parental strands during replication requires the DNA spinning at 3000 revolutions per minute. Thus, axis of rotation to prevent DNA to become positively supercoiled is required. The enzymes called ***DNA topoisomerases*** provide the required axes (swivel) of rotation during the replication of circular DNA in *E. coli*. This prevents the DNA from becoming tangled (positively supercoiled) ahead of the replication fork.

(ii) Continuous and Discontinuous Synthesis of Two DNA Strands

The synthesis of one DNA strand (*leading strand*) is continuous while the synthesis of second strand (*lagging strand*) is by a discontinuous mechanism.

The ***continuous replication*** is the synthesis of a nascent strand of DNA by the sequential addition of nucleotides to the 3′-OH terminus of the strand. This is the characteristic of ***leading strand*** (the strand being extended in the overall 5′ to 3′ direction).

The ***discontinuous replication*** is the synthesis of a nascent strand of DNA by the formation of short fragments of DNA (Okazaki small fragments – discovered by Reiji Okazaki and Tuneko Okazaki 1960s) and their subsequent covalent joining by DNA ligase. This is the characteristic of synthesis of the ***lagging strand*** which is being extended in the overall 3′ to 5′ direction.

The two modes of continuous and discontinuous replication can be distinguished experimentally. The continuous replication is indicated when the label is incorporated into *chromosome-sized DNA molecules*, on labelling the nascent DNA by exposure to ^{3}H thimidine for very short period. On the other hand, the discontinuous replication is indicated when the label first appears in *small pieces of nascent DNA*, prior to covalent joining, catalyzed by DNA ligase.

The results from studies in which intermediates in DNA synthesis were radioactively labelled by growing *E. coli* cells and bacteriophage T4- infected *E. coli* cells in the medium that contains ^{3}H-thymidine, indicated that the intermediates in DNA replications are the short DNA fragments rather than any other metabolic products. These short fragments were called Okazaki fragments. The lagging strand thus grows by the synthesis of short DNA fragments (Okazaki fragments) that are synthesized 5′ to 3′ direction and their subsequent covalent joining. The synthesis of the complementary strands of DNA at the molecular level occurs in opposite physical direction but both new strands are extended in the same 5′ to 3′ chemical direction.

(iii) Role of Primosome and Replisome

The ***primosome*** is a protein replication complex, contains DNA primase and DNA helicase activities, and catalyzes the initiation of Okazaki fragments during discontinuous DNA synthesis. It initiates to carry out the Okazaki fragments on the lagging strand. The primosome moves along the DNA molecule utilizing the energy of ATP. With its movement, the DNA helicase unwinds the parental double helix whereas the DNA primase synthesizes the RNA primers required to initiate the successive Okazaki fragments. The addition of deoxyribonucleotides by DNA polymerase III extends covalently the RNA primers. The transient breaks in the DNA are caused by the enzyme DNA topoisomerases. These breaks serve as swivels for DNA unwinding and keep the DNA untangled. The unwound pre-replicative DNA is coated by single-strand DNA binding proteins and keeps it in an extended state for DNA polymerase III. The DNA polymerase I replace the RNA primers with DNA and the DNA ligase sealed the single-strand nicks left by polymerase I. This sequence of events occurs at each replication fork during the semi-conservative replication in *E. coli.*

Both the DNA strands (leading and lagging strand) are replicated in a coordinate manner with the movement of replication fork along a parental double helix. The complete replication apparatus, present at a *replication fork*, moving along the DNA molecule is called the ***replisome.*** The ***replication fork*** is a Y-shaped structure where the two parental strands of a DNA double helix are unwound and are being used as templates for the synthesis of new complementary strands. Replisome carries out the semi-conservative replication of DNA. The replisome contains the DNA polymerase III holoenzyme, and two catalytic cores replicate the leading strand and the lagging strand.

The primosome unwinds the parental DNA molecule and synthesizes the RNA primers required for the discontinuous synthesis of the lagging strand. The replisome in prokaryotes contains 13 proteins. The lagging strand seems to form a loop from the primosome to the second catalytic core of DNA polymerase III to synthesize both the nascent leading and lagging strands by the two catalytic cores of the polymerase III holoenzyme.

(iv) Initiation of DNA Chain

The DNA chains are initiated with RNA primers. The *E. coli* chromosome initiates its replication at a unique sequence called *ori*C by forming the replication bubble (localized region of strand separation). The *ori*C by its interaction with *pre-priming proteins* forms the replication bubble (loops). Once a replication bubble is formed there should exists a mechanism to initiate (prime) the synthesis of new DNA chains. The testing results have proved that DNA synthesis is initiated by RNA primers. The ***RNA primer*** is a short segment of RNA (10 to 60 nucleotides) that is synthesized by the enzyme ***DNA primase*** and used to initiate the synthesis of a new strand of DNA. In prokaryotes the RNA primers are of 10 to 60 nucleotides long but these are shorter of only about 10 nucleotides in eukaryotes. The RNA primers provide the free 3′-OH essential for covalent extension of polynucleotide chains by DNA polymerases. The RNA primers are subsequently excised and replaced with

DNA chains by DNA polymerase I using the adjacent Okazaki fragments with its free 3′-OH as a primer in *E. coli.* After replacing the RNA primer with a DNA chain by DNA polymerase I, the 3′-OH of one fragment (Okazaki) is next to the 5′-phosphate group of the preceding fragment (Okazaki). The DNA ligase uses this product as an appropriate substrate to catalyze the formation of phosphordiester linkage between two fragments (Okazaki).

In brief, the synthesis and replacement of RNA primers during replication of the lagging strand of DNA occurs by the synthesis of a short RNA strand that provide a 3′-OH primer for DNA synthesis. The RNA primer is removed and replaced with DNA subsequently by 5′ to 3′ exonuclease and 5′ to 3′ polymerase activities of DNA polymerase I. The DNA ligase now covalently closes the nascent chain, catalyzing the formation of phosphodiester linkages between adjacent 3′-hydroxyls and 5′-phospates.

(v) Linking of Short DNA Fragments

The enzyme DNA ***ligase*** helps to link the DNA Okazaki short fragments together to produce the large DNA strands present in mature chromosome. The DNA ligase catalyzes the covalent closure of missing phosphodiester linkage (called ***Nicks***) in DNA molecules. This mechanism requires the energy to form the ester linkage by the DNA ligase and the source of energy is the ATP (adenosine triphosphate) or NAD (nicotinamide adenine dinucleotide). But the DNA ligase alone is not effective when the breaks in DNA are caused by missing of one or more nucleotides (called gaps). The DNA ligase by its combined action with DNA polymerase filled in and sealed the gaps.

(vi) DNA Proofreading and Error Correction

There is a mechanism of proofreading the newly synthesized DNA chain. This involves scanning the termini of nascent DNA chains for errors and correcting them. This is carried out by the 3′ to 5′ exonuclease activities of DNA polymerases. The ***proofreading*** is the enzymatic scanning of DNA for structural defects occurred in replication like mismatched base pair. The major replicative DNA polymerases are amazingly accurate but sometimes incorporate the incorrect nucleotides with an initial frequency of 10^{-5} to 10^{-10}. In case of an error (incorrect pair base or sequence of bases at the 3′ end of the primer), the 3′ to 5′ exonuclease activity of the DNA polymerase clips off the unpaired base or bases. On producing appropriate base paired terminus, the 5′ to 3′ polymerase activity of the enzyme starts re-synthesis by adding nucleotides to the 3′ end of the primer strand. The 3′ to 5′ exonuclease activity of DNA polymerase III catalyzes the proofreading of the nucleotides at the 3′-OH termini of DNA primer strands in the semi-conservative replication of DNA in prokaryotes.

DNA polymerase I of *E. coli* is monomeric enzyme in which the 3′ to 5′ exonuclease activity is built in while in multimeric enzymes the 3′ to 5′ proofreading exonuclease activity is often present on a separate subunit. The proofreading function in DNA polymerase III of *E. coli* is carried out by the ε subunit. No exonuclease activity is present in DNA polymerase IV of *E. coli*.

In eukaryotes, the DNA polymerase γ, δ, and ε contain 3′ to 5′ proofreading exonuclease activities while this activity is lacking in α and β polymerases.

The similarity in appearance among twins becomes less without proofreading. The changes due to errors in replication accumulate without proofreading in the genes during cell divisions from embryonic stage to adults. The DNA proofreading during replication and the activity of DNA repair enzymes decide the identity of the genotypes of identical twins. The DNA for various types of damage is scanned continuously by these enzymes and the errors are repaired before inheritance.

(vii) Rolling Circle Replication

The rolling circle replication is a mechanism for replicating circular DNA molecules. In this type of DNA replication one parental circular DNA strand is cleaved at the origin of replication while the other strand remains intact, and rolls or spins while serving as a template for the synthesis of a nascent complementary strand. The 5′ terminus of the cleaved strand is unwound and replicated discontinuously while continuous replication of the other strand occurs at the 3′ terminus with the intact circular as template. This type of DNA replication is used in many viruses to duplicate their genome, in bacteria to transfer DNA from donor cells to recipient cells during genetic exchange, and in amphibians to amplify extra-chromosomal DNA carrying clusters of ribosomal RNA genes during oogenesis.

This type of replication (Rolling-circle) can produce circular single-stranded progeny DNAs by site-specific cleavage of the single-stranded tails at the origins of replication and recircularization of the resulting unit-length molecules. The single stranded tails are used as templates for the discontinuous synthesis of complementary strands prior to cleavage and circularization to produce double-stranded progeny DNA molecules.

The DNA primase activity is not required to initiate the rolling circle replication. This is because this type of replication begins on cleaving the one strand of a circular DNA double-helix by an endonuclease. This cleavage forms a free 3′ – OH on one

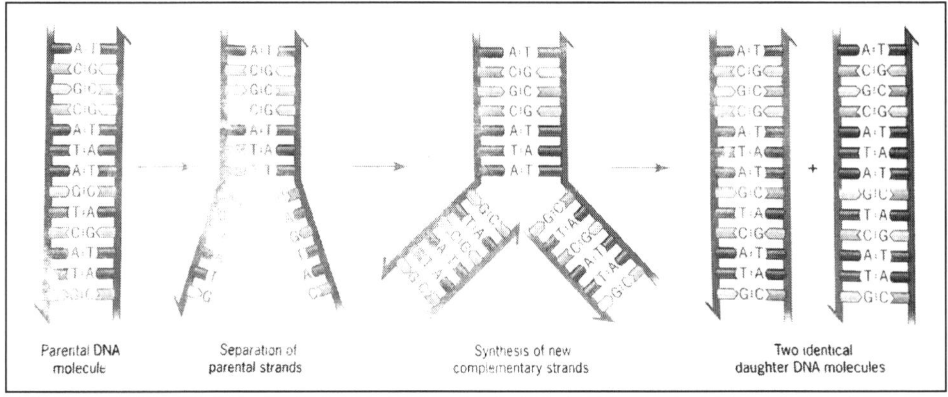

Figure 16.1: DNA Replication.

end of the cut strand and allows it to function as a primer. The DNA primase is required for the discontinuous synthesis of the lagging strand and it occurs on the single-stranded tail of the rolling circle. The reason is that the discontinuous synthesis needs the *de novo* initiation of each Okazaki fragments requiring DNA primase activity.

The different enzyme activities catalyzing the following steps in the semi-conservative replication of DNA in prokaryotes are as under:

Steps in DNA Replication	*Enzyme Activity*
(i) Formation of negative super-coils in progeny DNA molecules	DNA gyrase
(ii) Synthesis of RNA primer	Primase
(iii) Removal of RNA primers	5′ to 3′ exonuclease activity of DNA polymerase I
(iv) Covalent extension of DNA chains at the 3′ –OH termini of primer strands	5′ to 3′ polymerase activity of DNA polymerase III
(v) Proofreading of nucleotides at 3′ –OH Termini of DNA primer strands	3′ to 5′ exonuclease activity of DNA polymerase III

16.6 REPLICATION OF EUKARYOTIC CHROMOSOME: SPECIAL ASPECTS

The DNA replication in most of the aspects is similar in prokaryotes and eukaryotes with exception of some processes occurring in eukaryotes.

(i) Multiple Origin of Replication per Chromosome

The DNA molecules of eukaryotic chromosomes are of giant size (10^7 to 10^8 nucleotide pairs in general) *viz.* human genome have been estimated to have about 2.7 billion (2.7×10^9) nucleotide pairs containing about 25,000 to 30,000 genes, and about 6.5×10^7 nucleotide pairs are contained in the chromosomes of *Drosophila melanogaster*. The single replication fork cannot replicate the large DNA fast enough to permit the observed cell generation time. The DNA replication in *Drosophila* occurs at the rate of about 2600 nucleotide pairs per minute at normal temperature of 25°C. Thus, the replication of the DNA molecule in *Drosophila* will take about 17.5 days for a single replication fork, and 8.5 days with two replication forks moving bi-directionally from a central origin. But it has been estimated that the chromosomes of *Drosophila* embryos replicate within 3 to 4 minutes and the nuclear division takes place once every 9 to 10 minutes in early cleavage divisions. This makes it clear that giant DNA molecule must have many origin of replication (about more than 7,000 replication forks in *Drosophila*) distributed at equal intervals along the DNA molecule for its complete replication in 3.5 minutes.

The pulse-labelling experiment with Chinese hamster cells grown in culture with ^{3}H-thymidine for a few minutes by Joel Huberman and Arthur Riggs (1968)

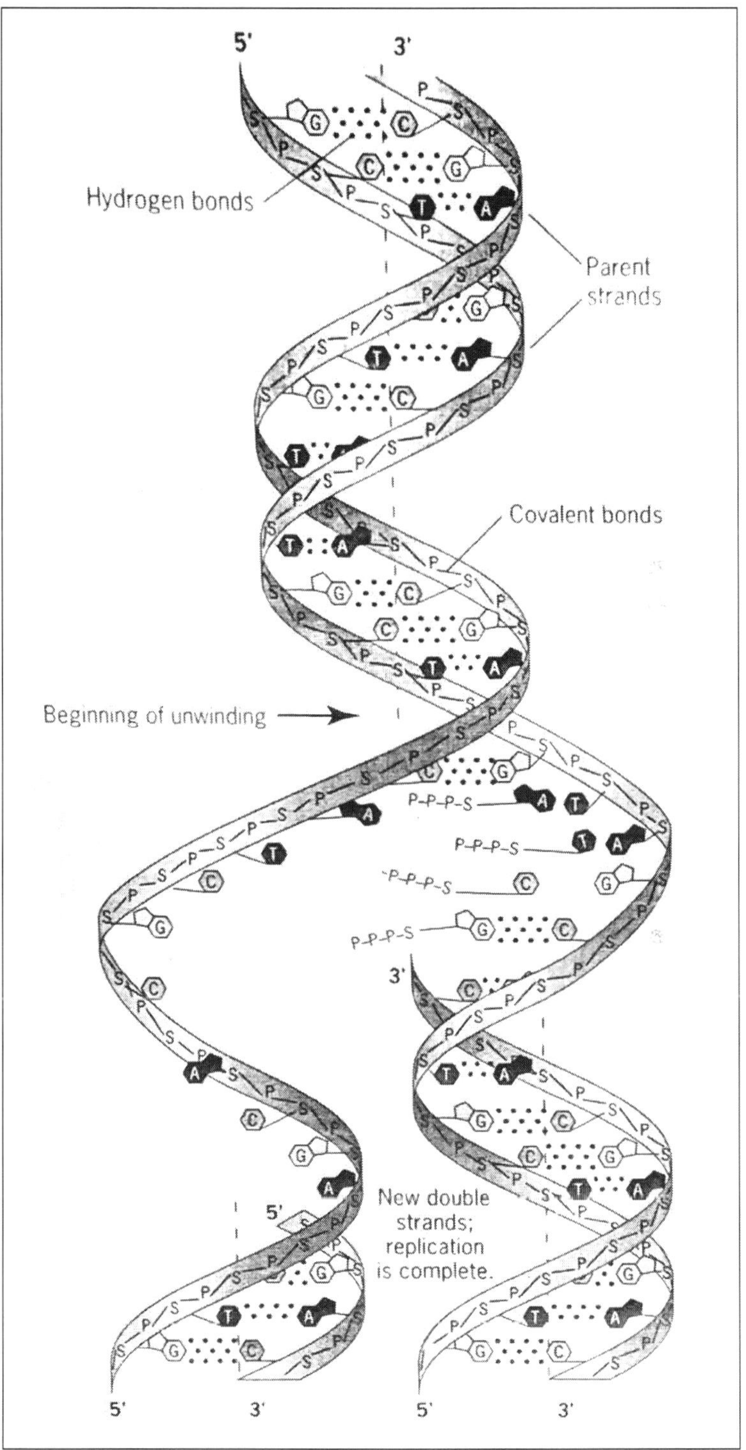

Figure 16.2: Semi-Conservative DNA Replication.

indicated that individual macromolecules of DNA contain multiple origins of replication and that the replication in eukaryotes is bidirectional like in most prokaryotes, as the replication forks move bi-directionally from central origins towards replication termini. Thus, the replication is initiated at more number of sites in each eukaryotic chromosome and this is called as multiple origin of replication. The DNA segment under the control of one origin of replication and two termini is called a ***replicon.*** Thus, there exist multiple replicons in each eukaryotic chromosome while in prokaryotic chromosome there is usually one replicon. The replication is initiated at more sites during very rapid cell division of embryogenesis compared to later ages.

(ii) More DNA Polymerases in Eukaryotes

The DNA topoisomerase and a DNA helicase are required for unwinding of the parental DNA strands in eukaryotes also like the prokaryotes. A single-strand DNA-binding protein called replication protein A keeps the unwound strands in the extended state. Three different DNA polymerases (α, δ, and ε) each with multiple subunits are present in each replication fork (replisome) in eukaryotes and all these are required for DNA replication. The eukaryotic replisome (replication fork) contains about 27 different polypeptides like 13 proteins are present in *E. coli* replisome. There have been identified 15 different polymerases (α, β, γ, δ, ε, κ, æ, η, θ, κ, λ, μ, σ, Φ, and Rev I) in eukaryotic organisms. These different DNA polymerases have different roles to play in DNA replication. The DNA polymerase γ is responsible for the replication of mitochondrial DNA.

(iii) Nucleosome Replication

The nucleosomes are about 11-nm beads in which the DNA of eukaryotic interphase chromosomes is packaged. Two turns of 166 nucleotide pairs of DNA are wound around an octamer of histone molecule of each nucleosome. However, it has been shown by electron micrographs of replicating DNA in *Drosophila* that the nucleosomes have normal structure and spacing on both sides of replication forks. Thus, there is same structure and spacing of nucleosomes immediately behind a replication fork (post-replicative DNA) as well as in front of a replication fork (pre-replicative DNA). This is indicative that nucleosomes must be disassembled to allow the replisome replicate the DNA involved in nucleosomes and then to reassemble resulting together the DNA replication and nucleosome assembly. However, the synthesis of histone proteins occurs throughout the cell cycle. The disassembly and assembly of nucleosomes during DNA replication in eukaryotes require a number of proteins. One of the proteins (called nucleosome assembly protein – 1) transports the histones from their place of synthesis (in the cytoplasm) to the nucleus while another protein (called chromatin assembly factor – 1) brought the histones to the sites of nucleosome assembly.

(iv) Telomerase Replication

The known mechanism for replication of linear DNA molecules is not enough to explain the replication of both strands of DNA at the ends of the molecules (telomeres). This is because DNA polymerases cannot replicate the terminal

DNA segment of the lagging strand (the strand being extended in the overall 3′ to 5′ direction) of a linear chromosome. Therefore, the telomeres of eukaryotic chromosomes must have either special structure or it should have special enzymes for replication. The evidences are available in support of both the alternatives. Thus, the telomeres have special structure which provides a mechanism for the addition of telomeres by an RNA-containing enzyme called ***telomerase.***

The enzyme *telomerase* was discovered by E. Blackburn and C. Greider (1985) while E. Blackburn and Jack Szostak discovered the mechanism of protection of telomeres from degeneration due to their special structure. All the three scientists shared the 2009 Noble Prize in Physiology or Medicine.

The enzyme telomerase adds the ends to the chromosomes. This mechanism of adding the chromosomes ends (telomeres) can be illustrated from telomeres of humans that contain tandemly repeated sequence of T T A G G G. The enzyme telomerase recognizes the Guanine rich telomere sequence on the 3′ overhang and extends it 5′ to 3′ one repeat unit at a time. This enzyme does not fill in the gap opposite the 3′ end of the template strand but it simply extends the 3′ end of the template strand. Uniquely the telomerase contains a built-in RNA template. The DNA polymerase catalyzes the synthesis of the complementary strand after the telomerase adds several telomere repeat units. The linear chromosome becomes shorter without telomerase.

There is little or no telomerase activity in most somatic cells. This results into the telomeres of the chromosomes of shorter length during each cell division. The chromosomes lost their telomeres if the somatic cells are divided in the absence of telomerase. This causes death of cell due to loss of essential genes near telomeres. Therefore, most of the somatic cells generally stop dividing after a limited number of cell divisions. The turning on (increase) the synthesis of telomerase, so that telomeres are not lost during the uncontrolled cell divisions of cancer cells, is one of the essential steps in conversion of a normal somatic cell to a cancer cell. The genes encoding telomerase are expressed in many cancer cells but these genes are not expressed in most somatic cells. It is therefore advisable for cancer treatment that telomerase inhibitors should be developed so as the telomeres are lost in the chromosomes in cancer cells resulting the cancer cells to die. However, this method of treating the cancer is not effective because some cancer cells do not have active telomerase.

Chapter 17

Gene Expression – Molecular Mechanism (Protein Synthesis) I. Transcription (RNA Production)

The phenotype of an organism is controlled by genes. It is the nucleotide sequences of genes that direct the growth and development of a cell, a tissue, an organ, and thus an entire body of the multi-cellular living organism. It is well known that the phenotype of a living individual is produced by the combined effects of all the genes by acting with the constraints imposed by the environment. It is also known that the number of genes varies among species depending on its developmental complexity. The subject matter of this chapter is thus to focus on the mechanisms by which the genes direct the synthesis of their products (RNAs and proteins) which in turn control the phenotypes of mature organisms.

17.1 GENE EXPRESSION (PROTEIN SYNTHESIS): A TWO STAGE PHENOMENON

The genome in the form of the DNA sequences (nucleotide sequences of genes) is organized into smaller units called *genes* and performs the important function of protein synthesis. Thus, the genes are expressed in the form of protein synthesis. The ***gene expression*** is the *phenotypic function* of genetic material. The *gene expression* is a process by which the genes produce RNAs and proteins and have their effect on the phenotype of a character of an individual. Therefore, the genes are expressed through production of RNA and synthesis of proteins which are made up of the amino acid sequences. Thus, the amino acids are called the structural stones of proteins. The different amino acids are assembled in different ways and form polypeptides to synthesize the different proteins. The gene expression is also called the functional property of gene as the gene produces its particular phenotypic effect on a character. The existence of one allele from the other is distinguished due to this functional property. The phenotype of an organism is the result of expression of genes. The genetic information contained in DNA is expressed in synthesis of a polypeptide chain (for protein synthesis) and called gene expression.

The amino acid sequences of proteins are synthesized from the genetic information stored in the nucleotide sequences of gene (part of DNA molecule). The genes transcribe (synthesize) the mRNA molecules which in turn are translated into their products (protein). The protein synthesis is thus one of the main functions of the genes and it is a two stage phenomenon *viz.* ***transcription*** and ***translation*** in both prokaryotes and eukaryotes.

The ***transcription*** means the RNA synthesis. This is the first step in gene expression. Thus, the process of the production (synthesis) of the mRNA molecule (along a DNA molecule) is called the ***transcription.*** The transcription involves the transfer of genetic information (message) stored in the sequences of nucleotide pairs in DNA (in the form of genes) to the nucleotides of RNA molecule. This RNA is produced (synthesized) as the unstable intermediaries and carries the message of information (hence called messenger RNA -mRNA), in eukaryotes, from the nucleus to the ribosome (sites of protein synthesis) in the cytoplasm. The transcription and RNA processing occur in the nucleus of the cell.

The ***translation*** is the second step in gene expression. This process of translation occurs in the cytoplasm on the ribosome and requires the use of many macromolecules. During translation, the message of genetic information carried by the sequences of nucleotides in mRNA molecules is translated (conveyed) to the ribosome in the cytoplasm and used to specify the nucleotide sequences of amino acids that are assembled together in polypeptide gene products (combined in different ways to synthesize the different proteins).

The facts of the RNA synthesis (*transcription*) occurring in the nucleus and protein synthesis (*translation*) occurring in the cytoplasm have been demonstrated. The techniques used in demonstrating these two processes at the respective places of their occurrence were the labelling of the RNA and protein precursors and the autoradiography.

17.2 THE CENTRAL DOGMA: TRANSFER OF GENETIC INFORMATION

There is a principle or doctrine of molecular biology that the genetic information stored in DNA is transmitted in every newly arisen living individual of every generation in the form of DNA (DNA to DNA) and for phenotypic expression of a character of living being in the form of DNA to RNA to protein (DNA to protein).

The genetic information is stored in nucleotide sequences of DNA. For phenotypic expression of a character of living being the DNA molecules are used to synthesize RNA molecules complementary to them (DNA to RNA) and this process is called *transcription*. Then RNA is used as a template to specify the incorporation of amino acids in the sequence of a polypeptide which forms proteins (called *translation*). Each amino acid in the polypeptide corresponds to a sequence of three nucleotides in the DNA. The triplet nucleotides that encode the different amino acids are called codons. The process of transcription and translation is called the ***Central dogma of biology.*** This is the usual flow of genetic information from generation to generation (DNA – its replication by DNA dependent DNA polymerase) and for gene expression to control the phenotype of a character through two stage process of transcription (DNA dependent RNA polymerase) and translation (mRNA molecules to polypeptides which synthesize proteins) which is a complex process involving ribosome, tRNAs, and other molecules. Therefore, the flow of genetic information in all the organisms according to the central dogma of molecular biology involves:

- ✰ *DNA replication* (synthesis of DNA from DNA – information flows from DNA to DNA),
- ✰ *Transcription of DNA to mRNA* – transfer of genetic information from DNA to RNA synthesis. This involves the synthesis of an RNA transcript complementary to one strand of DNA of a gene, and
- ✰ *Translation of mRNA to protein* – transfer of information from RNA to protein synthesis. This is the conversion of information stored in the sequence of nucleotides in the RNA transcript into the sequence of amino acids in the polypeptide gene product (protein) as per genetic code.

The flow of information in the process of synthesis of proteins is one way. This means that the genetic information flows from nucleic acids to protein (DNA to RNA to protein). The transcription is the first step of central dogma and does not involve a change of code due to complementary between DNA and mRNA. The second step (translation) involves a change of code from nucleotide sequence to amino acid sequences. The flow of genetic information is thus as shown here below:

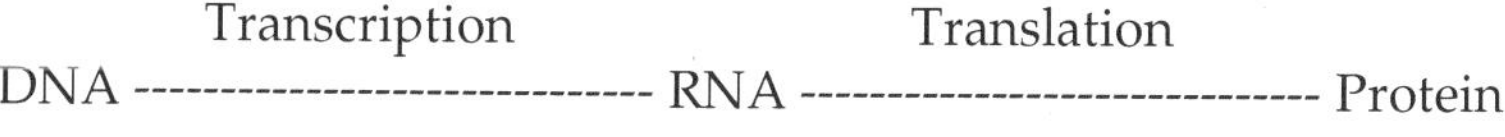

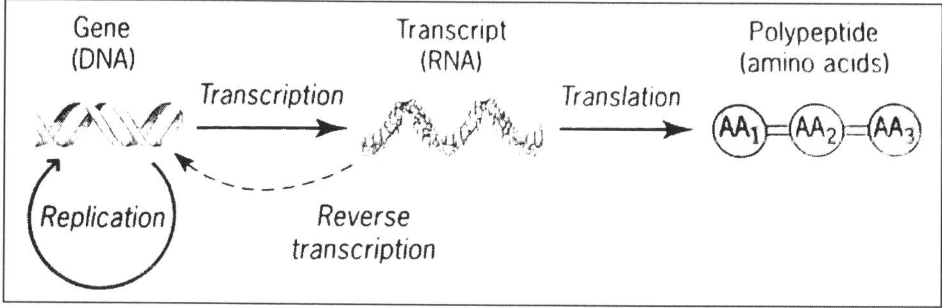

In other words, the information flows from genes (composed of DNA) through an intermediary (composed of RNA - the messenger RNA) to polypeptides (composed of amino acids – the proteins). It is thus clear that protein synthesis by genes (called the gene expression) is a two stage phenomenon of transcription (DNA to RNA - mRNA production, called *transcription* together with its movement in the cytoplasm) and translation (RNA to protein - protein production, called *translation*).

Exception to Central Dogma – Reverse Transcription

The transfer of genetic information from DNA to RNA is sometimes reversible (RNA to DNA) during the conversion of the genomes of RNA tumour viruses to their DNA pro-viral form. The RNA tumour virus store their genetic information in RNA and the information are copied into DNA by the enzyme ***reverse transcriptase*** after a virus infects a host cell. Thus, the discovery of RNA tumour viruses or retroviruses (retro means backwards flow of genetic information) provided an exception to the central dogma. But the transfer of information from RNA to protein is always not reversible.

The two steps involved in gene expression (protein synthesis) *viz.* transcription and translation have been discussed here.

17.3 TRANSCRIPTION (mRNA SYNTHESIS)

Some definitions -

The messenger RNA (mRNA) is produced by the DNA in the nucleus and it (mRNA) moves to the cytoplasm through nuclear pores to assist the ribosome in the cytoplasm for protein synthesis. The messenger RNAs are the RNA molecules that are translated on the ribosome.

The ***primary transcript*** is the RNA molecule produced by transcription (product of transcription) ***in prokaryotes*** is usually equivalent to the mRNA molecule. The ***primary transcripts in eukaryotes*** are the precursors to mRNA for which these are called ***pre-mRNAs*** and processed by excision of specific sequences and the modification of both the termini before their translation.

The ***transcription*** process starts by copying the information contained in DNA of the gene into mRNA molecule. The mRNA is assembled stepwise along one of the strand of DNA molecule (DNA template strand).

The RNA molecule produced by transcription of a gene is called a ***transcript*** or ***gene transcript*** or ***RNA transcript.*** Therefore, during transcription, one strand of DNA of a gene is used as a ***template*** to synthesize a complementary strand of RNA. The template is a pattern or model. DNA stores coded information and acts as a template from which information is copied into complementary strands of DNA or transcribed into mRNA.

A segment of DNA is called ***transcription unit*** that contains transcription initiation and termination signals and is transcribed into one RNA molecule.

The complete set of RNAs transcribed from a genome is called ***transcriptome.*** A protein that regulates the transcription of genes is called ***transcription factor.***

A locally unwound segment of DNA in which an RNA transcript is being synthesized is called ***transcription bubble.***

A protein that prevents RNA polymerase from terminating transcription at specific transcription-termination sequences is called ***transcriptional anti-terminator.***

The assembly of nucleotides occurs in such a way that A in the RNA pairs with T in the DNA, G of RNA pairs with C of DNA, C of RNA with G of DNA, and U in the RNA pairs with A in the DNA. Therefore, the nucleotide sequence of a template strand of DNA in the gene determines the nucleotide sequence of the mRNA. This can be understood by an example for the DNA strand. Suppose the DNA strand contains the nucleotide sequence AAA (3 units of adenine). This nucleotide sequence (AAA) of DNA is used as a template to produce the complementary sequence of UUU in the RNA transcript.

The mRNA produced/synthesized (*RNA transcript*) contains the required information for the synthesis of a polypeptide for protein synthesis and is separated from DNA template. Thus each of the gene's codon is present within the sequence of the mRNA to specify the incorporation of a particular amino acid into the polypeptide chain.

mRNA Synthesis

The transcription requires the help of mRNA which is synthesized in the nucleus by the coding strand of DNA. One strand of DNA acts as a template for the synthesis of mRNA.

Why mRNA is Required?

It is matter of great surprise to think about the process of control of the amino acid sequences, protein products of the genes, in view of the fact that the genes (DNA, chromosome) reside in the nucleus and the proteins are synthesized on the ribosome in the cytoplasm. It is logical to think that the genetic information stored in the sequences of nucleotide pairs in genes (located in the nucleus) must be transferred to the cytoplasm, the site of protein synthesis. This necessarily requires some mechanism of sending the message for transfer of genetic information from nucleus to the cytoplasm by crossing the barrier of nuclear membrane. The need of an intermediary or messenger in protein synthesis is more obvious in eukaryotes to cross the barrier of nuclear membrane. The evidences have indicated that there exists a short-lived (unstable) RNA molecule, called the messenger RNA (mRNA) to carry the message contained in the genes present in the nucleus to the ribosome in the cytoplasm where gene products (proteins) are synthesized. The mRNA acts this role of intermediary to carry (transferring), from nucleus to the cytoplasm, the specifications for the polypeptide formation for proteins.

Experimental Evidence of mRNA Synthesis

Such a messenger is most obviously required in eukaryotes but it is interesting that the first evidence for the existence of such a messenger (mRNA – an RNA intermediary in protein synthesis) came from the experiment on prokaryotes by Elliot Volkin and Lawrence Astrachan (1956) on bacteria (*E. coli*) infected with bacterial virus (bacteriophage T2). They observed by labelling RNA with the radioactive isotope ^{32}P that the newly synthesized RNA molecules after infecting

E. coli cells were unstable and similar in composition to the DNA of bacteriophage T2 and not to that of the DNA of *E. coli.*

Further evidence of an unstable mRNA synthesis in phage T 4 - infected cells came from the experiment of Sol Spiegelman and others (1961) wherein they had synthesized radioactive RNA in the bacteria (pulse-labelled bacteria with adding ^{3}H-uridine to the medium) after infection, incubated the infected cells for one minute and isolated total RNA from these cells (by breaking the cells) to determine hybridization of radioactive RNA molecules either with *E. coli* DNA or phage T4 DNA (the proportion of radio-active RNA hybridized with T4 DNA increased but decreased with *E. coli DNA* after infection). They found that most of the short-lived RNA molecules synthesized after infection were complementary to single strand of phage T4 DNA and not of *E. coli* DNA. This indicated that the RNA molecules were synthesized from phage T4 DNA templates rather than from *E. coli* DNA template.

Sydney Brenner and coworkers (1961) demonstrated that phage T4 proteins were synthesized on *E. coli* ribosome and thus the amino acid sequences of T 4 proteins were not controlled by components of the ribosome but the ribosome provided the workbench for occurrence of protein synthesis rather than providing the specifications for individual proteins. This supported the proposal put forth by Francois Jacob and Jacques Monod (1961) that the specifications for the amino acid sequences of individual gene products from the genes to the ribosome are carried by the unstable RNA molecules. The role of unstable RNAs (mRNAs) to transfer the genetic information from genes to the sites of protein synthesis in the cytoplasm was firmly established from subsequent research.

Common Characteristics of mRNA Synthesis

The mechanism of RNA synthesis is similar to that of the DNA synthesis but with the difference that:

- ✰ The precursors of RNA synthesis are the *ribo-nucleoside triphosphates* instead of the *deoxyribonucleoside triphosphate* for DNA synthesis,
- ✰ The synthesis of a complementary RNA chain uses only one strand of DNA as a template,
- ✰ The RNA chain synthesis does not require a preexisting primer strand as in case of synthesis of DNA but can be initiated *de novo,*
- ✰ The RNA molecule produced will be complementary and antiparallel to the DNA template strand (*transcribed strand of DNA* - used to produce a complementary strand of RNA) and identical (except that T is replaced by U) to the DNA ***non-template strand*** (non-transcribed strand of DNA). Only one strand of DNA acts as a template in the synthesis of a molecule of mRNA.
- ✰ The mRNA molecules are the ***coding strands*** of RNA which are also called the ***sense strands*** of RNA because their nucleotide sequences specify the sequences of amino acids in the protein gene product. The sense strand is a primary transcript or mRNA that contains a coding region (contiguous sequence of codons) that is translated to produce a polypeptide. Another

RNA strand which is complementary to the mRNA strand (produced from a gene) is called ***antisense RNA.***

- The RNA chain is synthesized in 5′ to 3′ direction like the DNA chains but by adding of ribonucleotides to the 3′- hydroxyl group at the end of the chain,
- The reaction involves a nucleophilic attack by the 3′- OH on the nucleotidyl phosphorus atom of the ribonucleoside triphosphate precursor and pyrophosphorus is eliminated, just as in DNA synthesis. This reaction is catalyzed by an enzyme called *RNA polymerase* in the nucleus of the cell, along one strand of double stranded DNA.

The RNA synthesis using only one DNA strand as template strand has been shown here in Figure 16.1 given below. This shows clearly that the RNA molecule produced (mRNA) is complementary and antiparallele to the DNA template strand, and identical to the DNA non-template strand (except U replaces T):

DNA molecule	3'-C G T A T G C T A G T C C G A T T G C G - 5' Template strand
(Double strand)	5'-G C A T A C G A T C A G G C T A A C G C - 3' Nontemplate strand
	↓ RNA synthesis
mRNA molecule	5'-G C A U A C G A U C A G G C U A A C G C -3' Sense RNA strand
(Single-strand)	

Figure 17.1: Showing the RNA Synthesis from only one DNA Strand of a Gene as Template.

In case the RNA molecule produced is mRNA, it will then specify (encode) amino acids in the protein gene product and hence the mRNA molecules are the coding strands of RNA, also called as *sense strand* of RNA. This is because the nucleotide sequences of sense strand "make sense" to specify sequences of amino acids in the protein synthesis.

In case of two DNA strands, the terms sense and antisense strands are not often used but the terms ***template strand*** and ***non-template strand*** are used for the *transcribed and non-transcribed DNA strands,* respectively. However, the strand of DNA used as the template for RNA synthesis is called the ***sense strand,*** the other strand is the ***anti-sense strand.*** The same strand is always not the sense strand throughout the entire DNA molecule or chromosome. The region of DNA actually transcribed into RNA is called the ***coding region.*** However, there are sequences preceding the actual coding region that are required for transcription. These sites, called ***promoters,*** are the sites of recognition and interaction between RNA polymerase and DNA that signal transcription to begin. Thus, the ***promoter*** is a nucleotide sequence to which RNA polymerase binds and initiates transcription. The promoter is also a chemical substance that enhances the transformation of benign cells into cancerous cells.

The RNA *polymerase* opens up a section of DNA strands to pair with complementary bases and thus provides a message of the same sequence (transcription). The RNA *polymerase* moves along the DNA template and the growing RNA strand separates allowing the hydrogen bonds between two DNA strands to rejoin. The RNA polymerases bind to specific nucleotide sequences (called ***promoters***) and initiate the synthesis of RNA molecules with the help of transcription factor (which is a protein) at transcription start sites near the promoters. RNA synthesis occurs within a locally unwound segment of DNA (sometimes called a ***transcription bubble***) produced by RNA polymerase.

The RNAs of all types are transcribed from a template strand of DNA, catalyzed by several enzymes collectively referred to as DNA-dependent RNA polymerase or simply *RNA polymerase.*

17.4 TRANSCRIPTION IN PROKARYOTES

The process of RNA production is known as ***transcription.*** The RNA molecule is produced by a segment of DNA. The segment of DNA used to transcribe in production of RNA molecule is called a ***transcription unit*** which may be equivalent to individual gene or several genes. The process of transcription in prokaryotes and eukaryotes has same basic aspects with some differences in ***promoter*** (specific sequences of nucleotides) region in DNA.

The RNA synthesis always occurs in the 5′ to 3′ direction. The regions (segments) of genes located towards the 5′ end and 3′ end of the transcript from some site in the mRNA molecule are the DNA sequences, often called as ***upstream*** and ***downstream regions***. There is convention of giving numbers to the nucleotide pairs (nucleotides) within and adjacent to the transcription units in relation to the transcription site (designated as + 1), the nucleotide pair corresponding to the first (5′) nucleotide of the RNA transcript. The nucleotide sequences (base pairs) in a unit of transcription preceding (is located 5′ to) the initiation sites are the ***upstream sequences*** and numbered with (–) prefixes. The base pairs following the initiation site (relative to the direction of transcription) are the ***downstream sequences*** and numbered with (+) prefixes. Thus, the *downstream sequence* is a sequence in a unit of transcription that follows (is located 3′ to) the transcription start site.

17.4.1 RNA Polymerase (Prokaryotes)

This is the enzyme that catalyzes the formation of RNA. The transcription process in prokaryotes (*E. coli*) is catalyzed by an enzyme RNA polymerase (catalyzes all RNA synthesis in prokaryotes). This enzyme is the complex multimeric protein. In *E. coli,* the enzyme with a molecular weight of about 480,000 contains 5 polypeptides, out of which two are identical. Thus, the complete RNA polymerase enzyme molecule (***holoenzyme***) has the composition of four distinct polypeptides (α_2, β, β′ and σ) -

- ☆ The α subunits hold the assembly of the *tetrameric core* (α_2, β, β′) of this enzyme,
- ☆ The β subunit contains the ribonucleoside triphosphate binding site,
- ☆ The β′ subunit harbors the DNA template-binding region, and
- ☆ The σ (sigma factor) is a subunit of prokaryotic RNA polymerase

responsible for the initiation of transcription at specific initiation. The sigma factor recognizes and binds RNA polymerase to the transfer initiation (promoter) sites in DNA. The σ factor plays no role in chain elongation but it is released after RNA chain initiation. In contrast to the core enzyme, the holoenzyme (σ present) initiates chains *in vitro at sites used in vivo.*

☆ The core enzyme (α_2, β, β′) catalyzes the chain elongation by the RNA synthesis from DNA templates *in vitro* and initiates RNA chains at random sites on both strands of DNA.

17.4.2 Stages of Transcription (Prokaryotes)

The ***transcription*** process in prokaryotes can be studied into the following three stages of initiation, elongation and termination of RNA chains -

(i) Initiation of a New RNA Chain

The initiation of synthesis of RNA chain is accomplished in three steps:

The *first step* involves the *binding of the RNA polymerase holoenzyme to a promoter region in DNA.* The binding of RNA polymerase to promoters in DNA is mediated by the σ factor. The holoenzyme remains bound during the synthesis of the first 8 – 9 bonds, after which the σ factor is released, and the elongation phase of RNA synthesis begins by the core enzyme. The short chains of 2 – 9 ribonucleotides are synthesized and released during initiation. The synthesis is stopped after chains of 10 or more ribonucleotides are synthesized and the RNA polymerase starts moving downstream from the promoter.

The *second step* is the localized *unwinding of the two strands of DNA* by RNA polymerase. The localized unwinding of DNA is facilitated by the AT- rich – 10 sequences which is an essential prerequisite to the synthesis of a new RNA chain. This provides a template strand free to base-pair with incoming ribonucleotides, and

The *third step* involves the *formation of the phophodiester bonds* between the first few ribonucleotides in the nascent RNA chain.

(ii) Elongation of RNA Chains

The RNA polymerase core enzyme catalyzes the elongation of RNA chain after the release of σ subunit. A locally unwound segment of DNA (*transcription bubble*) is the place within which the covalent extension of RNA chain occurs. Moreover, the RNA polymerase molecule performs both unwinding and rewinding activities of DNA. The RNA polymerase continuous unwinds the DNA double helix ahead of the polymerization site whereas the rewinding of complementary DNA strands occurs behind the polymerization site as it moves along the double helix.

On an average, the numbers of transcription bubble are about 18 nucleotide pairs in *E. coli* and the rate of incorporation is about 40 ribonucleotides per second into the growing chain. The new (nascent) RNA chain is displaced from the DNA template strand as the RNA polymerase moves along the DNA molecule. There is very short region of transient base-pairing (probably 3 bp length) between the growing chain and the DNA template strand. However, the base-pairing between the template strand of DNA and the new RNA is not concerned with the stability of the transcription complex but this stability is maintained primarily by the binding of the DNA and the growing RNA chain.

(iii) Termination of RNA Chain

The RNA polymerase gets a transcription -termination signal for termination of RNA chain elongation. The ***terminal signal*** is a nucleotide sequence that specifies RNA chain termination. As a result, the transcription complex dissociates releasing the nascent RNA molecule.

In *E. coli,* the transcription termination may or may not require the presence of a protein called ***rho***. The terminations are accordingly of two types *viz.* the *rho-dependent terminators* requiring the transcription terminator sequences in the presence of *rho* and *rho- independent terminators* not requiring the presence of *rho.*

The Rho-independent terminators are rich in GC region followed by 6 or more A-T bp with the adenines present in the template strand. The nucleotide sequence of GC-rich region contains inverted repeats in each DNA strand and these are inverted and complementary. On transcribing, these inverted repeat regions produce the single-stranded RNA sequences that can base-pair and form hairpin structures immediately after the synthesis of the participating regions of the RNA chain. This retards the movement of RNA polymerase molecules along the DNA and results into the termination of chain extension.

The two mechanisms of transcription termination (rho-dependent and rho-independent) have the following similarities -

- ✰ Both involve the formation of a hydrogen-bonded hairpin structure upstream from the site of termination, and
- ✰ The hairpins in both the cases impede the movement of RNA polymerase resulting it to pause.

On the other side, the two mechanisms of transcription terminators differ In that the rho-dependent terminators have two additional following sequences:

- ✰ A 50-90 nucleotide-pair sequence upstream from the inverted repeat sequences to produce an RNA strand with many cytosine (C's) but few guanine (G's) and hence forming no hairpins, or any secondary structure, and
- ✰ A sequence to specify a rho protein binding site. These sites are called *rut* because of *r*ho *ut*ilization near the 3′ end of the transcript.

The *rho* protein binds to the *rut* sequence in the transcript and moves 5′ to 3′ following RNA polymerase. On encountering the hairpin by the polymerase, it pauses, allowing *rho* to catch up, pass through the hairpin, and use its helicase activity to unwind the DNA/RNA base-pairing at the terminus and release the RNA transcript.

17.5 TRANSCRIPTION IN EUKARYOTES

The eukaryotes have a range of complexity from the single-celled yeasts to humans. The process of transcription (mRNA synthesis) though similar in prokaryotes and eukaryotes but is considerably more complex in eukaryotes. The *basic function of mRNA* is to carry the genetic message of DNA into cytoplasm where it is responsible for directing the synthesis of polypeptide chains. The mRNA is synthesized in the nucleus and must be transferred on ribosome in the cytoplasm for translation in encoding the proteins.

There is a difference in prokaryotic and eukaryotic mRNA. The prokaryotic mRNAs are multigenic containing the coding regions of two or more genes. On the other hand, the eukaryotic mRNAs (transcripts) are monogenic containing the coding region of a single gene, except in rare cases like in small worm (*Caenorhabditis elegans*) in which about ¼ of the transcription units (mRNAs) are multigenic.

17.5.1 RNA Polymerase (Eukaryotes)

The eukaryotes contain 3 to 5 different RNA polymerase, each with a distinctive function of catalyzing the transcription of specific class of genes. The 5 RNA polymerases are designated as ***RNA polymerase I, II, III, IV, and V.*** The first three polymerases are present in most of the eukaryotes and are more complex containing about 10 subunits

- ☆ *Polymerase I,* located in the nucleolus, synthesizes only rRNA and combined with ribosomal proteins. It catalyzes the synthesis of all rRNAs except to the small 5 s rRNA;
- ☆ *Polymerase II,* found in the nucleus (nucleoplasm), transcribes the nuclear genes to encode proteins and also synthesizes Hn RNA (heterogenous nuclear RNA, the nuclear pre-mRNAs) which is a precursor of mRNA;
- ☆ *Polymerase III,* also found in nucleoplasm, catalyzes the synthesis of only transfer RNA (tRNA) molecules, 5s RNA molecules, and small nuclear RNAs;
- ☆ *Polymerase IV,* present in nucleus of plants, synthesizes transcripts which are processed into short RNAs (called *small interfering RNAs,* ***siRNAs***) and act as important regulators of gene expression by interacting with other proteins to modify chromatin structure (condense or relax); and
- ☆ *Polymerase V,* present in nucleus of plants, synthesizes some siRNAs and antisense (non-coding) transcripts of genes regulated by siRNAs. The siRNAs seems to interact with non-coding transcripts and nucleosome-associated proteins to condense chromatin structure which cannot be transcribed.

The RNA polymerase IV and V play an important role to turn off the transcription of genes and this process of turning off the transcription of genes is through modifying the chromosome structure (called as ***chromatin modeling***). Why this modification is required need to be known. The *nucleosomes* containing the DNA of eukaryotes have the compact structure. In view of the compact structure of nucleosomes it requires the modification in their structure so as the genes contained in them are expressed. The change is needed to make available the promoters available to the proteins required for transcription. The genetic and biochemical approaches have shown that transcribed DNA is actually packaged into nucleosomes and in transcribed DNA the nucleosomes are changed by multiprotein complexes to ultimately facilitate the action of the RNA polymerase. This change in nucleosomes as a preparation for transcription is called ***chromatin remodeling.*** The chromatin remodeling are of different types and each type involves chromatin remodeling proteins, usually multimeric protein complexes.

17.5.2 Stages of Transcription (Eukaryotes)

In eukaryotes, like the prokaryotes, the transcription process is also completed in three same stages of initiation, elongation and termination:

(i) RNA Chain Initiation

In case of eukaryotes, all the RNA polymerases are helpless to initiate the transcription without the help of ***protein transcription factors***. These factors are represented A through F and these must bind to a promoter region in DNA to form a basal transcription initiation complex before the RNA polymerase binds and initiates the transcription. The RNA polymerases utilized different promoters and transcription factors. The RNA polymerase II initiates the synthesis of pre-mRNA to transcribe eukaryotic genes.

The initiation of the transcription requires the formation of a locally unwound DNA segment to provide a template DNA strand for the synthesis of a complementary RNA strand. This requirement of formation of locally unwound DNA segment is met by interaction of several transcription factors with specific sequences in the promoter for the transcription unit. The RNA polymerase II recognizes promoters which consist of short conserved elements located upstream from the transcription start point.

The *promoters of eukaryotic genes* transcribed by RNA polymerase II contain almost always two elements:

- ✰ One of the conserved elements (promoter sequence) that determines the transcription start site (position + 1) is called **TATA box.** This has a consensus sequence TATAAAA centered at about position – 30 and has an important role in positioning the transcription start point.
- ✰ The **CAAT box** is the second conserved element (nucleotide sequence) in eukaryotic promoters involved in the initiation of transcription. This is near position – 80 having the consensus sequence GGCCAATCT and increases the efficiency of transcriptional initiation.
- ✰ In addition, two more conserved elements are often present in RNA polymerase II promoters to affect the efficiency of a promoter in initiation transcription. These are *GC box* (consensus GGGCGG) and *octamer box* (consensus ATTTGCAT).

The nucleotide sequence that is present in the majority of genetic signals or elements that perform a specific function is called ***consensus sequence.***

The RNA polymerase II requires several ***basal transcription factors*** (proteins required for the initiation of transcription in eukaryotes) to interact with promoters to initiate transcription effectively and other regulatory sequences known as *enhancers* and *silencers* are required to modulate the efficiency of initiation. One of the basal transcription factors has helicase activity and travels with RNA polymerase II during elongation, unwinding the strands in the transcription region (*transcription bubble*).

The transcription is initiated by RNA polymerase I and III by similar but little simple processes compared to that used by polymerase II. The polymerase I and III transcribe the promoters of genes that are quite different from those utilized by polymerase II, though having some of the same regulatory elements. The RNA polymerase I promoters are bipartite. They have a core sequence extending from about – 45 to + 20 and an upstream control element extending from – 180 to about – 105. The sequences of both the regions are similar and GC-rich. The core sequence is enough for initiation and the efficiency of initiation is strongly increased by the presence of upstream control element.

There is a difference in the location of promoters of the genes transcribed by RNA polymerase III and those transcribed by RNA polymerase I and II. In fact, polymerase III promoters are of three types, of which promoters of most of the genes transcribed by RNA polymerase III are located within the transcription unit, downstream from the transcription start points instead of upstream as in units transcribed by RNA polymerase I and II while the promoters of rest of the genes transcribed by polymerase III are located upstream of the transcription start site like that of polymerase I and II.

(ii) RNA Chain Elongation

The RNA polymerases of prokaryotes and eukaryotes have quite similar key features and mechanisms of action, though they differ in substructures. Therefore, the eukaryotic RNA polymerases after being released from their initiation complexes catalyze the elongation of RNA chain following the same mechanism as in prokaryotes.

The added feature of RNA chain elongation is the addition of 7-methyl guanosine (7-MG) caps to the 5′ ends of eukaryotic pre-mRNAs when the growing chains are of about 30 nucleotides long. These caps contain an unusual 5′-5′ triphosphate linkage and two or more methyl groups. They are added co-transcriptionally, recognized by protein factors of RNA chain initiation, and protect the growing RNA chains from degradation by nucleases.

A protein complex facilitates chromatin transcription to remove histone H_{2A}/ H_{2B} dimers from nucleosomes so as the RNA polymerase II moves past nucleosomes. The same protein complex helps restoring the nucleosome structure by re-depositing the histone dimmers.

(iii) RNA Chain Termination

The transcription termination events occur at multiple sites located 1000 to 2000 nucleotides downstream from the site that become 3′ end (terminus) of mature transcript. The 3′ ends of RNA transcripts synthesized by RNA polymerase II are not produced by the termination of transcription but these are produced by endonucleolytic cleavage of the primary transcripts. The cleavage producing the 3′ end of a transcript usually occurs 11 to 30 nucleotides downstream from a polyadenylation signal having consensus sequence AAUAAA, and downstream from a GU-rich sequence near the end of the transcript.

The ***polyadenylation*** is the addition of poly (A) tails on eukaryotic gene transcripts (3′ ends of the eukaryotic mRNAs). The ***poly (A) tail (mRNA)*** is a polyadenosine tract of 20 to 200 nucleotides long at the 3′ ends of most eukaryotic mRNAs posttranscriptionally. The enzyme ***poly(A) polymerase*** adds the poly(A) tails to the 3′ termini of eukaryotic gene transcript (mRNA). This enzyme after cleavage adds poly (A) tails (tracts of AMP, adenosine monophosphate, of about 200 nucleotides long) to the 3′ ends of transcripts. The polyadenylation has the following requirements -

- A component to recognize and bind to the AAUAAA sequence,
- A stimulating factor to bind to the GU-rich sequence,
- An endonuclease, and
- The enzyme *poly (A) polymerase.*

The multimeric complex is formed by these proteins to carry out the cleavage and the polyadenylation. The poly (A) tail of eukaryotic mRNAs plays important roles in enhancing their stability and in their transport from nucleus to the cytoplasm.

The RNA polymerase I and III in contrast to RNA polymerase II, respond to discrete termination signals. The RNA polymerase I terminate transcription responding to an 18 nucleotide long sequence recognized by terminator protein while RNA polymerase III responds to a termination signal which is similar to the rho-independent terminator in *E. coli.*

During the process of transcription, there is a localized unwinding of the double helix, with transcription proceeding in the 5′ to 3′ direction from the single stranded region of the DNA template. This localized unwinding moves along the molecule followed by recoiling of the helix behind the newly synthesized RNA. The DNA molecule splits and a single strand of this molecule serve as a template for assembling of single strand of RNA with each base in the RNA strand being complementary to the bases on the DNA molecule strand. During formation of RNA strand, its each base takes up its proper position on the DNA strand having the base combination of A to U, U to A, C to G and G to C. The free ends of the bases in the RNA strand are connected with a new ribose, phosphate, base sequence. The single strand of RNA so produced is separated from the DNA template and passes into the cytoplasm.

17.6 PRIMARY TRANSCRIPTS AND mRNAs STRUCTURES

There is largest difference between mRNAs and primary transcripts in eukaryotes than in prokaryotes. The primary transcripts of eukaryotes undergo more extensive posttranscriptional processing than in prokaryotes. The eukaryotic transcripts are usually modified by -

- ☆ The excision of intron sequences,
- ☆ The addition of 7 – methyl guanosine caps to the 5′ termini of most eukaryotic mRNAs posttranscriptionally. This is called 5′ cap (mRNA),
- ☆ The addition of poly(A) tails (polyadenylation) to the 3′ termini, and
- ☆ The sequences of some eukaryotic transcripts are also modified by RNA editing processes.

In prokaryotes, the transcriptional processing is usually restricted to the excision of terminal sequences.

17.7 RNA EDITING AND ALTERATION OF INFORMATION

The genetic information in the mRNA intermediary is same as those present in DNA without any alteration. However, some exceptions have been discovered as per RNA editing. The information content of gene transcripts (mRNA molecules) is altered in RNA editing processes. The RNA editing are the posttranscriptional processes that alter the information encoded in gene transcripts (RNAs). There are two types of RNA editing.

The first type is the change brought by the changes in the structures of individual bases. This type of RNA editing is rare. The second type occurs by inserting or deleting the uridine monophosphate residues gene transcripts. This second type of RNA editing is more complex, occurs in the mitochondria of trypanosomes (flagellated protozoa - primitive single celled eukaryote, causing sleeping sickness in humans), and causes major changes in the polypeptides specified by mRNA molecules. This change is mediated by guide RNAs transcribed from distinct mitochondrial genes and contain partially complementary sequences to the pre-mRNA to be edited.

The RNA editing sometimes leads to the synthesis of two or more distinct polypeptides from a single mRNA. This contributes to protein diversity in eukaryotes However, the RNA editing is more important in gene expression of the mitochondria.

17.8 TRANSCRIPTION OF INTRONS IN EUKARYOTES

In contrast to the prokaryotic chromosomes which have continuous sequences of nucleotide pairs which specify collinear sequences of amino acids in the polypeptide gene products, the eukaryotic chromosomes have some noncoding intervening sequences, called as ***introns*** (intervening sequences). Thus, the nuclear genes of higher eukaryotes encoding the proteins have introns. These introns begin (5′) with GT and end (3′) with AG. Also, the 3′ subterminal A in the TACTAAC box is completely conserved and involved in bond formation during intron excision. These introns are present in between the expressed (coding) sequences of genes (called ***exons***, having biological information). It has been observed that mouse β- globin (one of two different proteins in haemoglobin) gene actually contains two introns.

Such genes having *introns* are called ***split genes*** or *discontinuous genes* or *mosaic genes*. The split genes are splitted into several distinct units separated by regions of non-coding DNA (introns). However, the entire sequences of the *split genes* are transcribed into pre-mRNAs and the intron sequences are subsequently removed by *splicing reactions* produced on *spliceosomes*, macromolecular structures.

In higher animals and plants, there are more common the interrupted genes compared to uninterrupted genes. However, there are some exceptions of genes in animals and plants lacking introns. There are as many introns as 50 in chicken 1α2 collagen gene. Moreover, the length of some of the introns varies in size. The collagen gene has 37000 nucleotide pairs but synthesizing an mRNA molecule of about 4600 nucleotide in length whereas the *Ubx gene* of *Drosophila* has an intron length of 70,000 nucleotide pairs. The largest gene in human contains 78 introns with a span of 2.5 million nucleotide pairs and causes one type of muscular dystrophy on mutation.

In view of the variation in length of introns it is logical to think that the introns may have some biological significance in regulating gene expression that may be in a positive and negative way. Some introns contain tissue specific promoters as well as the sequences to increase accumulation of transcripts. As per speculation, the exon-intron structure of eukaryotic genes has been the result of evolution of new genes by fusion of single exon ancestral gene and hence of evolutionary significance. However, many introns may have no biological significance.

Mechanisms of Introns Removal from RNA Transcript (Splicing)

The process that covalently join exon sequences of RNA and eliminates the intervening sequences (introns) is called ***splicing of RNA***. The intron (intervening) sequences are removed during RNA processing.

There have been reported the following three different types of intron excision mechanisms (splicing systems) from RNA transcripts:

(i) tRNA Precursor Splicing

The introns of tRNA precursors are excised by splicing reaction in two stages of making two cuts precisely by a nuclear membrane-bound *splicing endonuclease*, at the ends of the intron, and joining the two halves of the tRNA by a *splicing ligase* to produce the mature tRNA molecule. These reactions are the result of the conserved three-dimensional features of the tRNA precursors rather than of the nucleotide sequences.

(ii) Autocatalytic or Self-Splicing

There is automatic removal of the introns of some rRNA precursors through a reaction mediated by the RNA molecule itself, without requiring the involvement of any protein enzymatic activity. The reaction being catalyzed by an enzyme is indicated by altering the covalent bonds. There is no alteration of covalent bonds

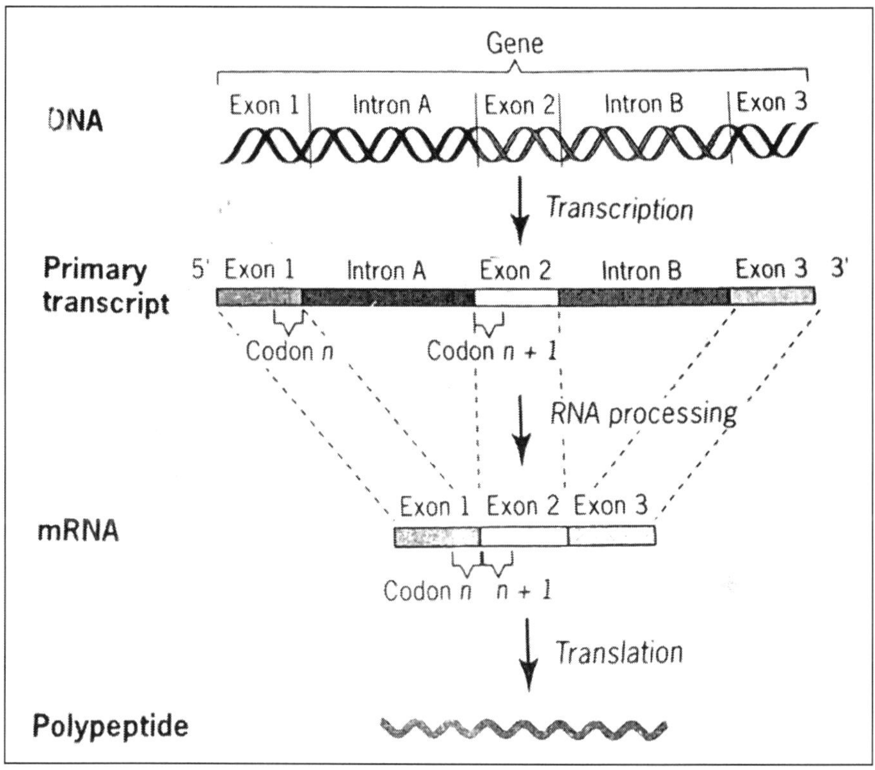

Figure 17.2: Removal of Intron Sequences from Primary Transcript.

in this case and hence it requires no involvement of protein enzyme activity. The splicing activity to excise the intron from rRNA precursor is intrinsic to the RNA molecule itself. This is known as *self-splicing* or *autocatalytic activity*. This self-splicing activity occurs in rRNA precursors of lower eukaryotes as well as in the precursors of rRNA, tRNA, and mRNA in mitochondria and chloroplasts of many species.

The self-splicing activity of excision of the intron in rRNA precursor needs no external energy source as well as no protein catalytic activity. However, this self-splicing involves a series of phosphoester bond transfers without any gain or loss of bonds. This self-splicing of intron excision requires two phosphoester bonds transfers so as the excise intron can circularize through another phosphoester bond transfer. This mechanism of self-splicing of rRNA precursors is due to the intron structure itself.

It was thought earlier as a dogma in biology that molecular reactions in living cells are catalyzed by enzymes composed of polypeptides (proteins). However, the self-splicing of RNA precursors (autocatalytic removal of introns of some precursor RNA molecules such as the tRNA precursors in Terrahymena) has demonstrated that RNA molecules can also contain catalytic sites, and hence the property of containing catalytic sites is not restricted only to proteins. This is because the self-splicing makes no involvement of any catalytic protein.

(iii) Pre-mRNA Splicing

The introns in nuclear pre-mRNA are excised by complex RNA-protein structures, called ***spliceosomes*** that are like small ribosomes in structure, containing a set (five) of small RNA molecules (snRNA, small nuclear RNA) and about 40 different proteins. These 5 snRNAs are involved in nuclear pre-mRNA splicing as components of the spliceosome. One of the snRNA is localized in the nucleolus and probably involved in ribosome formation. These snRNAs vay in size from 100 nucleotides to 215 nucleotides and some are even much larger in the yeast. The snRNAs are present in small nuclear RNA-protein complexes, called ***snRNPs*** rather than free molecules. The spliceosomes are made up from four different snRNPs and protein-splicing factors during the splicing process.

The nuclear pre-mRNA splicing is completed in two stages.

- ✰ The first stage of splicing involves cleavage at the 5′ intron splice site (UG-intron) and formation of an intramolecular phosphodiester linkage between the 5′ carbon of the G at the cleavage site and the 2′ carbon of a conserved A residue near the 3′ end of the intron. This cleavage stage occurs on complete spliceosomes and requires the hydrolysis of ATP.
- ✰ During the second stage of the splicing reaction, there is cleavage of the 3′ splice site of the intron, and two exons are joined by a normal 5′ to 3′ phosphodiester linkage. The spliced mRNA is exported to the cytoplasm and translated on ribosome.

Chapter 18

Genetic Code

All the proteins are synthesized by the cell. The synthesis of different proteins requires the arrangement of a different number of amino acids in a different sequential order. The sequence of amino acids in a protein molecule is determined by the linear arrangement of four nitrogen bases in DNA: two nitrogen bases are purines (adenine and guanine) and two nitrogen bases are pyrimidine (cytosine and thymine). These four nitrogen bases are represented by the respective four letters (English alphabets), taking the first alphabet of their name. These four letters are A, G, C, and T which represent the four nitrogen bases *viz.* adenine, guanine, cytosine, and thymine, respectively. Three nitrogen bases form one **nucleotide triplet** (called the ***genetic code***, a code word) and each code (nucleotide triplet) specifies a specific amino acid. Thus, the genetic code or codon is a set of adjacent *nucleotides in mRNA* which specifies the incorporation of an amino acid into a polypeptide chain or the *genetic code* is the sequence of triplet nitrogenous bases in mRNA molecule (that contains the information for protein synthesis). One specific amino acid of polypeptide chain is coded by a sequence of 3 nitrogenous bases (triplet) in DNA. This is known as triplet code which means a three letter code. Such triplet of bases (codon) is capable of selection and inserting a particular amino acid in a protein molecule. Therefore, the alphabets of just four letters (four nitrogen base pairs in DNA) contained the genetic information of living beings.

18.1 BASE AND IMPORTANCE OF GENETIC CODE

The order of arrangement of nitrogen bases is important, because the change in sequence order of nitrogen bases make a change in formation of a different amino acid. For example, the sequence of UUC codes for the amino acid *phenylalanine* whereas the sequence of CUU codes for the amino acid *leucine* and another sequence of UCU codes for the amino acid *serine*.

The information are though coded in the form of nitrogenous base sequence in DNA molecule but the code letters of RNA nitrogen bases are used for genetic code. This is due to the message from DNA is passed on to the cytoplasm by mRNA and the code on mRNA is translated into the sequence of amino acids.

The nitrogen bases in DNA molecule are A, G, C, and T, and the corresponding complementary bases in mRNA transcription are U, C, G, and A. This implies that:

if the base in DNA is A (adenine), the complementary base in mRNA will be U (uracil);

if the base in DNA is G (guanine) the complementary base in mRNA will be C (cytosine);

if the base in DNA is C (cytosine) its complementary base in mRNA will be G (guanine); and if the base in DNA is T (thymine), the complementary base in mRNA transcription will be A.

18.2 ESSENTIAL FEATURES OF GENETIC CODE

The genetic code has the following characteristics or properties:

(i) The ***code is triplet***, having three adjacent nitrogenous bases of mRNA in a specific sequence. There are 20 different amino acids that are incorporated into polypeptides for protein synthesis. Thus, at least 20 different codons are needed with these 4 bases in mRNA. The single letter code consisting only one nucleotide can provide only 4 codons or words *i.e.* one word for each nitrogenous base (A, G, C. and U are nitrogen bases in mRNA). The 4 codons are not sufficient to code for 20 amino acids. Similarly, the combination of two nitrogen bases (double letter code) could provide only $4^2 = 16$ codons or words which would have also not been sufficient to code for 20 amino acids. Three letter codons of 4 nitrogen bases ($4^3 = 64$ words) are sufficient to accommodate the code words for 20 amino acids.

The triplet codon (three nucleotide per codon) was supported by Francis Crick and colleagues (1961) on the basis of a genetic analysis of mutations induced by chemical proflavin (mutagenic agent that cause single base pair additions and deletions) at one locus (rII) of bacteriophage T4. The findings of Crick and colleagues were subsequently supported and established from the evidence of *in vitro* translation studies. The nucleotide triplets were found enough to stimulate specific binding of aminoacyl-tRNA ^{Phe} to ribosome. The comparison of nucleotide sequences of genes and mRNA with the amino acid sequences of their polypeptide products established the triplet (trinucleotides) nature of the genetic code.

(ii) ***Deciphering the genetic code***: This means to interpret the hidden writings. Before 1960s it was in the dark to know about – identification of specific codons to specify each of the 20 amino acids – the number of triplet codons out of 64 possible numbers are used – the manner the code is punctuated – the same or the different meaning of the codons in different species of organisms of plants, animals, bacteria, and viruses. The unfolding the genetic code to get the answers of these questions was a difficult and labourious work.

The findings of the following two types of experiments conducted on cell-free systems had been successful to reveal all the facts about the genetic code in helping to determine which aminoacyl-tRNAs were stimulated to bind to ribosomes activated with each of the trinucleotide message –

- ✰ Translation of synthetic mRNA molecules *in vitro* and determining which of the 20 amino acids were incorporated into proteins, and
- ✰ Activating the ribosomes with mini-mRNAs just 3 nucleotide long.

Marshall Nirenberg, Severo Ochoa, H.G. Khorana, and others combined the results of *in vitro* translation experiments conducted with synthetic mRNAs and trinucleotide binding assays, and worked out the meaning of all 64 triplet codons. They got 1968 Noble Prize in Physiology or Medicine for their work on genetic code.

(iii) The ***code is comma-less***. This means no punctuation is needed between any two words. This means that the coding regions of mRNA have no comma or other forms of punctuation and there is continuous reading of codons.

(iv) The ***code is non-overlapping***. This means that the same letter is not used for two different codons.

(v) The ***code is non-ambiguous:*** This indicates that a particular codon always codes for the same amino acid.

(vi) The ***code is degenerate*** (*Multiple codons*) ***and ordered:*** A particular amino acid is specified by more than one codon. This is called degeneracy. Thus, degeneracy of codon means that different codons can specify the same amino acid. The different codons have different nucleotides. Therefore, the nucleotide difference in the coding sequence of the gene has no effect on the amino acid sequence of the polypeptide. This is also called as ***silent polymorphism.*** Thus, degeneracy of genetic code produces the silent polymorphism. Most of the amino acids except two (methionine and tryptophan) can be coded by more than one codon. This is the multiple system of coding (multiple codons) which provides a protection to organism against many harmful mutations.

It is not random to use more than one codon for specific amino acid. A given amino acid specified by multiple codons differs by one base only. This different base (nucleotide) in multiple codons is the third or 3′ base of the codon. Thus, the different nucleotides can be present at third position without changing the amino acid that is specified. Therefore, the degeneracy is most pronounced in the third position of many codons.

The multiple coding systems are of two types, *viz.* complete and partial.

- ✰ *Complete degeneracy*: Any of the four bases may occur at the third position in the codon but it will still specify the same amino acid. There are eight such amino acids having all the 4 different bases at the third position, *viz.* valine, serine, proline, threnine, alanine, glycine, leucine, and arginine. The first 6 amino acids have 4 codons each containing all the 4 bases at third position whereas the last two amino acids (leucine, serine and arginine) have 6 codons each containing different bases at first position besides 4 different bases at third position.

☆ *Partial degeneracy*: In this type of degeneracy, the third base may be either of the two purines (A or G) or either of the two pyrimidines (C or U). In this case, the amino acid specified by the codon is changed with a change in third base from a purine to a pyrimidine or vice versa, *viz.* phe, isoleucine, Tyrosine, histidine, asperginine, lysine, aspartic acid, glutamic acid, cystine. Each of all these amino acids has two codons having different base at third position.

The genetic code is considered to be ***ordered*** in such a way that it minimizes mutational lethality. The multiple codons for any amino acid and the codons for amino acids with similar chemical properties are closely related with a difference of only a single nucleotide. The amino acid specified by the codon is not changed with the substitutions of most of the bases at the third position. The amino acids having similar chemical properties like leucine, isoleucine, and valine have different codons by only one base. Therefore, the substitution of one amino acid for another amino acid with similar chemical properties (*e.g.* valine for isoleucine) is the result of many single base-pair substitutions. Such of the conservative substitutions, in most of the cases, produce gene products that are active and minimize the effects of mutations.

(vii) The ***genetic code*** has ***initiation*** and ***termination codons:*** The codon AUG is the initiation codon to initiate the polypeptide chains, in both prokaryotes as well as in eukaryotes with rare exception of the use of GUG codon as the initiation codon. However, the initiation codon is recognized by an initiator tRNA ($tRNA_f^{Met}$) in case of prokaryotes and

$tRNA_i^{Met}$ for eukaryotes.

There are three codons for polypeptide chain termination. These termination codons are UAG, UAA, and UGA. These codons are recognized by protein release factors, instead of tRNA. In prokaryotes, the RF - 1 causes the polypeptide chain termination by responding to the codons UAA and UAG while the RF-2 terminates the chain by a response from the codons UAA and UGA. In case of eukaryotes, all the three termination codons are recognized by only a single release factor.

(viii) The ***code is universal*** - same genetic code is applied in all kinds of living organisms. The *in vitro* studies, mutations causing amino acid replacements, and the correlation between nucleic acid and polypeptide sequencing have provided the data to compare the meaning of all 64 codons in different species. On the basis of these data available from different sources it has been shown that the genetic code is nearly ***universal.*** This means that the codons in all the species with rare exceptions (mitochondria, yeast, and some other species) have the same meaning.

The mitochondria in mammals have their own chromosomes and protein-synthesizing machinery. But there are some differences in the codons of mitochondria and nuclear mRNA of mammals. These differences are -

- ✰ The UAG codon which is the chain termination specifies the amino acid tryptophan in the mitochondria,
- ✰ The AUA codon specifies methionine in mitochondria instead of isoleucine in nuclear mRNA,
- ✰ The two codons, AGA and AGG code the arginine in nuclear mRNA but these act as polypeptide chain terminator in mitochondria, and
- ✰ The rest of the 60 codons have same meaning in mammalian mitochondria as well as in nuclear mRNA.

The nuclear transcript of some protozoa and the mitochondria of other species have also rare differences in codon meaning. Since the differences are rare, it is considered that the genetic code is nearly universal.

18.3 TRIPLET CODES OF NITROGEN BASES FOR 20 AMINO ACIDS

The codes for 20 amino acids (each having 3 nitrogen bases – trinucleotides) have been given in the following Table 18.1:

Table 18.1: Triplet Codes of Nitrogen Bases for 20 Amino Acids

		Second Base Letter			
First Base	*U*	*C*	*A*	*G*	*Third Base Letter*
U	UUU Phe	UCU Ser	UAU Tyr	UGU cys	U
	UUC "	UCC "	UAC "	UGC "	C
	UUA leu	UCA "	**UAA****	**UGA****	A
	UUG "	UCG "	**UAG****	UGG Tryp	G
C	CUU "	CCU Pro	CAU His	CGU Arg	U
	CUC "	CCC "	CAC "	CGC "	C
	CUA "	CCA "	CAA Glun	CGA "	A
	CUG "	CCG "	CAG "	CGG "	G
A	AUU Ileu	ACU Thr	AAU Aspn	AGU Ser	U
	AUC "	ACC "	AAC "	AGC "	C
	AUA "	ACA "	AAA Lys	AGA Arg	A
	AUG * Met	ACG "	AAG "	AGG "	G
G	GUU Val	GCU Ala	GAU Asp	GGU Gly	U
	GUC "	GCC "	GAC "	GGC "	C
	GUA "	GCA "	GAA Glu	GGA "	A
	GUG * "	GCG "	GAG "	GGG "	G

* Chain initiation codon ** Chain termination codon.

18.4 TRIPLET CODONS OF AMINO ACIDS

Each of the 20 amino acid is trinucleotides which are called as DNA codes. Each code is transcribed into mRNA which is called codon. The DNA codes and mRNA transcription codons for all the 20 amino acids have been presented in the Table 18.2.

Table 18.2: Triplet Codons of Amino acids

Sl.No.	*Amino Acids*	*Abbreviation*	*DNA Code*	*mRNA Transcription (Codons)*
1.	**Alanine**	ala	CGA, CGG, CGT, CGC	GCU,GCC,GCA,GCG
2.	**Arginnie**	arg	GCA, GCT, GCC, TCT, GCG, TCC	CGU, CGC, CGA, CGG AGA, AGG
3.	**Aspargine**	asn	TTA, TTG	AAU, AAC
4.	**Aspartic acid**	asp	C TA, CTG	GAU, GAC
5.	**Cystein**	cys	ACA, ACG	UGU, UGC
6.	**Glutamine**	gln	GTT, GTC	CAA, CAG
7.	**Glutamic acid**	glu	CTT, CTC	GAA, GAG
8.	**Glycine**	gly	CCA, CCG, CCT, CCC	GGU, GGC, GGA, GGG
9.	**Histidine**	his	GTA,GTG	GAU, CAC
10.	**Isoleucine**	ilu	TAT,TAA, TAG	AUA, AUU, AUG
11.	**Leucine**	leu	AAT, AAC, GAA GAG, GAT,GAC	UUA, UUG, CUU CUC,CUA,CUG
12.	**Lysine**	lys	TTT, TTC	AAA, AAG
13.	**Metionine**	met	TAC	AUG*
14.	**Phenylalanine**	phe	AAA, AAG	UUU, UUC
15.	**Proline**	pro	GGA, GGG,GGT,GGC	CCU, CCC, CCA, CCG
16.	**Serine**	ser	AGA, AGG, AGT AGC, TCA, TCG	UCU, UCC, UCA UCG, AGU, AGC
17.	**Threonine**	thr	TGA, TGG, TGT, TGC	ACU, ACC, ACA,ACG
18.	**Tryptophane**	try	ACC	UGG
19.	**Tyrosine**	tyr	ATA, ATG	UAU, UAC
20.	**Valine**	val	CAA, CAG, CAT,CAC	GUU, GUC, GUA, GUG
	Terminating triplets		ATT, ATC, ACT	UAA, UAG, UGA
	Initiation codon		TAC	AUG

Codon: A set of three adjacent nucleotides in an mRNA molecule that specify the incorporation of an amino acid into a polypeptide chain.

***Anticodon*:** Three bases in a tRNA molecules that are complementary to the three bases of a specific codon in mRNA.

18.5 CODON – ANTICODON INTERACTION

The codons in mRNA molecules are recognized by aminoacyl-tRNAs during protein synthesis. This recognition is required for translation of a sequence of nucleotides in mRNA into the correct sequence of amino acids in the polypeptide product. As per the degeneracy of the genetic code the following two phenomena occur -

- The different codons specifying a given amino acid are recognized by several different tRNA. Several tRNA exist for certain amino acids and some tRNA recognizes more than one codon.
- The anticodon of a given tRNA is able to base-pair with several different codons.

Wobble Hypothesis - Codon-Anticodon Interaction

The base-pairing rules are strictly followed by the hydrogen bonding between the bases in the ***codons of mRNAs*** and the ***anticodons of tRNA.*** However, it is true only for the first two bases of the codon. But the base-pairing of the third base of the anticodon has some play (*wobble*) at this site which allows it to pair with more than one base according to Crick's hypothesis, called as ***wobble hypothesis*** which explains that one tRNA recognizes two codons. This allows several types of base-pairing (but not all types) at the third codon base during *codon-anticodon interaction.* According to the ***wobble hypothesis,*** the existence of at least two tRNA for each amino acid with codons that exhibit complete degeneracy has been proved to be true. Thus, a single tRNA can respond to two or more codons, as per *wobble hypothesis.*

The ***anticodon*** is constituted of three bases in a tRNA molecule that are complementary to the three bases of a specific codon in mRNA. According to *wobble hypothesis* the base-pairing between the 5′ base of the anticodons of tRNAs and the 3′ base of codons of mRNAs is as under:

Base in Codons of mRNAs	*Base in Anticodons of tRNAs*
A or G	U
C or U	G
G	C
U	A
A, U or C	I*

- Inosine, is the base, contained by several tRNAs, made from the purine hypoxanthine by posttranscriptional modification of adenosine, and when present at the 5′ end of an anticodon, it would base-pair with A, U or C in the codon.

The genetic code is not absolutely universal, even after mitochondria are excluded. There exist some variations in codon recognition and translation. The variations are due to the mutations in tRNA genes which change the anticodon and thus the codons recognized by the mutant tRNA. These mutations are ***suppressor mutations*** which are nucleotide substitutions and suppressed the effect of other mutations. A mutant tRNA is called ***suppressor tRNA*** that recognizes one or more of the termination codons and inserts an amino acid at a site where translation termination would normally occur.

One of the suppressor mutations that change tRNA specificity is the one that suppress UAG chain-termination mutation within the coding sequence of the gene. The mutations that produce chain-termination triplets within genes are known as ***nonsense mutations.*** These are mutations that change a codon specifying an amino acid to a termination codon. These mutations frequently arise from single base-pair substitution and result in truncated polypeptide. The position of these mutations within the gene determines the length of truncated polypeptide. The nonsense mutations produce completely nonfunctional polypeptide fragments. On the contrary is the ***missense mutation*** which changes a codon (triplet) specifying an amino acid to a codon specifying a different amino acid. The gene with missense mutation encodes a complete polypeptide but with an amino acid substitution in the polypeptide gene product.

EXERCISES- SOLVED

18.1 The following is given a short nucleotide sequence of a wild-type gene –

5′-ATGTCCGCATGGGGA -3′

3′-TACAGGCGTACCCCT -5′

(i) Write down the mRNA nucleotide sequence that will be produced after transcription of this gene segment, (ii) Write down the amino acid sequence that will be produced on translation of this mRNA nucleotide sequence.

Answer: (i) Transcription of above gene segment (DNA segment: 3′-TACAGGCGT ACCCCT -5′) will produce the following mRNA nucleotide sequence:

5′ –AUGUCCGCAUGGGGA -3′

(ii) Translation of the above mRNA produced by transcription of DNA segment will produce the following amino acid sequence –

Methionine-serine-alanine-tryptophan-glycine

18.2 The nucleotide sequence of template strand of a segment of a gene is 3′-GCT AAGC-5′. This gene sequence is transcribed into RNA. Find out the nucleotide sequence of RNA transcript.

Answer: The RNA transcript is complementary to the template strand of DNA and has the opposite chemical polarity. Therefore,

3′-GCTAAGC-5′ Nucleotide sequence of given DNA template strand

5′-CGAUUCG-3′ Nucleotide sequence of RNA transcript (To be formed)

18.3 The amino acid sequence reading from the amino terminus to the carboxyl terminus is methionine-tryptophan. Write down the sequence of nucleotide pairs in a gene in *Drosophila* that will encode this dipeptide (amino acid sequence).

Answer: The codon for methionine is AUG while for tryptophan is UGG. Therefore, the nucleotide sequence in the mRNA specifying the sequence metionine-tryptophan (dipeptide sequence) must be 5′-AUGUGG-3′.

The template DNA strand (from which the mRNA has been transcribed/ synthesized) will be complementary and antiparallel to the mRNA sequence. Thus, the template DNA strand will be 3′-TACACC-5′ and the other strand of DNA which must be complementary to this template strand (3′-TACACC-5′). Therefore, the complementary DNA strand will be 5′-ATGTGG-3′ and accordingly the synthesis of base pairs in the gene (DNA) must be:

5′-ATGTGG-3′ DNA strand complementary to template DNA strand

3′-TACACC-5′ *Template DNA strand which synthesizes mRNA

* This is the template strand of DNA which is complementary and antiparallel to mRNA strand (5′-AUGUGG-3′ which have specified methionine-tryptophan dipeptide sequence).

18.4 Given coding sequence of an mRNA as 5′-AUGUUUCCCAAAGGG-3′

(i) Name the amino acids that will be specified by this mRNA sequence on its transcription.

(ii) Find out the coding sequence of the template strand of the gene (DNA) from which the above coding sequence of mRNA has been transcribed.

Hint: (i) Use table 16.2 and find the answer as:

(Amino terminus) – methionine-phenylalanine–proline–lysine–glycine-(carboxyl-terminus)

(ii) The above coding sequence of mRNA (5′-AUGUUUCCCAAAGGG-3′) will be transcribed from the following coding sequence of template strand of DNA

3′-TAC AAA GGG TTT CCC -5′.

Chapter 19

Gene Expression – Molecular Mechanism (Protein Synthesis) II. Translation (Polypeptide Production)

The second stage (process) of the gene expression (polypeptide formation) is called as ***translation***. The translation means the synthesis of polypeptide chain and it occurs on 70S ribosome which dissociates into 30S and 50S subunits after completion of a polypeptide chain. The genetic information contained in DNA and transcribed into intermediaries mRNA molecules (gene's codons present in the sequence of mRNA) are translated (converted) into the amino acid sequences of polypeptides for protein synthesis according to the specifications of the genetic code. The mRNA acts as a template for the synthesis of a polypeptide. This implies that the sequence of nucleotides in mRNA specifies the incorporation of a particular amino acid into the polypeptide chain.

It is now important to understand about the ***structure of amino acids and proteins*** (See ***annexure 19.1 and 19.2***) and the mechanism by which the DNA (genetic material) in the form of nucleotides transfers the genetic information to specify the specific amino acid that are used to synthesize the different proteins.

19.1 RELATION BETWEEN GENES AND THEIR POLYPEPTIDE PRODUCTS

A gene's nucleotide sequence specifies a polypeptide's amino acid sequence. This needs that there exists a relation between genes and their polypeptide products and that relation should be co-linear. Thus, the sequences of nucleotide pairs in a gene and the amino acids in its polypeptide product are collinear. The classic genetic studies to support this co-linear relation have been discussed in *annexure 19.3*.

19.2 COMPONENTS REQUIRED FOR PROTEIN SYNTHESIS

The protein synthesis requires more energy compared to any other activities of metabolism and a large number of molecules that form about one-third of the total dry mass of the cell.

- ☆ The *E. coli* has about 200,000 ***ribosomes*** that form the major component of the metabolic machinery to the process of protein synthesis and constitutes 25 percent of the dry mass of each cell.
- ☆ In addition to ribosome, the RNA molecule known as ***tRNA***, and
- ☆ An enzyme called ***aminoacyl-tRNA synthetase*** to activate amino acids ise required.

The roles of these components required for protein synthesis have been discussed in *annexure 19.4*.

19.3 STAGES OF TRANSLATION (SYNTHESIS OF POLYPEPTIDES)

The sequences of nucleotides in an mRNA molecule are translated into the sequence of amino acids in its polypeptide product. Thus, the mRNA molecules provide the specifications for the amino acid sequences of the polypeptide gene products. This process of translation (protein synthesis) occurs in three stages, *viz.* polypeptide chain initiation, chain elongation and chain termination.

(i) Polypeptide Chain Initiation

The initiation of protein synthesis is complete with the formation of a peptide bond between the first two amino acids of the new polypeptide chain. The initiation of protein synthesis involves several aspects among which some are similar in prokaryotes and eukaryotes while others are different. Thus, it is required to discuss the initiation process separately in two types of organisms.

(a) Prokaryotes

The initiation process of forming the polypeptide chain in *E. coli* is complete with the completion of the following two stages:

The first stage of initiation of translation (polypeptide chain initiation) begins with the formation of complete 30S initiation complex. This 30S initiation complex is complete when the following two complexes are combined with each other as well as with protein initiation factor IF-1 and one molecule of GTP (Guanosine triphosphate). The *first complex* is formed by an interaction of a free 30S subunit of ribosome with an mRNA molecule in the presence of soluble protein initiation factors IF-3 to control the ability of the 30S subunit of ribosome to begin the initiation process. The *second complex* contains the special initiator tRNA (methionyl-tRNA $_f^{Met}$: f stands for formylated tRNA) and the soluble protein initiation factors IF-2.

In the final stage of initiation process, there is an addition of 50S subunit of ribosome to the initiation complex of 30S to produce 70S ribosome on which the translation occurs and also there is a release of the initiation factor IF-3 from the complex before joining the 50S subunit (50S subunit and IF-3 are never associated with the 30S subunit simultaneously). The addition of 50S subunit also requires energy from GTP and the release of other two initiation factors IF-1 and IF-2. The special tRNA (***tRNA*** $_f^{Met}$) is methionine tRNA. This specifies the initiation of the synthesis of polypeptide chains in prokaryotes in response to a translation initiation codon (AUG and sometimes GUG). Thus, all polypeptides synthesis begins with methionine.

The formation of the first complex (30S subunit and mRNA) depends in part on base pairing between a nucleotide sequence near the 3′ end of the 16S rRNA and a sequence near the 5′ end of the mRNA molecule and this base pairing plays an important role in translation. The mRNA in prokaryotes has a conserved hexamer of polypurine tract (consensus AGGAGG, called ***Shine-Dalgarno sequence*** after the discoverer) located about 7 nucleotides upstream from the AUG initiation codon. This conserved hexamer is complementary to a sequence near the 5′ terminus of 16S rRNA and is involved in the initiation of translation.

With the addition of the 50S subunit to the initiation complex, the special initiator tRNA (methionyl-tRNA $_f^{Met}$) takes its position in the peptidyl (P) site with the anticodon of the tRNA aligned with the AUG initiation codon of the mRNA. The methionyl-tRNA $_f^{Met}$ is the only aminoacyl-tRNA to bind directly to the P site without passing through the A site. The second codon of the mRNA is registered with the A site as the initiator AUG is positioned in the P site and dictates the aminoacyl-tRNA specificity at that site. Now, the stage is ready for the elongation phase of polypeptide synthesis to begin.

(b) Eukaryotes

The initiation of protein synthesis in eukaryotes is similar but involves several soluble initiation factors making the process more complex and different only in the following two features in initiation of translation:

- ☆ The amino group of the methionine on the initiator tRNA (methionine -tRNA $_i^{Met}$) is not formylated like that in prokaryotes, and
- ☆ The initiation complex is formed at the 5′ terminus of the mRNA and not on the Shine-Dalgarno/AUG translation start site.

The translation begins at the AUG nearest to the 5′ terminus of the mRNA molecule with the initiation sequence 5′ –GCC (A or G) CC**AUG**G- 3′. There is a special initiator tRNA (tRNA$_i^{Met}$: i for initiator) and this initiator (methionine- tRNA $_i^{Met}$) interacts with a soluble initiator factor and enters the P site directly like in *E. coli*. Thus, the ***tRNA***$_i^{Met}$ specifies the initiation of polypeptide chains in eukaryotes.

The initiation complex is formed at the 5′ terminus of the mRNA. This occurs on binding a cap-binding protein (CBP) to the 7-methyl guanosine cap (7 MG cap) and then binding other initiation factors to the CBP-mRNA complex, followed by 40S subunit of ribosome. This complex moves 5′ to 3′ along the mRNA molecule in search of an AUG codon. Now, the initiation factors dissociate from the complex, followed by the binding of 60S subunit to the complex of methionyl-tRNA/mRNA/40S subunit and forming the complete 80S ribosome. The elongation phase of polypeptide chain formation is ready to begin now.

(ii) Polypeptide Chain Elongation

This is similar in *prokaryotes and eukaryotes*. Each amino acid is added to the growing polypeptide chain following three steps:

- ☆ An aminoacyl-tRNA is bound to the A site of the ribosome. The mRNA codon in register with the A site provides the specificity. The nucleotides of the mRNA codon present at the A site pair with three nucleotides in the anticodon of the incoming aminoacyl-tRNA. This requires elongation factor Tu carrying a molecule of GTP. The binding of aminoacyl-TRNA at the A site requires GTP which is cleaved after peptide bond formation. The elongation factor Tu-GDP is released from the ribosome after the cleavage of GTP because the Tu-GDP is inactive, cannot bind to aminoacyl-tRNAs, and converted to elongation factor TU-GTP form which is active. The conversion is by another elongation factor Ts which hydrolyzes one molecule of GTP and also interacts with all the aminoacyl-TRNa except methionine-tRNA.
- ☆ There is transfer of the growing polypeptide chain from the tRNA in the P site to the tRNA in the A site. This is the result of the formation of a new peptide bond between the amino group of the aminoacyl-tRNA in the A site and the carboxyl terminus of the growing polypeptide chain attached to the tRNA in the P site and covalently joins the chain to the tRNA in the A site. The hydrolysis of GTP forms the peptide bond. An enzyme ***peptidyl transferase*** is built into the 50 S subunit of the ribosome (large unit of ribosome). The peptidyl transferase activity resides in the 23S rRNA molecule rather than in a ribosomal protein. The activity catalyzes the formation of peptide bonds between amino acids during translation. The enzyme ***terminal transferase*** adds nucleotides to the 3′ termini of DNA molecules.
- ☆ There is translocation of the growing polypeptide-tRNA present in the A site of the ribosome to the P site and departing of the uncharged tRNA from P site to the E site with the movement of ribosome 3 nucleotides towards the 3′ end of the mRNA molecule. Thus, the ribosome along the mRNA is translocated to position the next codon in the A site. The ribosome shuttles along the mRNA molecule getting energy from the hydrolysis of GTP. Thus, the translocation requires the GTP and the elongation factor G.

Now, after completion of third step, the A site is vacated after translocation of the peptidyl-tRNA from this A site and hence the ribosome is ready for the next cycle of chain elongation. Therefore, the above three steps are repeated in a cyclic manner during the entire elongation phase of polypeptide synthesis. The chain elongation is a rapid process requiring only about 0.05 seconds (*E.* coli) to add one amino acid to the growing chain. Most of the protein folds up on the surface of ribosome during synthesis and thus the attached to the ribosome the new polypeptide chain with increased length can be observed on scanning from the 5′ end of the mRNA to the 3′ end.

(iii) Polypeptide Chain Termination

The ***termination*** is the release of a complete macromolecule (DNA, RNA, or polypeptide) after the incorporation of the final subunit (nucleotide or amino acid). The polypeptide chain elongation gets terminated on entering at A site on the ribosome by either of the three chain termination codon (UAA, UAG, or UGA). The ***release factors* (*RFs*)** which are the soluble proteins recognize these termination codons.

In *E. coli*, there are two release factors (***RF-1*** and ***RF-2***). Two termination codons (UAA and UAG) are recognized by RF-1 while the codons (UAA and UGA) are recognized by RF-2. In eukaryotes, there is only one release factor (eRF) to recognize all the three termination codons.

The RF in the A site alters the ***peptidyl transferase activity*** by adding a water molecule to the carboxyl terminus of the new polypeptide. As a result of this reaction, the polypeptide is released from the tRNA molecule in the P site and triggers the translocation of the free tRNA from the ribosome.

The mRNA molecule is released from the ribosome coupled with the dissociation of the subunits of ribosome, on completion of termination process. And another round of protein synthesis is initiated by the ribosomal subunits, as discussed under initiation of polypeptide chain.

19.4 COMMON FEATURES OF SYNTHESIS OF DNA, RNA, AND POLYPEPTIDES

The three processes of synthesis *viz. DNA synthesis, RNA synthesis, and polypeptide synthesis* have in common the involvement of the synthesis of long chains of repeating subunits. Secondly, all these three processes can be divided into three stages of chain initiation, chain elongation, and chain termination.

19.5 SIMULTANEOUS OCCURRENCE OF TRANSCRIPTION, TRANSLATION AND mRNA DEGRADATION

In prokaryotes, there is simultaneous beginning of translation and degradation of an mRNA molecule before completion of its transcription (synthesis). All the three processes occur in the 5′ to 3′ direction and hence can occur simultaneously on the same RNA molecule. In prokaryotes, once the 5′ end of an mRNA molecule is newly synthesized it acts as a template for polypeptide synthesis because of no barrier of nuclear envelop between the polypeptide-synthesizing machinery and the site of mRNA synthesis. Therefore, in prokaryotes, the two stages of protein synthesis *viz. transcription* and *translation* are often occurred together. Oscar Miller and others developed the electron microscopy to observe the coupling of the two stages of protein synthesis in bacteria.

19.6 OVERVIEW OF PROTEIN SYNTHESIS

The process of translation (protein synthesis or polypeptide synthesis) is completed in three stages and governed by the specifications of the genetic code. The synthesis of polypeptide is stepwise (addition of one amino acid at one time) accompanied by reading the codons in order. Each amino acid in the polypeptide corresponds to a sequence of three adjacent nucleotides in the mRNA. A set of three adjacent nucleotides in mRNA molecule is called ***codon*** and specifies the incorporation of one amino acid into a polypeptide chain forming the protein. The different adjacent triplets of nucleotides (*codons*) encode the different amino acids. Thus, the genes encode amino acids to form polypeptides which ultimately synthesize the protein.

During translation, the sequence of nucleotides in the RNA transcript is converted into the sequence of amino acids in the polypeptide gene product under the control of the ***genetic code.*** For example, the UUU triplet in the mRNA transcript (formed from AAA of DNA) specifies the amino acid phenylalanine in the polypeptide gene product and this process is called translation which takes place (in the cytoplasm) on ribosomes, called intricate macromolecular machine (composed of 3 to 5 RNA molecules and different proteins varying from 50 to 90).

The polypeptide after its formation is disassociated from the mRNA. It is then folded into a precise three-dimentional shape before taking part in cellular functions.

The in-going information from DNA to RNA, the language (nucleotide sequence) remained the same, while the in-going information from RNA to protein, the language is changed from a nucleotide sequence to an amino acid sequence. The language of DNA available in the form of mRNA is translated into the language of protein. This process of using information contained in mRNA to synthesize a protein is called ***translation***. Thus, the sequence of nucleotides in mRNA is changed (translated) into the sequence of amino acids of a polypeptide chain. The sequence of triplets (codons) in mRNA determines the sequence of amino acids in the enzyme or other protein being synthesized on a particular ribosome.

The mRNA after it is synthesized in the nucleus, moves out of the nucleus to the cytoplasm and becomes associated with ribosome to form a complex called as polysome or polyribosome. The ribosomes are also composed of one type of RNA called as ribosomal RNA (rRNA) where the protein molecules are synthesized.

The ribosomes in the cell are the sites of protein synthesis and these are composed of proteins and rRNA. The ribosomes involved in protein synthesis form a group of ribosomes (called as polysomes or polyribosomes) by holding together by delicate strands of RNA. The polyribosomes perform two functions:

- ✰ To bind with mRNA which carries the coded message from DNA and
- ✰ To combine with tRNA which transfer the amino acids to the ribosomal assembly plant.

Chapter 20

Gene Expression – Regulation I. Prokaryotes

The growth of an organism from the single cell zygote to the mature adult and its every living activity is under the control of genes. The information for carrying out all the activities by an organism are encoded in the sequences of nucleotides of DNA molecules of the genome and the information are organized into smaller units of DNA molecule called ***genes.*** It is important to understand the mechanism of the regulation of gene expression.

Age and Gene Expression

All the proteins required by an organism are synthesized by the genetic information contained in the form of nucleotides of DNA molecule. The different kinds of proteins are required in specific amounts at different times of the life cycle and also with the change in environmental conditions. The evidences are available which have shown that different proteins are required to play their roles at different ages. The proteins that are required for carrying out the vital activities of an adult organism have no role to play during embryonic development but other proteins are required and hence synthesized for carrying out the activities during early ages of life. Therefore, the expression of different genes is required at different age of the organism. The expression of genes responsible for secondary sexual characteristics *viz.* udder development, onset of sexual heat, milk production and egg production in only in female animals; menstruation, ovary development and ovulation, and breast development in women; development of beard and moustaches, semen production, and baldness in men; and growth of puberty hairs only on attaining puberty in both men and women are age specific.

Environmental Conditions and Gene Expression

Secondly, the living organisms faced the diverse environmental conditions to which they are adapted, particularly the microorganisms. The specific sets of genes are able to turn on and turn off their expression in response to the changed environment. The particular gene's expression is turn on when required for growth and other activities but the gene's expression is turn off if not required for any work to carry out. A considerable energy is exhausted in turning on the gene expression in synthesizing the gene transcripts and translation products but this energy is saved and conserved in turning off the expression of genes, when the synthesis of gene transcripts and translation products is not required. Such a system of turning on and off the gene requires some mechanism to regulate the gene expression (flow of genetic information from DNA to protein synthesis) in response to change in age and the environmental conditions.

Mechanism Involved in Gene Regulation

Moreover, the regulation of gene expression or gene action or gene function requires the involvement of some mechanism as a control measure that which specific gene(s) is to be switched on to produce the required specific enzyme and which gene(s) is to be switched off whose enzyme production is not required by the cell at specific time. The DNA molecule contains the primary genetic information and expresses it by producing the mRNA. Thus, the *gene function* (expression) is regulated through the ability to control the mRNA production.

More clearly, the gene expression in all the types of organisms (prokaryotes and eukaryotes) is regulated/controlled/influenced by some factors. This means that the genes works (express)/come into action as directed by some genetic and environmental factors from time to time as per requirement of the organism under normal conditions.

Level of Regulation of Gene Expression

The gene expression is regulated at many levels. The different levels are the time or stages of gene regulation. These are transcription, mRNA processing, mRNA turnover, translation, and posttranslation level. The different ***levels of regulation of gene expression*** (pathway) are as shown below:

1.	2.	3.	4.	5.
Transcriptin	RNA Processing	RNA stability	Translation	Posttranslation
DNA →	RNA transcript →	mRNA →	Protein →	Function performed by protein

20.1 MECHANISM OF CONTROL OF GENE EXPRESSION

In prokaryotes, the control of transcription of DNA into RNA is the main aspect in regulating the gene expression. This means that a gene is not expressed if it is not transcribed. The transcription in prokaryotes requires the removal of negative regulatory molecules (like the repressor protein in *lac operon*) from the vicinity of a gene and the binding of a positive regulatory molecule (like the catabolic activator protein (CAP)/cyclic AMP complex) to the gene. These are the protein-DNA interactions and control the accessibility of a gene to the RNA polymerase (an enzyme that catalyzes the synthesis of RNA). Secondly, a mechanism that has been evolved in prokaryotes to control transcription, responds quickly to the environmental changes.

The gene expression in prokaryotes is not as complex as it is in case of eukaryotes. Gene expression in prokaryotes is regulated most commonly at the transcription level, though the fine-tuning often occurs at the translation level.

The mechanism of regulation of gene expression (action or function) has been more extensively studied in microorganism particularly the *E. coli.* The mechanism of the regulation of gene expression is little different in prokaryotes than in eukaryotes and hence has been dealt here separately under the following heads -

- ☆ Regulatory mechanisms of transcription,
- ☆ Gene expression is constitutive as well as inducible and repressible,
- ☆ Positive and negative control of gene expression,
- ☆ Operon models of gene expression
- ☆ *Two operons in E. coli viz. lac* operon and *trp* operon
- ☆ Regulation of gene expression at translational level, and
- ☆ Posttranscriptional regulatory mechanism

20.2 REGULATORY MECHANISM OF TRANSCRIPTION IN PROKARYOTES

The regulatory mechanism with the largest effect on phenotype acts at the transcription level, though the gene expression in prokaryotes is regulated at several levels of gene transcription, mRNA processing, mRNA turnover, translation, and post-translation. There may be various regulatory mechanisms of transcription but these are grouped in the following two categories -

- ☆ The first regulatory mechanism requires the rapid turn on and turn off the gene expression with a change in environment. Microorganisms achieve optimum growth and reproduction in a wide range of environmental conditions by adjusting their metabolic processes quickly and hence are adapted to changed environmental conditions.
- ☆ The second mechanism is the sequential expression of genes which is a genetically preprogrammed circuits or cascades of gene expression. Under this regulatory mechanism the gene products of one or more genes regulate the expression of other genes. They may turn off the transcription of first

set of genes or turn on the transcription of the second set of genes, and so on. Under this sequential expression the genes cannot usually be turn on out of sequence.

20.3 CONSTITUTIVE, INDUCIBLE AND REPRESSIBLE GENE EXPRESSION

On the basis of regulation of gene expression in prokaryotes, there are two types of genes:

(1) Constitutive Genes

These genes need no regulation but they are expressed continuously through production of certain enzymes by the organism irrespective of the presence or absence of substrate in the environment. The enzymes produced by these constitutive genes are called also the ***constitutive enzyme.*** Such enzymes are required all the times by the organism. The gene products like rRNA molecules, tRNA molecules, ribosomal proteins, RNA polymerase subunits, and the enzymes catalyzing the metabolic processes are the essential components of all the living cells to carry out the cellular functions. The genes specifying these products are expressed continuously. Therefore, such genes are said to be expressed constitutively and hence called as ***constitutive genes.*** Therefore, in prokaryotes, the genes that specify rRNAs, tRNAs, and ribosomal proteins, etc are expressed constitutively

(2) Regulated Genes

These genes are usually expressed only when their products are required. These genes encode the enzymes called ***regulated enzymes*** that are synthesized under some specific conditions and require some type of regulation of gene expression as and when required like cell growth. Some gene products are required for cell growth only under certain environmental conditions. The constitutive synthesis of such gene products is not required but the energy required would be wasteful which could be used for more rapid growth. Thus, a regulatory mechanism is required that could synthesize such gene products as and when they are required. This emphasize that the genes encoding the enzymes required for some activity of the cell should be turn on but if the enzyme is not involved then the genes encoding the enzyme should be turned off. Therefore, the enzymes that are synthesized in certain specific condition and require one or other type of gene regulation, are called ***regulated enzymes*** and the genes encoding these enzymes are called ***regulated genes.*** The regulated enzymes are thus synthesized as per demand of their biosynthetic products. The enzymes of most biosynthetic pathways for the synthesis of amino acids, purines, pyrimidine, etc are specified by the regulated genes.

The regulated enzymes or genes are of the following two kinds which exhibit two phenomena of induction and repression. The *E. coli* growing in different culture media exhibits these two phenomena of induction and repression.

(i) Inducible Enzymes

The gene(s) is induced to produce the enzyme. The enzyme which is synthesized only in the presence of its substrate in the environment is called the ***inducible***

enzyme and the substrate is called ***inducer.*** The inducer is thus a substance which induces gene expression (protein synthesis) on enzyme production. The genes whose expression is regulated in this manner (of producing an enzyme in the presence of an inducer) are called **inducible genes.** This process of turning on the expression of genes in response to a substance (inducer) in the environment to produce the required enzyme is called ***induction.***

The genes encoding enzymes of catabolic pathways are often expressed only in the presence of the substrates of the enzymes and their expression is *inducible.* Most of the bacteria grow in the presence of any one of several carbohydrates (glucose, galactose, lactose, sucrose, and arabinose) as a source of energy. For example, the *E. coli* grown in glycerol culture media produces in abundance the enzyme required for the breakdown of glycerol but the synthesis of other enzymes is minimal. But when the bacteria are grown by transfer on lactose containing medium, there is synthesis of two enzymes (β-galactoside permease and β-galactosidase) many times required for lactose utilization while the synthesis of other enzymes is considerably reduced. Thus, *E. coli* requires these two enzymes for lactose metabolism (lactose utilization by *E. coli* as a source of energy). The enzyme β-galactoside permease pumps (transport) the lactose into the cell and the second enzyme β-galactosidase catalyzes the hydrolysis of lactose (cleaving of the lactose) into its two simple sugar units of glucose and galactose. The glycerol and lactose are the substrate (substance in the growing medium) which acted as *inducer* for the synthesis of specific enzymes. This way the lactose (the substrate, the inducer) induces the synthesis of enzymes and hence the lactose is an inducer for enzyme synthesis or enzyme inducer or effector.

Likewise, the enzymes that are involved in catabolic (degradative) pathways (lactose, galactose or arabinose utilization) are inducible. However, the substrate and the inducer may not be identical. Thus all the substrate are not inducer as well as all the inducers are not substrate, *e.g.* the phenyl-β-D-galactoside is a substrate but it is not an inducer, and methyl-β-D-thiogalactoside is an inducer but it is not a substrate.

It should be remembered that induction occurs at transcription level. The induction changes the rate of enzyme synthesis but does not change the activity of the existing enzyme molecules. Secondly, the induction also differs from activation. The activation occurs when the binding of a small molecule to an enzyme increases the activity of the enzyme but does not affect its rate of synthesis.

(ii) Repressible Enzymes

An enzyme whose synthesis is diminished by a regulatory molecule is called repressible enzyme. Most of the organic molecules such as amino acids, purines, pyrimidines, and vitamins required for the growth of bacteria are synthesized by them. For example, there are 5 genes contained by *E. coli* to encode the enzymes required for catalyzing the biosynthesis of the amino acid tryptophan. Therefore, the tryptophan is not required in the *E. coli* growing medium for expression of these genes but these 5 genes must be expressed to provide the adequate amount of tryptophan in protein synthesis.

In view of the above example of biosynthesis of tryptophan in *E. coli,* it is clear that some enzymes are normally present in the cell and these are not synthesized in the presence of their end products in high concentrations. The synthesis of the tryptophan biosynthetic enzymes for optimal growth of *E. coli* in a medium containing enough tryptophan is not required and if added it would be a wastage of energy. In this situation when tryptophan is externally available in the growing medium, a regulatory mechanism is required in *E. coli* to turn off the synthesis of the tryptophan biosynthetic enzymes.

This process of turning off the gene expression in the presence of some signal (end products of the enzymes) is called **repression** and the gene whose expression is being turned off is called a ***repressed gene.*** A repressor gene encodes a repressor. The activity of gene(s) is suppressed in repression and hence the synthesis of protein is either stopped or reduced. The substance which stops or suppresses the protein synthesis is called ***repressor.*** The repressor is a protein that binds to DNA and turns off gene expression. The end product is called ***corepressor.***

The repressor on binding with the metabolite is structurally changed so as it can bind with the operator and prevents its transcription. This metabolite is called as *co-repressor* for the reason that it activates the repressor to inactivate the operator site. For example, the presence of histidine or tryptophan amino acid in high concentration in the medium starts acting corepressor. The histidine as a corepressor turns off the synthesis of 10 enzymes required in biosynthetic pathway to histidine. This type of repression is called ***coordinate repression***. A regulator gene produces a substance called ***aporepressor*** which unites with corepressor and form a functional ***repressor*** molecule. This repressor molecule or substance inhibits the synthesis of mRNA, by all the genes specifying enzymes in the biotic pathway. The genes encoding enzymes for anabolic pathways are usually turned off in the presence of the end product of the pathway (like the tryptophan) and their expression is *repressible.* On turning on the expression of the repressed gene is called to be ***derepressed*** and the process is ***derepression.*** The enzymes involved as the components of anabolic or biosynthetic pathways are called ***repressible enzymes.*** The repression also occurs at the transcription level like the induction. However, the gene regulation can occur at many levels but the most common level is the transcription.

The inducible and repressible enzymes of microorganisms can be distinguished by studying the synthesis or lack of synthesis of the enzyme in the cells grown on the medium containing that chemical. The inducible operons are turned off in the absence of the effector molecule while the repression operaons will be turning on. In other words, the synthesis of enzyme is probably ***inducible*** in the presence of a certain metabolite. The enzyme is probably ***repressible*** if the enzyme is synthesized in the absence (but not in the presence) of a particular metabolite.

20.4 POSITIVE AND NEGATIVE CONTROL OF GENE EXPRESSION IN PROKARYOTES

The regulation of gene expression in terms of induction (turning genes on) and repression (turning gene off) is controlled by both positive and negative control mechanisms. These two mechanisms (positive and negative) make the involvement of ***regulator genes*** to encode the products which regulate the expression of other genes. The product of a regulatory gene is required either to initiate or to shut down (turn off) the expression of one or more genes. The initiation of the expression of one or more structural genes by the product of regulator gene is called the ***positive control mechanism*** while the turning off the expression of one or more structural genes by the product of a regulatory gene is the ***negative control measure.*** Therefore, the positive control mechanism requires the regulatory protein(s) to turn on gene expression while in negative control mechanism the regulatory protein(s) is required to turn off gene expression. The ***structural genes*** are those which specify the amino acid sequences of enzymes or structural proteins.

A gene is expressed on binding the RNA polymerase to its promoter and synthesizing an RNA transcript. This RNA transcript contains the coding region of the gene. On binding the product of the regulator gene at the ***regulator protein-binding site*** (RPBS) adjacent to the promoter of the structural gene(s), the product of the regulator gene comes in action and the transcription of the structural gene(s) is turn on and it is the positive control mechanism. And it is the negative control mechanism when the transcription is turn off as a result of the action of the product of regulator gene after its binding at the RPBS adjacent to the promoter of structural gene(s).

The products of regulator gene required for activating the gene expression in positive control mechanism are called ***activators***. The activator is thus required to turn on the expression of the structural gene(s). On the contrary, the products of regulator gene required for repressing the gene expression in negative control mechanism are called ***repressors***. Thus, repressor is a protein that binds to DNA and turn off the expression of structural gene(s). The activators and repressors regulate the gene expression by binding to the sites adjacent to the promoters of structural genes.

However, the ***effector molecule*** in the cell (small molecules like amino acids, sugars, and like metabolites) plays an important role in binding a regulator protein to the RPBS. The effector molecule is a molecule that influences the behavior of a regulatory molecule, such as a repressor protein, thereby influencing gene expression. The binding occurs if the effector molecule is present in the cell otherwise not. Thus, the presence or absence of small effector molecules that form complexes with the regulator proteins decides whether or not the regulator proteins can bind to their binding sites. The effector molecules are accordingly of two types *viz.* those which involved in induction (turning on) of gene expression (inducible systems) called as ***inducers*** and those which are involved in repression (turning off) of gene expression (repressible system) called ***co-repressors.*** The co-repressors are the end products (metabolites).

In view of the above description, there are four mechanisms of gene regulation as:

- ✰ *Negative inducible control mechanism:* The free repressor binds to the RPBS and prevents the transcription of structural gene(s) in the absence of inducer. When inducer is present, it is bound by the repressor, and the repressor/inducer complex cannot bind to the RPBS and the RNA polymerase then binding to the promoter transcribes the structural gene(s).

- ☆ *Positive inducible control mechanism:* In this system, the activator cannot bind to the RPBS in the absence of inducer, and RNA polymerase cannot transcribe the structural gene(s) unless there is binding of activator/ inducer complex to the RPBS. This turn on the transcription of structural gene only in the presence of inducer.
- ☆ *Negative repressible control mechanism:* The transcription of structural gene(s) occurs in the absence of the co-repressor. The binding of repressor/ co-repressor complex to the RPBS prevents the RNA polymerase not to transcribe the structural genes. The free repressor cannot bind to the RPBS in the absence of co-repressor and hence the RNA polymerase transcribes the structural genes on binding to the promoter.
- ☆ *Positive repressible control mechanism:* The activator (product of the regulator gene) is bound to the RPBS so as the RNA polymerase is bound to the promoter to transcribe the structural gene(s). The co-repressor forms a complex with the activator protein which is unable to bind with the RPBS. This results into not to bind the RNA polymerase with the promoter and transcribe the structural gene(s).

There are some important differences among the above mentioned four mechanisms of gene regulation. These differences are as under:

(a) The regulator gene product (activator) takes part in turning on the gene expression in positive control system while the repressor (regulator gene product) takes part in turning off the gene expression in a negative control mechanism, and

(b) With both positive and negative control mechanism, the inducible or repressible gene expression depends on binding the free regulator protein or the regulator protein/effector molecule complex binds to the RPBS.

There are different effects of mutations in regulatory genes that produce non-functional products, in positive and negative control systems. The mutations cannot turn on the expression of the regulated genes in positive controls while these mutations cannot turn off the expression of the regulated genes in negative control system.

20.5 OPERON MODELS OF GENE EXPRESSION IN PROKARYOTES

According to the theory on gene functioning in microorganisms, the genes may be divided in two major groups as *structural genes* and *control genes*

The ***operon*** is a group of genes making up a regulatory or control unit. This unit includes an operator, a promoter, and structural genes. The operons in prokaryotes are the genes with related functions which frequently occur in coordinately regulated genetic units.

Francois Jacob and Jacques Monod (1961) proposed the operon hypothesis of negative control mechanism to explain the regulation of genes required for the utilization of lactose in *E. coli.* They studied the catabolism of lactose and suggested that the gene action is regulated at the transcription level by two phenomena of induction and repression. They discovered in their study of the *lactose* operon in *E. coli* that the genes for lactose metabolism were transcribed on adding the lactose to the cell growing medium. Thus, the lactose induced the gene transcription and hence it was an ***inducer*** of gene transcription.

They observed a group of three genes involved in synthesis of three enzymes which bring about the catabolism of lactose. The three enzymes they described are β-galactosidase, β-galactoside permease, and thiogalactoside transacetylase. The three genes encoding three enzymes are the structural genes which are closely linked and controlled in a coordinated manner.

Structure of an Operon

Each operon contains a set of contiguous structural genes and control genes. These two types of genes have close association. There are three control genes: a regulator gene, a promoter, and an operator. Thus, an operon is constituted of the following genes:

(i) Structural Gene

The structural genes are the DNA segments that code and control the sequence of amino acids during protein synthesis. These genes encode for the synthesis of various proteins that are grouped into three type *viz.* enzymes, non-enzymatic proteins such as haemoglobin, and repressor proteins which prevent the activity of other genes. The structural gene in the operon cannot be transcribed by RNA polymerase if the repressor is bound to the operator. On the contrary, if the operator is free of repressor, the RNA polymerase can transcribe the operon.

(ii) Control Genes

The control genes are to control the activity of structural genes either by induction or repression. The control genes are categorized as *regulator gene, promoter gene, and operator gene.*

(a) Regulatory Gene (r)

A gene that controls the rate of expression of another gene or genes. The regulator genes are the control genes to regulate the amount of protein to be produced. The regulator gene is considered to be present on the chromosome which is same or different on which are present the structural genes to produce a repressor (protein) which blocks the action of operator gene by not allowing the structural genes to produce proteins because they cannot produce mRNA.

Regulator gene produces specific enzyme which acts as a repressor substance. The regulator gene, in case of *lac* operon, encodes a protein which binds strongly to the operator gene and suppresses its activity. The *lacI* gene produces a protein that controls the expression of the structural genes of the *lac* operon in *E. coli.* The repressor substance is converted by a depressor substance (substrate or hormone) into an inactive compound which allow the operator gene to function and the structural genes to produce mRNA. The repressor substance if present, combine with the operator site and prevent the structural genes to produce mRNA.

(b) Promoter Gene (p)

This is a DNA segment where the RNA polymerase binds and initiates transcription. Thus, the promoter is a nucleotide sequence and the binding site for RNA polymerase. The transcription of the structural gene is initiated by this promoter gene and controls the rate of mRNA synthesis. The structural as well as regulator genes have their promoters.

(c) Operator Gene (o)

The operator is a part of operon that controls the expression of one or more structural genes by serving as the binding site for one or more regulatory proteins. This is also a DNA segment located adjacent to the structural gene on the same chromosome and control the synthetic activity of adjacent structural gene to produce mRNA (transcription) by acting like a switch to make them *on* and *off*. The operator is a part of operon that controls the expression of one or more structural genes by serving as the binding site for one or more regulatory proteins. The repressor substance produced by regulatory gene binds with operator gene. Thus, the operator is the binding site for a regulatory gene (called repressor).

An operator with the structural genes under its control is called an *operon*. The adjacent DNA cistron is initiated by operator gene to produce mRNA. The repressor substance is converted by a depressor substance (substrate or hormone) into an inactive compound which allow the operator gene to function and the structural genes to produce mRNA. The repressor substance if present, combine with the operator site and prevent the structural genes to produce mRNA.

20.6 TWO OPERON IN *E. COLI*

These are for the lactose utilization (*lac* operon) and the regulatory mechanism of tryptophan biosynthesis (*trp* operon) have been discussed as under:

20.6.1 Lactose (Lac) Operon in *E. coli*

The *lac operon* contains three structural genes (*lacZ, lacY,* and *lac A*), three operators (O_1, O_2 and O_3), and a promoter (P). The *lac* operon is a negative inducible and catabolic repressible system operon.

(i) Induction

It is the process of *'turning on'* the expression of a gene or set of genes by an ***inducer*** which is a substance of low molecular weight that is bound by a repressor to produce a complex that can no longer bind to the operator. Thus, the presence of inducer turns on the expression of gene(s) controlled by the operator. A gene that is expressed only in the presence of a specific metabolite (the inducer) is called an ***inducible gene.*** An enzyme that is synthesized only in the presence of the substrate that acts as an inducer is called ***inducible enzyme.*** The ***three structural genes*** in the *lac operon* (*lacA, lacY, and lac Z*) are expressed only in the presence of lactose and absence of glucose, and encode the three enzymes β-galactosidase, β-galactoside permease, and thiogalactoside transacetylase, respectively. The function of third enzyme is not known.

The ***lac* operator** functions as a binding site of repressor. A repressor (360 amino acids long) is encoded by the *lac* regulator gene. The *lac* repressor, in the absence of inducer (lactose), binds to the *lac* operators and prevents RNA polymerase from initiating (catalyzing) the transcription of the three structural genes (operon). The blocking of the transcription of the structural genes of the operon involving the repression in the lactose operon is the *negative regulatory mechanism*. The inducer of the operon, *allolactose,* is derived from lactose by a reaction catalyzed by the enzyme β-galactosidase. This allolactose is bound by the repressor and causes the release of the repressor from the operator. Thus, the transcription of the three structural genes is induced by allolactose.

The ***lac* promoter** contains two units: One is the RNA polymerase binding site and another is a binding site for another protein (called ***catabolite activator protein,*** CAP) that prevents the induction of *lac* operon in the presence of glucose. The glucose is utilized as a source of energy.

The *lac**I*** gene, *lac* operator O_1, and the *lac* promoter were identified from mutant strains that showed changed expression of the *lac* operon genes. The mutations in **I** gene and the promoter mostly causes the constitutive synthesis of the *lac* gene products. The $\mathbf{I}^-$ and $\mathbf{O}^c$ constitutive mutations can be distinguished from their behavior in partial diploids in which they (regulatory elements) are located in *cis* configuration (***coupling phase-*** two linked genes coming from same parent) to the regulatory genes or *trans* configuration (***repulaion phase*** double heterozygote – two genes coming from different parent) to them (regulatory genes or elements) relative to the mutations in *lac* structural genes. A *cis*-acting element has its effect on the expression of the genes when present in *cis* configuration while a *trans-* acting element will have its effect in either the *cis* or in the *trans-* configuration.

(ii) Catabolite Repression

The glucose prevents the induction of the *lac* operon and also other operons of carbohydrate catabolism. This is known as ***catabolite repression*** or ***glucose effect*** which assures glucose metabolism. The catabolic repression of the *lac* operon and several other operons are mediated by a regulatory protein called ***catabolic activator protein (CAP)*** and a small effector molecule called ***cyclic AMP*** (adenosine-3′, 5′ –monophosphate, cAMP). The CAP/cAMP complex exerts positive control over the transcription of the *lac* operon. Thus, the CAP-cAMP is an example of *positive regulation mechanism*. This is because this complex has a positive effect on the transcription of the *lac* operon. This complex in the *lac* operon promotes the transcription of the structural genes of the operon. Its effect is opposite to the repressor binding to an operator. The cAMP acts as the effector molecule.

The catabolic repression has its biological significance. The phenomenon of catabolic repression has evolved to assure the use of glucose as a carbon source when it is available rather than less efficient energy sources.

20.6.2 Tryptophan (trp) Operon in *E. coli*

Charles Yanofsky and colleagues analyzed the functions of the five structural genes and the adjacent regulatory sequences of the *trp* operon in *E. coli.*

Structure of trp operon is that it contains 5 five structural genes and the *trp*L regulatory region. The length of the five genes (A to E) is 804, 1191, 1353, 1590, and 1560 nucleotide pairs. These five genes have intergenic distances of 2, 14, 6, and 2 bp, respectively between two genes starting from *trp*A gene.

Organization of the trp operon of *E. coli* indicates that –

- ✰ All these 5 genes (*trp*A to *trp*E) are located adjacently to each other;
- ✰ The *trp*R gene is not closely linked to the *trp* operon and encodes the *trp* repressor;
- ✰ The operator (O) region of the *trp* operon lies within the primary promoter (P_1) region;
- ✰ There is a weak promoter (P_2) at the operator-distal end of the *trp* D gene. This P_2 promoter increases the basal level of transcription of the *trp*A, *trp*B, and *trp*C genes;
- ✰ The two sequences of transcription (t) and termination (t′) are located downstream from *trp*A gene; and
- ✰ The *trp*L region specifies a 162 nucleotide long mRNA leader sequence.

Pathway of biosynthesis of tryptophan is shown below –

The tryptophan amino acid is produced as a result of the conversion of chorismic acid by three enzymes produced from the five structural genes (*trp A to E*) as:

Chorismic acid → 1 Anthranilic acid → 1 PRA 2 → CDRP → 2 InGP → 3 Tryptophan

1 = Antranilate synthetase ($\delta_2\ \varepsilon_2$);
2 = Indole glycerolphosphate synthetase;
3 = Tryptophane synthetase ($\alpha_2\beta_2$);
PRA = phosphoribosyl anthranilate; CDRP = carboxyphenylamino-deoxyribose phosphate;
InGP Indole-glycerol phosphate.

The *biosynthetic functions* of the five *trp* genes are:

- ✰ The *trp*A gene synthesizes the α polypeptide,
- ✰ *The trp*B gene synthesizes the β polypeptide,
- ✰ Gene *trp*C to Indole glycerolphosphate synthetase,
- ✰ Gene *trp*D synthesizes δ polypeptide, and
- ✰ Gene *trp*E synthesizes ε polypeptide.

Levels of Expression of trp Operon

The repression and attenuation are two levels for regulating the expression of *trp operon*. The ***repression*** controls the initiation of transcription whereas the ***attenuation*** controls the premature transcript termination.

(i) Repression

The ***repression*** is a process of *'turning off'* the expression of a gene or set of genes in response to some signal. A protein that binds to DNA and *'turns off'* the gene expression is called ***repressor.*** A gene that encodes a repressor is called ***repressor gene.*** An enzyme whose synthesis is diminished by a regulatory molecule is called ***repressible enzyme.***

The *trp* operon of *E. coli* is a negative repressible operon which controls the synthesis of the enzyme that catalyzes the biosynthesis of the amino acid tryptophan. The transcription of five structural genes in the *trp* operon is repressed in the presence of tryptophan in high concentration. The RNA polymerase binds to the promoter region in the absence tryptophan (a derepressed state, the co-repressor) and transcribes the structural genes of the operon. On the contrary, the co-repressor/ repressor complex binds to the operator region in the presence of tryptophan (repressed state) and prevents the initiation of the genes in the operon by the RNA polymerase. Absence of tryptophan increases the transcription rate of the *trp* operon 70 times more compared to that occurs in the presence of tryptophan.

(ii) Attenuation

The attenuation is the second mechanism for regulating gene expression by the premature termination of transcription in the leader region of a transcript in prokaryotes. This mechanism encodes enzymes involved in amino acid (tryptophan) biosynthetic pathways of tryptophan operon. Thus, the attenuation is the premature termination of the *trp* operon transcription. There are also other operons (thr, leu, phe, his, and ilu) which are regulated by this mechanism (*attenuation*).

The presence or absence of the end product (tryptophan) determines the occurrence of attenuation In case of tryptophan operon in *E. coli*. The attenuation decreases the synthesis of the tryptophan biosynthetic enzymes to the extent of 10 times.

The attenuation occurs only in the presence of tryptophan-charged tRNA ^{Trp} at a site near the end of the mRNA leader sequence (the sequence 5′ to the coding region) when tryptophan is present in the growing medium of bacteria. On occurrence of attenuation (premature termination), a truncated *trp* transcript of 140 nucleotides is produced.

The nucleotide sequence in the 5′ region of a prokaryotic gene (or in its RNA) controls the phenomenon of attenuation resulting in premature termination of transcription possibly by forming a secondary substance and hence called the ***attenuator.*** The nucleotide sequence of the attenuator is capable to terminate *trp* operon transcription. There is a bp sequence in the attenuation region (leader region of mRNA) and this sequence is identical to the transcription-termination signals at the end of operons in most of the bacteria. Thus, this sequence can base pair to form alternative hairpin structures, one of which is a typical transcription termination signal. The formation of hairpin depends on the translation of a leader peptide containing two tryptophan residues. This bp sequence contains a G:C -rich palindrome followed by several A:T base pairs. With the transcription of these termination signals a new RNA is produced which form a hydrogen-bonded hairpin structure followed by several uracils. As a result of formation of the hairpin structure there is a conformational change in associated RNA polymerase which causes the termination of transcription within more weakly hydrogen-bonded (A:U) region of DNA-RNA base-pairing. This could be explained on the basis of the followings –

- ✰ In prokaryotes, the two process of protein synthesis (transcription and translation) occurs simultaneously and so the translation events occurring can affect transcription. The ribosomes start translating the mRNAs during the time of their (mRNA) synthesis and hence translation events may affect transcription, leading to end of transcription,
- ✰ The mRNA leader sequence of 162 nucleotide long *trp* operon also contains sequences identical to the transcription-translation signals for the base-pairing to form hairpin structures (as explained above). There are 4 leader regions of nucleotides (nucleotides 60-68, 75-83, 110-121, and 126-134) to base-pair in forming the hairpin structures. The nucleotide sequences of these 4 regions can base pair in any combination. But, the base pairing of region 3 and 4 nucleotide sequences produces the transcription termination hairpin, and
- ✰ The leader sequence contains an AUG translation initiation codon, followed by 13 codons for synthesis of amino acids, and then contains the translation termination codon (UGA).

In the low concentration or absence of tryptophan, the translation of leader sequence stall at one end of the *trp* codons. This (stalling) will result the base pairing of leader regions 2 and 3 and will prevent region 3 from pairing with region 4. The base pairing of region 3 and 4 form the hairpin to stop transcription. Therefore, when there is base pairing of 2 and 3 nucleotide sequences it will not form the transcription termination hairpin structure. This is because the base pairing of 3 and 4 regions will not occur (region 1 and 4 will remain unpaired). Therefore, the transcription will continue passing the attenuator to the *trp*E gene (transcription will proceed through the entire *trp* operon and will stop at the *trp* codon which prevents the formation of the transcription-termination hairpin) in the absence or low concentration of tryptophan.

On the contrary, in the presence of sufficient tryptophan, the translation will proceed past the *trp codons* to the translation-termination codon. This process will disrupt the first hairpin (disrupting the base pairing between leaders region 2 and 3, leaving free the region 3 to base pair with region 4 to form hairpin). This forms the transcription-termination hairpin and to occur the attenuation by stopping the transcription at the attenuator sequence. This reduces the amount of mRNA for the *trp* structural genes and hence the transcription is stopped premature.

20.7 RELATION OF GENE EXPRESSION AT TRANSCRIPTION LEVEL

The fine-tuning of the gene expression is often regulated at the second stage of protein synthesis (*translation*) by modulating either the rate of initiation of polypeptide chain initiation or the rate of polypeptide chain elongation.

The mRNA molecules in prokaryotes are mostly multigenic, having for several genes the coding sequences. For example, the *lac* operon in *E. coli* has mRNA nucleotide sequences encoding three proteins (enzymes). The genes are co-transcribed and so the three genes encoding three gene products (proteins - enzymes) must be turned on and turned off together at the transcription level. However, these three gene products (enzymes) are synthesized in unequal amounts. The lactose in the growing medium of *E. coli* is used as the sole source of carbon. The *E. coli* cell on lactose rich medium contains different molar quantities of the three enzymes *viz.* 3,000 molecules of β-galactosidase, 1500 molecules of β-galactoside permease, and 600 molecules of thiogalactoside transacetylase. These different molar quantities of these different proteins (enzymes) per *E. coli* indicated their posttranscriptional control. The mRNA molecule is involved usually in all the three processes of transcription, translation, and mRNA degradation and they all occur simultaneously in prokaryotes. Therefore, the following mechanism could be responsible for different quantities produced from the same transcript (mRNA) –

- ☆ The ATG initiation codon of different genes *have unequal efficiencies of translational initiation,*
- ☆ It is quite common that intergenic regions of a transcript *altered the efficiencies of ribosome movement*. The hairpin or other forms of secondary structures that impede ribosome migration along the mRNA molecule often results into decreased translation rates, and
- ☆ The specific regions of mRNA molecules also occur at *differential rates of degradation.*

20.8 POSTTRANSCRIPTIONAL REGULATORY MECHANISMS IN PROKARYOTES

The feedback inhibition is a posttranscriptional regulatory mechanism. The ***feedback inhibition*** of gene action is different from repression. The feedback inhibition is the *end product inhibition* whereas in repression the mRNA synthesis is checked. The feedback inhibition occurs when the end product of a biosynthetic pathway is in high concentration and inhibits the activity of the first enzyme in the pathway so as the biosynthesis of the end product is arrested rapidly. The synthesis of end product also results in its arresting (blocking) if it is added to the medium.

However, the synthesis of the enzyme is not affected by this regulatory mechanism of feedback inhibition. The inhibition of the synthesis of the enzyme occurs as a result of loose binding of the end product (present in high concentration) of a biosynthetic pathway with the first enzyme in the pathway. The end product of a biosynthetic pathway often binds to and arrests the activity of the first enzyme in the pathway, which quickly blocks the synthesis of the end product. The binding modifies the tertiary structure of an enzyme and hence inactivates the catalytic site. This inhibits enzymatic activity and prevents the over production of the end products and their intermediate metabolites. For example, the amino acid isoleucine is the end product of a five step conversion of threonine (amino acid) as:

Threonine → α-ketobutyrate → acetohydroxybutyrate → dihydroxyisoleucine → α-ketoisoleucine → Isoleucine

The addition of isoleucine in the culture medium of *E. coli* blocks the threonine to isoleucine pathway because the *E. coli* uses the added isoleucine and hence the synthesis of the isoleucine in the *E. coli* is stopped.

The feedback inhibition of gene-product activity applies to the inhibition of the synthesis of another amino acid ***histidine***. When histidine is added to the growing medium of *E. coli,* its synthesis is stopped quickly long before the stopping of the synthesis of the histidine biosynthetic enzymes. The addition of histidine to the growing medium, besides turning off the synthesis of the histidine biosynthetic enzyme, also inhibits the activity of the first enzyme (N′-5′-phosphoribosyl-ATP transferase) in the histidine biosynthetic pathway by feedback mechanism.

This feedback inhibition also applies well in arresting (blocking) the synthesis of ***tryptophan*** (biosynthetic pathway) in *E. Coli.* The tryptophan is an end product of biosynthetic pathway of chorismic acid. This end product (tryptophan) is bound by the first enzyme in the pathway (anthranilate synthetase), completely stops its activity, and arrests the synthesis of tryptophan (see *trp operon*). The feedback inhibition-sensitive enzymes contain an end-product binding site(s) in addition to the substrate binding site(s). On binding the end-product, such enzymes undergo *allosteric transitions* that reduce their affinity for their substrate. The ***allosteric transition*** is a reversible interaction of a small molecule with a protein molecule that causes a change in the shape of the protein and a consequent alteration of the interaction of that protein with a third molecule. Such proteins undergoing allosteric transition are called ***allosteric proteins.***

The feedback inhibition occurs when the end product of a biosynthetic pathway is not utilized. This accumulates the end product inside the cell, causes the excess of end product, and stops the further synthesis of that substance. This results in binding of the accumulated end product (isoleucine) to the enzyme. This causes the enzyme inactivated. This inhibition phenomenon at the enzyme level is called as ***allosteric interaction.***

Chapter 21

Gene Expression – Regulation II. Eukaryotes

The gene expression (protein synthesis) in both the prokaryotes as well as in eukaryotes involves the transcription of DNA into RNA with subsequent translation of RNA into polypeptides to form proteins. However, the gene expression in prokaryotes and eukaryotes differs in the mechanism evolved.

21.1 OCCURRENCE OF PHENOMENON IN REGULATION OF GENE EXPRESSION

The different events occur in ***chronological orders*** are as under:

(i) Transcription of a gene, splicing of an RNA molecule, migration of an mRNA molecule into the cytoplasm, polypeptide synthesis, and degradation of an mRNA molecule.

(ii) The phenomena of regulation of gene expression that *occur in the **nucleus***: Stimulation of gene expression by a transcription factor, alternate splicing of the primary transcript of a gene, polyadenylation of a gene's primary transcript, silencing of gene expression by heterochromatin, and whole chromosome inactivation.

(iii) The phenomena of regulation of gene expression that *occur in the **cytoplasm***: Translation of mRNA, inhibition of translation by a microRNA binding to mRNA, degradation of mRNA induced by a short interfering RNA, and binding of a peptide hormone to its receptor.

(iv) The phenomenon of "binding of a steroid hormone to its receptor" in the regulation of gene expression may takes place in *the nucleus or cytoplasm*, depending on the particular steroid hormone.

(v) The phenomenon of histone acetylation, locus control region (human genes for β-globin), GAL4 protein (transcription factor in yeast which regulates two adjacent genes, *GAL1 and GAL10* by binding DNA sequence between them), and DNase I sensitivity (human genes for β-globin) are associated with gene activity;

(vi) The phenomenon of DNA methylation, histone methylation, and heterochromatin are associated with gene inactivity.

The term ***gene regulation*** is little bit creates confusion in mind that how it is different from *gene action* or *gene expression*. Actualy the action or expression is at the phenotypic level generalled called gene action, while the gene expression particularly is the way the genes express their action at phenotypic level which is by way of protein synthesis (Molecular genetics) through biochemical pathways (Biochemical genetics), and the gene regulation means the way the gene action or expression is controlled or regulated by various factors.

The gene regulation in eukaryotes is under the control of some structural, genetic and environmental factors. Therefore, the eukaryotic gene expression has been discussed in view of those factors controlling or regulating the gene expression under the following heads:

- ☆ Control of transcription of eukaryotic genes under some structural complexities,
- ☆ Regulation of eukaryotic gene expression in relation to chromatin organization,
- ☆ Regulation of eukaryotic gene expression in relation to Sex chromosomes,
- ☆ Regulation of eukaryotic gene expression in relation to RNA related factors,
- ☆ Regulation of eukaryotic gene expression in relation to environmental factors,
- ☆ Regulation of eukaryotic genes at transcription level,
- ☆ Regulation of eukaryotic genes at posttranscription level.

21.2 STRUCTURAL COMPLEXITIES IN CONTROL OF TRANSCRIPTION IN EUKARYOTES

The expression of eukaryotic genes is regulated in different ways from prokaryotic genes. The eukaryotes have more complexities in their body and cell structure which influence the gene regulation. The control (regulation) of gene expression in relation to those structural complexities is discussed here as under:

(I) Differences in Body Structure

The eukaryotes are mainly multi-cellular. This multi-cellular structure of eukaryotes becomes a great hurdle in intercellular communication in transcriptional regulation. The environmental signals have to pass through layers of cells to have an effect on the transcription of genes (DNA) in a specific tissue.

The eukaryotes being multi-cellular organisms have many *different types of cells viz. blood cells, nerve cells, muscular cells, skin cells, epithelial cells, brain cells, etc.* These cells are further organized into different tissues and organs. Moreover, there is an elaborate system of membranes in eukaryotic cells for which these cells are compartmentalized and thus subdivided into separate organelles, like nucleus, the mitochondria, endoplasmic reticulum (ER), and the chloroplasts (in case of plants). Such a division of eukaryotic cells into organelles with a membrane system bounds them and physically separates the events of gene expression.

All these organelles are involved in different cellular functions *viz.* the nucleus contains the genetic material, mitochondria and chloroplasts converts and store energy and known as power house of the cell, and the ER functions in transporting the materials within the cell. The different genes are expressed in different cells and hence the genes have opposite expression profile and regulated in a spatial dimension. The difference in gene expression of such multi-cellular organisms is created by their spatial regulation and underlies the complexity in their anatomy and physiology.

(II) Difference in Cell Structure

The genes are present in the nucleus which is located in between the cytoplasm and the cell surface, in eukaryotes. The environmental signals are usually received by the cell surface from where these are to be passed on to the nuclear membrane through the cytoplasm, and then to the chromosomes to have an effect on the level of transcription. This cellular structure requires more fairly elaborate internal signaling systems in controlling the transcription of DNA.

21.3 REGULATION OF EUKARYOTIC GENE EXPRESSION IN RELATION TO CHROMATIN ORGANIZATION

The DNA and protein are equally present in eukaryotic chromosomes and often called ***chromatin***. However, different chromatin parts (regions) are not only chemically different but they have different organization. The main portion of the protein part of chromatin is constituted of histones which are acetylated in some regions while the nucleotides in the DNA are metylated in other regions. Moreover, the packaging proteins (nucleosome structure) may also have a role in gene regulation.

21.3.1 Density of Chromatin Region (Euchromatin and Heterochromatin)

The transcription occurs preferably in loosely organized chromatin. The chromatin within the nucleus of the cell has variation in its density for which it causes differential staining of different portions of chromosomes. On this basis the chromatin parts are called ***heterochromatin*** which stains deeply/darkly throughout the cell cycle and the ***euchromatin*** which is lightly staining counterpart during interphase. The heterochromatin is rich in repeated DNA sequences and in transposable elements while the euchromatin may contain repeated sequences and transposons but not usually to the extent of heterochromatin. The heterochromatin has few protein-coding regions while euchromatin has many protein-coding genes.

The euchromatin part has vast majority of eukaryotic genes while the heterochromatin part is said to be genetically inactive. Not only this, but also the functional ability of the euchromatic genes is impaired by their transposition to a heterochromatic part, the genes after transposing to heterochromatin region function either abnormally or they do not function at all in some cases. This impairment in functional ability creates a mixture of normal and mutant characteristics in the same individual. This variability in phenotype is the result of the change in position of the euchromatin gene to the heterochromatin region. Such a variable condition is called as ***position-effect variegation.*** This effect is the result of changing the position of euchromatic gene and hence this term is used.

The inversion and translocation of genes or DNA segment move the euchromatic gene into the heterochromatin. Such examples of *position-effect variation* have been discovered in *Drosophila, e.g. white mottled allele* in X chromosome. There is rearrangement of wild type *white* gene by inversion with one break near the euchromatic *white* locus and other break in the heterochromatin portion. This rearrangement interfere the normal phenotype of *white* gene causing mottled-eye phenotype and produces the variegated eye colour phenotype of *Drosophila.* Thus, the euchromatic *white* gene in the heterochromatic environment (region) cannot function normally.

The position-effect variegation changed the gene expression without changing the nucleotide sequence of the gene. Further, it was observed that white patches appeared in the eye and these were clonally inherited with cell division. Such a condition is ***epigenic*** ("epi" means "above" in Greek). This is because this heritable state involving some aspects of chromatin organization near the repositioned gene other than the actual sequence of the gene regulates the gene expression. The ***epigenetic*** is a term used to the non-genetic causes of a phenotype.

It is thus obvious that the heterochromatin represses the transcription (gene function), even of a normal euchromatic gene in heterochromatic environment. The heterochromatin is associated with the repression of transcription. This is because the transcription machinery is not accessible to its condensed form (characteristic of heterochromatin). This is well evidenced from the epigenic regulation of gene expression in position-effect variegation. Thus, position-effect variegation is an example of the ***epigenetic regulation of gene***.

21.3.2 Sensitivity of Chromatin to Nuclease Enzyme

The transcriptionally active DNA is more open, sensitive, and more accessible to digestion with DNase I enzyme (nuclease attack) than nontranscriptional DNA. This nuclease sensitivity of transcriptional active genes is associated with the rate of mobility of two small nonhistone proteins during gel electrophoresis. These proteins are HMG14 and HMG17 (HMG stands for high mobility group) which have high mobility. The removal of these proteins with high mobility from the chromatin there is a loss in nuclease activity which is restored again on adding these proteins.

The sensitivity of DNA in chromatin is measured by the action of pancreatic deoxyribonuclease I (DNase I) enzyme that cleaves DNA molecules and degrades them into their constituent nucleotides. It was demonstrated by Mark Groudine and Harold Weintraub (1976) that transcriptional active DNA is more sensitive to this enzyme DNase I than non-transcribed DNA. They conducted an experiment by partially digesting the extracted chromatin from chicken RBC with DNase and analyzed the residual chromatin material for sequences of two genes. These two genes were β-globin which is actively transcribed in RBC and ovalbumin gene which is not transcriptional active. The β-globin DNA was found to be digested by DNase I enzyme to the extent of over 50 percent while the ovalbumin DNA was digested to only 10 percent. This showed that actively transcribed gene was more open (accessible) to nuclease digestion. The DNA is cleaved at a few sites by treating the isolated chromatin with a very low concentration of this enzyme. These sites are called DNase I *hypersensitive sites* some of which are present upstream of transcriptional active genes in either promoter or enhancer regions.

The human β-globulin genes are of 15-kb-long, reside in a cluster spanning 28 kb on chromosome 11, contain several DNase I hypersensitive sites that are present upstream of the genes themselves and called *locus control region* (LCR). Each of the genes in the cluster encodes slightly different polypeptides. The different genes of this cluster are expressed at different ages. The gene ε is expressed during embryonic development, two γ genes in foetal age, the δ gene in infants, and β gene is expressed in adult age. This sequential expression of genes is as per requirement of different kinds of haemoglobin at different ages of human development. Such a requirement of different kinds of haemoglobin at different ages is due to the differences in oxygen requirement, different circulatory systems, and different physical environments during embryonic, foetal, infants, and adult age. This temporal expression of β-globin genes is thus an adaptation to the changed conditions.

There are binding sites for transcription factors in the LCR of human β-globin gene cluster. These sites preactivate the individual genes for transcription as detected by an increase in the sensitivity of the DNA within the LCR to DNase digestion with its low concentration. The transcription factors that bind to specific enhancers in this β-globin gene complex stimulate the transcription of the β-globin genes. However, the sequences in the LCR decide the tissue and temporal specificity of β-globin gene expression.

The LCR as indicated from studies on transgenic mice must be present upstream of the β-globin genes as well as in its natural orientation so as to properly control the gene expression. The function of LCR is thus in a manner of an orientation-dependent whereas the function of enhancers is an orientation-independent and also in different positions relative to a gene's promoter. It is also important to know that the LCR can control the expression of β-globin gene on inserting the entire gene cluster (LCR + β-globin gene) in a different chromosomal position whereas the enhancers cannot function on transposing to a different chromosomal position. The LCR owing this property may insulate the β-globin gene from the orientation and position effects of chromatin around them.

21.3.3 Nucleosome Structure – Chromatin Remodeling

The differential sensitivity of chromatin (to digestion with nuclease enzyme DNase I) raises doubts about the transcriptional ability of DNA packaged in nucleosomes, whether the nucleosomes are open or closed when the RNA polymerase passes along the DNA template. In case if it is transcribed what could have been the structural changes in the nucleosome during transcription.

The genetic and biochemical studies together have cleared these doubts by showing the following changes in nucleosomes in preparation for transcription:

- ✫ The nucleosomes contain the already transcribed DNA, and
- ✫ The nucleosomes in transcribed DNA are changed by multiprotein complexes to facilitate the action of RNA polymerase.

This change in nucleosomes making them prepare for their transcription is known as the ***chromatin modeling.***

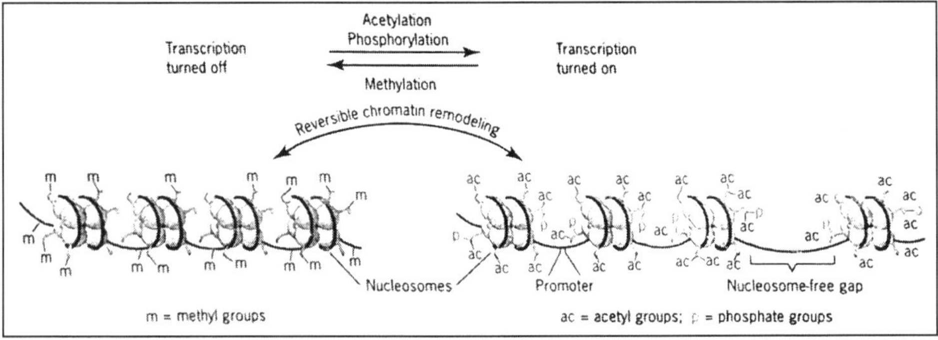

Figure 21.1: Methylation of DNA and Histones, Acetylation and Phosphorylation on Chromatin.

The chromatin is remodeled by multiprotein complexes during transcriptional activation. The ***chromatin-remodeling*** are of the following two general types -

- ✫ ***Modifications of histone H4***: There are two modifications of histone H4 to make open the chromatin for increased transcriptional activity:
  - **(a)** ***Acetylation of histones***: The enzymes (*Histone acetyl transferase, HATs*) transfer acetyl groups to the amino acid lysine at specific position in the histones of the nucleosomes. This is called acetylation of histones and it increases the gene expression, for the reason that this acetylation loosens the binding of DNA to histone octamer of nucleosome. This histone acetylation is also considered to be an *epigenetic modification* of chromatin, though its transmission pattern through cell division is not clear.
  - **(b)** ***Phosphorylation***: The enzyme *Kinases* seems to have an important role together with these chromatin-remodeling complexes to transfer phosphate groups to molecules (phosphorylation). The acetylation

of lysine-14 in histone H4 often occurs before phosphorylation of serine-10 in that molecule.

- ☆ ***Disruption of nucleosome structure*** near gene's promoter: The chromatin-remodeling complexes that disrupt nucleosome structure are the SWI/SNF complex found in baker's yeast and named after two types of mutations (switching inhibited and sucrose nonfermenter) that have discovered its constituent proteins. The humans and other eukaryotes have been observed to have the related complexes in their cells. There are at leat 8 proteins found in SWI/SNF complex. The gene regulation is controlled by the complex through sliding the histone octamers along the associated DNA in the nucleosome or the complex can transfer the octamer to other positions on a DNA molecule. Thus, there is nucleosome shifting catalyzed by this complex (SWT/SNF) and provide an access of the DNA to the transcription factors which (TF) in turn initiate the gene expression.

Reverse Remodeling of Chromatin

Like the chromatin activation it can also be remodeled into inactive chromatin. This is the reverse remodeling and it involves two biochemical modifications to the histones in nucleosome. These are -

- ☆ *Deacetylation:* It is catalyzed by the *histone deacetylases* (*HDACs*), and
- ☆ *Methylation:* It is catalysed by the *histone methyl transferase* (*HMTs*)

21.3.4 DNA Methylation

The regulation of gene expression in some of the eukaryotes particularly the mammals is important in view of chemical modification of nucleotides. There are about 40 percent G:C base pairs of the total about 3 billion bp in a particular mammalian genome out of which about 2 to 7 underwent to chemical modification. The modification is by an addition of a methyl group (CH_3) to one or more of the nucleotides in a nucleic acid (DNA or RNA). This addition of methyl group to nucleotide is called ***methylation***. The methylated cytosine are found in base-pair doublets with structure as:

5′ mCpG 3′
3′ GpCm 5′

where,

mC = Methylcytosine,
P = Phosphodiester bond between adjacent nucleotides in each DNA strand.

The restriction enzymes which are sensitive to chemical modifications of their recognition sites are used to digest DNA so as to detect the methylated CpG dinucleotides. This is because the methylated and unmethylated DNAs produce different patterns of restriction fragments on digesting with this enzyme. The restriction enzyme (Hpa II) recognizes and cleaved the sequence CCGG but on methylation of second cytosine in this sequence, this enzyme fails to cleave the sequence.

The CpG rich segments are of about 1 to 2 kb long and called ***CpG islands.*** These are clusters of cytosines and guanines that often occur upstream of human genes. There are about 30,000 CpG islands mostly near the transcription start point in human genome and the cytosines in these islands are rarely methylated. It is to remember that unmethylated condition is conducive to transcription whereas the ***methylated DNA*** is associated with transcription repression (turning off the expression of gene). The DNA near CpG island is hypersensitive to digestion with DNase, with somewhat different nucleosome than present elsewhere in the genome, with less histone H1, and acetylated some core histones

The transcriptional repression is observed in female mammals in case the inactive X chromosome is extensively methylated. The chromatin region with repeatable sequences and also rich in transposable elements are also methylated. This property provides a way to protect from adverse effect of transposon expression and movement. Most probably, two proteins that repress transcription bind to methylated DNA and one of them (meCP2) cause changes in chromatin structure. It is thus possible that methylated CpG dinucleotides bind specific proteins forming a complex which prevent the transcription of nearby genes. The methylation of DNA is associated with gene silencing in mammals.

The DNA methylation is transmitted in every round of DNA replication, though the methylated state is transmitted clonally through cell division but when a DNA

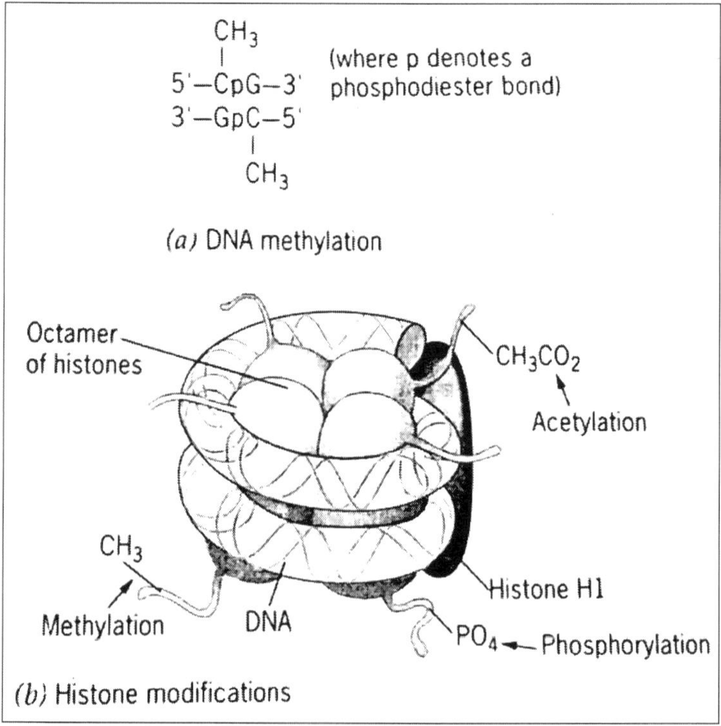

Figure 21.2: Chemical Modifications of (a) DNA and (b) Histones in Chromatin Modelling.

sequence is methylated both strands of the sequence acquire methyl groups. The DNA replication produces one methylated parental strand and one unmethylated strand. However, the enzyme methyl transferase recognizes this asymmetry and adds a methyl group to the unmethylated DNA strand. Thus, DNA methylation is an ***epigenetic modification*** of chromatin.

In this context of epigenetic modification, it should be noted that the genetically identical twins with their origin from a single fertilized egg (monozygotic twins) also become epigenetically different to the extent to which they share life experiences. Two types of ***epigenetic modifications*** (*DNA methylation* and *histone acetylation*) were examined in the chromatin of WBC of identical twins in Spain (Fraga and coworkers, 2005). The studies have indicated that about 1/3 of the total identical twins studied had notable differences in the overall levels of DNA methylation and histone acetylation and the differences increased along age and among pairs who shared less of their life together or those having different health histories. The differences in DNA methylation were distributed throughout the genome but localized to the telomeres and gene-rich regions like long and short arms of chromosome 1, short arm of chromosome 3, and the long arm of chromosome 8. The twins with the same genotype can have different "epigenotypes" which lead to epigenetic differences, probably due to their different life histories (person' experience – diet, social and physical activities, medical treatments, exposure to different environments and so on, may play their role in shaping the "epigenome" which decides the way the genome is expressed. Another project on "Epi-twin" is in progress since 2010 to study epigenetic modifications.

21.3.5 Imprinting – Sex of Parent Transmitting the Gene

The imprinting is a process that alters the state of a gene without altering its nucleotide sequence, which is often associated with methylation of specific nucleotide in the gene. The altered gene is established in the germ line and is transmitted to the offspring where it may persist throughout the offspring's life.

In some unusual cases, the gene expression is controlled by the sex of the parent which transmitted that gene or say that the gene expression is controlled by its parental origin, *i.e.* whether the gene under expression has been transmitted by male or female parent. For example, in mice, the ***Igf2 gene*** (which encodes an insulin –like growth factor) is expressed if transmitted by the male parent (father) rather than from female parent (mother). Likewise another gene designated as ***H19*** is expressed if transmitted by the mother and not from the father. In this way a gene is altered and it is said that the gene has been ***imprinted*** which indicates that from which parent the gene has come in the progeny. Thus, the gene is marked in some way that from which parent the gene has come.

The DNA methylation in mammals is also responsible for such an unusual expression of gene. The mark that conditions the expression of a gene is methylation of one or more CpG dinucleotides near the gene. Initially the parental germ line forms these methylated dinucleotides. Therefore, the gene is methylated in the opposite parental germ line. For example, the Igf2 gene which is expressed for being transmitted from the father means that this Igf2 gene is methylated in the female germ line but remained unmethylated in male germ line. The embryo at fertilization contains one methylated and one unmethylated allele and this state is preserved during RNA replication. The developing animal will express the paternally transmitted Igf2 gene because the gene contributed maternally is methylated and hence remain silent without its expression. On the contrary, the H19 gene is methylated in male germ line while the gene is unmethylated in female germ line. The number of such imprinted genes identified in mice and humans have reached more than 20 for each of which the methylation imprint has been established in the parental germ line. However, the methylation imprints are reset each generation depending on the sex of the animal. Thus, a methylated gene inherited from one sex can be unmethylated if it passes through an offspring of the opposite sex. The sex-dependent methylation of gene means that sex-specific factors control the methylation machinery.

21.4 REGULATION OF EUKARYOTIC GENE EXPRESSION IN RELATION TO SEX CHROMOSOMES: DOSAGE COMPENSATION MECHANISMS

There are normally two dosage of each gene except for sex-linked genes (the genes present on sex chromosomes). Two members of the sex chromosome are different in two sexes, in organisms having XX/XY or XX/XO sex determination system. The two sex chromosomes are not genetically identical and hence not homologous. The female of these organisms have two dosages of X-linked genes due to having two X-chromosomes whereas the males have a single dose of sex-linked genes because of having only one X-chromosome. Thus, there is an imbalance in the number of genes in the two sexes and hence the animal development is uaually sensitive to this difference of dosage of genes. This imbalance due to deviation from normal condition of two dosages of each gene can cause abnormality in either way of developing good or bad phenotype of the individual having one extra or one less X chromosome. The loss or excess of chromosomes may be in the autosomes as well as in the sex chromosomes.

The rarely occurred conditions of one extra or lesser chromosome in human, *Drosophila,* and other species, ard their consequences for the development of abnormal phenotypes (syndromes) in such individuals has been discussed in chapter 11.

The reason of one extra or one less X chromosome lies in the sex determination mechanism that females have two dose of X-chromosome against single dose of X-chromosome in males. The mammals, flies (*Drosophila*), and nematodes (*C. elegans*) have XY chromosome mechanism of sex determination and hence face a problem of numerical difference of X-linked genes between two sexes.

The problem of development of abnormal phenotype due to unequal numbers of X-linked gene dosage could be solved to compensate this numerical difference in X-chromosomes by adapting either of the following mechanisms to increase or decrease the activity of X-linked gene:

☆ One copy of each of X-linked gene to become genetically *inactive* in females,

- ✰ Each X-linked gene to become genetically *twice more active* (increase in activity), and
- ✰ Each of two X-linked genes to become *partially inactivated* genetically.

Actually this problem has been solved by nature in different ways, called as the ***dosage compensation mechanisms*** of X-linked genes. The *dosage compensation* is a phenomenon in which the activity of a gene is increased or decreased according to the number of copies of that gene in the cell. There are three dosage compensation mechanisms, *viz. inactivation, hyperactivation, and hypoactivation* of X-chromosome in different species.

21.4.1 Inactivation of X-chromosome in Mammals

In mammals one of the two X - chromosomes in females (XX) becomes inactivated randomly in the somatic cells during early stage of development. The X - chromosome inactivated once remain inactivatedin all the descendants of that cell. This equalizes the number of transcriptionally active X-linked genes. The mechanism of inactivation was proposed by a British geneticist Mary Lyon in 1961 based on the studies on mice and hence called as ***Lyon's hypothesis***.

One of the two X chromosomes looks and acts differently from other chromosomes. This condenses into a darkly staining mass associated with the nuclear membrane and this mass of chromatin is called the ***Barr body*** after Canadian geneticist Murray Barr, its discoverer. Secondly, this X chromosome is genetically inactive. The inactive X chromosome is easily identified in mammalian cells due to its condensation. This Barr body of condensed mass of X chromosome is found in the nuclei of placental mammals. However, the inactivated chromosome in germ cells is reactivated during meiosis for meeting the requirement of pairing for oogenesis. Thus, it decondenses during S phase of cell cycle so as the inactive X chromosome is replicated. But, there is late replication of inactive X chromosome than other chromosome due to the reason that decondensation is time taking. This shows that this inactive X chromosome has somewhat different chromatin structure than other chromosomes. The chemical analysis has indicated that the DNA of this inactivated X chromosome is modified by the addition of numerous methyl groups.

There is a particular site of inactivation in X chromosome in mammals, called the X *inactivation Center* (XIC). This particular site starts spreading in opposite directions towards the ends of the chromosome. However, all the genes are not inactivated but one gene remains active and this is called XIST (X inactive specific transcript) which is present near the XIC.

The XIST gene in humans encodes a 17-kb transcript which has no significant open reading frames and hence it may not encode for a protein. But the functional product of this XIST gene is the RNA itself which though polyadenylated is restricted to the nucleus and remains localized specifically to inactivated X chromosome. Thus, this RNA is not associated with any active X chromosome either in male or female.

The homologue of human XIST gene in female mice is said to be transcribed during early age at low level from both of the X chromosome. However, the transcripts from each of a female mouse's **Xist** genes are not stable but remains linked with their genes. With the advances in age of mice, the transcript from one of the genes is stabilized enveloping the entire X chromosome having that gene. There is disintegration of the transcripts from other *Xist* gene and hence its transcription is repressed as a result of methylation of nucleotides in the promoter of the gene. Thus, in female mouse, one X chromosome (whose *Xist* gene continues to be transcribed) becomes coated with *Xist RNA* while the other is not affected. Any of the two X chromosomes may become coated randomly and its mechanism is not known. The coating results into repression of most of the genes of the coated chromosome and hence turning this chromosome as genetically inactive. The X chromosome repressing its *Xist* gene remains active in this mammalian dosage compensation system.

21.4.2 Hyperactivation of X-chromosome in *Drosophila*

Another kind of mechanism for dosage compensation occurs in *Drosophila* but it occurs in males than in females, contrary to that among mammals. The single X chromosome in male flies becomes genetically more active (hyperactive). This is acheived by transcribing the genes present on the single X chromosome in male *Drosophila* more vigorously (increase in activity of gene) so as to compensate the output of the genes present on two X chromosomes in female *Drosophila*. The genes present on single X chromosome in male *Drosophila* is hyperactivated so that its genes are as active as the double dose of X-linked genes located on two X chromosomes of females.

The dosage compensation needs the gene products (proteins) of five different genes called the dosage compensation genes or male-specific lethal (***msl***) loci. The gene products of these genes are called as MSL proteins. Each of the MSL proteins binds specifically only to the X chromosome in males but do not bind to other chromosomes either in the male or any chromosome in the female's genome. This binding is allowed by two types of RNA molecules (called roX1 and *ro*X2, indicating RNA on the X chromosome) which are transcribed from genes on the X chromosome. The **ms*l*** gene is not functional in females.

A complex MSL proteins joined with *ro*X RNAs is formed and binds at 30 – 40 sites on the male' X chromosome. The MSL/*ro*X complex spreads bidirectionally on the X chromosome and involves in chromatin remodeling required for the process of hyperactivation. One of the MSL proteins is a histone acetyl transferase and the acetylated form of histone H4 is exclusively associated with hyperactivated X chromosome. Thus, the RNA-protein complex through binding at many sites on single X chromosome in male *Drosophila* mediates its hyperactivation and stimulates the transcription of its genes more vigorously.

21.4.3 Hypoactivation of X-chromosome in Nematode

There is another mechanism present in nematode (*C. elegans*) for dosage compensation of unequal numbers of X – linked genes. This nematode differs with respect to X chromosomes distribution between sexes. This is because the individuals with two X chromosomes (XX individuals) are hermaphrodites, functioning as both male and female whereas the XO individuals are males. The dosage compensation mechanism for X-linked transcriptional activity equalizes these two genotypes by partial repression of the genes on both of the X chromosome of somatic cells of hermaphrodites. The two X chromosomes (XX) in hermaphrodite worms are hypoactivated.

The products of several genes (proteins) seem to be involved in this mechanism through their binding specifically to the X chromosomes, though they may bind when both X chromosomes are present in a hermaphrodite state but do not bind either to the single X chromosome or any of the autosomes (males or hermaphrodites). This mechanism is thus exactly opposite that involved in *Drosophila*. The hyperactivation of the two X chromosomes in this worm's hermaphrodites is mediated by proteins that bind to these chromosomes and reduce the transcription of their genes. Thus, a protein complex binds to the X chromosomes and represses instead of enhancing the transcription.

21.5 CONTROL OF EUKARYOTIC GENE ACTION IN RELATION TO RNA RELATED FACTORS

The primary event of gene expression is the transcription of DNA into RNAs (mRNAs) which occurs in the nucleus. Some factors related to RNA have their effect on regulation of genes:

21.5.1 RNA Processing: Modification in RNA

The prokaryotic RNAs do not undergo the terminal and internal modifications like those in eukaryotic cells. The eukaryotic RNA is processed before its translation. This processing of RNA of the eukaryotes includes:

- ✰ Capping of RNA at its 5′ end,
- ✰ Polyadenylation at its 3′ end (addition of poly A tails to eukaryotic gene transcript, RNA), and
- ✰ Change made internally by losing its non-coding sequences (*introns*).

The RNA transcripts (mRNA) undergo modification in the nucleus, called as RNA processing of eukaryotes *viz.* capping, polyadenylation, and removal of introns. This resulting messenger RNA are then exported to the cytoplasm to associate with the ribosomes, many of them are present on ER membrane. Now, the mRNAs after associated with ribosomes, are translated into polypeptides. Thus, the regulation of gene expression occurs at different locations in the cell as a result of physical separation of the events of gene expression. The gene regulation can occur in the nucleus at either the DNA or RNA level or it may occur in the cytoplasm at either the RNA or polypeptide level. Therefore, the eukaryotic gene expression can be regulated at different levels of the transcription, processing, or translation.

Similar to prokaryotes, the protein-DNA interactions become mediators in regulation of gene transcription in eukaryotes. The specific regions of the DNA are bound by the positive and negative regulator proteins in order to either stimulate or inhibit the gene transcription. Therefore, these proteins are called ***transcription factors***. These transcription factors (proteins) interact with DNA to control the transcription in eukaryotes. These proteins (transcription factors) are of many types and have some special characteristics by which they interact with the DNA.

21.5.2 Differential Splicing Pattern of RNA – Removal of Introns

The introns are the noncoding regions possessed by most of the genes in eukaryotes. These introns interrupt the nucleotide sequences in not to specify the amino acids of a polypeptide. Therefore, the removal of these introns from RNA transcript of a gene is essentially required so as the nucleotide coding sequences are expressed properly. The process of removing the introns is known as ***splicing*** of RNA and it involves the precise covalent joining of the coding sequences (exons, expressed sequences) into mRNA as discussed under section 16.6. Three types of intron excision mechanisms (splicing systems) from RNA transcripts have been discussed there.

Alternate Splicing

The way of interaction of the splicing machinery with the RNA decides the removal of introns individually or in combination. The removal of two introns together will automatically remove the exons in between them and hence there are chances of modification of coding sequence of RNA due to deletion of exon. The transcripts of larger genes are splitted in different ways (*alternate splicing*) to create a large array of mRNAs and making it possible for a single gene to code different but related polypeptides. This contributes to the variability of cell action due to the different forms of the spliced gene. The transcription of the gene for troponin T (a protein found in the skeletal muscle of vertebrate having 150 to 250 amino acids) is an example of alternate splicing. The troponin T gene in rat is of more than 16 kb long containing 18 exons. On splicing the transcript of this gene in different ways produce a large array of mRNAs. Many different troponin T polypeptides are produced on translation of these mRNAs. These different forms of troponin T function in slightly different ways within the muscle.

21.5.3 Differential Stability of mRNA

The mRNAs are synthesized from DNA template in the nucleus from where they ate transported through nuclear pores to the cytoplasm. These serve as template for polypeptide synthesis in the cytoplasm. Here in the cytoplasm, a particular mRNA is translated by several ribosomes which move along it in sequential way. Now, it is the turn for the degradation of mRNA after the translational assembly. The mRNA degradation during the process of gene expression is another control point. The stability or longevity of different mRNAs is different depending on the number of rounds of polypeptide synthesis. Some mRNAs support multiple rounds and called as long-lived mRNAs while others are short-lived which cannot take multiple rounds of polypeptide synthesis.

In order of continuous synthesis of the polypeptide encoded by the rapidly degraded mRNA, it is essential that it is replenished (filled up again) by additional transcript. However, the polypeptide after exercising its effect is no longer required because of its continuous synthesis may be harmful. Therefore, in such cases, the rapid degradation of mRNA is reasonable to prevent the synthesis of undesirable polypeptide. The stability or longevity of mRNA is affected by some cytoplasmic factors -

- ☆ *Poly (A) tails*: The mRNAs seem to be stabilized by poly (A) tails,
- ☆ *Sequence of 3′ untranslated region, preceding a poly (A) tail:* These influence the mRNA stability. Several short-lived mRNAs have a sequence AUUUA which is repeated several times in their 3′ untranslated regions. The longer lived (stable) mRNAs become unstable on artificially transferring this highly repeatable sequence to the 3′ untranslated region of more stable mRNAs,
- ☆ *Chemical factors*: The stability of mRNA seems to be affected by hormones. The steroid hormone estrogen transcriptionally activates a gene (*vetellogenin*) in the toad *Xenopus laevis* as well as increases the stability of its mRNA besides inducing the transcription of this gene,
- ☆ *Small noncoding RNA molecules* (siRNAs or miRNAs): The stability of mRNAs and their translation into polypeptides has also been recently revealed to be regulated by the small noncoding RNA molecules that are small interfering RNAs (siRNAs) or micro RNAs (miRNAs). These are small RNA molecules of about 21 to 28 nucleotides long and produced from longer and double stranded RNAs in many eukaryotes like animals, plants, and fungi. The siRNAs target mRNA molecules which are devoid of introns. Thus, if siRNA were made from double-stranded RNA derived from an intron, it would be ineffective against an mRNA target. These small RNA molecules base-pair with sequences in specific mRNAs. On base pairing, these small mRNAs molecules act in two ways. They either cause the cleavage and subsequent degradation of mRNA or prevent the mRNA to translate them into polypeptide. The small RNA molecules have their important role to play in both plants and animals. They provide in plants the critical defense against RNA viral infection and also regulate in plants and animals the gene expression during maturation and development.

21.6 GENE REGULATION IN RELATION TO ENVIRONMENTAL FACTORS

Attempts have been made to identify the specific inducers of eukaryotic gene expression following the research findings on *lac* operon of *E. coli* by Jacob and Monod (1961). The findings have indicated that the effect of environmental and nutritional factors on induction of eukaryotic genes was not to the extent as it was in case of prokaryotic genes. The ***environment*** is the aggregate of all the conditions and influences that affect the life and development of an organism. The effects of heat shock, hormones, and other proteins that are not hormones in transcriptional activity of eukaryotic genes have been cited below:

21.6.1 Temperature Effect: Heat Induced Transcription

Sometimes the organisms face the heat stress. Under the stress of high temperature, the organism respond to stabilize the internal cellular environment by synthesizing a group of proteins, called as *heat-shock proteins.* These proteins are found in both prokaryotes and eukaryotes with about 40 to 50 per cent identity in amino acid sequences of these heat-shock proteins in *E. coli* and *Drosophila* and these proteins are among the most conserved known polypeptides.

The heat stress specifically induces the transcription of the genes (heat-shock genes) encoding the heat-shock proteins. Thus, the expression of these proteins is regulated at the transcription level. A family of genes has been found to be present in two nearby clusters on one of the autosomes in *Drosophila* and encode one of the heat-shock proteins called *HSP* 70 (heat-shock protein with molecular weight of 70 kilodaltons). The *hsp 70* gene has its 5 to 6 copies in two clusters and induced by heat stress. Each of the genes in cluster is transcribed into RNA when the temperature exceeds 33°C. The RNA transcript is exported to the cytoplasm and translated to produce HSP 70 polypeptides. There is present a polypeptide called heat-shock transcription factor (HSTF) in the nuclei of *Drosophila* cells. This polypeptide (HSTF) mediates the heat induced transcription of the *bsp* 70 genes. The HSTF is altered chemically under heat stress by phosphorylation. This alteration in HSTF results in its binding specifically to the nucleotide sequences upstream of the *bsp* 70 genes. The nucleotide sequences of *bsp* 70 genes to which the phosphorylated HSTF binds are called *heat-shock response elements* (*HSEs*). The binding between the two (*HSEs* and *phosphorylated HSTF*) makes the genes more accessible to RNA polymerase II. This enzyme is responsible to transcribe the most protein-encoding genes.

21.6.2 Hormones Induced Signals

In eukaryotes there is a system of sending inter-cellular signals by secreting a ***hormone.*** The hormones through their circulation in the body come in contact to the specific target cells and then regulate the expression of particular genes through initiating a series of events. There are two types of hormones secreted in animals, *viz. steroid hormones* and *peptide hormones.*

(a) Steroid Hormones

These are small, with lipid nature, and lipid-soluble molecules derived from cholesterol. So they have little or no trouble to pass through cell membranes. In this group of hormones are the:

(i) Female hormones *viz.* estrogen and progesterone that play important roles in female reproductive cycles,

(ii) Male hormone *viz.* testosterone for male differentiation and behavior,

(iii) Glucocorticoids that are involved in regulating the level of blood sugar, and

(iv) Ecdysone, a hormone to control developmental events in insects.

These hormones after entering into the cell interact with the cytoplasmic or nuclear protein, called ***hormone receptors***. These hormone receptors or complexes interact with DNA and act as transcription factors to regulate the expression of certain genes.

(b) Peptide Hormones

These are the linear chains of amino acids, encoded by genes, *e.g.* ***insulin*** (regulate blood sugar levels), ***somatotropin*** (growth hormone), and ***prolactin*** (target tissues in the breast of female mammals). These hormones cannot pass freely through cell membranes because of their large size and hence their signals are transmitted to the interior of cells by *membrane-bound receptor proteins.* The peptide hormone interacts with its receptor and causes a conformational change in the receptor which leads to bring changes in other proteins inside the cell. Such changes activate the hormonal signaling system to regulate the expression of certain genes through the cytoplasm into the nucleus (called ***signal transduction***).

The specific nucleotide sequences in the DNA called *hormone response elements, HREs, are* analogous to *HSEs,* mediate the hormone-induced gene expression, located near the genes they regulate, and serve to bind the specific proteins, which then act as transcription factors.

(c) Proteins that are not Hormones

There are other kinds of proteins that are not hormones (because they are not produced by a particular gland or organ) also induce the transcriptional activity. These are the secreted, circulated molecules like nerve growth factor, epidermal growth factor, and platelet-derived growth factor, and other non-circulating molecules associated with cell surface or with the matrix between cells. However, the general mechanism to induce transcription by these proteins resembles to that of the peptide hormones.

21.7 REGULATION OF EUKARYOTIC GENES AT TRANSCRIPTION LEVEL

The transcription is the first stage in gene expression and hence it is the fundamental level to control the gene expression in both prokaryotes and eukaryotes. The DNA sequences within or near the genes interact with proteins to regulate the transcription of eukaryotic genes.

21.7.1 DNA Sequences Involved in Transcription

The gene contains a region called *promoter,* the place for initiation of transcription and recognized by RNA polymerase. The initiation of transcription requires several accessory proteins or ***basal transcription factors.*** The binding of each of these proteins to a sequence within the promoter is needed in order of proper alignment of the RNA polymerase on the template strand of DNA. There are some *special transcription factors* like those involved in heat- shock and hormone-inducible genes, to control the transcription of eukaryotic genes. The transcriptional activity of a gene is regulated when these special transcription factors bind to response elements (the sequences called ***enhancers*** present near the gene) and interact with the basal transcription factors and the RNA polymerase (which bind to the promoter of a gene).

The ***enhancers and promoters are different.*** The ***promoter*** is a nucleotide sequence to which RNA polymerase binds and initiates transcription. The promoters are present immediately upstream of the gene and function only in one orientation. The ***enhancer*** may be a major or modifier gene that increases a physiological process; or it may be a DNA sequence that affects transcription of a nearby gene. The enhancers have three properties to act over a considerably large distances (up to several thousand bp from their regulated genes) and their effects on gene expression are neither influenced by their position (position-independent: upstream, downstream or within an intron of a gene) or by their orientation (orientation-independent: they function normally in both normal as well as in inverted orientation) within the DNA to regulate transcription from a gene promoter. The transcription factors recognize and bind to specific sequence within enhancers.

Moreover, the enhancers are relatively long (several hundred bp long) containing sometimes repeated sequences and most enhancers function in a tissue-specific to stimulate the transcription only in certain tissues. The example of tissue specificity can be cited of the *yellow* gene in *Drosophila*. This gene produces pigmentation in many parts of the body (wings, legs, thorax, and abdomen). This yellow gene is regulated by several enhancers and each enhancer activates transcription in a different tissue. The mutations alter the transcription of the yellow gene in some tissues producing different colouration in some tissues but not in others.

21.7.2 Transcription Factors Involved in Transcription

A large number of eukaryotic proteins, called ***transcription factors*** have been observed to stimulate transcription in eukaryotes. Most of these proteins have two important chemical regions. One is a DNA-binding and another is a transcriptional activation region. These two domains (regions) may either be located on separate parts of the molecule or may be overlapped.

The DNA-binding domain in *yeast* is located near the amino terminus of the polypeptide in the ***GAL4*** transcription factor while one of the two transcription activation regions is in the middle and other is near the carboxy terminus. The transcription factors in animals are the steroid hormone receptor proteins. They have the DNA-binding region in the centre while the transcriptional activation region that extends towards the amino terminus seems to be overlapped by DNA-binding domain. There is also a third domain (region) in steroid hormone receptors to specifically bind the steroid hormone.

The transcriptional factor that is bound to an enhancer has important role to induce the transcriptional activation and to make easy the way for RNA polymerase to initiate transcription for conformational changes in the assembled proteins. The transcription activation domain of the factor follows either of the two ways – one by contacting with one or more proteins at other enhancers and second by interacting directly with proteins which are bound in the promoter region.

Structural Motifs

There are characteristic predominating features in the structure (***structural motifs***) of many eukaryotic transcription factors. These motifs are the polypeptides formed as a result of associations between amino acids within their polypeptide chains. The different structural motifs of transcription factors are called *zinc finger,* *helix-turn-helix, leucine zipper, and helix-loop-helix.* These motifs are the short peptide loop or stretch of amino acids. These are:

- ☆ *Zinc finger motif* is a short polypeptide loop formed by jointly binding a zinc ion with two cysteins in one part of polypeptide and 2 histidines in another part. These finger motifs have their role in DNA binding,
- ☆ *Helix-turn-helix motif* is an extension of three short helices of amino acids separated from each other by turns. The helical segment close to the carboxy terminus is needed for DNA binding while other helices form protein dimers. This motif coincides with a highly conserved region of about 60 amino acids called ***homeodomain*** due to their encoding by the homeotic genes of *Drosophila.* The mutations in the homeotic genes change the developmental fates of a group of cells (*antennae* are caused to develop as *legs*). This is a bizarre (odd) phenotype, an example of homeotic transformation (substitution one body part for another during the course of development). Each homeotic gene in *Drosophila* encodes a protein *with a homeodomain* and these proteins bind to DNA. The homeodomain proteins stimulate the transcription of a particular genes during development,
- ☆ There is a stretch (extension) of amino acids with a leucine at every seventh position in transcription factors. The polypeptides with this structural feature (motif) called *Leucine zipper* form dimmers by interactions between the leucines in each of their zipper regions. The zipper sequence is adjacent to a positively charged stretch of amino acids. On interacting two zippers the charged regions form a surface to negatively charged DNA,
- ☆ *Helix-loop-helix* is a fourth structural motif which is an extension of two helical regions of amino acids separated by a nonhelical loop. These proteins are denoted *basic HLH* (*helix-loop-helix*) *or bHLH proteins.*

The transcription factors with dimerization motifs like zipper or HLH form homodimers by combining with polypeptides like themselves or heterodimers when combined with different polypeptides. This later combination achieves the complex patterns of gene expression. The activation by a heterodimer decides the transcription factor of a gene in a particular tissue. This heterodimer is formed only in case its constituent polypeptides are synthesized in that tissue.

21.8 REGULATION OF EUKARYOTIC GENES AT POSTRANSCRIPTION LEVEL

Some posttranscriptional mechanisms have also been found to be involved in regulating the expression of eukaryotic genes. The small noncoding RNA molecules (*See Section 13.4.1* (*II, e*) that are small interfering RNAs (siRNAs) or micro RNAs (miRNAs) are involved in the phenomenon of RNA interference.

These small RNA molecules in the cytoplasm base-pair with target sequence in mRNA molecules (complementary or partially complementary mRNAs) and interfere in gene expression by either causing their (mRNAs) degradation or repression of their translation. This is called ***RNA interference*** (***RNAi***) of posttranscriptional gene regulation. Thus, the short noncoding RNAs interact with mRNAs produced by these genes and regulate the expression of eukaryotic genes. The interaction is mediated by base-pairing between the single strand RNA in the RNA-protein complex and a complementary sequence in the mRNA molecule. The RNA-protein particle is called an **RNA-Induced Silencing Complex** (*RISC*) because this interaction prevents the expression of gene (that produced the mRNA). On base-pairing between the RNA within the RISC and the target sequence in the mRNA, the RISC cleaves the mRNA in the middle of base-paired region. The cleaved mRNA is then degraded. The RISC behaves like a catalyst and is capable repeatedly to target and cleave mRNA. The translation of mRNA is inhibited even when the base-pairing between RNA within RISC with its target sequence is imperfect because the mRNA is not usually cleaved. The RISC –associated RNAs with this effect of inhibition of translation of mRNAs are called ***microRNAs.*** This phenomenon has been observed in many eukaryotic organisms like humans, *Drosophila,* Arabidopsis, and *Caenorhabditis elegans* (nematodes).

Chapter 22

Gene Expression – Biochemical Pathway (Biochemical Genetics)

The study of genetics with biochemistry to explain the nature of metabolic pathways and their control is called as *biochemical genetics.* Thus, Biochemical Genetics is the study of biochemical pathways of gene function.

The biochemical (metabolic or biosynthetic) pathway constitutes all the steps involved in transforming a precursor to its end product for expression of a trait and each step of the path is catalyzed by a specific enzyme which is synthesized under the control of a gene. There is a long path between gene and final product, the primary gene product is the mRNA which is complementary to the DNA and controls the assemblage of amino acids to form enzymes at the surface of ribosomes. Therefore, the phenotypic expression of any character is not a direct effect of a gene (portion of DNA) but it is accomplished by the developmental and biochemical processes through the synthesis of proteins which are under the direct control of genes. Among the proteins synthesized by the genes, some are enzymes and control biosynthetic pathways. Therefore, the genes control the expression of characters by controlling the developmental and biochemical activities of the cells through the enzymes which are synthesized by genes. It was shown by Beadle and Tatum (1941) that the genes express themselves through the synthesis of ENZYMES. For example, a dominant gene which is the wild type (original gene) synthesizes the enzyme required for the expression of a normal character whereas a recessive gene is unable to synthesize that functional enzyme and so unable to express that phenotype but behaved differently expressing the modified phenotype.

22.1 BIOCHEMICAL PATHWAY OF GENE ACTION

The best known example of gene-enzyme relation is the metabolism of the amino acids, phenylalanine and tyrosine, in man. The phenylalanine is an essential amino acid of human dietary proteins and it may be incorporated into cellular proteins or converted to phenylpyruvic acid or tyrosine. The following metabolic and inherited disorders are caused by the improper functioning of the enzymes involved in the metabolism of phenylalanine and tyrosine (defective metabolism), as a result of mutant genes which are autosomal recessives in homozygous condition. These disorders are caused by mutations in genes encoding the necessary enzymes that control steps in single metabolic pathway of phenylalanine-tyrosine metabolism.

The ultimate result of gene expression is the development of a character in terms of its phenotype. The main function of genes to produce phenotype is through protein synthesis which involves a series of the chemical reactions controlled by enzymes. Thus, there is involvement of several chemical reactions in carrying out the functions of a cell.

Enzyme Production

The production of enzymes/proteins is controlled by genes. The genes produce enzymes mainly as their way of functioning. These enzymes are involved in different steps of metabolism. All these chemical reactions need specific enzymes to work as catalysts for performing the reaction.

The chemical reaction has two requirements of the presence of a catalyst and the energy.

- ☆ The enzymes act as catalysts in initiating the chemical reaction and the energy acts as the power to perform and complete the chemical reaction. The specific reaction requires specific enzyme. The enzymes are proteins composed of amino acid subunits. Each enzyme is a specific protein and is composed of a particular number and sequence of amino acids. The number and sequence of amino acids are different for different enzymes. It is the enzyme that make possible for an individual that which type of reaction is needed to proceed for performing a particular function.
- ☆ The adenosine-triphosphate (ATP) is a single energy level compound, in all living organisms, which react with innumerable compounds and causes them to take part in reaction. The ATP molecule is like a nucleotide molecule in the sense that ATP consists of adenine, ribose sugar but three phosphate groups instead of one phosphate group as in case of nucleotide. The second and third phosphate groups are bound by a high energy bond. The ATP has one low and two high energy phosphate bonds, depending on the amount of energy liberation. An individual utilizes high energy bond between the second and third phosphate group in chemical reaction.

The genes determine the sequence of amino acids in a polypeptide chain of protein molecule. The polypeptide chain contains the information in the form of genetic code which is the triplet sequence of nitrogen bases in mRNA molecule which has copied the same from DNA molecule. The mechanism of gene action (function) has been explained based on two theories of *one gene one enzyme* and *one gene one polypeptide.*

(i) One Gene One Enzyme Theory

Beadle and Tatum (proposed this theory based on their work on red mold (*Neurospora crassa*) and got Noble Prize in 1958. They proposed that each gene in an organism controls the production of a specific enzyme. This organism Neurospora grows on minimal medium of sucrose, salts and one of the vitamin B (biotin). All other complex substances of the culture medium are synthesided by this organism. Specific enzymes are involved in carrying out the biochemical synthetic reactions.

The asexual spores of this organism were exposed by them to UV rays (mutagen). These mutated ascospores failed to grow in the minimal medium and required the addition of ***thiamine*** for the normal growth. The mating of the mutated forms with a normal form produced asci which had 4 mutated and 4 normal ascospores. These were grown in a minimal medium containing thiamine and transferred (after their multiplication and establishment their colonies) to tubes without having thiamine. All of the transferred spores devoid of thiamine in the tubes failed to grow. This showed that the mutant form in which some specific gene has mutated could not synthesize thiamine necessary for the enzyme production.

Beadle and Tautam in their controlled experiment have shown that thiamine synthesis from simple substance of minimal medium is completed in a number of steps, requires the presence of a specific enzyme at each step, and each enzyme is produced by a separate gene. Synthesis of this vitamine involves many chemical reactions each of which is controlled by a specific enzyme produced by a specific gene. This way, the requirements to produce the final products are the raw material in the medium, genes to synthesize the enzymes and the intermediated products. These geneticists, by adding intermediate compounds (precursors) to the medium, were able to locate the particular step in thiamine synthesis which was blocked in the mutant strain in which specific enzyme was not produced. Thus, they presented this theory of 'one gene one enzyme' which could explain some of the human hereditary diseases described earlier by Garrod (1908) as *inborn errors of metabolism, e.g.* Alkaptonuria (urine of patients of this hereditary disorder turns black on exposure to air) and phenylketonuria (PLU) which is a diseases of phenylalanine accumulation in the blood.

(ii) One Gene One Polypeptide Theory

This theory states that one gene controls the synthesis of one polypeptide chain instead of complete enzyme or protein molecule is based and it is based on 'sickle-cell anemia observed specially in Negroes. In this disease the RBCs become sickle shaped in venous blood, due to lower concentration of oxygen, causes the repture of cells, and severe hemolytic anemia. It was observed that this diseases is the result of mutation of β chain of haemoglobin A which causes difference in arrangement of amino acid molecule in haemoglobin which is a protein having about 600 amino acids arranged in four polypeptide chains (2 identical α-chains and two identical β- chains). The sickle-shaped haemoglobin (Hb ^{S}) differs from normal haemoglobin (Hb ^{A}) in the presence of valine in place of glutamic acid in peptide number 7 of the β- chain. (See chapter on mutation). Thus, the sickle anemia is produced by a single change in two β polypeptide chains out of the total four polypeptide chains as a result of a single mutation in one gene. This shows that one gene controls the synthesis of one polupeptide chain and not the complete protein.

Starch Formation

The example of starch formation from glucose may be cited to understand the process of gene function (action). The starch is a polymer made up of monomer units of glucose molecules. The glucose is first converted into glucose phosphate by ATP and it is reduced to adenosine-diphosphate (ADP). The glucose phosphate molecule takes part in reaction with the help of catalyzing agent (enzyme) and starch is formed. Likewise, the ATP also takes part in other reaction.

Pigment Production

Another example of gene action that can be cited is the production of a pigment, melanin. One of the common components of many proteins is the phenylalanine, an amino acid found in blood and it is metabolized by converting into another amino acid, called tyrosine. The conversion of phenylalanine into tyrosine requires the presence of an enzyme (phenylalanine hydroxylase) which is controlled by a gene (P). In the absence of gene P, the enzyme will not be produced and hence the phenylalanine will not be converted into tyrosine. It will result improper metabolism of phenylalanine and it causes a disease called phenylketonuria (PKU) which is associated with mental retardation.

The amino acid tyrosine is the major precursor of melanin. The tyrosine is metabolized into *melanin* (pigment) under the control of an enzyme, *tyrosinase,* which is under the control of a gene (C). Thus, gene C in the form of genotype CC, synthesizes the enzyme tyrosinase so that melanin pigment is produced. The melanin is produced in part due to the enzymatic action of gene C. In the absence of this dominant gene (C), the recessive genotype (cc) is produced at this locus and the enzyme tyrosinase is not produced and hence melanin is not produced. Consequently no pigment (melanin) is produced. The deficiency of melanin results *albinism* (no colour).

(a) Normal Metabolism

P. hydroxylase (Gene, P) Tyrosinase (Gene, C)

Phenylalanine .... Tyrosine .... DOPA ...... Melanin

(dihydroxyphenylalanine)

(b) Abnormal Metabolism

Phenylalanine....No gene P, no enzyme (no tyrosine) = PKU;

Tyrosine .... no gene C, no enzyme (tyrosinase) = Albinism (no melanin).

The melanin is the basic pigment and source to produce various colours of skin, hair, and eyes of animals. After the production of melanin, requires the production of specific enzyme to produce specific colour of farm animals. The synthesis of different enzymes to produce different colours requires different genes.

The melanin is also further acted (metabolized) upon by an enzyme controlled by another gene *e* and produces a yellow pigment. The enzyme tyrosinase that catalyzes the production of melanin will be absent in the individual with recessive genotype (cc) and hence the melanin will not be synthesized. Therefore, in the absence of melanin (absence of gene C and presence of genotype cc), the yellow pigment cannot be produced, even though the gene *e* is present. The recessive gene c does not allow the production of melanin, so it is epistatic gene. The gene c in homozygous condition (cc) has stopped the action of gene e at another locus and hence enzyme e is not produced. This process of epistasis (gene interaction) has been represented digrammetically as:

(a) Normal Pathway

Gene C Gene e

(Enzyme C) (Enzyme e)

Tyrosine .... Melanin .... Yellow pigment

(b) Gene Interaction (Epistasis between gene c and e)

Genotype cc Gene e

(No enzyme C) (Enzyme e)

Tyrosine .... No melanin .... No yellow pigment

Multiple Genes

The final expression of a single character requires many steps (biochemical reactions). This constitutes the involvement of multiple genes (G_1, G_2, G_3, etc) in the biochemical pathway. A specific enzyme is involved in controlling each step of a specific gene. There is stepwise conversion of one substance (called precursor) into another (called product) involving biochemical reaction in such cases. The end product acts as a precursor for the next step till the final and end product is formed. This constitute biosynthetic pathway of different steps of biochemical reactions. An example of multiple genes is of the biochemical pathway of ***amino acid tryptophan*** in *E. coli* which synthesizes this tryptophan amino acid from substance ***chorismic acid***. This is a 4 step action expression of character (production of end product tryptophan amino acid from substrate chorismic acid) as shown below:

Gene G_1

E_1

Substrate: ***Chorismic acid*** Anthranilic acid

E_2 Gene G_2

End product: ***Tryptophan*** Indole glycerol phosphate Carboxyphenylamno deoxyribose phosphaate

E_4 E_3

Gene G_4 **Gene G_3**

22.2 HUMAN BIOCHEMICAL GENETICS

A change in the code sent by DNA causes the production of a different protein in the ribosomes, resulting into a mutation (mutant allele) which causes malfunctioning of gene. Thus, defects are caused by mutant genes as result of blocking a particular step in biochemical reactions. These can be studied when an error in the metabolic pathway due to mutant gene is observed in the form of a defect or disease in an organism. The effect of abnormal gene (mutant) helps to know the normal gene function. The various studis have shown that the function of gene is chemical in nature which means that specific gene controls the specific chemical reaction.

Some inborn errors of metabolism in man have been studied. Bateson (1902) reported the inheritance of a rare human defect (alcaptonuria) as a recessive trait. A book "Inborn Errors of Metabolism" was published in 1909 by Garrod, A.E., English Physician when he noted that some of the hereditary diseases in man are due to the effects of mutant genes on the metabolic system.

As a result of gene mutation, the enzyme responsible to produce normal phenotype is not produced but another enzyme is produced. This alternate enzyme of the biochemical pathway determines the alternate phenotype that may be abnormal. Thus, the normal metabolic pathway is blocked and causes abnormal phenotype (disease). The following are some of the examples:

(1) Phenylketonuria (PKU) or Folling' Disease

It is a autosomal recessive disorder of amino acid phenylalanine-tyrosine metabolism. This disease is hereditary and metabolic, caused by a recessive gene in homozygous condition. It occurs by the absence of an enzyme (phenylalanine hydroxylase) which converts phenylalanine to tyrosine. As a result there is accumulation of toxic substance (phenypyruvic acid) in the brain, damages the brain tissues affecting the brain development and causing mental disorders (idiocy – impairment of mental ability). In normal person the phenylpyruvic acid is converted into hydroxy-phenylpyruvic acid as a result of catalysis of the enzyme (phenylalnine hydroxylase) controlled by normal gene. The presence of phenylpyruvic acid in the urine is the symptom of this condition. The enzyme phenylalanine hydroxylase is necessary for the normal metabolism of amino acid, phenylalanine which is ingested in the diet. The phenylalanine is not toxic itself and but it is metabolized into other substances.

When a defective gene (mutant) is produced, the children have recessive genotype ***pp***. Such children with recessive genotype fail to produce the normal enzyme in the liver (phenylalanine hydroxylase) and hence the normal metabolism is disturbed. There is an accumulation of the amino acid phenylalanine, derived from the breakdown of proteins, due to inactivation of specific liver enzyme (phenylalanine hydroxylase) which prevents the metabolism of phenylalanine to tyrosine. In the absence of normal enzyme there is no conversion (break down) of the phenylpyrivic acid into hydroxyphenylpyruvic acid. As a result the phenylpyruvic acid accumulates in the blood and causes damage of brain tissues. Such persons fail to break down the phenylpyruvic acid into hydroxyphenylpyruvic acid and suffered with a disease known as *phenylketonuria* (PKU). This disease can be diagnosed in newborn babies. The phenylketonuria children are mentally retarded and known as *phenylpyruvic idiots*. However, the environmental factor, ***diet***, can manipulate to modify a phenotype. There is no serious mental impairment in infants who are fed low phenylalanine diets.

(2) Alcaptonuria

This is the first studied inherited disorder of the phenylalanine-tyrosine metabolic pathway. This disease is thus hereditary (autosomal recessive mutation) and metabolic. The mutant allele inactivates the enzyme homogentisic acid oxidase. It is caused due to the presence of a substance, called alcapton (homogentistic acid), in the urine. The enzyme homogentistic acid oxidase is required to covert alcapton (homogentistic acid) into aceto-acetic acid. In the absence of the catalase enzyme in the person suffering from alcaptonuria, the homogentistic acid is not converted into aceto-acetic acid and passed out in the urine and turns black on exposure to air. The persons carrying the recessive mutant gene may not synthesize the required enzyme and hence the step in the normal degradation of alcapton (homogentistic acid) is blocked. Thus, due to accumulation of alcapton in the patients, the urine turns black after coming in contact with air. This disease is also characterizes by the hardening and blackening of the cartilage of the bones. The mutant allele causing the alkaptonuria had played an important role to bring insight into the concept of the gene.

(3) Albinism

It is the absence of pigmentation in the skin, hair, and eyes. The absence of melanin pigment causes albinism. This is due to the autosomal recessive mutation which blocks the conversion of tyrosine to the dark pigment melanin in individuals which are homozygous recessive for this mutant allele whereas the heterozygotes for this mutant allele usually have normal levels of pigmentation. The melanin is produced from tyrosine as a result of catalysis of the enzyme *tyrosinase*. The person with recessive mutant genotype fails to produce this enzyme required to convert dihydroxyphenylalanine into melanin and hence no pigment is formed. The persons are albino lacking the pigment melanin in their hairs, skin and eyes. The absence of enzyme tyrosinase that catalyzes the first step in the synthesis of melanin from tyrosine causes one type of the albinism. The blocks in subsequent steps in conversion of tyrosine to melanin result in other types of albinism.

(4) Tyrosinosis

This disorder is very rare, also inherited like an autosomal recessive trait and results from the lack of the enzyme tyrosine transaminase required to degrade tyrosine to CO_2 and H_2O. The tyrosine is accumulated in the blood and urine of persons having recessive gene in homozygous condition (tt). The individuals with tyrosinosis also have various congenital abnormalities. This disorder is due to lack of conversion of hydroxypyruvic acid into dihydroxyphenyl pyruvic acid and the persons suffer with tyrosinosis.

(5) Tyrosinemia

This is also a metabolic and inherited disorder caused by mutation in recessive condition. The individuals with tyrosinema have higher levels of both tyrosine and p-hydroxyphenyl pyruvic acid in their blood and urine. This causes the liver failure and consequently the newborns suffering with this disorder die within 6 months of their age. This disorder is the result of lack of the enzyme p-hydroxyphenyl- pyruvic acid oxidase which catalyses the tyrosine into CO_2 and H_2O.

Both tyrosinosis and tyrosinema are caused by mutations in genes encoding the enzymes required for the catabolism of tyrosine. The degradation of tyrosine into CO_2 and H_2O require the presence of two enzymes (tyrosine transaminase and p-hydroxyphenyl- pyruvic acid oxidase). The tyrosinosis and tyrosinema result from lack of these two enzymes due to mutations in genes encoding these enzymes.

(6) Goitrous Cretinism

The conversion of tyrosine into thyroxin (thyroid hormone) is required and the persons lacking the required enzyme for conversion are deficient in thyroid hormone which causes goitrous cretinism. This results into the physical and mental retardation and hypertrophy of thyroid gland.

Other examples: There are certain genetic defects, observed in humans and also in animals, which are perhaps the result of the failure to produce a specific protein or due to the production of abnormal protein. The examples are as under-

(7) Sickle Cell Anemia

This disease occurs in human population of central Africa, Greece and south India. The RBC of patients become sickle shaped instead of normal round shape. The RBC of normal persons contain haemoglobin A (Hb^A) whereas sickle-shape RBC contain an abnormal haemoglobin called haemoglobin C (Hb^C). The persons that are homozygous for haemoglobin S ($Hb^S Hb^S$) suffer from anemia characterized by sickle shape of erythrocyte. This disease is fatal in early age. The haemoglobin of homozygote is of the abnormal types. On the other hand, the heterozygote does not suffer from anemia. The selective advantage of heterozygote has been shown to be associated with their resistance to malaria. The sickle cell homozygote ($Hb^S Hb^S$) is anemic severely, having sickling of RBC but resistant to malaria while the normal homozygote ($Hb^A Hb^A$) is not anemic, have normal haemoglobin but susceptible to malaria and the heterozygote is mild anemic but resistant to malaria for which the heterozygote has advantage over both homozygote.

It has been found that both the normal as well as abnormal haemoglobin contain same types of amino acids but different in the amount of one of the polypeptides. The normal haemoglobin contains two glutamic acid units and one valine whereas the abnormal haemoglobin contains one unit of glutamic acid and two units of valine. Thus, one unit of glutamic acid is replaced by the valine unit and this change creates mutation which results in the production of abnormal protein. This gave the evidence that gene carries the code to control the synthesis of a particular protein molecule.

(8) Agammaglobulinemia

This is a genetic defect in human body when the gamma globulin (protein) is not produced in the body. This protein is received by new born baby from its mother and gradually decreases with age reducing to zero at 4 months of age and its production is started at about 3 weeks of age. The absence of this protein increases the susceptibility to bacterial infection.

(9) Tay-Sacs Disorder

It is a lethal autosomal recessive disorder in humans. The affected individuals have neurological degeneration and death in early childhood. This disease is a lipid storage disorder and is one of the most tragic human diseases caused by autosomal mutant gene in homozygous condition (autosomal recessive mutation). Warren Tay (1881) described this disease but its biochemical basis is recently known for about 30 years. The mutation causing this fatal disease occurs in HEXA gene (autosomal) that encodes the enzyme hexosaminidase A. The disease is caused due to absence of this enzyme. However, this mutation is rare. The Ashkenazi Jewish population of central Europe carries the mutant gene. This mutant gene is present in about one in 30 adults in heterozygous condition but the occurrence of the disease among their children is in about one in 3600.

This disease occurs during infancy. The infants carrying the mutant gene in homozygous condition are normal at birth but within few months of their age they show some early symptoms of the disease like that they become hypersensitive to loud noises and develop cherry-red spot on the retina of the eye. Such children between 6 to 12 months of age undergo progressive neurological degeneration leading to mental retardation, blindness, deafness, general loss of control of body functions, and by their 2 years of age they are paralyzed and suffer with chronic respiratory infections. At the age of 3 to 4 years death occurs in these children.

There is no treatment of this disease for the reason that the enzyme supplied for treatment cannot penetrate the barrier between brain cells and circulatory system. Moreover, the method has not so far been established to introduce genes into neurons so as to provide the functional copies of the defective gene to somatic cells (somatic-cell gene therapy).

The Tay-Sacs mutation can be detected during fetal development by the following two procedures:

- ☆ ***Amniocentesis:*** The procedure to obtain a small amount of amniotic fluid from a pregnant lady. This involves removing the fluid from the cavity surrounding the developing foetus through a needle inserting into abdomen of pregnant lady. The cavity surrounding the foetus is called amniotic sac which is enclosed by a membrane. The liquid content of the amniotic sac containing cells of the embryo is called amniotic fluid. Both fluid and cells are used for diagnosis of genetic abnormalities of the embryo or fetus.

☆ *DNA test*: Recently, a DNA test has also been developed to detect the mutant gene. This DNA test involves screening the 8-cell pre-embryos produced by *in vitro* fertilization and taking only one cell for DNA test. This method is important to allow heterozygous parents to have children without risk because after making the test only the normal embryos (not having mutant gene in homozygous state) are implanted into the uterus of the mother. The 7-cells of the embryo after taking one cell for DNA test retain the capacity to develop into a normal embryo after implantation.

The nerve cells are coated by a complex lipid called *ganglioside* (G_{M2}) which insulates them from the events occurring in neighbouring cells so that there is speeding up of nerve impulses. The enzyme hexosaminidase acts on ganglioside G_{M2} and cleaves it into a smaller ganglioside G_{M3} and N-acetyl-D-galactosamine. In the absence of this enzyme the *ganglioside* (G_{M2}) accumulates and suppresses the nerve cells. As a result of buildup of complex lipids on neurons blocks their action, causing the deterioration of the nervous system and finally ending in paralysis of the patient.

(10) Lack of Sex Drive (Libido)

This is an inherited defect in bulls wherein there is failure of the production of a particular hormone by anterior pituitary gland.

22.3 BIOCHEMICAL GENETICS OF OTHER ANIMALS

(1) *Drosophila*: Mutants of Eye Colours

The eye transplantation experiments were conducted by Beadle, G.W. with his fellow worker on Drosophila in Europe. They studied the development of pigment in transplanted eyes.

The eye discs from larvae of mutant colours were transplanted in wild type or vice versa. The wild types were used as host eye colour and vermilion and cinnabar as donor's eye cour and vice versa. Moreover, both the mtant types (Vermilion and cinnabar) were taken as host eye colour and donor's eye colour

On the basis of the results of eye transplantation they suggested the biosynthetic pathway along with the steps in eye pigment formation.

(2) Neurospora: Biochemical Mutations

The Neurospora is a unicellular fungus widely used for biochemical mutations affecting amino metabolic pathways, synthesis of molecules of nucleic acids and vitamins. The study of biochemical mutations has suggested the biosynthetic pathways of arginine and tryptophan synthesis in Neurospora.

Chapter 23

Techniques of Molecular Genetics – Recombinant DNA Technology

Man has been continuously making efforts since the beginning of cultivation of plants and domestication of animals during ancient period, to meet his various requirements through improving the production from plants and animals and by way of forming the societies and construction of colonies, villages and cities. In this direction, numerous technologies have been developed. Human knowledge on natural sciences has been since long in the direction to develop technologies to make human life comfortable and welfare. Technologies, engineering and industries have been the major contributions of physics and chemistry in this direction.

23.1 VARIOUS TECHNOLOGIES

However, the knowledge of biological sciences or life sciences have also been of major utility primarily as a source of food and then in the field of human health (medical science) too. Twentieth century has been a boon to human welfare by providing new bio-techniques in the field of molecular biology (known as *biotechnology*). These technologies include the techniques required for engineering the various tools (non-living matter) and the techniques used in the following areas:

- Mechanical, electrical, chemical and civil engineering,
- Technologies related to general and industrial microbiology,
- *Enzyme technology* (making suitable change for improving in the activity and usefulness of either existing enzyme or in creating new enzyme activity by making suitable changes in its amino acid sequence),

- ☆ *Food and beverages biotechnology* through agriculture and animal production as well as their conversion into useful products like fermented food (Idli,beer, yoghurt, whey, cheese, rice wine), use of enzymes in food technology (fruit juice and wine, beer); production of single cell protein (SCP) by use of bacteria, fungi, yeast and algae,
- ☆ *Fuel biotechnology* for industrial and other uses by inventing methods of utilizing biomass from energy crops which convert CO_2 and H_2O through solar energy into biomass (wood, sugar and starch crops, and hydrocarbon prodcing crops like *Euphorbia lathyrus, milk weed* (*Asclepia speciosa*) *and tree legumes* (Capaifera multijuga) produce hydrocarbons,
  - (*i*) *Production of biogas* (mixture of gases - about 60 per cent methane, CH_4) produced by anaerobic bacterial digestion of organic matter. Biogas consist mainly methane and CO_2 plus traces of hydrogen (H_2) and other gases. Biogas is produced from waste of industrial, agric, A.H., domestic and municipal origin,
  - (*ii*) *Bioethanol* (ethanol produced by microorganisms - *Saccharomyces cerevisiae*) from biomass. Bioethanol has more latent heat, burnt completely, higher flash point than petrol. But bioethanol is highly hydrophilic (absorb moisture) and hence poses starting problem, use about 10 per cent more fuel than petrol. Bioethanol can be obtained from sugar and starch crops, cellulosic material,
  - (*iii*) *Biodiesel* from lipids accumulated in plants and algae or from hydrocarbons (Carbon and hydrogen containing compound only),
  - (*iv*) *Biohydrogen* when hydrogen is generated by biological means (anaerobic bacteria and photosynthetic algae), and
- ☆ *Environment biotechnology* includes the study of sources and hazards of wastes and pollutants. This also includes the waste treatment (removal/ destruction) like land filling, aerobic and anaerobic waste water treatment, biodegradation of xenobiotic compounds

Likewise, man has also made tremendous improvement in plants and animals for their increased productivity by genetic manipulation. With the advancements of the subject of *genetics* the techniques have been developed for manipulation of genes after knowing about the genetic (hereditary) material (DNA) constituted of many genes and have also progressed for manipulation of whole genome.

23.2 BIOTECHNOLOGY: RECOMBINANT DNA TECHNOLOGY (GENETIC ENGINEERING)

The applications of molecular genetics techniques for gene manipulation to human welfare cover important and integral part of separate subject called ***biotechnology*** which is combination of ***bio*** + ***technology***. There has been tremendous growth of this subject (***biotechnology***) emerging in its two separate branches *viz.* Animal Biotechnology and Plant Biotechnology. It is important at this place to know about biotechnology in brief.

The ***biotechnology*** has been defined differently on depending the approach, content and emphasis. Gibbs and Greenhalgh (1983) defined it as the use of living organisms (Bacteria, algae, fungi, yeast, cells of higher animals and plants or subsystems of any of these or isolated components from living matter) in systems or processes for the manufacture of useful products.

Or the *biotechnology* is the controlled use of biological agents for beneficial use (U.S. National Science Foundation).

Or the biotechnology is the integrated use of biochemistry, microbiology and engineering sciences in order to achieve technological application of the capabilities of micro-organisms, cultured cells/tissues and parts thereof (European Federation of Biotechnology).

The ***biotechnology*** involves the processes for the large scale production of products using live organisms, cells or enzymes. The biotechnology uses genetically modified organisms to produce gene products (functional protein) and to make a suitable formulation for their large scale production and marketing. This field was started after learning the chemistry of DNA and construction of recombinant DNA. This is the key process in biotechnology and is called recombinant DNA technology or ***genetic engineering***. The biotechnology has changed the daily life of human beings because its products have made qualitative improvement in food production and health for human and other species beneficial to human beings.

The definition of biotechnology may be taken in different ways. However, the main emphasis to them is laid for utilization of biological entities (micro-organisms, cells of higher organisms which may be living or dead) and their components like enzymes to generate some useful products or service for welfare of human. The biotechniques may include the production technologies related to agriculture including horticulture and animal husbandry for production of useful products by utilizing the biological entities (plants and animals). But the agriculture and animal husbandry are old and separate disciplines, but use of plant and animal cells cultured *in vitro* to generate products and services constitute an integral part of biotechnology. The ***Biotechnology*** is a very old area itself but the term biotechnology is of recent origin and has now become a separate discipline.

☆ ***Biotechnology*** *– an old field*: Man has been using micro-organisms (yeast) to make vinegar, curd, wine, and beer since long even before 6000 BC; sewage treatment using microbes; production of acetone, butanol, and glycerol since 1900, genetic engineering, monoclonal antibodies for disease diagnosis since 1981, use of insulin and interferons produced by genetically engineered microbes since 1983 – 1984.

The technology for production of glycerol (used in manufacture of explosives) was developed during First World War by Germans whereas British resorted to acetone-butanol fermentation by use of *Clostridium acetobutylicum*. The technology for citric acid production by use of *Aspergillus niger* was developed during this period of War. Fleming (1930) discovered the production of antibiotic penicillin from *Penicillium notatum* but its commercial production was begun during Second World War.

- ☆ ***Biotechnology*** – *a new area of research* as a new discipline is the Recombinant DNA technology (genetic Engineering). This technology was developed as a result of continuous effort of man to make capable the micro-organisms for novel processes to create them highly valuable, *e.g.* human gene producing insulin (used in treatment of diabetes) was transferred and expressed in bacterium *E. coli*. Likewise, many useful products from animal and plant cells are used to produce valuable products. This recombinant DNA technology is being used to create new and highly useful traits in crop varieties and animals.

The subject matter of ***biotechnology*** is now the ***recombinant DNA technology*** and other similar techniques come under. In this way, *biotechnology* in addition to recombinant DNA technology covers *hybridoma technology, enzyme technology and enzyme engineering, uses of micro-organisms* to convert simple organic molecules (sugars) into more useful products (alcohol, acetic acid) and to produce unique biochemicals (antibiotics).

Thus, *biotechnology is multidisciplinary* in nature encompassing several disciplines of basic science (microbiology, chemistry, biochemistry, physiology, genetics, molecular biology, immunology, cell and tissue culture) and engineering (chemical and biochemical engineering) forming the basis of large scale production of micro-organisms and cells and their recovery processing. The 5 major operations involved in biotechnological process are:

- ☆ Strain or culture choice and improvement,
- ☆ Mass culture,
- ☆ Optimization of cell responses,
- ☆ Process operation, and
- ☆ Product recovery.

The ***important areas of biotechnology*** in which it is making significant contributions to human welfare are as under:

- ☆ Plant Biotechnology: Agriculture, Horticulture and floriculture, and forestry,
- ☆ Animal Biotechnology: Animal husbandry including dairy, food processing and beverages, animal as well as human health and medicines, fisheries and acquaculture,
- ☆ Industrial biotechnology: Chemicals and biochemicals
- ☆ Medical biotechnology
- ☆ Population control
- ☆ Crimes and parentage disputes
- ☆ Environment biotechnology
- ☆ Mining
- ☆ Renewable energy and fules

23.3 BIOTECHNOLOGY IN INDIA

The 69 th session of Indian Science Congress held at Mysore in 1982 considered the importance of biotechnology and constituted a National Biotechnology Board for the purpose of encouraging and coordinating research activities in this area. Subsequently a separate *Department of Biotechnology* (DBT) was set up under the Mininstry of Science and Technology.

The *biotechnology research centres* were started at 3 *National Institutes* working under ICAR. The three National Institutes are:

- ☆ IARI, New Delhi;
- ☆ NDRI, Karnal; and
- ☆ IVRI, Izatnagar, Bareilly.

Among these centres, the IARI centre was named as NRC for Plant Biotechnology which came into operation in 1993.

Later on, the DBT started funding for optimum development of facilities at 7 more centres with the mandate to exploit biotechnological approaches for cropm improvement. These centres are:

- ☆ Madurai Kamraj University, Madurai (TN);
- ☆ T.N. Agril. Universiity, Coimbatore;
- ☆ Osmania University, Hyderabad;
- ☆ Bose Institute, Calcutta;
- ☆ National Botanical Research Institute, Lucknow;
- ☆ JNU, New Delhi;
- ☆ Delhi University (south campus), New Delhi.

Besides above, the research activities in the area of biotechnology are being promoted by ICAR and CSIR, New Delhi.

The ICAR has created several *biotechnology wings* at different crop research institutes under its working. Generous support to these centres is being extended by the DBT. These are:

- ☆ Indian Pulae Research Institute, Kanpur;
- ☆ IGFRI, Jhansi.

A National Facility for *Plant Tissue Culture Repository* for clonally propagated crops has been organized at NBPGR, New Delhi with the attention of DBT being ficussed on the conservation of germplasm through the approaches of biotechnology and to fulfil this mandate.

Three *National Gene Banks*, in addition to the conventional seed and field gene bank, with the facilities of tissue culture repository and cryobank (using liquid nitrogen at – 196 ° C) are having these facilities. These three gene bank centres also having the facilities for providing training to the other member states of G – 15 are as:

- ✰ National Gene Bank at NBPGR, New Delhi for medicinal and aromatic plants,
- ✰ Central Institute of Medicinal and Aromatic Plants (CIMAP), Lucknow, and
- ✰ Tropical Botanical Garden and Research Institute (TBGRI), Trivandrum

Several *Indian Biotechnology Companies* have their base of micropropagation (rapid clonal propagation) for exporting all the plantlets under contact with foreign companies. Three pilot plants with the mandate for large scale micropropagation of forest trees (teak, eucalyptus, poplar, etc) and fruit trees for augmenting afforestation are being funded by the DBT. These are

- ✰ Tata Energy Research Institute (TERI), New Delhi'
- ✰ Natinal Chemical Laboratory (NCL), Pune, and
- ✰ J.N. Vyas University, Jodhpur.

United Nations Organization (UNO) has established an International Centre for Genetic Engineering and Biotechnology (ICGEB) with 2 centres located at Trieste (Italy) and New Delhi which started operating in 1987.

DBT has also initiated *two teaching programmes* for manpower development in the area of biotechnology. These two programmes are

- ✰ Master's level [M.Sc./M. Sc. (Ag)/M. Tech] training at 19 centres located in different universities for with eligibility of admission for graduates in Science, Agriculture and Engineering, and
- ✰ Post-doctoral training at 3 centres.

The *private sector* has also taken up biotechnological research. Some companies have developed biotechnology wings and have also released diagnostic kits for some diseases.

23.4 MOLECULAR ANALYSIS

The eukaryotic genetic elements (genes, DNA, chromosomes, and genomes) are made up of macromolecules. The analysis of the structure and functions of these molecules is known as *molecular analysis*.

The big size of these molecules of eukaryotes makes their molecular analysis difficult. Secondly, the crossing among the divergent species in eukaryotes is not possible due to their genetic isolation which has caused the reproductive isolation and makes impossible to create new genetic variation for exploitation.

On the contrary, in case of prokaryotes (Bacteria), the genetic elements are of smaller size and the genetic recombination occurs as a result of transfer of genetic material from one bacterial cell to another cell of different origin (species).

The foreign DNA segment of divergent origin is introduced into a chromosome of bacterial cell by genetic recombination mechanism. This knowledge and technique gave insight to the development of recombinant DNA technology, gene cloning, and other techniques like molecular hybridization techniques and has solved the problem of genetic isolation, molecular analysis of large size genes, DNA molecules, RNA molecules, Protein molecules, and chromosomes as well as of the genetic recombination. These techniques are called the ***techniques of molecular genetics.*** The genes and other segments of large chromosome can be isolated, replicated, and studied by using the nucleic acid sequencing techniques, electron microscopy, and other analytical techniques.

23.5 IMPORTANT DISCOVERIES AND TECHNIQUES OF MOLECULAR GENETICS

The following ***important discoveries*** for the techniques of molecular genetics including genetic engineering have made feasible the molecular analysis of large genetic elements (genes, DNA, chromosome, genome, and cell) -

1. Restriction Endonucleases – annexure 23.2
2. Gene isolation - annexure 23.4.1
3. Gene synthesis – annexure 23.4.2
4. Construction and screening of DNA libraries – annexure23.4.1
5. PCR techniques of gene amplification/multiplication (gene cloning) – annexure 23.4.3 and 23.7
6. Biological tools (Enzymes, vector DNA, and passenger DNA) used in genetic engineering. Annexure 23.1, 23.3 (vector)
7. DNA transfer technique (Integration) – transformation and transduction- annexure 23.5
8. Introduction of cloning vector in to host – annexure 23.5 – chapter **23**, 3rd point of producing recombinant DNA molecule
9. Probes – annexure 23.8
10. Gel electrophoresis - annexure 23.10
11. Autoradiography – annexure 23.9
12. *In situ* colony hybridization – annexure 23.6
13. Somatic cell hybridization. – annexure 23.11
14. Hybridization techniques (Southern blot, Northern blot, and Western blot for molecular analysis of DNA, RNA, and Proteins, respectively) – chapter **23**
15. Genome mapping: Molecular analysis of genes and chromosomes for physical maps of DNA molecules (RE sites and nucleotide sequencing as physical maps) – chapter **25**
16. Microarrays and gene chips technology – see Cell Genetics and ***genomics***: TOMAR and TOMAR, 2018
17. DNA sequencing procedures – see Cytogenetics and ***genomics***: TOMAR and TOMAR, 2018

The various *techniques of molecular genetics* have been categorized into the following three major groups and dealt in this chapter as under –

☆ ***Genetic engineering*** used for the production of recombinant DNA molecules (*recombinant DNA technology*) and its amplification, often referred as *gene cloning.*

  (i) The ***recombinant DNA molecule*** is a DNA molecule produced *in vitro* by joining all or parts of two different DNA molecules by the incorporation of a gene of interest into a self-replicating DNA molecule.

  (ii) The ***gene cloning*** is the amplification (multiplication) of the resulting recombinant DNA molecule. This can be done *in vivo* (appropriate host cell) or *in vitro.*

Recombinant DNA technology includes following three steps:

I. Production of Recombinant DNA Molecule

(a) Gene identification and isolation: Gene isolation from organism, from gene synthesis (chemical and enzymatic synthesis), amplification/ multiplication (gene cloning) *in vitro* (PCR) and *in vivo;*

(b) Insetion/integration of isolated gene in a suitable vector (passenger DNA + vector DNA)

(c) Introduction of cloning vector into a suitable host

II. Gene Cloning

Amplification/multiplication of recombinant DNA:

(a) Selection of recombinant clones

(b) Cloning of recombinant DNA: Amplificatio/multiplication of DNA insert (DNA to be inserted) into host genome (*in vitro* by PCR and *vivi*)

III. Somatic Cell Hybridization

☆ ***Electrophoresis and hybridization techniques*** for the molecular analysis of DNA, RNA, and Proteins. and

☆ ***Molecular mapping of genome*** (***restriction fragment sites and nucleotide-pair sequencing techniques***) for the molecular analysis of genes and chromosomes.

23.6 LANDMARKS IN MOLECULAR TECHNIQUES

The history of *important landmarks in the DNA sequencing research* started with the discovery of J. F. Miescher (1868) for an acidic substancc (in human pus cells) to which he called nuclein (nucleic acid – DNA). (Levene, 1869-1940) in 1940s documented the presence of polynucleotide chains in this acidic substance, nuclein (nucleic acid) and this nucleic acid could get importance only after this discovery of Levene.

The second footstep in this direction was the research conducted by Avery *et al.* (1944) who established the role of nucleic acid in storing and transmitting the genetic information (declaring DNA as the genetic material). The third most important step was the discovery of double helix structure of DNA by Watson and Crick (1953).

The ***nucleic acid sequencing*** became a major target of early molecular biologists following Rosalin Franklin's confirmation of the helical structure of DNA, and Fred Sanger's determination of the amino acid sequence of insulin in 1955. Sanger received the 1958 Noble Prized in Chemistry for this work. With the above inventions, the DNA sequencing work of genomes was started.

Ochoa received the 1959 Noble Prize for his discovery of ***RNA polymerase***. Francis Crick and colleagues (1961) published the first strong evidence in support of a ***triplet code*** (3 nucleotides per codon).

Marshall Nirenberg and Philip Leder revealed the triplet nature of the genetic code and were able to determine the sequences of 54 out of 64 codons in their experiments. Nirenberg and Khorana shared the 1968 Noble Prize in Physiology or Medicine for their work on genetic code with Robert Holley.

Rober W, Holley and colleagues (1964) published the first nucleic acid sequence, the ribonucleotide sequence of alanine transfer RNA (yeast tRNA) using RNA digestion and chromatography methods which required large quantities of sample.

Wu (1970) sequenced lambda cohesive end DNA using primed synthesis concept and 2-D electrophoresis and less material was required. Walter Fiers and his team (1972) of the University of Ghent (Belgium) was the first to determine the sequence of a gene for Bacteriophage MS2 coat protein. They expanded the work and determined the complete nucleotide-sequence of bacteriophage MS2-RNA in 1976 (whose genome encodes just four genes in 3569 base pairs) and Simian virus 40 in 1978.

F. Sanger and Alan Coulson (1975) published a sequencing procedure using DNA polymerase with radio-labelled nucleotides that they called the *Plus and Minus technique*. This involved two closely related methods that generated short oligonucleotides with defined 3′ termini. These oligonucleotides could be fractionated by electrophoresis on a polyacrylamide gel and visualized using autoradiography. The procedure could sequence up to 80 nucleotides in one attempt and was a big improvement, but was still very laborious.

Frederick Sanger (1977) discovered dideoxy termination sequencing procedure. He and his group (1977) was able to sequence most of the 5,386 nucleotides of the single-stranded bacterophage Φ174, completing the first fully sequenced DNA-based genome. The refinement of the *Plus and Minus* method resulted in the Sanger's chain-termination method which formed the basis of the techniques of DNA sequencing, genome mapping, data storage, and bioinformatics analysis.

Gilbert (1977) developed the chemical degradation sequencing protocol. Frederick Sanger and Walter Gilbert shared half of the 1980 Nobel Prize in chemistry with Pal Berg (recombinant DNA) for independently developing methods for the sequencing of DNA. With the development of the chain termination and chemical degradation concepts and use of polyacrylamide gel electrophoresis to separate DNA tracts, the DNA sequencing efficiency was increased to about 1000 – 1500 bp per person per year.

Walter Gilbert and Allen Maxan (1977) of Harvard University independently developed the Maxam-Gilbert *method* (also known as the *chemical method*) of DNA sequencing. This method involves the preferential cleavage of DNA at known bases, a less efficient method.

Walter Goad (1979) from New Maxico was encouraged by the advancements in sequencing research and proposed the idea for a database which should contain all available DNA sequences. He with his team during 1982 to 1992 incorporated sequences into the database which became the GenBank and maintained at Los Alamos National Laboratory (New Mexico).

Messing (1980) developed the cloning vectors from *E.coli* filamentous bacteriophage M13 to get single-strand copies of cloned DNA, with DNA sequencing efficiency of 15,000 bp per year per person.

Kary Mullis (1985) developed polymerase chain reaction (PCR) technique for gene amplification. Hood (1986) developed partially automated sequencing system and computer assisted data handling was started.

23.7 PROGRESS OF DNA SEQUENCING

The ***Human Genome Project*** was initiated in 1990 under the chairmanship of Watson by which time the DNA sequencing efficiency increased to about 1, 000, 000 bp/person/year.

The first bacterial genome was sequenced by Venter (1995) using automated fluorescent sequencing instruments and introducing the PCR sequencing concept. The first eukaryotic genome of yeast was sequenced in 1996 by International consortium of scientists. Fully automated 96-capillary sequencer was developed making available the electrophoresis sequencing system (PerkinElmer, 1998). The efficiency of DNA sequencing increased to 150, 000, 000 bp/machine/year. Complete sequence of a worm's genome, *Caenorhabditis elegans* in 1998 and of euchromatic sequence of *Drosophila* genome, and of *Arabidopsis thaliana* genome in 2000 was done.

First draft of the sequence of human genome was published in 2001 by International Human Genome Sequencing Consortium and Celera Genomics Scientists and first draft of sequence of the mouse genome was published in 2002 by Mouse Genome Sequencing Consortium. International Human Gene Sequencing Consortium came out with 99 per cent of euchromatin sequence of human genome in 2004. Next generation-454, Illumina, SOLiD- sequencing machine came up and by the year 2010 sequence of over 60 per cent of the ***Neanderthal genome*** was published.

The fully automated machines at present have the DNA sequencing efficiencies up-to 25 billion bp/day. The geneticists have progressed to the extent that the expression of all the genes of the entire genome can be studied in a single experiment.

23.8 GENETIC ENGINEERING: RECOMBINANT DNA TECHNOLOGY

Meaning

The manipulation of genes by man is called ***genetic engineering***. The *genetic engineering* means reconstructing of a cell's genetic organization which is accomplished by the recombinant DNA technology. This includes artificial synthesis, modification, removal, addition, and repair of genetic material (DNA) for the purpose to change the phenotype at will.

The genetic material (gene or DNA segment) from organisms of quite diverse origins with little DNA sequence homology can be attached into an appropriate vector and introduced into a host cell for multiplication and expression. The DNA molecules are *isolated* from two different species, *cleaved* (excised) with a restriction enzyme, *mixed* under annealing conditions, *and covalently joined* (ligated) by treatment with DNA ligase. The DNA molecules are joined into a suitable vector - small bacterial chromosome - plasmid) which can then be grown in large amounts (clones) in *E. coli*.

This field is of great interest and also be of a great importance or advantage for the benefit of human particularly to set right the disease causing genes, may also be a great surprise one day to create life, and thus may change the traditional concept of "***Grace of God***".

Principle

A piece of DNA transferred into an alien organism may not multiply itself in the progeny cells of the organism. But it may multiply as well as inherited along with the host DNA provided the piece of DNA is integrated into the genome of the recipient. Now this integrated DNA has become part of a chromosome which is capable to replicate due to the presence in the chromosome, a specific DNA sequence which is called as ***origin of replication*** and this point is responsible to initiate replication. Therefore, any alien piece of DNA in an organism needs to become a part of a chromosome(s) which has a specific sequence "origin of replication". Thus, an alien (different nature) piece of DNA can replicate and multiply itself in the host organism, after it is linked with the "origin of replication". This is the principle of getting multiple copies of any template DNA and this multiplication is called as ***amplification*** or ***gene cloning***.

Purpose of DNA Technology

This recombinant DNA technology has a purpose of multiplication (amplification or cloning) of the desired gene. Thus, the technology is a two stage process *viz.* production of a joint DNA molecule (called ***recombinant DNA molecule***) obtained by joining together two or more DNA segments (fragments) from organisms of different origins; and then multiplication of this joint or recombinant DNA molecule in an appropriate host, usually a bacterium. The purpose of multiplication of recombinant DNA molecules is accomplished with one of the following three objectives:

- To get large numbers of copies of specific DNA fragments,
- To integrate the desired gene into the chromosome of a host to express itself, or
- To recover large quantities of the protein produced by the concerned gene.

The completion of first objective of obtaining large numbers of copies of the desired gene, is essential to complete the second and third objective

The recombinant DNA molecule production technology involves some biological tools (enzymes, Vector DNA and Passenger DNA – ***Annexure 23.1***). The details of the specific enzymes – **restriction endonuclease** have been given in **annexure 23.2**. This enzyme recognizes specific DNA nucleotide sequences and cleave (cut) the DNA molecules at these specific sites into suitable pieces called restriction fragments (or DNA fragments), inserting these DNA fragments (DNA sequences) into cloning vector (small self-replicating DNA molecule – plasmids and bacteriophages), and join together the appropriate fragments with DNA ligase (*ligation*). This recombinant DNA molecule is subsequently introduced into living cells (host – bacteria) by transformation and amplified by replication *in vivo* so as to get its million-fold copy (amplification or cloning).

Importance of Recombinant DNA and Gene Cloning

The recombinant DNA and gene-cloning techniques have played major roles in the progress in the field of biology and have proved very useful to study the genetic control of essentially all biological processes.

- These techniques are useful to isolate essentially any gene or DNA sequence of interest and to characterize it structurally and functionally.
- Large quantities of a gene can be obtained to determine its nucleotide-pair sequence (sequencing of gene).
- The amino acid sequence of any polynucleotide encoded by the gene can be predicted based on the nucleotide sequence and the knowledge of the genetic code.
- The oligonucleotides can be synthesized based on the predicted amino acid sequence of a polynucleotide encoded by a gene, and
- These oligonucleotides can be used to raise antibodies which in turn can be used to identify the actual product of the gene and localize it within cells or tissues of the organism.

Difference between Recombinant DNA Molecule and Mutation

New genetic variability in the cell is introduced in both cases by adding or changing only one gene or a small fragment of DNA to the genome. The majority of the genes remain the same. The recombinant DNA molecules coming from different species results in a novel functional gene product in the cell and it is more analogous to duplication mutations (extra chromosomal segment) than other types of mutations.

Techniques of Genetic Engineering

The ***hybridization*** (crossing of parents homozygous for different alleles at a locus, *viz. AA x aa* will produce hybrid progeny of the genotype Aa) is the oldest and most widely used technique of genetic engineering to change the genotype and phenotype of the hybrid progeny. The genetic material can now be manipulated by new techniques of genetic engineering developed during the last half of 20th century.

The techniques of genetic engineering primarily include the followings:

I. Recombinant DNA technology

II. Gene cloning

III. Somatic cell hybridization or protoplast fusion.

I. Recombinant DNA Technology

The recombinant DNA is the DNA of an organism which integrates into itself a segment (piece) of DNA from other organism by virtue of the *denaturation* and *renaturation* properties of DNA. The separation of two strands of DNA by breakdown of hydrogen bond on heating is called ***denaturation*** whereas the reunion of complementary strands to form DNA duplex on cooling is the ***renaturation***. The single strands of DNA from different organisms can join provided the segments have complementary base pairs.

The first instance of construction of an artificial recombinant DNA molecule emerged from the possibility of linking a gene (DNA piece) responsible for antibiotic resistance with a native ***plasmid*** (autonomously replicating circular extra-chromosomal DNA) of a bacterium *Salmonella typhimurium.*

Paul Berg (1972) of Stanford University produced first recombinant DNA molecules. The recombinant DNA molecule contained phage lambda gene inserted into the small circular DNA molecule of Simian virus 40. A Noble Prize in chemistry in 1980 was shared by Paul Berg for this work.

Another team also from Stanford University (Stanley Cohen and Herbert Boyer, 1972) inserted an *EciRI* restriction fragment from one DNA molecule into the cleaved *EcoRI* restriction site of a self-replicating plasmid. This recombinant plasmid after introducing into *Ecoli* cells by transformation, showed autonomous replication like an original plasmid. This team performed the linking through isolation of the antibiotic resistance gene by cutting out a piece of DNA at specific location which was made possible with the discovery and help of the ***restriction enzyme*** (known as *molecular scissor*). The cut piece of DNA was then linked with the plasmid DNA which acted as ***vectors*** to transfer the piece of DNA attached to it. This is just like the insect which acts as a vector to transfer the malaria causing parasite into human body. Similarly to this, a plasmid can be used as a vector to transfer an alien piece of DNA into the host organism. The enzyme DNA ***ligase*** made it possible the linking of antibiotic resistance gene (alien DNA piece) with the plasmid. This is because the enzyme ligase acts on cut DNA molecules and joins their ends making a new combination of circular DNA (which is self replicating) created *in vitro*. This new combined DNA produced by using this whole procedure is called as ***recombinant DNA***.

This recombinant DNA, on transferring into *E. coli*, could replicate to make its multiple copies using the new host's DNA polymerase enzyme. This ability of multiplying the copies of antibiotic resistance gene in *E. coli* was called ***gene cloning*** of this antibiotic resistance gene.

In vitro Production of Recombinant DNA Molecule

The DNA molecules from two different sources (species) are both digested with a restriction endonuclease. This enzyme recognizes a specific DNA sequence (*palindromic*) of any species of either animals or plants or microbes, catalyses the cleavage of this specific sequence of nucleotide pairs of the DNA, and makes staggered cuts in the two strands. The digestion of DNA by restriction endonuclease, *e.g. EcoRI* (*cleavage of DNA*), produces DNA fragments with the same complementary single-stranded 5′ - AATT -3′ ends irrespective of the source of DNA.

The resulting fragments have complementary single-stranded ends. These two DNA fragments of any two species are paired by the complementary ends and join by the addition of DNA ligase (*ligation*). Thus, two DNA fragments can be covalently fused and produce the recombinant DNA molecule. For example, an *Eco RI* fragment of human DNA can be joined with *Ecoli RI* fragment of *E.coli DNA* or two *EcoRI fragments* of human DNA. The production of recombinant DNA molecule has been shown as under:

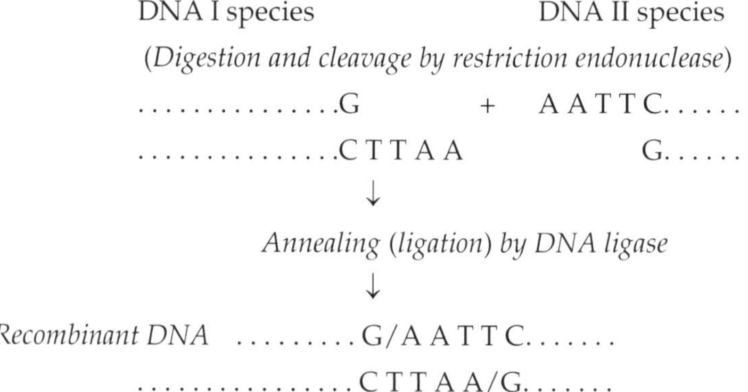

23.8.1 Production of Recombinant DNA Products

This is the production of foreign gene products which is the aim of DNA technology (to produce a desirable protein by expression of alien piece of DNA). The alien DNA is multiplied after its insertion into a cloning vector and its transfer into a bacterial, plant or human/animal cell. However, this foreign or alien gene (recombinant DNA) must be expressed which is possible only under optimal conditions (temperature, pH, substrate, salts, vitamins, oxygen). The large scale production of gene product (protein) is required after the gene of interest is cloned and the conditions to induce the gene expression for production of target protein (***recombinant protein***) are optimized.

The cells of cloned gene may be grown in the laboratory on a small scale and the desired protein may be extracted from the culture. This can then be purified by using any one of the separation techniques. This small volume culture is not sufficient in producing the required quantities of products to sell in the market on commercial scale. Therefore, the cells of cloned genes can also be multiplied on large scale to get larger biomass leading to more yields of desired protein. The continuous culture system is used for the purpose. In this continuous system the medium used is drained out from one side and adding the fresh medium from other side to keep the cells in their physiological active phase. For this purpose of large scale production the ***bioreactors*** that are vessels can be used to process large volume (100 – 1000 litres) culture. In these bioreactors the raw material is biologically converted into required specific products (proteins, enzymes, *etc.*).

Next steps are the processes involving separation and purification. The product so produced needs to be formulated with suitable preservatives followed by clinical trials if the product is a drug. This also needs the quality control testing of the product.

The recombinant DNA technology (genetic engineering) requires the *production of recombinant DNA molecules* (A DNA molecule containing DNA fragments from two sources of different origin) and then obtaining their multiple copies (*gene cloning* or gene amplification) for further use. These two processes (production of recombinant DNA molecule and its cloning) are completed in the following steps –

The industrial scale production of biopharmaceuticals and biologicals using genetically modified microbes, fungi, plants, and animals are essentially dealt in biotechnology.

The technique of genetic engineering to combine DNAs from different sources to produce hybrid molecule of heredity has been perfecting by a number of laboratories in the world. The recombinant DNA molecules are produced by following 3 steps:

(i) Identification and isolation of the desired gene, and cutting of DNA by enzyme,

(ii) Insertion or integration of isolated gene (DNA insert) in a suitable vector, and

(iii) Introduction of cloning vector into a suitable host.

(i) Isolation of DNA of interest

The biological tools used in recombinant DNA technology are the enzymes, vector DNA, and passenger DNA (See ***annexure 23.4***).

The desired gene or DNA molecules (DNA insert) may be identified and obtained (gene isolation) by either of the following sources:

(*a*) ***Gene Isolation*** - from an organism or from the DNA libraries *viz.* cDNA library and genomic library, or screening DNA libraries to identify gene (genetic selection and molecular hybridization – colony hybridization wit plasmids and cosmid vectors; plaque hybridization with phage lambda vector (see ***annexure 23.4.1***), (b *Gene synthesis* - chemical or enzymatic synthesis of gene (see ***annexure* 23.4.2**),

(c) ***Amplification of isolated/synthesized Gene*** - *in vivo* or *in vitro* by PCR technique (see ***annexure* 23.4.3**).

(ii) Integration of Passenger DNA to Vehicle DNA (Passenger DNA + Vehicle DNA = Production of Recombinant DNA)

This is the Insertion of isolated gene in a suitable vector. After having isolating the source DNA as well as the vector DNA with a specific restriction enzyme, the DNA segment of source DNA is integrated (inserted, tranferred) into the vector DNA at appropriate site. The integration means the joining of source DNA with vector DNA. The two DNA fragments are mixed and the enzyme *ligase* is added for their leagasing (annealing). This results in production of recombinant DNA molecule. (***Annexure* 23.5**)

Thus, the recombinant DNA is formed by integrating the passenger DNA (*synthetic* and *cDNA*) to vehicle or *vector DNA*. This is done in the following steps -

(a) Dissolving (opening up) the cell wall of an organism (bacterium) with a suitable enzyme (*lysozyme*) to take out the DNA for use as vehicle or passenger. The DNA of this cell is isolated from cell contents by ultracentrifugation and thus purified.

(b) Integration of the passenger DNA to vehicle DNA by one of the following ways:

- ☆ By using *restriction* enzyme – the same restriction endonuclease is used to cleave both the passenger and vehicle DNA so as they have complementary sticky ends which pair on mixing under suitable conditions and are sealed with joining enzyme (*ligase*) to produce recombinant DNA. Thus, the DNA fragments are ligated with a vector.
- ☆ By *extending tails* (ends) – used in case of having different restriction sites or lacking the restriction sites by one or both DNAs. The procedure of producing the recombinant DNA involves - adding the single-stranded complementary ends (tails) to duplex DNAs, pairing of these complementary tails, and sealing the gaps with enzyme *ligase*.
- ☆ By using the *linkers* – used in case of lacking the restriction sites by passenger DNA. The procedure to form recombinant DNA involves – attaching to the ends of passenger DNA the short segments (linkers) of synthetic DNA having restriction sites similar to those of vehicle DNA and joining the sticky ends of passenger and vehicle DNAs.

(iii) Introduction to Recombinant DNA (Passenger DNA + vehicle DNA = cloning vector) into Host Cell/Organism

The recombinant DNA (ligated DNA) is introduced into the host (recipient cell) to produce hybrid cells so as to give rise to new species. The host for recombinant DNA had been earlier the *E. Coli* bacterium but now another bacteria (*Bacillus subtillis*) and yeast are also used. The host bacteria should not have the plasmids.

The cell wall of bacteria is treated with calcium chloride or lysozyme to make it permeable. The recombinant DNA is added to the growing culture of bacteria so that the bacteria take up this recombinant DNA along with nutrients. The recombinant DNA replicates on division of bacteria and express the characters of both the parent DNAs. Thus, if the recombinant DNA bears a gene resistant to an antibiotic (*e. g.*, ampicillin) is transferred into *E. coli* cells, the host cell (Bacterium) becomes transformed into ampicillin-resistant cells.

When the bacterium is host organism it is not possible to take up the plasmid through cell membrane of bacterium because the DNA is a hydrophilic molecule. Some treatment is thus required so as the bacterial cell may take up plasmid DNA. A specific concentration of a divalent cation such as calcium is required to treat the host cells (bacteria). This treatment with calcium increases efficiency to enter the DNA to the bacterium through pores in its cell wall. The cells with recombinant DNA are incubated on ice, followed by heat shock at 42° C, and again to give them on ice treatment. The recombinant DNA is taken up by the bacteria by this treatment. (See ***annexure*** ***23.5*** for gene transfer techniques).

Another method is that of micro-injection which is used to introduce alien DNA into host cells. In this method the recombinant DNA is directly injected into the nucleus of an animal cell.

Still another method called as *Gene gun* or *biolistics* is mostly suitable for plants. The cells are bombarded with high velocity micro-particles (gold or tungsten) coated with DNA. This method uses the 'disarmed pathogen' vectors which on infecting the cell, transfer the recombinant DNA into the host.

Prospects of Genetic Engineering

The important prospects are as under:

- ☆ The gene therapy has been developed for treating hereditary diseases (genetic defects) like haemophilia
- ☆ The traits of animals and plants may be tailored as desired by adding genes and hence the species may be improved
- ☆ Use of bacteria to synthesize vitamins, hormones, and antibodies by introducing the gene fot these substances/molecules
- ☆ N_2 fixing genes may be transferred from bacteria (legume crops) to other grain crops to enhance crop production without using chemical fertilizers
- ☆ Genes of interest may be located on chromosomes and it can be ascertained the time and location of enzyme to be formed.

23.8.2 Procedure of Gene Cloning: Amplification of Recombinant DNA

The *gene amplification* or *gene cloning* which is different from animal cloning is the multiplication of gene of interest (Desired DNA insert or recombinant DNA molecule). The gene cloning needs the following two steps:

(1) Selection of recombinant clones, and

(2) Cloning of recombinant DNA molecule (Amplification of DNA insert) in host genome - gene cloning by PCR *in vitro* and *in vivo*.

The molecular analysis of genes or DNA molecule needs its identification and isolation in essentially pure form in sufficient amount.

It is often thought of preserving a peculiar genotype. This means to counteract the death so that the specific genotype is not lost. The cloning of a genotype is the answer of preservation of life. The cloning means the production of a clone which is a population of genetically identical individuals or cells produced by vegetative propagation or tissue culture technique.

The production of many copies of a gene or specific DNA sequence is called ***gene amplification*** (*multiplication*). The techniques for the analysis of genes and other DNA sequences require their sufficient quantities in pure form. The desired gene in pure form needs its selection among the cells containing the desired recombinant DNA molecules and its sufficient quantity needs its multiplication in suitable host.

The term ***clone*** is used for asexual progeny derived by vegetative propagation from a single cell or individual or gene. Thus a clone carries genetic material identical to that from which it has been derived (gene, DNA segment, cell, or individual). The ***cloning*** is the production of many copies of a gene or specific DNA segment (sequence). The technologies used in cloning these asexual progenies are respectively called as cell cloning, animal cloning/plant cloning, and gene cloning.

The ***gene cloning*** is a process carried out by incorporation of a gene of interest into a self-replicating DNA molecule and the amplification of the resulting recombinant DNA molecule in an appropriate host cell. Thus, *gene cloning* is a two stage process comprising inserting a gene of interest in a vector (self-replicating DNA molecule) and the gene multiplication (amplification).

(1) Selection of the transformed host cells containing recombinant clones: The isolation of the clones that are transformed by the recombination vector from those that contain the unaltered vector is done.

(2) Multiplication of DNA insert in the host: The desired DNA insert after its identification is multiplied to get sufficient number of copies. The multiplication (amplification) of a desired gene is done for one or more of the following purposes:

- Structural analysis of the gene, like sequencing,
- Production of protein by introducing the desired DNA insert into a bacterium like *Bacillus subtilis* which secretes proteins into the medium,
- Investigation of the function of the gene, and
- Introducing the desired gene into the host genome to produce transgenic animals and plants.

Approaches of Amplification

The genes or DNA sequences can be amplified using two approaches which are the *in vitro* (PCR) and *in vivo* (*cloning vector*).

(*See* ***Annexure 23.4.3*** *for details*)

The cloning of foreign DNA segments takes the advantage of restriction endonucleases that produce complementary single-stranded ends. These enzymes produce identical complementary ends on cleaved foreign DNAs and on the vector DNAs into which the foreign DNAs are inserted. A foreign DNA cloned using an enzyme that produces single-stranded complementary ends can always be excised from the cloning vector by cleavage with the same restriction enzyme that was originally used to clone it. For example, a gene of interest is inserted into the enzyme (*HindIII*) site in the polycloning region of the cloning vector (Bluescript) with DNA ligase, have amplified the plasmid containing the gene of interest in *E.coli*, and have isolated a large quantity of gene or Bluescript DNA. In this situation the gene of interest (*Hind III fragment*) from the cloning vector can be excised by digestion of the cloning vector (Bluescript) with endonuclease *HindIII.*

23.8.3 Somatic Cell Hybridization or Protoplast Fusion

The process of somatic cell hybridization or protoplast fusion had overcome the impossibility of hybridization between different species and genera. Harris, H. and Watkins, J.F. (1965) in Oxford first reported to form viable hybrid cells by fusion of cells of different animal species (man and mouse). In this case the nuclei of hybrid cells contain chromosomes from both cells for which these hybrid cells are called ***heterokaryons.***

Later on, many reports have come for the fusion of cells from different animal species. However, such a hybrid cell could not produce any hybrid animal for the reason that the animal cells do not differentiate in a culture medium.

Technique of somatic cell hybridization: See ***annexure 23.11***

The technique of ***protoplast fusion*** has produced two inter-specific plant hybrids *viz.* hybrid *tobacca* and hybrid *Petunia.*

- ☆ Carlson *et al.* (1972) produced the hybrid tobacco with a diploid genome of 42 chromosomes by fusion of cells of two tobacco species (N. *glauca* with 2n = 24 and N. *Langsdorfil with 2n = 18*).
- ☆ Power *et al.* (1976) produced a hybrid between two different species of *Petunia.*

The plant protoplasts and animal cells have also been fused. Cocking *et al.* (1975) have reported the fusion of yeast protoplast and hen erythrocytes while Dudits *et al.* (1976) have reported the fusion of human cells with carrot protoplasts.

Hybridization with somatic protoplast fusion does not involve the fusion of gametes which is the sexual reproduction and hence such hybridization is called ***para-sexual hybridization.***

Prospects of the Protoplast Fusion

This type of hybridization has overcome the problem of sexual barriers and hence provides a new technique of genetic manipulation. Thus, this technique of protoplast fusion is able to mix up the genetic materials of sexually isolated organisms.

23.9 SOUTHERN BLOT HYBRIDIZATION: MOLECULAR ANALYSIS OF DNA

The molecular analysis of DNA means to investigate the structure of gene. This requires the following steps:

- ☆ The DNA samples are subjected to gel electrophoresis for separation of macromolecules (DNA) with different sizes and charges,
- ☆ Transfer of DNA molecules on a membrane (Nylon or nitrocellulose) – Southern blot,
- ☆ Denaturation either prior to or during transfer by placing the gel in alkaline solution,
- ☆ Drying or UV irradiation or baking in vacuum to fix (immobilize) the DNA on the membrane,
- ☆ Hybridization of immobilized DNA with a radioactive DNA probe,
- ☆ Washing of the film to wash off the non-hybridized probe, and
- ☆ X-ray photograph of the film to develop autoradiogram (bands – Southern blots).

The details of the above steps are as under:

The ***electrophoresis*** is the migration of suspended particles in an electric field. The ***gel electrophoresis*** is a powerful technique in this respect (***Annexure 23.10***).

Southern, E.M. (1975) devised a method to identify the location of genes and other DNA segments on restriction fragments separated by gel electrophoresis. The DNAs are dissolved in buffer with density greater than that of the electrophoresis buffer so as to settle the DNA samples to the bottom instead of their diffusion in the electrophoresis buffer. The DNA buffer also contains a dye so as the migration rate of molecules through the buffer is monitored.

The transfer of DNA molecules on a membrane after their separation by gel electrophoresis is an important and essential feature of this technique. Therefore, the DNA molecules after their separation are transferred onto nitrocellulose or nylon membrane. The transfer of DNA fragments from an electrophoretic gel to a cellulose or nylon membrane by capillary action is called ***Southern blot.*** This technique was developed by the scientist E.M. Southern. The procedure for transfer of DNA from gel to the nitrocellulose filter resembles blotting and hence this process is also called as ***Southern blotting.*** It is the DNA-DNA hybridization technique.

The ***DNA is denatured*** in this technique, either prior to or during transfer by placing the gel in an alkaline solution. The transfer solution (20 X *SSC* or 0.4 M

NaOH) carries the DNA from the gel to the membrane. The SSC stands for *sodium chloride and sodium citrate*. The DNA binds to the membrane on contact.

The ***DNA is immobilized*** on the membrane by drying or UV irradiation or baked under vacuum to affix the DNA firmly prior to hybridization.

Hybridization (*in situ*) is performed between a radioactive DNA probe containing the desired sequence and the immobilized DNA on the membrane. The hybridization takes place between a probe and the DNA sequence containing the nucleotide sequence complementary to the sequence of the probe.

The membrane is then washed so as the non-hybridized probe is washed off. The X – ray film of washed off membrane is developed to detect the presence of the ***radioactivity.*** The dark bands on the film indicate the positions of DNA sequences that have hybridized with the probe.

This technique is very useful to detect an autosomal mutant gene causing cystic fibrosis which is the most commonly inherited disease in newborn babies, particularly in northern European people. The positional cloning has been successful to identify the gene causing this disorder.

The nucleotide-pair sequences of both the normal and mutant gene are known. The labelled oligonucleotides can be synthesized and used as hybridization probes to detect the presence of each allele (normal and mutant causing harmful effect). Each probe under hybridization condition will hybridize only with the normal allele that has perfect complementary to self. AS the sequences of the normal gene flanking the mutant site are known, oligonucleotide PCR primers can be synthesized and used to amplify this segment of the DNA obtained from small tissue. This explains the carrier of mutant allele.

The amplified DNAs can then be separated by agarose gel electrophoresis, transferred to nylon membrane, and hybridized to the respective labelled oligonucleotide probes, and the presence of normal allele can be detected by autoradiography. The mutant gene can be detected in heterozygote as well as homozygote.

23.10 NORTHERN BLOT HYBRIDIZATION: MOLECULAR ANALYSIS OF RNA

The RNA molecules like the DNAs are separated by agarose gel electrophoresis and can be transferred from agarose gel to a cellulose or nylon membrane for hybridization studies. The transfer of RNA molecules from an electrophoretic gel to a cellulose or nylon membrane by capillary action is called the ***Northern blots*** simply because this transfer of RNA is analogous to the Southern blotting technique.

The RNA molecules are sensitive to degradation by RNase and hence required their protection from these enzymes. The RNA molecules should be denatured during electrophoresis for their separation based on their size because they have secondary structures. The RNA molecules are denatured by adding formaldehyde to the electrophoresis buffer. Some other chemical denaturant in place of formaldehyde may be used.

The RNA blots after transfer to the membrane are hybridized to either RNA or DNA probes just like Southern blot.

This technique has proved useful in the study of gene expression, to determine when and where a particular gene is expressed. However, this technique only measures the accumulation of RNA transcripts without providing information of the reason of accumulation.

RNA Analysis by Reverse Transcriptase-PCR Method

The RNA molecules can also be detected and amplified by reverse transcriptase-PCR. The synthesis of DNA strands complementary to RNA templates (cDNA) is catalyzed by the enzyme reverse transcriptase and it can be used *in vitro*. The DNA strand so synthesized is converted to double-stranded DNA by different methods (like synthesis of double-stranded cDNAs from mRNA molecules), including the use of a second primer and the heat-stable *Taq* polymerase. These double-stranded DNA molecules are now amplified by PCR technique.

The first strand of DNA (called ***cDNA*** as it is complementary to the mRNA) can be synthesized by use of either:

- ☆ An oligo (dT) primer that anneal to the 3′-poly (A) tails of all mRNAs, or
- ☆ Gene-specific primers (sequences complementary to the RNA molecule of interest).

Construction of cDNA Libraries

The 3′-poly (A) tails of mRNA means the mRNA strand at its 3′ end at the site containing adenine base (A). This is because most mRNA molecules contain 3′ poly (A) tails. The expressed DNA sequences can be identified more easily by complementary DNA libraries. The poly (T) oligoprimers can be used to prime the synthesis of complementary DNA strands. The synthesis is catalyzed by reverse transcriptase. The synthesis of DNA strand starts from 3′ strand of mRNA strand forming 5′ strand of DNA. Now, the RNA-DNA duplexes are converted to double-stranded DNA molecules by the combined activities of ribonuclease (RNase) H, DNA polymerase I, and DNA ligase. The ribonuclease (RNase) H degrades the RNA template strand into short fragments which serve as primers for DNA synthesis. The DNA polymerase I catalyze the synthesis of the second DNA strand and replicates RNA primers with DNA strands. The DNA ligase seals the remaining single-strand breaks in the double-stranded DNA molecules.

The double-stranded cDNAs so produced form the construction of cDNA libraries. These cDNAs can be used to insert into plasmid or phage lambda cloning vectors by adding complementary single-stranded tails to the cDNAs and vectors.

[The specific gene transcripts are amplified by first using reverse transcriptase to synthesize a single-stranded DNA complementary to the mRNA of interest. The synthesis is initiated with a gene-specific oligo-nucleotide primer that only anneal to the mRNA of interest. The complementary DNA strand is then synthesized by using a reverse primer and Taq polymerase. Large quantities of double-stranded cDNA are subsequently synthesized by PCR in the presence of both the gene-specific and reverse PCR primers].

The gene-specific oligo-nucleotide primers are selected to anneal to sequences in the 3′-noncoding regions of the mRNAs. The gene specific primers can be used in reverse transcriptase PCR to amplify a specific gene transcript. The products of gene transcript obtained from amplification are analyzed by gel electrophoresis. The products appear in the gel is an indication that the sample under analysis contained the mRNA. Thus, it is quick and easy way to know the transcription of a specific gene.

Modification of RT-PCR method has been developed for quantitative estimation. The relationship between RNA input and DNA output can be determined by the analysis of known amount of the RNA. This relationship is helpful to know the amount of RNA initially present in the sample on the basis of the quantity of DNA generated by the experimental sample.

23.11 WESTERN BLOT HYBRIDIZATION: MOLECULAR ANALYSIS OF PROTEINS

The protein analysis also requires the transfer of proteins from electrophoretic gel to a cellulose or nylon membrane by means of an electric force. This transfer of protein is called ***western blot*** as the procedure is analogous to Southern blotting technique.

The polyacrylamide gel electrophoresis is used to separate and characterize the proteins. The individual polypeptides (two or more subunits) contained by many functional proteins are separated by electrophoresis run in the presence of detergent sodium dodecyl sulfate (SDS) which denatures the protein. The proteins after electrophoresis are detected by staining with Coomassie blue or silver stain. Alternately, the separated polypeptides are transferred from gel to the nitrocellulose membrane for detecting individual proteins with antibodies. The transfer is done by using an electric current which allows the proteins to move from the gel to the surface of the membrane.

The specific protein is identified by placing the membrane with the immobilized proteins in a solution containing antibody to the protein. The presence of initial (primary) antibody is detected by placing the membrane, after washing off the non-bound antibodies from membrane, in a solution containing a secondary antibody. This secondary antibody reacts with immune-globulins in general. The immune-globulins is the group of proteins comprising all antibodies. The secondary antibody unites to either a radioactive isotope for autoradiography or to an enzyme that produces a visible product on adding the proper substrate.

23.12 MOLECULAR ANALSYIS (MAPPING) OF GENES AND CHROMOSOMES

The recombinant DNA technologies have been of great use to determine the structure of genes, chromosomes, and complete genome. The physical map of gene, chromosome or genome is its nucleotide sequence. The restriction enzyme cleavage sites and nucleotide sequences of genes and chromosomes are used to construct physical maps.

23.12.1 Restriction Enzyme Cleavage Sites – As the Physical Map

The DNA molecule is cleaved by restriction enzymes at some specific cleavage sites and these cleavage sites can be used to construct physical maps of the chromosomes. The polyacrulamide or agarose gel electrophoresis is used to determine the size of the restriction fragments. The DNA has an essentially constant charge per unit of mass for the fact that it is made up of the subunits of nucleotides each of which have one phosphate group. This decides the rate of migration of DNA fragments during electrophoresis depending on their length. The rate of migration is inversely proportional to the length of fragments.

A set of DNA markers with different length of known size (nucleotide pairs) is used to estimate the size of DNA restriction fragments. The set of DNA molecules may be of size 1000 nucleotide pairs and multiple thereof. The DNA molecule is cut at different sites producing two DNA fragments of different sizes on cleavage by different restriction endonucleases. For example, a DNA molecule of 6 kb = 6000 nucleotide pairs will produce two fragments of 4000 and 2000 bp on cutting by *Eco RI* but the same DNA molecule of 6 kb will produce two fragments of sizes 5000 and 1000 bp (nucleotide base pairs) on cleaving by *HindIII restriction endonuclease.* However, the relative positions of cleavage sites by two enzymes do not provide any information about the location of the two cleavage sites relative to one another on the DNA molecule. Therefore, in order to establish the relative positions of two cleavage sites to each other, the DNA molecule is then simultaneously digested by both these enzymes to produce three fragments of sizes 3000, 2000, and 1000 nucleotide pairs. This is just like the two- and three-point cross data in linkage studies in locating the relative position of genes on the chromosome.

In order to construct the more extensive maps of restriction sites, several different restriction enzymes are used. Thus, detailed maps of entire chromosomes can be constructed by using large numbers of restriction enzymes. These are called the *restriction maps* which reflect the true physical distances along the DNA molecule whereas the genetic maps based on linkage studies do not reflect the true physical distances.

The physical maps of entire genome can be constructed by use of computer assisted restriction mapping with other molecular techniques. The construction of physical map of entire genome was first constructed for a worm (*Caenorhabditis elegans*) which is the multicellular eukaryote. This worm has also been used for studies on the genetic control of development and whose physical map was correlated with its genetic map.

23.12.2 Nucleotide-Pair Sequence – As the Physical Map

The nucleotide-pair sequence, complete with a chart of all nucleotide-pair changes that alter the function of that gene or the chromosome, provides the ultimate physical maps of DNA molecules (specific gene or the chromosome). It has now become a routine of laboratory work to sequence the entire genome of an organism after 1976 when the entire 5386-nucleotide-long chromosome of phage **Φ174** was sequenced. The DNA sequencing was performed using the sequencing protocols of 1977 (published by Sanger and colleagues) which depended on the generation of a population of DNA fragments having one common end of same nucleotide and terminate at all possible positions at the other end.

Sanger's procedure of sequencing uses the *In vitro* DNA synthesis in the presence of specific chain-terminators to generate populations of DNA fragments ending at A, G, C and T, respectively. The Sanger's procedure of chain terminator has been replaced by new methods.

The DNA sequencing work is performed now by the automated DNA sequencing machines. The new second generation sequencing machines can sequence up to 25 billion nucleotide pairs in one day.

One of the procedures is called *pyro-sequencing* for the reason that on adding a nucleotide to the end of a primer strand releases the pyrophosphate which is detected by this procedure.

Another procedure called *454 sequencing* utilizes a laser beam for recording the addition of fluorescently labelled nucleotides during the extension of primary strands bound to tiny beads in a water-oil mixture.

Still another procedure called *Illumina sequencing* (formerly Solexa sequencing) uses reversible terminators to detect single nucleotide for their adding to growing strands. The sequencing machines use this procedure. Large numbers of reactions occur simultaneously for which it is often called *massively parallel sequencing*.

Chapter 24

Applications of Molecular Genetics – Genome Manipulation

There are biotechnological applications in agriculture for increasing food production, *viz.* agro-chemical based agriculture, organic agriculture, genetically engineered crops.

In future the biotechnology may progress in the direction of understanding the molecular basis and pathway of learning and memory as well as the aging process, and the mechanism of regulating the cell division in the direction to use this knowledge in preventing and curing the human cancer and other life-threatening diseases.

Animal biotechnology covers the study including the various techniques of animal genetics and breeding (covering cytology including cell culture, cytogenetics, molecular genetics, and genomics), animal reproduction, animal nutrition, and animal health including human health along with their applications for animal improvement programmes.

24.1 AREAS OF ANIMAL IMPROVEMENT

The different areas of animal improvement are:

(1) ***Animal Genetics and Breeding*** to exploit genetic variability for the permanent improvement of livestock and evolving new breeds of livestock and poultry. The genetic composition of an individual can be altered. The new combination of genes can be produced either using the conventional

breeding methods or by using the recent genetic engineering technologies, known as transgenesis (the process of manipulating the DNA of an organism and expressing an extra - foreign gene). The transgenesis has altered/manipulated the genes of plants, bacteria, fungi, and animals. Such organisms with manipulation of their genome are called ***genetically modified organisms***. The development of molecular based technologies such as recombinant DNA technology (genetic engineering), and gene cloning have provided new avenues for genetic improvement of animals and plants.

These include the various techniques used in classical/basic genetics, cytology, cytogenetics, molecular genetics, biochemical genetics, immuno-genetics, developmental genetics (Organogenesis), and genomics.

The various applications of the techniques of molecular genetics for improvement of livestock and poultry species are:

(i) DNA finger printing,

(ii) Transgenesis,

(iii) Animal Cloning,

(iv) Genome maps, Next chapter 25, and

(v) Stem cell technology – See "*Cell Genetics* and *Genomics*" Tomar and Tomar, 2018

(vi) Cell culture product – These include virus vaccines and useful biochemicals (enzymes, hormones, cellular biochemicals like interferrons and immunological compounds including monoclonal antibodies, hybrid antibodies, and recombinant proteins. see "Cell Genetics and Genomics" by Tomar and Tomar (1918).

(2) ***Animal Reproduction*** for augmenting the reproductive rate and related areas: The various reproductive biotehnologies include the A.I., frozen semen technology, ETT, production of IVF embryos, embryo cryopreservation, sexing of sperms or embryos, and embryo splitting. See "*Sustainable Livestock and Poultry Breeding*" by Tomar and Tomar (2016), published by Daya Publishing House, Darya Ganj, New Delhi.

(3) ***Animal nutrition*** to provide better food material that comes from plants which have the ability to capture the solar energy and to make its use in production of vegetative matter and food grains. The vegetative part of plants is used as green and dry roughages and food grains are used as concentrates for animals to provide them energy for performing various body functions. The regular supply of food to animals in the form of roughages and concentrates is the only factor for their continuous functional behavior and optimum production of various animal products like milk, meat, eggs, wool, *etc.*

In view of harvesting the optimum production from animals various quality feeds and feed processing techniques, mixed feed technology, bypass nutrients (proteins and fats) including genetic manipulation of rumen microbes have been developed. See *"Sustainable Livestock and Poultry Breeding"* by Tomar and Tomar (2016), published by Daya Publishing House, Darya Ganj, New Delhi.

Recent developments have been made in the area of *"Nutrigenomics and Proteomics"*. See "Cytogenetics and Genomics" Tomar and Tomar (2018), published by Daya Publishing House, New Delhi.

(4) ***Animal management*** to provide comfort to the animals: Efforts have been made in this direction through amelioration of heat and cold stress by various techniques of housing with heat reducing cooling systems, various feeding practices (change in animal diet, grain feeding, dietary fat, protein feeding, mineral feeding, feed additives, antioxidant feeding), and change in the breeding strategies. See *"Sustainable Livestock and Poultry Breeding"* by Tomar and Tomar (2016), published by Daya Publishing House, Darya Ganj, New Delhi.

(5) ***Animal Health Care*** is very important aspect of sustainable animal breeding and affects the survival of people which rests on survival of animals in various ways. The animals are the richest source of food, cloths, medicines, draft power, great companion of man, and so on. See *"Sustainable Livestock and Poultry Breeding"* by Tomar and Tomar (2016), published by Daya Publishing House, Darya Ganj, New Delhi.

The various techniques have progressed to search the *defective genes* (mutants) responsible for causing the diseases in human. This has been possible by comparing the nucleotide sequences of normal and mutant alleles causing human diseases. The biotechnology has its applications including therapeutics, diagnostics, waste and pollutant treatment, and energy production.

The animal and human health care includes the production of Mono clonal antibodies used in disease diagnosis like veneral diseases, hepatitis B and other viral diseases, cancer, etc; DNA probes also used for disease diagnosis, recombinant vaccines like human hepatitis B virus, E. coli vaccins for pigs, rabies virus, *etc.*; valuable drugs like human insulin, human interferrons, human and bovine growth hormones.

Gene therapy has been developed to cure genetic diseases like Huntington's chorea, cystic fibrosis. Likewise babies of desired sex through A.I. with X or Y carrying sperms, DNA finger printing.

The various aspects of human health care are:

(*i*) *Disease Prevention* (viral vaccine produced as a cell culture product),

(*ii*) *Disease Diagnosis* (*Molecular diagnosis includes inherited human diseases* and *Molecular tests* for diagnosing human diseases),

(*iii*) *Disease Treatment* (Molecular technique of treatment includes *Gene therapy*), forensic medicines.

These have been discussed with a greater detail under these heads in chapter 8 of the book of authors (2018) *"Cytogenetics and Genomics"*.

24.2 DNA PROFILING/TYPING OR GENOTYPING

This is the record of patterns of DNA polymorphisms in human genome and provides strong evidence of an individual's identity or nonidentity to distinguish individuals for which this was originally called as DNA identification analysis or ***identity testing.*** The DNA sequence data when used in personal identity cases is called ***DNA profiling*** and earlier it was known as ***DNA fingerprinting.*** *It is the procedure of developing the DNA fragment band (alleles) patterns which characterizes one or more rare features of an individual's genome (hereditary make up). The* ***DNA fingerprinting*** (DFP) is the DNA-DNA hybridization technique giving a unique individual specific pattern and has played a great role in human identity cases for decades. The basis of fingerprinting is that no two individuals have identical prints and also their genomes do not have the same nucleotide sequences, except identical twins.

It is very important tool in cases of uncertain identity, like paternity, murder, rape, and for identifying the mutilated bodies after tragedies such as explosion, crashes, *etc.* This technique is used to identify bodies and body parts recovered from debris. The DNA profils are prepared from minute amounts of blood, semen, hair bulbs or other cells by extracting DNA from these cells and amplified by PCR. The STRs are characterized by PCR using fluorescent primers, capillary gel electrophoresis, and fluorescence detectors.

The concept of fingerprinting was laid down by Wayman and White (1980) based on the observation of a polymorphic DNA locus which was characterized by a number of variable length restriction fragments called as restriction fragment length polymorphism (RFLPs). However, the history of DNA fingerprinting is more recent after the work of Jeffreys *et al.* (1985) who discovered a region having 33 bp sequences that was replicated 4 times within an intervening sequence. They detected a complex ladder of DNA fragments which was unique for each individual.

It is well known that the DNA has 4 nitrogen bases (2 purines – adenine and guanine, and 2 pyrimidine bases – cytosine and thymine) which form DNA sequences in different ways. These sequences vary in number in different individuals, called repetitive sequences which generally comprise 2 – 250 base pairs of a specific sequence and repeated from a few to several thousand times. The multiplicity of lengths of the segments is called length polymorphism which is hyper-variable repeats (HVRs) or variable number tandem repeats (VNTRs). The variable number tandem repeats (VNTRs, also called ***minisatellites*** are composed of repeated sequences 10 to 80 nucleotide pairs long. The second type of DNA polymorphisms is the sort tandem repeats (STRs, also called ***microsatellites*** which are composed of repeated sequences 2 to 10 nucleotide pairs long.

The bands of DNA profile are inherited in a simple Mendelian fashion and behave as co-dominant. Both the maternal and paternal derived variants at any given locus are detectable. The band patterns also behave like independent loci. The DNA fingerprinting is most important among various genome markers and like RFLP *there are genetic loci for which every individual is unique and different from others.* Therefore, an individual inherits one or the other of the allelic status of each marker from each parent whereas another individual of the same parents inherits different marker set. However, *two offspring may have some markers in common but other markers as different but the unrelated individuals have no markers in common*. The probability of two DNA samples matching by chance is very low (10^{-6} to 10^{-15}).

The numbers of variable bands which appear in DNA fingerprints depend upon combination of enzyme and probe (nucleotide sequence capable of hybridizing with its complementary chain sequence). The patterns of DNA fingerprints in an individual have the characteristics to remain same without showing any change:

- ☆ Irrespective of source of DNA from any tissue of the body (WBC, semen, hair bulbs etc).
- ☆ Irrespective of fresh, frozen or dried tissues provided the tissue is not contaminated.
- ☆ Irrespective of age of individual (from birth to death) except mutation which may cause loss or appearance of one or more bands.

Methodology of DNA Fingerprinting

This involves the following steps:

(i) Isolation of DNA, mostly from blood and semen.

(ii Digestion of DNA, by restriction endonucleases (HaeIII, HinfI, AluII, etc). This is done in a reaction mixture containing DNA, enzyme, buffer, BSA and distilled water.

(iii Separation of different fragments, according to size, by electrophoresis.

(iv) Transfer of size separated DNA fragments, on nitrocellulose or nylon membrane. This is done by using the capillary method or vacuum transfer method.

(v) Probe labelling: The probes are labelled with ^{32}P radioactive labelled nucleotide.

(vi Hybridization: The labelled probe DNA is hybridized with complementary sequences located on nylon membrane. This involves the incubation of nylon membrane with labelled probe in hybridization solution and washing the membrane repeatedly in a series of solutions to remove non-specific binding.

(vii) Autoradiography: This is a technique used to detect the sequences in genome. This involves the alignment of hybridized nylon membrane with X-ray film and incubation at low temperature (-70° C).

(viii) Analysis and interpretation of band patterns by comparing the position of bands and band sharing tendency. This can now be done with computer software.

Applications of DNA fingerprinting (DFP) are as under:

1. Individual identification
2. Pedigree analysis and parentage verification
3. Zygosity testing (twins)

4. Sex determination
5. Conservation of genetic resources (identification of genetic relatedness).
6. Demographic studies (estimation of individual and population homozygosity, effective population size, population sub division, relatedness, social organization and kin selection)
7. Identification of loci controlling quantitative traits or disease resistance
8. Pathogen identification
9. Detection of source of tissues, particularly in meat industry to avoid adulteration
10. Detection of somatic mutation or cancer
11. Taxonomical tool
12. Quality control of cell banks.

Paternity Test

The blood type test comparisons of child and its parents have been earlier used in case of uncertain paternity. Now DNA profiles have replaced the blood type tests for more and sure accuracy in identifying the true or genuine individual/father.

In conducting the paternity test the DNA samples are obtained from the cells of child and from both the parents to prepare DNA profiles. On comparing the profiles, all the bands in the child's DNA profile should be present in the combined DNA profiles of the parents. About half of the DNA bands or peaks in the child's DNA profile result from DNA sequences of the mother and another half from DNA sequences of the father.

Forensic Applications

The DNA profile was first used in 1988 as evidence in criminal case in Florida against an accused rapist. This test involves the matching of DNA profile prepared from the bloodstain at the crime scene with the DNA profile of the suspect. The DNA profiling is a powerful tool in personal identity cases. The DNA profiles provide strong evidence of individual identity in case of paternity and forensic cases.

Sex Determination by Sexing of Semen and Embryos

The sex of the new born offspring can now be determined before fertilization by sexing of semen. The sperm containing X or Y chromosome are separated and the female is inseminated to produce desired sex. The separation is done using staining procedure and detecting by laser beam with the help of standard flow cytometry equipment.

Another approach of sexing is to determine the sex of the embryos. The following methods are used:

(a) Enzyme activity method - the activity of certain X -linked enzymes is measured. This is twice in case of female embryos than male because the females have two X chromosomes. This method has the limitation of embryonic mortality and not being 100 per cent accurate.

(b) H - Y antigen detection - Male specific antigen known as H- Y antigen is immunologically detected. However, it gives an accuracy of 85 per cent.

(c) DNA probing - One cell from an early embryonic stage is extracted and the sex is determined by localization of DNA sequences present on Y chromosome. The DNA of the biopsed cell of the embryo is hybridized to a labelled sequence of the DNA specific to Y chromosome. The presence of Y chromosome in the biopsed cell is indicated by the positive hybridization. This method has also the limitation of reduced viability of biopsed embryo.

(d) Karyotyping - some cells of an embryo are taken to examine the metaphase chromosome and karyotyped for two X chromosome or one Y chromosome.

(e) Polymerase chain reaction (PCR) method - This technique is more accurate (95 per cent), rapid and does not affect embryo viability. It involves amplifying Y chromosome specific DNA sequences directed by primers with a thermostable DNA polymerase from a small amount of DNA of one or more blastomers.

24.3 TRANSGENESIS – GENE TRANSFER TECHNOLOGY

The animals can be modified by introduction of foreign DNA into their genome such that all the cells of an animal including germ cells are genetically changed. The genes can be changed so as to change the characteristics of an animal. This extra gene may be introduced in an embryo and this gene can knock out the functioning of another gene in the embryo. A foreign or modified gene that has been introduced into an organism is called *transgene*. The animal whose genetic composition is deliberately modified by introducing foreign (exogenous) DNA molecule into them is said to be ***transgenic*** or transgenic animal. This process is called the ***transgenesis*** or ***transgenics***. This technique was applied first on mice (Gorden and Ruddle, 1982) because of its small body size, liter size and low generation interval. The technique of transgenesis was afterward used in rats, rabbits, sheep, pigs and birds.

This technology produces the animals of specific characteristics and hence it is purpose specific. The purpose of this technique in farm animals is to produce genuine human proteins of pharmaceutical value in large amount. The DNA gene for protein drug of interest can be transferred into another organism that will produce large quantity of protein. The foreign or modified gene that has been introduced into an organism is called ***transgene***. In dairy animals the purpose is to change the protcin composition of milk. The transgenesis may allow the production of animals resistant to diseases.

Steps Involved in Transgenesis

The transgenesis involves the technique of recombinant DNA technology and cloning completed in the following steps:

- ☆ Isolation of the gene of interest on a strand of DNA,
- ☆ Cutting of DNA at specific points by restriction enzymes,

☆ Joining the cut DNA with a vector which may be virus or part of bacterial cell (plasmid), and

☆ The gene of interest is carried by the vector into the organism that will produce the protein.

Methods of Producing Transgenic Animals – Gene Transfer Method

The transgenic animals by use of recombinant technology for gene transfer are produced by three methods *viz.* DNA microinjection, embryonic stem cell mediated gene transfer and retrovirus mediated gene transfer.

(*i*) *DNA microinjection*: This procedure involves surgically removal of the eggs from female parent and then fertilizing the egg *in vitro*. The microinjection of gene of interest or DNA from another animal of same species or from a different species is performed into the pro-nucleus (haploid nucleus of sperm prior to nuclear fusion) of the fertilized ovum. The manipulated fertilized ovum is transferred/implanted into the oviduct of a recipient female (Foster mother). However, the insertion of DNA is a random process that the inserted gene may not insert itself into a site on the host DNA that will permit its expression. Therefore many copies of genes are injected. The injected DNA molecules are integrated at random sites in the genome. This method has been used to produce transgenic pigs, sheep, cattle, and other domestic animals.

(ii) *Embryonic Stem Cells* (*ESC*): The method of producing transgenic animals involves the introduction of genetically engineered ESC into an early stage developing embryo (blastocyst stage) which is implanted in foster mother. The ES cells come from blastula stage of embryos. These cells are cultured *in vitro*, transfected or injected with DNA, and then introduced into another developing embryo.

(iii) *Vector mediated method*: The gene transfer is mediated by means of a vector (virus or plasmid). Commonly the retrovirus is used as vectors to transfer genetic material in to host cell. The retrovirus infects the cells of an early embryo prior to implantation into a recipient female. This results in a chimera with diverse genetic constitution. This method involves removal of 8-cell stage embryo and its infection by virus carrying foreign gene. The virus penetrates the cells but may not replicate because it is made defective. This transformed embryo is implanted in foster mother. The transgenic line is established by mating.

Applications of Transgenesis

The transgenic (gene transfer) livestock production research remained limited to increase the growth of animals by introducing genes responsible for growth hormones regulation, disease resistance of animals (influenza resistance is caused by M_x gene), and to improve the quality and quantity of animal products like wool quantity and quality of sheep, meat in pigs, and milk quantity and composition in cattle/buffaloes.

The transgenesis is used to produce human drugs (animal pharming). The successful production of transgenic animal can produce pharmaceutical proteins in its blood and excretions (milk, urine, sperm or egg) and can grow rejection-resistant organs for transplant. The pharmaceutical proteins/drugs may be used for treatment of certain diseases like cystic fibrosis, hemophilia, thrombosis, wound healing in sheep; thrombosis and haemophilia in pigs; thrombosis in goats; hemophilia and wound healing in cows, *etc.* Monoclonal antibodies used in vaccine production can also be produced from transgenic animals. A number of human proteins have been found expressed in transgenic animals. These are human haemoglobin, human serum albumin, fibrinogen, lactferrin, human fertility hormones, monoclonal antibodies *etc.*

The other areas of research to apply this technique of transgenics are to produce the lines of animals *resistance to diseases, modification of performance traits* and *Xeno-transplantation* (transplantation of animal organs, tissues or cells in to humans).

- ☆ To study gene regulation and normal functions of the body and its development. This is done by introducing genes from other species that alter the formation of complex factors involved in growth as insulin like growth factor.
- ☆ The transgenic animals are designed to serve as models for human diseases like cancer, CF, rheumatoid arthritis and Alzheimer's and to study the way the genes contributes to the development of disease.
- ☆ The transgenic animals to produce useful biological products can be produced by the introduction of the part of DNA or gene which code for a particular product like human protein (α-1- antitrypsin) used to treat the disease (*emphysema*) as well as for the treatment of other diseases like Phenylketonuria (PKU) and CF. The first transgenic cow, Rosie, in 1997, produced had human protein-enriched milk containing α- lactalbumin.
- ☆ Transgenic mice in place of monkeys are produced for use in testing the safety of vaccines like polio vaccine for use by humans.
- ☆ Transgenic animals are produced to carry genes which make them sensitive to toxic substances compared to non-transgenic animals. These animals are then exposed to the toxic substances and to study their effects in a less time. This known as toxicity/safety testing like that used for testing toxicity of drugs.

24.4 ANIMAL CLONING - NUCLEAR TRANSFER TECHNIQUE OR REPRODUCTIVE CLONING

The cloning is the production of genetically identical organisms. In other words, the cloning is to produce duplicate organisms. This is also called ***reproductive cloning***.

The first cloned animal in the world was a sheep named *Dolly* which was produced by Dr. Ian Wilmut in 1997 at Roslin Institute, Edinburgh (Scotland). The cloning is based on the fact that every somatic diploid cell (differentiated cell) has the genetic material (DNA)/genetic information required to develop/make an exact copy of the original body. The progeny of a single cell is called a *"clone"*. This has proved that differentiated cells have the genetic potential to direct development.

The ***Dolly sheep*** was produced by fusing an egg of ewe of a Blackface breed (called egg cell mother) with a cell from the udder of ewe of Fin Dorset (genetic mother). The nucleus of an egg (ovum) in Blackface ewe was removed before fusing the egg with the udder cell. Thus, the genetic material of an egg (ovum) taken from Blackface ewe was replaced with the nucleus from a cell taken from the udder of an adult female sheep of Fin Dorset. The newly formed egg was subsequently stimulated to divide to produce an embryo and this embryo was implanted in the uterus of another Blackface ewe (surrogate or gestational mother). This embryo was allowed to grow and develop in the uterus of surrogate mother till full term of pregnancy when the ***Dolly*** was born. This way, the Dolly had no father but three mothers (egg cell mother, genetic mother, and surrogate mother).

The cloning involves the fusion of a donor cell (embryonic or somatic) to an oocyte or zygote (of the recipient) following its enucleation (removal of genetic material). Thus, the genetic material of the donor cell (Fin Dorset – genetic mother) is transferred to the enucleated recipient cell (Blackface ewe – egg cell mother). This recipient cell from egg cell mother) is usually a secondary oocyte which can be obtained following ovulation *in vivo* or by *in vitro* maturation of oocytes. The enucleation (removal of nucleus of egg mother cell) is accomplished either by splitting the oocyte or by removing the chromosomes by aspiration.

Clones have been produced using embryonic, foetal and adult cells. The cloning has been successfully achieved in animals using early embryonic source material (sheep, cattle, pig), nuclear transplantation, embryonic cultured cell line and somatic cells of adult animals (Dolly sheep and cattle).

The reproductive cloning encounters some problems. Reproductive cloning if not performed from a normal nucleus it may lead developmental abnormalities resulting short lifespan. The cloned animal may not thrive well but shows lack of vigour. This suggests that the somatic nuclei are different from zygotic nuclei produced by fertilization. The reasons may perhaps be that the somatic nucleus has accumulated mutations or may have undergone changes associated to genetic imprinting or chromosome inactivation (may be methylation of some nucleotides, acetylation of histones, and so). Therefore, this technique of reproductive cloning in humans is not safe and hence not recommended.

24.4.1 Types of Animal Cloning

The animal cloning is of the following types:

(*i*) ***Embryo cloning*** wherein one or more cells are removed from embryo to develop one or more duplicate embryo. It is the medical technique to produce monozygotic twins (identical) or triplets. One or more cells of fertilized embryo are removed and allow developing into one or more duplicate embryos. This produces twins or triplets with identical DNA.

(*ii*) ***Adult DNA cloning*** wherein the DNA from an embryo is removed and replaced with the DNA of an adult animal. This embryo is the implanted in a womb to develop into a new animal – like Dolly sheep. This technique is known as *"**nuclear transfer**"* and often referred to as *"**reproductive cloning**"*. This technique produces a duplicate of an existing animal.

(*iii*) ***Therapeutic cloning*** wherein the stem cells are removed from the embryo to produce a tissue or whole organ for transplanting back into the patient who supplied the DNA. The therapeutic cloning is done with the purpose to produce a healthy copy of a patient's tissue or organ for transplant. The tissue or organ has patient's original DNA. This technique of cloning is useful to clone various organs to replace the diseased/damaged organs like in case of liver failure, kidney failure, lungs, heart' attack as well as to correct/treat various diseases like leukemia by cloning bone marrow, cystic fibrosis, spinal cord injury, Down's syndrome, Tay-Sachs disease, diabetes, heart disease and cancer.

The technology used in the isolation or synthesis and joining together the unlike pieces of DNA to make the biologically active recombinant DNA molecules which can be introduced into bacteria or yeast where they can replicate and function, is called the ***recombinant DNA technology*** or ***genetic engineering***.

The propagation of a piece of DNA (Eukaryotic or prokaryotic) in another cell is the ***molecular cloning*** or ***DNA cloning***. All the cells derived from the original cell into which the foreign DNA has been introduced, contain exactly the same genetic information including the piece of foreign DNA. The bacterial cells are used for cloning for the reason of their fast growth rate, though eukaryotic cells (yeast) can be taken.

For the propagation in bacteria, the eukaryotic DNA fragment is spliced (inserted) *in vitro* into a plasmid (extra-chromosomal circular DNA molecule which can replicate independently of the bacterial chromosome) or bacteriophage cloning vector and the resulting recombinant plasmid is reintroduced into the bacterium where it replicates and passed on to the daughter cells on dividing the bacterium.

24.4.2 Production of Cloned Calves/Kids in India

The world first cloned buffalo calf by cloning technique was produced in February, 2009 and second cloned buffalo calf "Garima" in June, 2009 at NDRI, Karnal. The cloned buffalo calves 'Garima' and 'Garima-II' were born using a foetal and ESC as the donor cell, respectively.

A male buffalo calf 'Shresth' was produced in August, 2010 from a cloned embryo frozen at – 196° C for one week in liquid nitrogen and its thawing at room temperature to bring it back to life.

A first female calf 'Mahima' was born from cloned buffalo Garima in January, 2013. Another female cloned Murrah buffalo calf 'Lalima' was born in May, 2014 at NDRI, Karnal. A cloned male calf 'Rajat' was produced in July, 2014 from the somatic cell recovered from seminal plasma of frozen semen of a PT bull which was died 10 years ago.

The first cloned Pashmina goat was successfully produced at Sher-e-Kashmir University of Agricultural Sciences and Technology.

24.4.3 Applications of Livestock Cloning

The cloning technology (nuclear transfer) has the following promises -

- ☆ Cloning is useful in propagation of an infinite number of a proven valuable farm animal at faster rate and hence increase the rate of genetic gain and accuracy of selection,
- ☆ Induce genetic modifications in animal cells and multiplication of the modified cells *in vitro* and their use in producing transgenic animals used in production of pharmaceutical (therapeutic) proteins,
- ☆ Production of tissues/organs for xenotransplantation: The cloning combined with transgenics in pigs may overcome the shortage of human organs for transplantation if certain known and effective genes from pig genome are added or removed because this will reduce the ability of the human immune system to reject a transplanted pig organ. Some companies are genetically developing the modified pigs and the modification remained so far limited to only by adding genes. The nuclear transfer may also allow deletion of genes from pigs, α – galactosyl transferase gene codes for an enzyme that creates carbohydrate groups attached to pig tissues and responsible for the immediate rejection of an organ from a normal pig by a human patient,
- ☆ Cloning can be used for creation of thousands of precise duplicates of genetically engineered animals (identical offspring using embryonic cell lines) in a single generation,
- ☆ Cloning offers novel opportunities for tissue regeneration and development of targeted embryonic stem cells for therapeutic applications. Cell transplants may be used to correct genetic diseases (disorders) by replacing the mutant genes, called as *gene therapy*. This may also be done by use of complementary piece of DNA or RNA to disable the mutant or harmful gene, called as *antisense genetics*. This neutralizes the activity of harmful gene. The cell based therapy can be done by cell transplants. The rejection of transplanted cells by the patient can be avoided by deriving the type of required cells from the patient.
- ☆ It is much simpler and effective means of conservation of breeds. Skin biopsies, hair follicles and blood samples might be suitable sources of cells to grow in the laboratory and frozen for long term storage,
- ☆ It may be used to increase population size,
- ☆ It may use the embryos cloned from cells of high performing F_1 individuals to retain heterosis.

The somatic cell cloning through nuclear transfer to produce cloned animals though remarkable but is highly inefficient and prone to epigenetic errors due to high rate of mortality which limit the acceptability of somatic cell cloning.

24.5 PRODUCTION TO EUKARYOTIC PROTEINS IN BACTERIA: NUTRITION AND HEALTH

The valuable proteins are isolated from eukaryotes only in small amounts and at higher cost. Earlier the insulin used for diabetes was used to be extracted from pancreas of slaughtered cattle and pigs which caused to some patients to develop allergy or any other reaction to this foreign protein.

The insulin contains two short polypeptide chains (A and B) linked together by disulphide bridges and it is synthesized as a pro-hormone in mammals containing an extra stretch (C peptide) and hence needs processing.

Now, the recombinant DNA technologies by producing the genetically engineered bacteria (GEB) and other microbes can be used:

- ☆ To produce human insulin, human growth hormone, and other valuable eukaryotic proteins (entire family of interferons).
  - (*i*) ***Human insulin*** – a protein produced in microorganism was first used in the field of pharmaceuticals in 1982 for diabetic patients and became the commercial success of the recombinant DNA technologies. Two DNA sequences of A and B chains of human insulin were prepared and introduced in plasmids of *E. coli* to produce insulin chains. The human insulin was formed by producing two chains separately, extracted and combined by creating disulphide bonds.
  - (*ii* ***Human growth hormone*** (hGH) is a protein deficient in some type of pituitary dwarfism. The hGH is a single polypeptide chain of 191 amino acids in length, required for normal growth, and is produced in *E. coli*. The HGH synthesized in *E. coli* is fully active in humans. The hGH became the second genetically engineered pharmaceutical best suited and approved for use by humans by the U.S. Food and Drug Administration,
- ☆ To produce the ***antibiotics,*** antifungal drugs, amino acids, vitamins, to provide metabolic machinery for the detoxification of pollutants, and to convert biomass to combustible compounds,
- ☆ To synthesize valuable ***enzymes*** like proteases from *Bacillus licheniformis* and other bacteria and used as cleaning aids in detergents, as meat tenderizers and as digestive aids in animal feeds. Likewise, the enzyme amylases and glucose isomerase are manufactured by microbiological processes. The amylase is used in breaking down the complex carbohydrates such as starch to glucose and the enzyme glucose isomerase is used to convert glucose to fructose used as a sweetener.

Since the production of insulin during 1982, the bacteria have been used to synthesize other human proteins of medicinal value. These are the:

(i) ***Blood clotting factor VIII*** which lacks in persons of one type of hemophilia,

(ii) ***Plasminogen activator*** which is a protein which disposes blood clots, and

(iii) ***Rennin*** production commercially by genetically engineered bacteria which was earlier produced (extracted) from fourth stomach of calf.

The recombinant microorganisms as well as transgenic plants and animals will be used in future to produce many more proteins including enzymes for use in industrial applications.

24.6 METHODS OF GENETIC DISSECTION OF BIOLOGICAL PROCESSES

The research in last century has well established that every biological process is under the control of genes. There are two approaches to know the pathways of biological processes for their control by genes.

24.6.1 Classical Genetic Approach

This is also known as ***mutational dissection approach.*** The basis of this approach is to characterize the mutant gene causing abnormal phenotypes. In order to determine the effect of mutation, the comparative molecular studies are made on wild-type and mutant organism. The genes are identified based on the products encoded by the genes and responsible for biological process of interest. Biologists also got success in some cases to know the sequence of events occurring in completing the process. However, the advancement of newer techniques in molecular genetics has replaced this old approach.

24.6.2 Reverse Genetic Approaches

The new approaches have come to know the details of events occurring in completing a biological process what is known as the *genetic dissection of biological processes.* These newer approaches are known as ***reverse genetics.*** This approach makes use of the nucleotide sequences of genes which become known earlier than actually knowing the function of the gene.

The nucleotide sequences of genes are used in reverse genetic approaches to devise the procedures in either of the two ways *viz.* isolating null mutations in them or shutting off their expression. The organisms lacking functional product of the gene are used to know the function of a specific gene.

The followings are the three important reverse genetic approaches. These approaches involve inhibition of expression of specific genes by -

- ☆ Insertion of foreign DNA to produce the ***"knockout" mutations*** in mice,
- ☆ T-DNA and transposon insertions in plants, and
- ☆ RNA interference.

(a) Knockout Mutations in Mice

A mutation that completely abolishes or disrupts the function of a gene is called ***knockout (null) mutation.*** The procedure of insertion of foreign DNA in mice is used to produce transgenic mice. The transgenes are inserted at random sites into the genome. However, the foreign DNA inserted may contain a homologous sequence to that of the mouse gene and may be inserted into that sequence through homologous recombination. In this case the insertion of foreign DNA into the gene disrupt (knockout) its function.

The knockout mutation involves the construction of a gene-targeting vector which is potential to have homologous recombination with one of the chromosomal copies of the gene. The knockout mice are very useful in the study of development, physiology, neurobiology, immunology in mammals, and a number of inherited human diseases like sickle-cell anemia, heart disease, and cancer. In view of the value of knockout mice in relation to human health, a project to produce knockout mutations in mouse genes has been initiated in 2006 at National Institutes of Health. The knockout strains are being produced and distributed for research work.

(b) T-DNA and Transposon Insertins

T-DNA is the segment of DNA in the Ti plasmid of *agrobacterium tumefaciens* that is transferred to plant cells and inserted into the chromosomes of the plant. The Ti plasmid is large plasmid in *A. tumefaciens* responsible for the induction of tumours in plants with crown gall disease and is an important vector for transferring genes into plants, especially dicots. The T-DNA after inserting into a gene disrupts its function.

Second are the transposon genetic elements which have the ability to move from one location in the chromosome to another and disrupt the function of the gene into which it gets inserted. Thus, T-DNA and transposons introduce *insertional mutagenesis* and called as ***null mutation*** or ***knockout mutation*** and this insertional mutagenesis is basically the same produced by the insertion of foreign DNA into genes. Both T-DNA and transposon are used for *reverse genetic analysis*.

(c) RNA Interference

The ***RNA interference*** is a phenomenon in which double-stranded RNA prevents the expression of a gene homologous to at least part of the RNA. This (***RNAi***) is the third reverse genetic approach discovered by Andrew Fires and others (1998) and shared 2006 Noble Prize in Physiology or Medicine. The RNA interference (RNAi) can block gene expression with double-stranded RNA (dsRNA) which in turn can be used to know the genetic (molecular or biochemical) pathway of biological processes by inhibiting the functions of specific genes.

Andrew and others injected double-stranded RNA (***dsRNA***) into *C, elegans* and this interfered with or shut off the expression of the genes containing the same nucleotide sequence. It is known that double-stranded DNA is important to prevent the expansion of populations of transposable genetic elements, preventing the viral infections and fight against human diseases, and in regulating the gene expression. Thus, the RNAi is used as silencer genes to turn off or turn down their expression in *C. elegans, D. melanogaster,* and many other plants.

It is very easy to perform RNAi in *C. elegans* to effective gene silencing and this can be done in either of the three ways *viz.* microinjection of the worms with dsRNA, soaked in media contain ing the dsRNA or feeding bacteria synthesizing the dsRNA of interest.

The most important requirement of gene silencing is the presence of dsRNA carrying at least a portion of the nucleotide sequence of the gene whose function in the organism or cell is to be turn off. This requirement can be fulfilled in two ways. One is the synthesis of dsDNA *in vitro* and microinjection into the organism. Second is the introduction into the organism by transformation or transduction, the gene-expression cassette carrying two copies of at least a portion of the gene of interest in inverse orientation. RNA molecule is that encode complementary and forms a partially double-stranded stem-and-loop or hairpin structure. The dsRNA in both ways of introduction stimulate RNA-induced gene silencing.

The studies of RNAi of gene silencing have provided useful information about the functions of hundreds of genes and hence the RNAi has become a powerful tool to know genetic pathway of biological processes. There are hundreds of genes to encode ***microRNAs*** which **form** dsRNAs *in vivo*. The microRNAs have regulatory functions. The therapeutic applications of RNAi and their commercial use are awaited like their use to inhibit the reproduction of virus (such as human immunodeficiency virus, HIV) or to shut off the expression of ***oncogenes*** (cancer causing genes).

Application in medicine: production of insulin, gene therapy.

24.7 REPRODUCTIVE BIOTECHNIQUES

The different different reproductive biotechnologies are like A.I., Frozen semen technology, IVF, ETT, Embryo cryopreservation, and Embryo splitting. These have been discussed with a greater detail under these heads in chapter 24 of the book of authors (2016) "*Sustainable Livestock and Poultry Breeding*" published by Daya Publishing House, New Delhi.

24.8 CELL CULTURE PRODUCTS

The different products obtained from animal cell culture are *viral vaccines, interferons, recombinant proteins, hybrid antibodies and monoclonal antibodies.* These have been discussed with a greater detail under these heads in chapter 6 of the book of authors (2018) "*Cytogenetics and Genomics*". Published by the same publishers.

24.9 GENOME MAPS

The various topics described under genome maps are: *Genome projects, Molecular marker*, Chrosome jumping and walking, and FISH - Fluorescence *in situ* hybridization, Microsatellite (STR) mapping including Somatic cell hybrids, and Genetic and physical maps. These have been described in next chapter 25.

Chapter 25

Markers and Genome Maps

Different species of organisms have different number of chromosomes *viz.* bacteria has only one chromosome whereas the higher organisms (plants and animals) have more number of chromosomes. The man, farm animals, lab animals, birds are diploids in which the chromosomes are present in pairs. The sum total of chromosomes in an organism is called the ***genome***. A detailed schematic description of the structural and functional organization of all the chromosomes in the genome of an organism is called the ***genome map***.

Each chromosome has many gene loci which influence the expression of different phenotypic, biochemical, physiological, and behavioural characters of organisms. This means the genes are located and linked on chromosomes at their different positions or locations which are called ***gene loci***. These gene loci are linearly organized on the chromosomes.

Gene and Chromosome Mapping

The ***gene mapping*** is a method to identify the genes responsible for specific traits. The location of genes and other molecular markers on the chromosome is called the ***chromosome mapping***.

The genes on the chromosomes can be mapped based on recombination frequencies (linkage maps or genetic maps), positions relative to cytological features (cytological maps), or physical distances. The information about the location of genes in the genome has been one of the important contributions in genomic research. This information has been helpful to identify and isolate gene with a known phenotypic effect and called *positional cloning*. The positional cloning has been used to identify the genes responsible some human inherited diseases caused by mutant alleles (genetic disorder) like cystic fibrosis and Huntington's disease.

The purpose of developing (constructing) the detailed maps of genome are:

- ☆ To correlate the genetic and physical maps with markers as well as with cytological maps of the chromosomes that are constructed on the basis of banding patterns, and
- ☆ Ultimate goal is to identify and isolate the genes based on their location in the genome.

The detailed maps of the chromosome regions near the genes of interest decide the utility of positional cloning. This focused on developing the detailed maps of human chromosome as well as the genome of other model organisms.

25.1 GENOME PROJECTS

The National Institute of Health and Department of Energy, U.S.A. jointly administered by many countries had undertaken a genome project to acquire complete knowledge of the organization, structure, and function of the human genome. The aim of the project was to find out all the genes in each of the humans chromosomes and then of other organisms to determine their function and to know the mechanism of forming the complete organism.

The strategy of this genome project includes mapping, sequencing and functional analysis of all the genes in the genome of humans.

25.1.1 Genome Mapping

To prepare high resolution or saturated genetic and physical maps of human genome and of other organisms by using molecular markers.

25.1.2 Sequencing

This is the second goal of the project. It is to sequence the entire genomic DNA of humans.

25.1.3 Functional Analysis

This is the ultimate objective of the genome project. It is the most challenging task to know the function of each of the genes (app 50,000 to 100,000) in human genome by mutation approach. However, the approach of site directed mutagenesis available at present is labour-intensive and hence nedds to evolve new methods. Therefore, this work of functional analysis is long lasting taking centuries together.

(See for details the book "Cytogenetics and Genomics" by Tomar and Tomar, 2018).

25.2 TYPES OF MARKERS

The different markers are of the following 4 types:

(i) *Morphological* or *anatomical* or *classical markers:* These are inherited variants which are morphological (pigmentation like flower colour and other physical characters) or anatomical in origin. The genes controlling these characters are useful markers but still these are not ideal because the genes are widely spaced out with large gaps between them. These markers have low degree of polymorphism (heterozygosity) for which these are not so useful for genome analysis.

(ii) *Chromosomal markers:* Some of the chromosomal abnormalities (structural or numerical variations) also serve as markers. They have low degree of polymorphism and hence not so useful for genome analysis.

(iii) *Biochemical markers* (isozymes): These are observed due to variation in the macromolecules present in the body fluids (milk, urine, blood, saliva) and tissues which are detectable by immunological methods (Blood groups, MHC, etc) and electrophoretic method (isozymes, milk protein, blood proteins etc). Biochemical markers though have low to high polymorphism but these are controlled by certain genes with pleiotropic effect and dominance effect which make the genotypes indistinguishable at the phenotypic level. The gene expression may be sex limited and the genes may be sex linked. Moreover, these markers reflect the variability in the coding sequences which is less than 10 percent of the total genome.

(iv) *Molecular* or *genomic markers:* The conventional markers have their limitations of exhibiting low level of polymorphism and affected by environment, besides that they represent only the coding regions of genome which is only 5 – 10 per cent of the complete genome.

The DNA technologies have shown a large number of genetic polymorphisms (variations) at the DNA sequence level. These polymorphisms at DNA level (nucleotide level) are used as markers and known as molecular markers or genomic markers which detect or reveal the genetic variability at DNA sequence level. The molecular or DNA marker is any DNA fragment or gene which is free of environment effect. The examples are RFLPs, mini-satellite/VNTR, microsatellite. These markers are used for evaluation of the genetic basis for observed phenotypic variability. In fact the parts of genome that are not genes are called DNA markers. Therefore, the molecular markers do not affect performance traits but they only mark the chromosome segment having genes controlling the performance traits.

The molecular or genomic markers (DNA based markers) can be measured in both the sexes at any age and possess unique genetic properties. They are numerous, distributed throughout the genome, follow Mendelian inheritance, usually express in codominant fashion, often multi-allelic giving mean heterozygosity of more than 70 percent, unaffected by environmental factors without pleiotropic effect on QTL, and may also explain some of the within family genetic variation. The molecular markers have the added advantage that DNA samples can be taken not only from blood but also from any tissue like sperm, hair follicle. The DNA samples can be stored for long period and DNA analysis can be done at any age irrespective of sex.

25.3 GENETIC MARKERS

The *genetic marker* is defined as any stable and inherited variation that can be measured or detected and can be used to detect or identify the presence of a specific genotype or phenotype other than itself which is otherwise non measurable or difficult to detect. Thus, the ***genetic marker is a character*** whose inheritance pattern can be followed at the morphological, chromosomal (cytological), biochemical or DNA level. These characters are called markers because these are used to get the information about the genetics of other characters.

Each of the polymorphism serves as a genetic marker. These markers are often multi-allelic and multi-loci and hence have high PIC (Polymorphism information content – a measure of the usefulness of a marker for linkage studies). Thus, *the variations (polymorphisms) occurring in non coding regions are used indirectly as markers for linkage analysis.* However, the association between the marker and QTL is the function of distance between these two (marker and target trait). The close linkage (association) is required for successful MAS.

The DNA sequencing is used to identify variations at a locus but it is expensive and labourious. The polymorphisms in DNA sequences are detected by means of certain enzymes (called restriction enzymes) which cleave double stranded DNA molecules. A number of techniques have been developed to visualize DNA sequence polymorphism. The markers of various types are used to evaluate DNA polymorphism.

25.4 TYPES OF MOLECULAR MARKERS

The electrophoretic variants of enzymes (*Isozymes*) and DNA sequences are used as ***molecular markers*** in chromosome mapping. The molecular marker is a DNA sequence because it can be located at a specific site in a chromosome.

25.4.1 Defined and Anonymous Markers

The molecular markers can be classified in two groups on the basis of whether their function or specific features are known (*Defined marker*) or not known (*Annonymous marker*).

- ✰ The ***anonymous markers*** are a cloned random DNA fragment whose function or specific features are unknown.
- ✰ On the other, ***defined markers*** may contain a gene or some specific features like restriction sites for rare cutting RE, *etc*. These defined markers are polymorphic having different structures in different individuals of a species and hence known as ***polymorphic markers***. The differential mobilities of different markers detectable in gel electrophoresis indicate the structural differences.

(*a*) ***Anonymous polymorphism***: This covers and reveals arbitrary polymorphism which is developed on a purely random basis. These include minisatellite, microsatellite, and RAPD (Random Amplified Polymorphic DNA) markers.

(*b*) ***Defined polymorphic markers*** are kept in four types: (i) RFLP, (ii) RAPD, (iii) VNTR DNA (minisatellite and microsatellite), and (iv) CpG islands. See below for more detais.

(*i*) ***Restricted fragment length polymorphism (RFLP):*** The RFLP is the fragments of DNA and used as a marker. The first technique utilizing the concept of the use of genetic variation at DNA level as a molecular marker is the RFLP in viruses (Grodzicker *et al.*, 1974) and in the human globin gene cluster (Jeffreys, 1979). The DNA polymorphism is detected by hybridizing a chemically labelled DNA probe to a Southern blot of DNA digested bt restriction endonuclease (RE).

The RFLPs are variation in the length of DNA fragments produced by cleaving (cutting) the DNA molecule with specific restriction endonuclease (restriction enzymes). The digestion of DNA with particular restriction enzyme results restriction fragments of different sizes called as RFLPs. This is because the restriction enzymes cut DNA at recognition sites.

An alteration in a single nucleotide (mutation) creates or destroys a restriction site causing variation in the number of sites. Thus, the variation (polymorphism) occurs among individuals in the positions of cutting sites and the length of DNA between the sites. This results in the restriction fragments of different sizes. As a result of change even in a small proportion of the restriction sites yield a large number of potential DNA markers because there are millions of nucleotides in the genome. The range of fragment lengths is different for different restriction enzymes. There exists a large battery of restriction enzymes which cut DNA at specific sequences; these recognition sites may be 4-8 bases long. If an enzyme cuts the DNA of some but not all animals at a particular site then a polymorphism is inferred in at least one of the bases in the recognition site.

The DNA is digested with restriction enzymes and the resulting fragments are separated by gel electrophoresis, transferred to a filter by Southern blotting, probes are hybridized to the filter and sequences in genome bound with hybridized probe are then visualized as hybridization bands. The individuals carrying different allelic variants for a locus will show different banding patterns.

The hybridization can be carried out with genomic probes (cDNA, cloned genes, genomic DNA sequence) and with genome derived cloned probes of different families of hyper-variable repetitive DNA sequences (minisatellites, VNTR, microsatellites) and synthetic oligonucleotides.

(*ii*) ***Random Amplified Polymorphic DNA (RAPD):*** This is useful in DNA polymorphism analysis with high level of detectable polymorphism. It is the polymorphic DNA which is amplified randomly by PCR analysis. This procedure involves the use of single primer of arbitrary nucleotide sequence in PCR for amplification of DNA to detect nucleotide sequence polymorphism. When the primer is short, the priming may take place at several sites in the genome that are located within amplifiable distance. This does not require any information on gene sequence. The polymorphisms are usually noted by the presence or absence of an amplification product from a single locus because the RAPD polymorphisms results due to either a nucleotide base change that changes the primer binding site or an insertion or deletion within the amplified region. The technique is rapid requiring less time, efficient, and less expensive but it is less efficient to RFLP and DFP.

(iii) Variable number of Tandem Repeats (VNTRs): These are made up of a variable number of end-to-end duplications of identical or almost identical sequence of 2 – 80 bp each. These are distributd in the entire genome. The polymorphisms is these markers is usually associated with the number of repeats which means that different numbers of repeat units at a given locus in a chromosome are different in different individuals and these differences constitute the alleles of VNTR loci. The variations in the distribution patter of repeated sequences in the different alleles also cause polymorphism. This is especially in case of minisatellite DNAs and this is analysed by MVR-PCR technique. The VNTRs are further grouped as minisatellite and microsatellite DNAs which together constitute the ***hypervariable region*** or DNA.

Minisatellite and Microsatellites: They are the regions of repetitive DNA and are highly polymorphic spots on non-coding regions characterized by repeating DNA blocks each of which contains up to several hundred of base pair in size.

(*a*) *Mini-satellites*: They are tandem repeats of short sequences (15 - 60 bp long), inter-spread in the most chromosomes. The changes in the number of repeats caused by unequal crossing over between homologous tandem repeats or due to gain/loss of repeat units at a particular locus as a result of slippage during replication create hyper-variability of mini-satellites. These are called hyper-variable repeats (HVRs) which are tandem repeats of DNA sequences. The HVRs are also called as mini-satellite or VNTRs. This change in DNA sequence continues over many generations and hence each such locus represents a variety of alleles with different number of tandem repeats. Therefore, these loci in the population have *Variable Number of Tandem Repeats* (VNTR) and hence called as VNTR loci. The VNTRs define the length of the individual-specific 'alleles' which can be examined by Southern Blot or PCR techniques. Some of the HVR loci have more than 10 alleles and the frequency of hetero-zygotes in the population may exceed 90 per cent. The probability that two unrelated individuals have identical lengths of DNA at a particular HVR is very low.

(b) ***Microsatellite:*** The microsatellites are short DNA fragments of usually less than 100bp which are tandem repeats of 2- 5 nucleotides length for which these are called as short tandem repeats (***STR***), simple sequence repeats (***SSR***) or simple sequence length polymorphism (SSLP) or *sequence tagged microsatellite repeats* (STMR). A tandemly repeated unit in DNA of only 1 to 6 nucleotides long is also called ***simple tandem repeat***. They are randomly distributed throughout the genome showing variation in number of repeats, highly polymorphic, and non-functional. These are multi-loci markers and of choice for linkage analysis. However, these are expensive and time consuming.

The term microsatellite was coined by Litt and Luty (1989) to characterize the simple sequence repeats (SSR) amplified by PCR. The short length of microsatellites makes them emenable to amplification by PCR and subsequent separation on PAGE (Polyacrylamide gel electrophoresis). They occur at a high frequency (one lakh DNA) with their abundant number (50000 -100000) in mammalian genome and display a high degree of polymorphism (PIC value of 0.6 or more) in eukaryotic genome. Polymorphism arises from differences in number of times the simple sequence motif is repeated. The microsatellites are now considered the most powerful genetic markers for biodiversity evaluation for their high heterozygosity.

(iv) CpG islands: These are stably unmethylated in human genome constituting about 1 per cent of the human DNA. Mostly these islands are associated with genes. For the purpose of genome mapping these are the sequences whch can be used as powerful markers.

25.4.2 Other Classifications of Molecular Markers

The molecular markers are classified in the following different ways:

(I) Technique based markers:

(a) PCR based markers: RAPDs, STS, AFLP, SSR;

(b) Hybridization based markers: RFLPs.

These are further divided into single and muti loci. The single locus marker is derived from a single locus in the genome like allozyme, most RFLPs and the typical microsatellite markers. The multi loci marker screen many loci *e.g.* RAPD

(II) (a) Site directed polymorphism: RFLPs, sequence specific oligonucleotides; and

(b) Anonymous polymorphism: minisatellite like VNTR; microsatellite like SSR, STRs, STMR; and RAPDs.

(III) (a) First generation markers: RFLPs and RAPDs;

(b) Second generation markers: VNTRs (minisatellite and microsatellite), and AFLPs; and

(c) Third generation markers: SNPs and Expressed Sequence Tags (short cDNA sequences used to link physical and genetic maps).

(IV) (a) Length variation based markers: SSRs, *etc.*; and

(b) Sequence variation based markers: RFLPs, RAPDs, AFLPs, and SNPs.

(V) Dekkers (2004) classified the markers as:

(*a*) *Direct markers:* Loci that code for the functional mutation;

(*b*) *Linkage disequilibrium markers:* loci that are in population wide linkage disequilibrium with the functional mutation; and

(*c*) *Linkage equilibrium markers:* loci that are in population wide linkage equilibrium with the functional mutation in outbreed populations.

The linkage disequilibrium refers to the non-random association of alleles between two loci.

(VI) The different types of molecular markers can also be categorized as:

(a) Isozymes,

(b) Restriction fragment length polymorphic DNA (RFLP),

(c) Random amplified polymorphic DNAs (RAPD),

(d) Variable number of tandemly repeated (VNTR) DNA, and

(e) Short tandem repeats (STR) DNA which includes minisatellite DNAs of about 0.2 to 2 kb long and microsatellite DNAs less than 100 bp made up of tandem repeats of 2 to 7 bp for which called STR, SSR (simple sequence repeats and SSLP (simple sequence length polymorphism.

I. Classification

(a) Polymerase Chain Reaction (PCR) Based Markers

The followings are some of the PCR based markers:

(i) ***Sequence Tagged Sites (STS)****:* This is alternative to RAPD primers. The RAPD primers often identify repetitive DNA sequences while STS primers identify single or low-copy DNA sequences because the STS primers are designed from mapped low-copy number sequences on a known sequence of specific region of genome. The STS is a short and unique sequence to identify a known location on the chromosome. But the STS primers are longer than RAPD primers for which they are more stable than RAPD primers. The RAPD markers can be converted into STS markers. The STS markers, in comparison to RAPD markers, require sequence analysis before primers can be designed.

(ii) Amplified Fragment Length Polymorphism (AFLP)*:* This technique is PCR based developed by Vos *et al.* (1995). AFLP targets specific restriction fragments for amplification. The technique involves the digestion of DNA with two different restriction enzymes. It combines the advantages of

RFLP and PCR technique. It is rapid and more efficient but expensive.

(iii) ***Simple Sequence Repeats (SSR):*** The SSR are the micro-satellite repeats. These are also called as short tandem repeats (STR) and sequence tagged microsatellite repeats (STMR).

(b) Hybridization Based Markers

The DNA profiles are visualized by hybridizing the restriction enzyme-digested DNA, to a labelled probe, which is a DNA fragment of known sequence or origin. The techniques include RFLP analysis.

Second Classification

This is another classification of genetic markers.

(*a*) ***Site directed polymorphism***: This involves searching the known sequences or genes for polymorphism. These include restriction enzyme polymorphism (RFLP), sequence polymorphism, sequence-specific oligonucleotides and conformational polymorphism.

(i) *Sequence polymorphism*: All methods of describing differences between the DNA of animals depend upon detecting differences in the nucleotide sequence. This method is more efficient to determine the sequence of a specific gene.

(ii) *Restricted fragment length polymorphism* (*RFLP*): Already described above.

(iii) *Sequence specific oligonucleotides*: These are sets of PCR (Polymerase Chain Reaction) primers which function in an allele specific manner.

(iv *Conformational polymorphism*: They are used to detect polymorphism in specific locations which relies upon detecting sequence-specific mobility of PCR products under electrophoresis

(*b*) ***Anonymous polymorphism***: This covers and reveals arbitrary polymorphism which is developed on a purely random basis. These include minisatellite, microsatellite, and RAPD (Random Amplified Polymorphic DNA) markers.

II. Classification: Single-Nucleotide Polymorphisms (SNPs)

These are third generation markers, and also the sequence length based molecular markers.

The *single nucleotide polymorphisms* (SNPs) are DNA sequence polymorphisms (variations) which occur when a single nucleotide in the genome sequence is changed and varies in a population. The SNP occurs when a single nucleotide replaces either one of the other three nucleotides due to single nucleotide substitutions (transitions, transversions) or single nucleotide insertions/deletions. Thus, the schange of the base sequence of DNA segment causing SNP leads to a change in protein composition. The SNP has high polymorphism information content (PIC). The SNPs may occur in both coding and non coding regions.

The SNPs provide a powerful alternative form of allele specific PCR markers (which are mainly designed from previously mapped single or low copy sequences). The SNPs have the advantage that the exact nature and location of allelic variation are known. However, the SNPs are time consuming and costly to develop. But once the primers are developed and tested, their sequences can be used by others.

An international project, called ***Human HapMap Project*** was initiated with the goal to characterize the similarities and differences in human genomes based on the identification and map SNPs from DNA samples of different human populations. The idea behind this collaborative enterprise was the value of *SNP haplotypes* to study ancestry and evolution in human populations, and to work out disease association.

Large amount of genetic variation has been observed in human genome. These genetic variation besides other causes in human genome also result from the followings:

- ✰ Gross changes in the range of 1 kb to 1 mb (deletions, duplications, inversions, and translocations),
- ✰ Small changes by insertions or deletions of one or a few nucleotide pairs which are more frequent, and
- ✰ Single nucleotide-pair substitutions like A:T to G:C or its reverse (G:C to A:T substitutions) which are the most common changes in human genome and have produced a large number of ***single-nucleotide polymorphisms(SNPs)***.

The occurrence of SNPs in human genome by comparing the nucleotide sequence in the same chromosome of two individuals has shown that on an average, one SNP is present in every 1200 nucleotide pairs. The SNPs are mostly not present in the coding regions of genes and also do not produce the changed or mutant phenotype.

The SNPs can be detected by the microarray hybridization or gene-chip technique. The details have been given in chapter 24.

The individual SNPs show population variation not only in their frequencies but also in their absence in some population. These are produced by a single mutation in an individual and then spread in the population. Each SNP is associated with other SNPs. The closely linked SNPs on a chromosome are inherited together as a genetic unit and called as a ***haplotype.*** The haplotype as a unit of closely linked SNPs are inherited together because there is little chance of crossing over and to form their new combinations. The haplotypes are undoubtedly modified by mutation while crossing over generates new haplotypes in evolution.

The SNPs and haplotypes are of great value in the followings:

- ✰ Valuable molecular markers because of their frequency and distribution throughout the human genome.
- ✰ Provide information about the human evolution,
- ✰ Provide information about the relation among different groups (ethnic groups), and

☆ To identify genes causing human diseases like breast cancer, glaucoma, and rheumatic arthritis by finding the association between the SNPs and a particular disease. Therefore, the SNP or haplotype help to identify the real gene responsible for a particular disease and so to know the risk of developing that disease in an individual.

25.5 SELECTION OF IDEAL MARKER

It is essential to identify and select the ideal marker and secondly the association between marker and economic trait should also be clearly known. The following approaches to select the ideal marker can be used:

(*i*) *Shot gun method:* There is random selection of a set of markers and association of particular marker with performance records is checked. This method has lost its value with the recent improvement in the advancement of information on markers and genome map.

(*ii*) *Candidate gene method:* It is well known that mutation creates phenotypic variation in the trait. In order to know the variation in the particular gene, the gene or its parts are sequenced in a number of animals and its association with particular trait is tested. This method has certain limitations *viz.* candidate genes affecting a trait are more, sequencing and association studies in large number of animals for all the candidate genes become tedious, occurrence of mutation in non-coding region of gene creates complications which also increases the cost of genotyping, and difficulty to identify all the candidate genes for a particular trait because no prior information about candidate gene which has mutation may cause no selection of particular marker.

(*iii*) *Genetic mapping method:* Most of the economic characters of farm animals are polygenic which have pleiotropic effects and linked to each other. The genetic markers can be used to map linked loci affecting quantitative traits. The genetic variability in a polygenic trait can be accounted by quantitative trait loci (QTL). Anderson (2001) has defined the QTL as a chromosomal region that contains one or more genes which influence the polygenic trait of economic importance. The QTL can be detected by mapping studies (mapping of genes by linkage) showing significant differences in performance trait among the individuals having different QTL alleles.

Among the three types of markers, the direct markers and, to a lesser extent, LD markers are able to select on genotype due to association between genotype and phenotype. The LE markers are used to select for different linkage phases between markers and QTL from family to family. Many SNP dense markers are now available for exploiting linkage disequilibrium in mapping QTL. The extent and pattern of linkage disequilibrium throughout the genome is important in gene mapping which is enabled by the high throughput SNP genotyping technologies.

25.6 APPLICATIONS OF MOLECULAR MARKERS

The polymorphisms observed at the DNA sequence level have been playing a major role in human genetics for the following aspects:

(I) Short range or immediate applications:

1. Parentage determination
2. Individual identity
3. Genetic distance estimation and evolution
4. Determination of twin zygosity and freemartinism
5. Identification of disease carrier (heterozygous) animals
6. Sex determination

(II) Long range applications

7. Gene mapping
8. Breeding programme (Marker assisted selection, Genome selection)
9. DNA fingerprinting
10. Transgenic breeding.

25.7 TYPES OF CHROMOSOME MAPS

The gene maps **or chromosome maps** are of three type *viz.* genetic maps or linkage maps, physical maps, and cytological maps. The detailed genetic and physical maps of the genomes of many organisms have been constructed, including the human genome.

25.7.1 Genetic Maps

The recombination frequencies between markers are the basis of constructing genetic maps of chromosomes. The genetic map is a diagram of a chromosome with distances based on recombination frequencies (centiMorgan). The genetic map showing the relative position of genes on a chromosome based on genetic analysis is called *linkage map*. **The genetic map is constructed from linkage relationship which decides the recombination frequencies between markers (frequency of meiotic exchange among linked traits).** ***In humans, 1 cM is equivalent to about 1 mb of DNA, on an average.*** These genetic maps locate the genes responsible for traits and they show the relative orders and distances between loci on the chromosome. Linkage analysis requires the segregation of alleles for which there should be 100 per cent heterozygosity in parental generation like the F_1 generation in crosses between inbred lines or different breeds.

The conventional genetic maps are constructed for those genes which are expressed showing distinct phenotypic effects. Such maps have the following limitations:

- ☆ The number of active genes is less and limited,
- ☆ The mapping of these genes is tedious and time consuming, and
- ☆ The QTL controlling the quantitative characters may not be mapped.

In view of the above limitations in gene and chromosome mapping, attempts have been made to use the molecular markers having differences among strains at the molecular level, like DNA and protein. The genetic markers which may be any Mendelian character require for mapping any genome. All genetic markers can be used for linkage mapping.

Approaches of genetic mapping: There are two approaches for genetic mapping *viz.* saturation or random mapping and targeted mapping.

(a) The ***saturation or random mapping method*** involves the generation of large number of markers to cover the whole genome so that the trait of interest lies near to at least one marker. This is done by using either of the technique of RAPD, STS (Sequence Tagged Sites), AFLP, RFLP, SSCP (Single Stranded Conformational Polymorphism) and the microsatellite analysis.

(b) The ***targeted mapping method*** involves the isolation of markers in a specific region or for a specific trait. This is carried out by different techniques including EST (Expressed Sequence Tags), subtractive hybridization.

RFLPs Maps

The genetic maps are constructed by use of the molecular markers such as restriction fragments of different lengths, known as *restriction fragment length polymorphism* (*RFLP*). This is the existence of two or more genetic variants detectable by visualizing fragments of genomic DNA that were obtained by digesting the DNA with a restriction enzyme. The DNA fragments are usually fractionated by electrophoresis, transferred to a membrane by Southern blotting, and then visualized by autoradiography after hybridization to a labelled DNA probe.

The restriction enzyme does not recognize the cleavage sites as a result of mutation when the mutation changes the nucleotide sequences in the restriction enzyme cleavage site. But other mutations may create new restriction sites. As a result of mutation the variation is produced in the length of the DNA fragments by digestion with various restriction enzymes. This creates the restriction fragment length polymorphism (*RFLP*). The RFLP is of great use in constructing the detailed genetic maps which in turn can be used in positional cloning. A linear or circular physical map of a DNA molecule showing the sites that are cleaved by different restriction enzymes is called *restriction map.* The DNA sequence that is cleaved by a restriction enzyme is called *restriction site.*

The DNA of different ecotypes (strains adapted to different environmental conditions) or the different lines of a species or even different relatives have many RFLPs which can be used in constructing genetic maps. The RFPL shows Mendelian inheritance segregating in crosses like co-dominant alleles (markers), The RFLPs themselves are phenotypes used to classify the progeny of crosses as parental or recombinants. The RFLP segregate with the restriction fragments from both the homologous chromosomes visible in gels or detected on auto-radio-grams of Southern blots produced from the gels. Some RFLPs can be visualized directly when the fragments in DNA digest are separated by agarose gel electrophoresis after staining with ethidium bromide and viewed under ultraviolet light. The other categories of RFLPs can be detected only by using specific cDNA or genomic clones as radioactive hybridization probes on genomic Southern blots.

The RFLP are of value in mapping the human chromosomes. The procedure of RFLP was used in mapping the chromosome to construct an early map of about 2000 RFLPs on the human genome.

Short Tandem Repeat (STRS) Maps

The most useful RFLP in humans involve short sequences present as tandem repeats. The number of these short sequences is highly variable. Thus, these are called *variable number tandem repeats* (*VNTR*), also called *minisatellites*) and *short tandem repeats* (*STRs, also called* microsatellite). These are highly polymorphic. These both (VNTR and STR) vary in length due to the:

- ☆ *Differences in the number of copies of the repeated sequences between the restriction sites and not due to differences in the positions of restriction enzyme cleavage sites.*

The high-density maps of eukaryotic chromosomes (including humans) are constructed by using the STRs which are polymorphic tandem repeats of sequences of small size (2 – 5 nucleotide pairs long). The STRs are composed of polymorphic tandem repeats of the dinucleotide sequence AC/TG (AC in one strand and TG in the complementary strand) are useful markers.

A comprehensive map of 5264 (AC/TG) STRs in the human genome was published in 1996 and these STRs defined 2335 sites with an average distance of 1.6 cM or about 1.6 mb between adjacent markers. A large international consortium by 1997 had used RFLPs to map over 16000 human genes (ESTs and cloned genes) and they had integrated their map with the physical map of human genome. In this study over 20,000 STSs were mapped to 16, 354 distinct loci. These genetic maps of RFLP markers (VNTRs, and STRs) were useful to identify and characterize mutant genes responsible for causing many human diseases.

25.7.2 Physical Maps

The physical maps such as the restriction maps discussed under section 21.10.1 are constructed based on the molecular distances (distance in base pairs) separating the markers on the big DNA molecules of the chromosome *viz.* base pairs (bp), kilo bases (kb = 1000 bp), mega bases (mb = 1 million bp). The physical maps often contain locations of overlapping genomic clones (*contigs*) and unique nucleotide sequences called *sequence-tagged sites* (STSs).

The physical maps relate genes and markers to the actual location on a specific chromosome. In other words, they relate traits to actual chromosomal location. These maps can be cytogenetically or molecularly based,

Physical mapping is done using the techniques such as somatic cell hybridization, radiation hybrids, fluorescence in situ hybridization (FISH).

The RFLP maps are the genetic maps, have made possible the positional cloning, and supplemented with the physical maps of chromosomes. The overlapping clones can be identified and the physical maps of not only of the chromosomes but also of the entire genome can be constructed by isolating and preparing the restriction maps (genetic maps) of large numbers of genomic clones, though it is not so easy task especially for large genomes.

Vast amounts of data need to be searched for overlaps and for construction of physical maps of entire genome. Even though, the detailed physical maps have been prepared and become available including the human, *D, melanogaster*, *C. elegans* (Worm used for developmental genetics), and *A. thaliana*.

Some useful traits affected by major genes have been identified in different species like

Cattle: Horn development gene on chromosome I,
Muscular hypertrophy gene on chromosome 2, and
Obesity gene on chromosome 6.

Sheep: Booroola fecundity gene on chromosome 6,
Obesity gene on chromosome 4 and
Muscular hypertrophy gene on chromosome 18.

Goat: Horn development gene on chromosome I,
Dominant white coat colour gene on chromosome 8,
with major effect on muscle glycogen content
Meat quality on chromosome 15, and
Calcium release channel gene on chromosome 6.

25.7.3 Cytological Maps

The cytological maps are constructed based on the banding patterns of chromosomes observed in microscope after treating with various stains. The genetic and physical maps can be correlated with *cytological maps* based on banding pattern of the chromosomes.

The *cytogenetic maps* are based on the location of markers within or near cytological features of chromosomes observed by microscopy. The *in situ* hybridization allows the knowledge of the positions of genes and clones on the cytological map of the chromosome, in some species. The following examples may be cited:

(a) The giant polytene chromosomes in the salivary glands are present in *Drosophila.* The banding patterns of these chromosomes allow high-resolution maps of the chromosomes. The position of a clone of unknown genetic content can be known on the cytological map with considerable precision.

(b) The position of specific DNA sequence on chromosomes in mammals including humans can be determined by fluorescent *in situ* hybridization (FISH) stained by any of several chromosome-banding protocols.

If RFLPs can be identified that overlap with these sequences, they can be used as STS sites that anchor genetic maps of chromosomes to cytological maps, producing *cytogenetic maps*. In case these sequences find position on the physical maps by Southern blot hybridization experiment, they can also be used to tie the physical maps to both the genetic and cytological maps of the chromosomes.

The high-density maps have been constructed for many chromosomes including all of the human chromosomes. This is performed by integrating the genetic, physical, and cytological maps.

25.8 MAP POSITION-BASED CLONING OF GENES

Regarding the rate of gene expression, there are some genes which are expressed at very high levels in specialized cells but most of the genes are expressed at moderate or low levels. The maps of these two types of genes can be constructed using the following two different approaches:

- The gene to be cloned should be expressed at very high levels in specialized cells or tissue, like the protein haemoglobin synthesized in mammalian ***reticulocytes*** (young RBC) to the extent of about 90 percent. Thus, the reticulocytes can be used to isolate easily the α- and β-globin mRNAs and used to prepare radioactive cDNA probes for genomic library screens.
- *Positional cloning*: This is another approach for the genes that are expressed in moderate or low levels require their mapping precisely. This technique requires searching for a clone of the gene depending on its location in the genome. This approach called ***positional cloning*** is used to identify any gene.

Positional cloning: It is the isolation of a clone of a gene or other DNA sequence based on its map position in the genome. The genetic crosses or pedigree analysis in humans with large families helps in positional cloning. The gene is first mapped located in a specific region of the chromosome from genetic cross or from family data in case of humans. The gene is localized on the physical map of that region of the chromosome. The gene after identifying by physical mapping is isolated from mutant and wild type individuals and sequenced to identify mutations that have resulted in a loss of gene function. The positional cloning has been used to identify the genes responsible for causing inherited disorders in humans, *e.g.* cystic fibrosis and Huntington's disease.

In case of species in which transformation, the copies of the wild-type allele, are introduced into mutant organism to know the reappearance of wild phenotype of the character. The appearance of wild type phenotype in the mutant organism indicates that the wild-type allele introduced is the desired gene.

25.9 CHROMOSOME WALKING AND JUMPING

These two are the techniques used for the construction of restriction maps of genomes. The detailed genetic, cytogenetic, and physical maps of chromosomes allowed the isolating of genes by chromosome walks and chromosome jumps. The gene can be usually isolated by chromosome walks or chromosome jumps if the molecular marker (such as RFLP, VNTR, or STR) maps close to a gene.

The positional cloning is accomplished by mapping the gene, identifying RFLP, VNTR, STR or other ***molecular marker*** near the gene and then walking or jumping along the chromosome until the gene is reached. The chromosome walks and chromosome jumps depends on the distance between the molecular marker and the gene of interest.

These two techniques enable the identification of contigs which are the contiguous fragments. The ***contig*** is a set of overlapping clones that provide a physical map of a portion of a chromosome. They contain neighbouring DNA fragments having an overlapping region. The basis of these techniques is the possession of overlapping region. The contigs facilitate mapping and so the correct alignment of base sequence data.

25.9.1 Chromosome Walking

This is a procedure that uses overlapping clones to move sequentially down a chromosome from one site to another site. This technique is more convenient used to prepare restriction maps of small parts of chromosomes. This technique is applicable for much smaller DNA fragments. The chromosome walk starts when the distance is low between molecular marker (RFLP or known gene clone) and the gene of interest. This technique helps to identify the DNA fragments with overlapping regions and so to locate two or more fragments containing a large sequence of interest *e.g.* parts of a single large gene as in case of eukaryotic large genes over 1000 kb long. The chromosome walking is a conventional cloning technique used to obtain DNA fragments and to prepare restriction maps of small regions of chromosome. This technique is easy in species having small genome and little repetitive DNA. The walking procedure is very difficult in species with large genomes and with abundance of dispersed repetitive DNA.

This technique of chromosome walking is a positional cloning of a gene. The chromosome walk starts by selecting (identifying) a molecular marker (RFLP or known gene clone) close to the gene of interest/isolating a DNA fragment containing a known gene or nearby gene and use this clone as hybridization probe to screen a genomic library for overlapping sequence. This fragment is used as the starting point or called reference point in the genetic map. The restriction map of this fragment (overlapping clones identified in the library screen) is prepared and one end of this fragment is isolated and subcloned. The end segment is used as a probe to locate a neighbouring overlapping fragment in the genomic library having complementary sequence for this probe. The restriction map of this new fragment is prepared and the sequence at the other end of this new fragment is used as a probe to locate the next overlapping neighbouring fragment. This process of chromosome walking is repeated continuously to produce successive fragments till the other end of the chromosome (gene of interest) is reached. Isolating a series of overlapping genomic clones repeatedly allow to walk along the chromosome. It is essential that one end of each of new fragment should be complementary to the probe used to identify it.

The verification of the isolation of the clone of a gene of interest is performed. This is performed in *Drosophila* and *Arabidopsis* by introducing the wild type allele into the organism having mutant allele and to see whether the organism show the wild type phenotype. In humans, verification is done by determining the nucleotide sequences of the wild-type allele as well as several mutant alleles and observing that the coding sequences of the mutant alleles are defective and unable to produce the functional products.

25.9.2 Chromosome Jumping

This is a procedure that uses large DNA fragments to move discontinuously along a chromosome from one site to another site. The chromosome jumping is the technique used in case of the large distance between the closest molecular marker and the gene of interest. Thus, it is used for large DNA fragments usually of several hundred kb in size. The chromosome jumping is thus a long walk in which each jump can cover a distance of 100 kb or more. This technique is also started like a chromosome walk by initiating a jump using a molecular probe (RFLP, VNTR, or STR) as a starting point. Large DNA fragments are prepared by partial digestion of genomic DNA with a restriction endonuclease. Endonuclease is an enzyme that breaks strands of DNA at internal positions.

This technique uses jumping and linking libraries generated by a rare cutting enzyme (*Not I* for humans). The jumping library and linking library clones are prepared. The genomic DNA is digested with *Not I* and the fragments are separated by pulse field gradient electrophoresis to construct the physical map of chromosome. All the DNA fragments so obtained are hybridized with each clone from two libraries (jumping and linking). Each clone should hybridize with two fragments containing the sequences represented in the clone. The correct order of various DNA fragments (produced by *NotI* enzyme digestion) in the organization of different chromosomes in the genome is determined by pooling the data from both the libraries.

The chromosome jumping is useful for large genomes like the human genome. This technique has been used to identify the gene responsible for causing cystic fibrosis in humans.

25.10 FISH: FLUORESCENCE *IN SITU* HYBRIDIZATION

(See *annexure 25.9*)

25.11 MICROSATELLITE (STR) MAPPING

The STR sequences are too short and hence cannot be mapped by FISH technique but are mapped by the following two techniques:

25.11.1 Somatic Cell Hybridization

These are man-mouse somatic-cell hybrids. This can also be used to assign the genes to specific chromosome. Somatic cells of different types can be fussed to obtain the hybrid cells. These hybrid cells are useful in the following ways:

(i) To map the gene or chromosome,

(ii) To study the control of cell division and gene expression, (*iii*) Production of ***monoclonal antibodies*** by producing ***hybridoma.*** The hybridoma is a hybrid cell between an immortalized cell and an antibody producing lymphocyte. A hybridoma is obtained by fusing a – **B** lymphocyte with usually a tumour cell of the antibody forming system. The tumour cells are called ***myelomas,***

(iv) To study malignment transformations, and

(v) To obtain viral replication.

The chromosome mapping by somatic cell hybridization is based on fusion of human and mouse cell lines. The human chromosomes are preferentially eliminated by fusing the somatic cells of man and mouse. Each of the hybrid-cell will contain a single human chromosome. Amplification is performed by PCR using a human-specific microsatellite sequence as primer. Only the cell line which has the human chromosome having this sequence will be amplified. This enables the location of the given sequence to a specific chromosome.

(See ***annexure*** *25.**10***)

25.11.2 Individual Chromosome Preparation

By use of a fluorescence activated cell sorter (FACS) all the human chromosomes can be separated from each other except 9, 10, 11, and 12. The procedure is to arrest the mitotic cells at metaphase by use of colchcine and the cells are disrupted so as to come out of the chromosomes from the cell. These are then stained C:G rich sequence. These stained chromosomes are passed one by one through the FACS which separates them based on their size and the amount of fluorescent from each of the two dyes. The sorting out upto 2000 chromosomes/second is possible. There are other suitable approaches to separate chromosome number 9, 10, 11, and 12. About 300-500 specimens of each chromosome are sufficiently enough for PCR approach for use of microsatellite sequences as primers.

Part 3

Genetic Statistics

Chapter 26

Probability Rules

In genetic studies, a number of different crosses are made to know the genetic basis of a character on the basis of the outcome (s) of the cross. Making a cross is a process and its outcomes (results) are the events. The frequency of an event is expressed in terms of probability. The event is the outcome (result) of a process or happening. The process or happening may be the tossing of a coin, drawing of a card from a pack of 52 playing cards, making a specific cross of two individuals of opposite sex, production of a progeny from a cross. The event may be the chance of getting a head or tail on a coin toss, getting an ace, king, or queen from a deck of cards, or getting a dominant or recessive homozygote from a mating between two heterozygotes. There are a number of possible outcomes (events) of the process and all possible outcomes (events) of the process are considered in estimating the frequency of a particular event. The collection (record) of all events of a process is called the *sample space.* For example, tossing a coin is a process and its sample space has two events *viz. tail* and *head*. Similarly, drawing a card is a process whose sample space is 52, one for each card. The frequency of an event is the probability of that event. The joint occurrence of two events together (*i.e.* A *and* B events) are independent to each other or the occurrence of one event is influenced by the occurrence of other event (they may depend on each other, *i.e.* either A or B occurs). Here, in probability theory, the independent means that one event provides no information about the other.

Once the genetic basis of a trait is known, the outcomes (results) of the particular cross may be predicted on the basis of the expected frequency from the inheritance pattern of the character. The agreement between the results obtained and the results predicted on the basis of genetic hypothesis can be tested by a statistics, known as the chi-square test. The subject matter of this chapter is thus the probability and the use of the chi-square test.

26.1 EVENTS AND THEIR PROBABILITIES

There is sometimes a doubt about the certainty of any statement. Further, the degree of doubt is different in different cases as there is no surety of any statement. Therefore, the statement of less definite nature is made in terms of probability or chance or likelihood.

The probability is thus a measure of the degree of doubt in making a statement, expressed in terms of chance or likelihood and measured as ratio. The probability is concerned or related with the repeated events. An event is the result (outcome) of a trial (experiment), expressed in different forms. The different forms (results or outcome) are termed as the events. An event occurred if the result of the trial is one of the outcome (form) which makeup that event. Some of the examples are -

- ✰ Tossing a coin is a trial and the result (outcome) of trial will have two forms: one result (outcome) is that the coin has the head upside and the second is for the tail to be upside. Thus, there are two events: one event is that head is up and the second event is that tail is up. Both these events are likely to happen with equal chance or probability which is ½ for each event.
- ✰ Similarly, in a trial to draw a card of particular colour (red and black) from the pack of 52 cards have two events *viz.* Black colour card and red colour card, each of the events have an equal probability of ½.
- ✰ Further, in a trial to draw a card of particular type (spade, club, heart, and diamond) from a pack of 52 cards, the probability of getting one type of card is ¼.
- ✰ The birth of a male child is an event if the result (outcome) of pregnancy termination leads to the birth of a male child. However, there are two outcomes or results *viz.* birth of a male child or a female child. Thus, the probability of a male child to be born is ½ and the probability of a female child to be born is also ½.
- ✰ A six sided dice when thrown may show any of the numbers from 1 to 6 face upward. Thus, these six are the outcomes or results. The probability of any number facing upward (event) is $\frac{1}{6}$.

26.2 TYPES OF EVENTS

The events are classified as under:

(i) Simple and Compound Events

The occurrence of a single event is known as *simple event* whereas the joint occurrence of two or more of the single events in connection with each other is called the *compound event.* The single event is one result or outcome of a random experiment which cannot be divided further.

The composite or compound event is a combination of more than one outcome (result) and can be divided into simple events. For example, to get a specific number of a die is a simple event whereas to get odd or even numbers of a die *viz. 1, 3, 5* or 2, 4, 6 is a compound event. Similarly, from a pack of 52 cards, a king is drawn and then a queen is drawn, each of these events (drawing of a king or queen is called simple event) and the event of the joint occurrence of both (drawing of a king and a queen both) will be called a compound event.

(ii) Exhaustive Events

The events include all the possible cases (outcomes) of a trial. A combination of all possible simple events from the total results (outcome) of a random experiment is called exhaustive event. For example, head and tail from a toss of a coin are two simple events which form exhaustive events. Likewise, from tossing of 2 coins make up 4 simple events as HH, HT, TH, TT, and these form together exhaustive event.

(iii) Independent and Dependent Events

The events are said to be dependent or independent accordingly as the occurrence of one event does or does not affect the occurrence of the other. Two or more events out of which the occurrence of one event does not affect the occurrence of other event are said to be independent but when the occurrence of one event affect the occurrence of the other event, these are then said to be dependent events.

For example, to pass an examination by two students are two events but these are independent because to pass the examination by one student does not affect the other student to pass the examination. Similarly, formations of 2 gametes by heterozygous parent are two independent events. Sometimes, the independence of events is not clear. In this case the independence is decided by the multiplication law of probability as:

Two events (A and B) of a trial of random experiment will be independent if P (AB) = P (A) × P (B). For example, the probability to draw a red card from the pack of 52 playing cards is $\frac{26}{52} = \frac{1}{2}$. This is event A with probability as ½ *i.e.* P (A) = $\frac{1}{2}$. The probability of one ace is $\frac{4}{52} = \frac{1}{13}$. This is event B with probability as $\frac{1}{13}$, *i.e.* P (B) = $\frac{1}{13}$. The combined probability of A and B events (red card being ace in this example) is $\frac{2}{52} = \frac{1}{26}$ ($P_{AB} = \frac{2}{52} = \frac{1}{26}$) or P (A) × P (B) = P (AB)= $\frac{1}{2} \times \frac{1}{13} = \frac{1}{26}$. This is the joint or combined probability of two independent events. Thus, the probabilities of independent events are multiplied when combined. Therefore, the probability of the simultaneous occurrence of two or more independent events is equal to the product of the probabilities of each event.

(iv) Equally likely Event

When the probability of occurrence of all events is equal to each other, the events are called as equally likely events.

For example, the chance of occurrence of head or tail of coin on land after its throwing in the air is equal. Thus, these two events (head and tail) are equally likely events. Thus, P (H) = P (T) = ½. Similarly, the probability of occurrence of any number out of 1, 2,, 5, 6 of a six faced dice is equal and it is $\frac{1}{6}$. Formation of 2 gametes by heterozygous parent (Aa) for single gene pair are equally likely events. The formation of 2 gametes (carrying *A* allele and carrying ***a*** allele) are also two independent events.

(v) Mutually Exclusive Events or Incompatible Events

Both the events cannot happen together (simultaneously). Thus, the occurrence of one event prevents the occurrence of other event.

For example, the birth of a male child in a gestation (for single birth) excludes the possibility of the birth of a female child. It is not possible for two events (male and female birth) to occur simultaneously.

The combined probabilities of mutually exclusive events are obtained by adding their separate probabilities. This is known as addition law of probability or Laplace's 2nd principle. In case of coin throwing either head or tail of the coin will be seen upward.

On the contrary, when two or more events occur together they are said to be *compatible e.g.* in drawing a card from a pack of playing cards, the card drawn may be of red colour and at the same time it will have some number *viz.* Ace, king, queen, *etc.* Similarly, a married person may also be an educated person. Marriage is one event and education is second event, and the occurrence of these two events is compatible events.

26.3 PROBABILITY DEFINED

The probability can be defined in the following two ways:

(i) Mathematical Definition

If a random experiment has *N* exhaustive, mutually exclusive and equally likely outcomes (events) out of which *m* are favourable to an event *A*, then the probability of occurrence of the event *A* is $\frac{m}{n}$.

$$\text{Thus, } P(A) = \frac{m}{n} = \frac{\text{Number of favourable outcomes or cases}}{\text{Total number of cases}}.$$

If an event can happen in *a* ways and fails in *b* ways, the chance or probability of its happening is $\frac{a}{(a+b)}$ and of its failure is $\frac{b}{(a+b)}$. This is known as Laplace's first principle.

(ii) Statistical Definition

The probability is the limit of the relative frequency of success in an infinite sequence of trials. If any random experiment is repeated N times under similar conditions and the outcome (event) *A* occurs *m* times, then the probability of occurrence of the event A is $\frac{m}{n}$ provided N goes to infinite.

Thus, the probability of event A is defined as a ratio and expressed as $P(A) = \frac{m}{n}$

where,

m = Number of favourable cases (outcomes or events), and

N = Total number of exhaustive, mutually exclusive and equally likely cases.

26.4 CHARACTERISTICS OF PROBABILITY

1. If the occurrence of an event A is certain to happen, then its probability is 1. P (A) = 1.
2. If occurrence of an event A is uncertain to happen, then its probability is zero. P (A) = 0.
3. Probability is concerned with a group of events and not to a particular or single event.
4 Probability concerns a proposition (formal statement).
5. Certainty is the limiting form of probability.
6 There are degrees of probability.
7 Degree of probability depends on the amount of evidence (number of favourable and unfavourable cases of an event to occur).

26.5 RULES OF CALCULATING PROBABILITY

The probability has the following fundamental rules of counting and combinations:

(1) Fundamental Rules of Counting

There are two fundamental rules of counting or laws of compositions of events. These are as.

*First law – **probability of both events***: If an event can happen in *m* ways and the second event in *n* other ways, then both the events will happen in *m x n* ways. For example, if there are 4 ways to enter in a house and 3 ways to come out of the house, then the total numbers of ways to enter and come out of the house are 4 × 3 = 12.

*Second law – **probability of either event:*** If two events happen in *m* and *n* ways, respectively, then either one of the event will happen in m + n ways. In the above example, a man can enter the house or come out of the house in 4 + 3 = 7 ways.

(2) Rule of Combinations (^nC_r)

Number of ways to select *r* trials out of total *n* trials is taken as ^nC_r and it is calculated as -

$$\textit{Number of ways} = {}^nC_r = \frac{n!}{r!(n-r)!}$$

where,

^nC_r = the number of combinations of n things (objects) taken *r* at a time or the number of different samples of size *r* that can be taken from *n* objects.

n! = factorial ***n*** which is estimated from the product (multiplication) of numbers starting from 1 to the number factorial. Factorial ***n*** = n (n-1) (n -2) (n -3). 1. Thus the factorial means the multiplication of the numbers by all integers down to 1. For example, if n =5, then n! = 5! = 5 × 4 × 3 × 2 × 1 = 120. The factorial zero = 1.

26.6 LAWS OF PROBABILITY

26.6.1 Additive Theorem of Probability

This is also called as Laplace's 2nd principle. This principle is applied for ***mutually exclusive events*** that do not occur simultaneously. This principle states that:

If an event can happen in 2 or more different ways which are mutually exclusive, the chance (probability) that it will happen is the sum of the probabilities of its happening in these different ways, or

The probability that one of the several mutually exclusive event will occur is the sum of the probabilities of the event happening in different ways.

For example, in a trial of drawing a card from a pack of 52 cards, the two events E_1 the card being *diamond* and E_2 the card being *heart* are mutually exclusive (both events cannot happen together). The card being of red colour (E_3) is their combined probability. Thus, the combined probability of the red card will be equal to -

Red coloured card = Diamond card + Heart card

$$P(E_3) = P(E_1) + P(E_2)$$

$$= \frac{13}{52} + \frac{13}{52}$$

$$= \frac{1}{4} + \frac{1}{4} = \frac{1}{2}$$

This means that in half of the cases the card will be of red colour (either diamond or heart).

26.6.2 Multiplication Theorem of Probability

This is called as Laplace's 3rd principle and applied for ***independent events*** or ***equally likely events***. The theorem states that -

The probability of simultaneous occurrence of 2 or more independent events is equal to the product (multiplication) of their separate probabilities. Thu, if p_1, p_2, p_3, p_n are the probabilities of happening of *n* independent events, then the probability of happening of all the events simultaneously is

$P = p_1\, p_2\, p_3 \cdot p_n.$

For example, the formation of 2 gametes by a heterozygous parent (Bb) is independent to each other, *i.e.* both the gametes (B and b) will be formed. The probability of forming B gamete is ½ and of forming b gamete is also ½. Thus, if ½ of the gamete from female parent had B allele and ½ of the gamete from male parent had B allele, then the combined probability of uniting 2 gametes of opposite sex for forming BB zygote is $\frac{1}{2} \times \frac{1}{2} = \frac{1}{4}$.

26.7 DISCRETE PROBABILITY DISTRIBUTION

Variable vs Attributes

The characteristic of a population which takes different values and can be represented numerically is called the ***variable*** or ***variate*** *e.g.* height, age, weight, milk yield, number of children in a family, number of fruits on a tree, crop yield, *etc.* The variable is denoted by **X**. The various values of **X** like X_1, X_2, X_3, ... X_i forms the distribution of **X** variable/variate.

On the contrary, a characteristic of a population which takes different values but cannot be represented numerically is called ***attribute*** *e.g.* beauty, colour of flowers.

Types of Variables

A variable/variate is of two type *viz. random* and *non-random variable.*

(1) The ***random variable*** is also called chance variable or stochastic variable/variate. The random variable is the one when its values differ on different individuals of a population depending on the chance according to the law of predetermined probability.

(i) The random variable may be ***continuous variable*** which take any values within the range like height, age, weight, milk yield, crop yield, *etc.* The random continuous variables are measured in quantitative terms *e.g. gm, kg, cm, meters, days.* The distribution of the values of continuous variables is called continuous distribution or ***normal distribution*** and it shows a *bell shape curve* on plotting the values on a graph.

(ii) The random variable may also be ***discrete variable*** or discontinuous variable when it takes some of the values within the range *e.g.* number of children in a family, number of fruits on a tree, number of pods/fruits per branch of a tree, number of tillers per plant, number of accidents, *etc.* The discrete variable is measured in numbers and represented by the probabilities (p_i) of discrete variables (X_i) of different groups (X_i = 1, 2, 3, ..., i, etc). The distribution of discrete variables is called discontinuous distribution or discrete variable distribution. The distribution of the sets of X_i values of discrete variables grouped according to their different numbers together with their probabilities (p_i) constitutes the probability distribution of random discrete variable **X** or ***discrete probability distribution***.

(2) The ***non-random variable*** is the one whose values for different individuals are not determined by probabilistic law but determined according to some deterministic law, *e.g.* salary of an employee which is decided under the pay rules as per qualification, work basis, *etc.*

The ***discrete probability distribution*** is shown by the probabilities, p_i, of different groups (X_i). This can be made clear by an example of drawing a card from a pack of 13 cards of particular type (spade, club, heart, and diamond) and assigning them different values as:

Knaves = 1, Queens = 2, kings = 3, aces = 4, and other cards = 5.

Thus, the X_i values are 1, 2, 3, 4 and 5 with their probabilities as:

$$p_1 = p_2 = p_3 = p_4 = \frac{1}{13}, \text{ and}$$

$$p_5 = \frac{9}{13}, \text{ since excluding the first 4 types of cards are left 9 out of 13.}$$

These 5 values (p_i = 1 to 5) constitute the probability distribution of X discrete variables.

The ***mean*** of these different X_i values is estimated as:

$$X = E(X) = \Sigma\, p_i X_i$$

$$= 1 \times \frac{1}{13} + 2 \times \frac{1}{13} + 3 \times \frac{1}{13} + 4 \times \frac{1}{13} + 5 \times \frac{9}{13}$$

$$= \frac{1}{13} + \frac{2}{13} + \frac{3}{13} + \frac{4}{13} + \frac{45}{13}$$

$$= \frac{55}{13} = 4.23$$

This is the expectation or *mean* of random discrete variable used to characterize its probability distribution.

The ***variance*** of X is given as:

$$V(X) = \Sigma\, p_i (X_i - X)^2$$

$$= \frac{1}{13}(1-4.23)^2 + \frac{2}{13}(2-4.23)^2 + \frac{3}{13}(3-4.23)^2 + \frac{4}{13}(4-4.23)^2 + \frac{45}{13}(5-4.23)^2$$

$$= 0.8025 + 0.765 + 0.3491 + 0.0163 + 2.0523$$

$$= 3.9852$$

Types of Discrete Probability Distribution

This type of distribution is of the following three types:

- ☆ Binomial Distribution
- ☆ Multinomial Distribution, and
- ☆ Poisson Distribution.

26.8 BINOMIAL DISTRIBUTION

An expression having two terms separated by either + or – sign is called the binomial expression or simply binomial *e.g.* $(a+b)$, $(a-b)$, $(3a+b)$, $(a-4b)$ *etc.*

In $(p + q)^n$, the ***p*** and ***q*** represent the probabilities of alternative independent events and the power or exponential ***n*** represents the number of trials. The sum of the two terms in binomial must be one *i.e.* $p + q = 1.0$

Binomial Theorem

The multiplication process gives the following results:

$(p + q)^2 = p^2 + 2pq + q^2$

$(p + q)^3 = (p^2 + 2pq + q^2)(p + q) = p^3 + 3p^2q + 3pq^2 + q^3$

$(p + q)^4 = (p^2 + 2pq + q^2)^2 = p^4 + 4p^3q + 6p^2q^2 + 4\,pq^3 + q^3$

$(p + q)^5 = (p^2 + 2pq + q^2)^2(p + q) = p^5 + 5p^4q + 10p^3q^2 + 10\,p^2q^3 + 5pq^4 + q^5$,

and so on.

The multiplication process has expanded the binomial and hence it is called as binomial expansion which becomes harder and labourious with the increase in exponential of $(p + q)$. This can be easily solved with the help of binomial theorem which provides the expansion of $(p + q)^n$. Thus, the theorem which gives the expansion of $(p + q)^n$ is called the ***binomial theorem***. This produces a series of terms which is called binomial series.

The binomial expansion can be obtained for higher powers but with great difficulty and time taking. Therefore, a ***short cut method*** for expanding $(p + q)^n$ may be obtained as:

$$(p + q)^n = {}^nC_0p^n + {}^nC_1p^{n-1}q + {}^nC_2p^{n-2}q^2 +. + {}^nC_rp^{n-r}q^r +. + {}^nC_nq^n$$

$$= \Sigma\, {}^nC_rp^{n-r}q^r \text{ with } p + q = 1.0 \text{ and the summation is made from } r = 0 \text{ to } n$$

Where, ${}^nC_r$ is the coefficient of binomial expansion representing the number of combinations of ***n*** things taken ***r*** at a time, or the number of different samples of size ***r*** (number of male or female births) that can be chosen from ***n*** objects (total gestations). The ${}^nC_r$ is calculated as described under ***section 26.5*** (Law of combination).

The ***numbers of ways*** or combinations (${}^nC_r$) to obtain 2 males in 3 gestations are:

$${}^nC_r = {}^3C_2 = \frac{3!}{(3-2)!\,2!} = \frac{(3\times2\times1)}{(1\times2\times1)} = 3$$

And the 3 combinations or 3 ways to get 2 males will be male – male – female, male-female-male, and female - male – male.

The number of ways or combinations (^nC_r) is used to obtain the coefficients in a binomial expansion which is important in solving problems in genetics because the coefficients represent the number of ways in which the condition of each term may be satisfied. For example, the probability of occurrence of one event (take success) taken as ***p*** and the probability of occurrence of its alternate event (failure of ***p* = *1* – *p* = *q***) taken as ***q***. Now, the probability that in ***n*** trials a success will occur ***s*** times and a failure will occur ***f*** times may be obtained as:

$$\left(\frac{n!}{s!f!}\right)p^sq^f$$

Where, n!/s!f! = Number of ways which satisfy the condition of each term, and

Probability = No. of ways × p^sq^f

$$=\left(\frac{n!}{s!f!}\right)p^sq^f \text{ or } \frac{n!}{r!(n-r)!}$$

To understand this, see examples 26.6 (b) and 26.8

26.9 Characteristics of Binomial Theorem

I. ***Number of terms in the expanded form of binomial***: The fully expanded binomial will have n + 1 terms. This means that the number of terms in the binomial is one more than the power of the expansion.

II. ***Coefficients:*** The coefficients of the terms have the following characteristics:

(*a*) The coefficients are symmetrical about the middle term of the expansion. This means that the coefficients of the terms are equidistant from the beginning and the last are equal in magnitude.

(*b*) The coefficients of the first and last term: These are 1 and hence not written.

(*c*) The coefficient of each succeeding term: These are obtained by the following 3 methods:

(*1*) They are obtained by multiplying the coefficients of the present term by the power of ***p*** and divided by the number of the present term represents in the series. That is the coefficient of next term is obtained by multiplying the coefficient with the exponent of the preceding term and dividing by the number of preceding term. The coefficient of each term represents the number of ways in which the conditions of each term may be satisfied.

Taking with n = 3, the binomial can be expanded as:

$$(p + q)^3 = p^3 + 3p^2q + 3pq^2 + q^3$$

Here, 1 st term (p^3) represents 3 males and may be obtained by one way,

2 nd term ($3p^2q$) represents 2 males and 1 female and

3rd terms ($3pq^2$) represents 1 male and 2 females which may be obtained by 3 ways or combinations, and

4th term (q^3) represents 3 females which may be obtained by only 1 way or in one combination.

(2) *Secondly*, the coefficients may be find out by the formula C = n!/a! b!,

Where, n! is the factorial n which is itself the power of the expansion,

a! is the exponent of p (first term), and

b! is the exponent of q (second term).

For example, the coefficient of the 4th term in the binomial expanded to the seventh power (n = 7) will be obtained as:

C = n!/a! b! = 7!/4! 3! (Since 4 [th] term will be $p^4 q^3$).

$$7! = 7 \times 6 \times 5 \times 4 \times 3 \times 2 \times 1 = 5040$$

$$4! = 4 \times 3 \times 2 \times 1 = 24$$

$$3! = 3 \times 2 \times 1 = 6$$

And hence $\frac{7!}{4!3!} = \frac{5040}{24} \times 6 = \frac{5040}{144} = 35$

(3) *Thirdly*, the coefficients for any expanded binomial can be obtained by use of ***Pascal's triangle***, when any coefficient is the sum of the nearest two numbers in immediately above row (Table 26.1).

III. ***Power of the binomial (n):*** It has the following two characteristics:

(a) The power of the first factor (***p***) is n and that of the second factor (***q***) is zero which is equal to 1.0. The power of ***p*** decreases by one while power of ***q*** increases by one in each succeeding term of the expansion. Thus, the power or exponents of ***p*** (first factor) begin with the power to which the binomial is raised (***n***) and decreases one by one to zero whereas the exponent of ***q*** (second factor) begin with zero and increased to the power to which the binomial is raised (***n***).

Table 26.1: Bionomial Coefficients Obtained by Pascal's Triangle

Sample Size (n)	*Binomial Coefficients*
n	1
1	1 1
2	1 2 1
3	1 3 3 1
4	1 4 6 4 1
5	1 5 10 10 5 1
6	1 6 15 20 15 6 1
7	1 7 21 35 35 21 7 1
8	1 8 28 56 70 56 28 8 1
9	1 9 36 84 126 126 84 36 9 1
etc.	

(*b*) The sum of powers (exponential or indices) of **p** *and* **q** for any term is ***n***. To find out any term in the binomial expansion the following method is used –

The value of ***r*** is taken as the number of the term minus one *e.g. suppose* it is required to find out the 6 th term of the expansion $(P + q)^{10}$. The power of ***q*** which is represented by ***r*** starts from zero in the first term and increases by one in each succeeding term. Thus, the 6 th term will have q^5 and $r = 5$. Therefore, the 6 th term will be obtained as:

$$\left({}^{n}C_{r}\right)\left(p^{r}\,q^{n-r}\right)=\left[\frac{n!}{r!(n-r)!}\right]\left(p^{n-r}\,q^{r}\right)$$

$$=\frac{10!}{(10-5)!5!}\left(p^{10-5}\,q^{5}\right)$$

$$=\frac{10!}{5!5!}p^{5}q^{5}=252\,P^{5}\,q^{5}$$

Thus, the 6 th term of $(p + q)^{10}$ binomial is $252\,P^5 q^5$.

The characteristics of binomial expansion theorem may be summarized as under:

Term	*Coefficients*	*Exponential of*	
		p	*q*
1	1	n	0
2	$\frac{n(1)}{1}$	n - 1	1
3	$\frac{n(n\quad 1)}{1.2}$	n – 2	2
4	$\frac{n(n\quad 1)(n\quad 2)}{1.2.3}$	n – 3	3
.	.	.	.
.	.	.	.
n – 1	1	0	1

In the example of n =3 (*i.e.* 3 births), the probability of getting 3 males or 3 females is $\frac{1}{8}$, of getting 2 males and 1 female is 3/8, of getting 1 male and 2 female is $\frac{3}{8}$. And the sum of all these probabilities is 1.0 *i.e.* $\frac{1}{8}+\frac{3}{8}+\frac{3}{8}+\frac{1}{8}=1.0$.

The above procedure may be followed for frequencies of the two terms other than ½ and ½ like p = ¾ and q = ¼. But it will affect the shape of distribution curve. If p = q = ½ the binomial distribution is symmetrical otherwise skewed.

26.10 MEAN (EXPECTATION) AND VARIANCE OF BINOMIAL DISTRIBUTION

The probability distribution with ***n*** trials (samples/tests) and ***p*** probability, the expectation or mean of the distribution of the number of success (***r***) is:

E (X) = X = np

And the variance of ***X*** is:

$V_X = \sigma^2 = np\ (1 - p) = npq$ and $\sigma = \sqrt{npq}$

When the results are presented in terms of the successes (***r/n***) proportion,

The mean (X) = p, $\sigma^2 = \frac{pq}{n}$, and $\sigma = \sqrt{\frac{pq}{n}}$

26.11 EFFECT OF N, P, AND R ON PROBABILITY

The probability distribution is clearly the function of ***n*** and ***p***. The probability increases as ***r*** increases from 0 up to a largest whole number less than (N + 1)p, after which the probability decreases as ***r*** increasesfrom maximum to ***n***. This can be shown as:

I Set: n = 10 and p = ½.

In this case the highest value of ***p*** is obtained when ***r*** is the largest whole number less than (10 +1) x 0.5 = 5.5 Thus, the largest whole number for ***r*** is 5. The value of

$p = \frac{10!}{5!5!} (½)^5 (½)^5 = 0.246$,

but if ***r*** = 4, then $p = \frac{10!}{4!6!} (½)^4 (½)^6 = 0.205$ and

if ***r*** = 3, then $p = \frac{10!}{3!7!} (½)^3 (½)^7 = 0.117$.

Now, if ***r*** exceeds 5, say 6, then $p = \frac{10!}{6!4!} (½)^6 (½)^4 = 0.5$ and

if ***r*** = 7, then $P = \frac{10!}{6!4!} (½)^7 (½)^3 = 0.117$.

II Set: n = 10 and p = 0.2.

In this case largest number for ***r*** is (10 + 1) 0.2 = 2. Therefore, $p = \frac{10!}{2!8!} (0.2)^2 (0.8)^8 = 0.302$.

If ***r*** = 3, then $p = \frac{10!}{3!7!} (0.2)^3 (0.2)^7 = 0.2013$.

And if ***r*** = 5, then $p = \frac{10!}{5!5!} (0.2)^5 (0.2)^5 = 0.0247$

Further with the increase in n, the probability decreased or vice versa. Taking r equal to largest whole number = (n + 1) p and p = q = ½, then the probability is o.1762, 0.246, 0.312 and 0.375 for n = 20, 10, 5 and 3, respectively.

26.12 MULTINOMIAL DISTRIBUTION

The binomial distribution deals with only two possible alternatives for each event. For example, male or female birth in a gestation, head or tail of a coin, Aa or aa offspring, *etc.*

(1) Trinomial Distribution

e.g. for genes showing co-dominance at a locus.

There may be more than two possibilities of an event like a third type of offspring is born. This can be dealt with by using a polynomial raised to the appropriate higher power. In this case, an additional term is added to the binomial. The addition of third term results the expansion term to a ***trinomial distribution***. This is expressed as $(p + q + r)^n$, where p, q and r represent the probabilities of the three different types of offspring or event, respectively. The probability of *trinomial combinations* is calculated as:

$$\frac{n!}{\left[W!X!Y!Z!(p^W q^X r^Y s^Z)\right]}$$

where, X, Y, and Z are the number of offspring of each type with p, q, and r probabilities.

(2) Multinomial Distribution

The distribution with more than three types of phenotypes also occurs and is covered under ***multinomial distribution***. For example, 4 phenotypes appear when a dihybrid cross is made with their frequencies as p, q, r, and s with W,X,Y and Z number of offspring Now, the formula becomes as under –

$$\frac{n!}{\left[W!X!Y!Z!(p^W q^X r^Y s^Z)\right]}$$

where, X, Y, and Z are the numbers of offspring of each type with p, q, and r probabilities.

Thus, the binomial distribution may be generalized to accommodate any number of variables. For example, if k number of events $(e_1, e_2,,e_k)$ occur with their probabilities as $p_1, p_1, p_2,. p_k$, respectively, then the probability that $e_1, e_2,.,e_k$ occur $k_1, K_2,.,k_n$ times, respectively is

$$\frac{N!}{(k_1, k_2, k_n)(p_1^{k_1} p_1^{k_2} \ldots\ldots p_n^{kn})}$$

where, $k_1 + K_2,. + k_n = N$

26.13 USE OF PROBABILITY

Laws of probability are useful to solve a number of problems related to human life. The different uses have been given here as under:

1. Law of Statistical Regularity and Inertia of Large Numbers

This law has its base in the principle of probability. Thus, the theory of probability is the base to the future plans. Besides this, the L.I.C. and business of gambling are based on the principles of probability.

- ☆ According to the first law if the data on a population are available in sufficient numbers, then the data represent the characteristics of the population.
- ☆ According to the second law the change in the characteristics of a population is slow.

The above mentioned both the laws based on the theory of probability indicate that sample of a population is enough to study the population and the properties of the sample represent the properties of the population, and these properties will exist in future for a long time.

2. Use of Probability in Genetics

The principles of probability have the following definite use of probability:

(i) Predicting the Genetic Ratios

The genetic law of segregation and recombination is based on laws of probability. The genes are expected to segregate in the form of gametes during meiosis in all the possible combinations due to chance. Secondly, when crosses are made among individuals of different genotypes, the genes in the gametes are expected to recombine at fertilization in all possible combinations due to chance.

(a) Single Factor Segregation and Recombination

The use of the law of probability in heterozygous mating for a single gene segregation (Aa × Aa) is given as under:

Each heterozygote for a single gene pair (Aa) is expected to produce two kinds of gametes, one containing *A* allele and the second containing the allele *a*, each occurring with the probability ½. The male gamete containing the allele *A* or *a* is independent of the female gamete containing the allele *A* or *a*. Therefore, the probability of uniting the male gamete *A* with the female gamete *A* at fertilization is ½ × ½ = ¼. This is because these two events are independent and hence their separate probabilities will be multiplied to get their combined probability. Similarly, the probability of uniting two gametes of opposite sex containing the allele *a* is also ½ × ½ = ¼.

A monohybrid cross (Aa × Aa) produce a heterozygote offspring in two ways – one way is the union of male gamete *A* with the female gamete *a*, and second is the union of male gamete *a* with female gamete *A*. Each of the 2 ways has the probability of ¼ as:

	Males (Aa)		Females (Aa)	
Kinds of gametes produced	A	a	A	a
Probability of gamete production	½	½	½	½
Probability of uniting two gametes (Aa)	½ × ½ = ¼		½ × ½ = ¼	

In this manner, the occurrence of one event excludes the occurrence of the other event. So the probability that a heterozygote will be produced from a monohybrid cross is ¼ × ¼ = ½.

The theoretical genotypic ratio of 1:2:1 obtained from a monohybrid cross represents the numeration of fractions associated with the probabilities of the 3 expected genotypes: ¼ AA: ½ Aa: ¼ aa.

(b) Two or more Factor Segregation and Recombination

The law of probability can be applied to crosses involving two or more pairs of genes.

The expected results of the two monohybrid crosses within the dihybrid cross can be combined based on the law of probability as under:

I[st] *Monohybrid Cross*		*2*[nd] *Monohybrid Cross*		*Dihybrid Cross*	
Phenotype	*Probability*	*Phenotype*	*Probability*	*Phenotype*	*Probability*
Starchy	¾	Green	¾	Starchy green	¾ × ¾ = 9/16
		White	¼	Starchy white	¾ × ¼ = 3/16
Sugary	¼	Green	¾	Sugary green	¼ × ¾ = 3/16
		White	¼	Sugary white	¼ × ¼ = 1/16

(ii) Testing the Carrier Individual for Recessive Allele

It is important to know the probability of individuals in the population carrying the recessive allele particularly when it controls a lethal or objectionable trait. This can be determined by use of laws of probability.

(a) Test Cross

A test cross is made to detect the heterozygote individual by mating the heterozygote with recessive (Bb × bb). If the individual under test is homozygous dominant (BB) it will not produce any progeny with recessive trait but if it was a heterozygous dominant (Bb) it will produce offspring with recessive trait (bb). However, the individual may be heterozygous dominant (Bb) and due to chance no gamete bearing recessive allele (b) was involved in fertilization process and hence no progeny with recessive trait will be produced. Thus, the conclusion will be wrong that the individual under test is homozygous dominant.

The important point to consider is that how many successful mating are required to test the individual to have recessive allele. The law of probability is helpful to answer this question as under -.

(b) Other Crosses

The law of probability can also be used to determine the number of progeny required for testing an individual to carry recessive allele under other conditions like when it is not practical to perform the test cross because the individual showing the recessive trait is unable to breed, *e.g.* a type of recessive dwarfism in cattle (Snorter dwarfism) which have high mortality and low fertility. In such a case, mating of an individual under test is made with known heterozygous individual. The second situation is when sufficient numbers of known heterozygous individuals are not available for mating. In this situation the daughters of known heterozygous could be used. However, in both the cases, the number of mating required for testing are more compared to test cross.

26.14 APPLICATIONS OF BINOMIAL THEOREM IN GENETICS

The probability which in other words is the average tends to become closer to its real expected value with the increase in sample size. However, it is much more likely that some deviation from the expectation may occur in any sample data with the result that different ratios will be observed in different sets of data. It is then important to test whether the observed deviation agree with the proposed explanation (*Hypothesis*). A geneticist is interested to determine the ratios and to test them how closely they agree to the expectation. The two laws of combined probabilities form the basis of the binomial distribution in testing the genetic ratios.

(1) To Know the Number of Ways

(i) The first use of binomial theorem has been shown to find out the number of possible ways to get a particular type of individual with its probability.

  (a) With equal probability of 2 alternative events ($p = q = ½$). In other words, it is used to determine the probability of progeny showing a given heritable trait in a particular family.

  (b) With unequal probabilities of 2 events *i.e.* $p \neq q$.

(ii) The binomial theorem can be used to know the different kinds of mating.

(2) Testing Genetic Ratios

The determination of genetic ratios derive essentially from two basic laws of probability for mutually exclusive or alternative events which do not occur together (additive law for combined probability) and for two or more events that occur together (multiplicative law for combined probability). The formation of two gametes by a heterozygous parent is independent of each other. The probability of forming both the gametes (Events) is ½ or 50 per cent and their combined probability (*i.e.* both the gametes will be combined together) is ½ × ½ = ¼.

SOLVED EXERCISES - PROBABILITY RULES

Example 26.1

How many will be the numbers of ways or combinations (^nC_r) to obtain 2 heads in 3 tosses of a coin?

Solution

$$^nC_r = {^3C_2} = \frac{3!}{2!(3-2)!}$$

$$= \frac{(3\times2\times1)}{2\times1\times1} = \frac{6}{2} = 3$$

The 3 ways in 3 tosses to obtain 2 heads will be as:

Tossing	Orders of getting 2 heads		
1	H	H	T
2	H	T	H
3	T	H	H

Example 26.2

How many and what ways will be to get 2 objects out of 3 objects A, B, and C.

Solution

$$^nC_r = {^3C_2} = \frac{3!}{2!(3\quad 2)!}$$

$$= \frac{(3\times2\times1)}{2\times1\times(1)} = \frac{6}{2} = 3$$

The 3 ways to get 2 objects out of 3 objects will be AB, AC, and BC.

To select *r* trials out of total *n* trials, the event will occur *r* times and will not occur *n-r* times, the chance (probability) of happening of the event in every one of these *r* trials and failing in the remaining *n* – *r* trials will be $p^r q^{n-r}$.

Where, p is the probability of an event to happen in a single trial,

q is the probability of not happening the event so that q = 1 – p.

A set of *r* trials can be selected in ^nC_r ways. The required chance that the event happens in *r* trials and fails to happen in the remaining *n* – *r* trials is $^nC_r p^r q^{n-r}$.

Example 26.3

Find out the probability that out of 5 births (sib-ship of 5 offspring) 3 will be males and rest 2 will be females.

Solution

Probability = $^nC_r p^r q^{n-r}$

$$= \frac{n!}{r!(n-r)!} p^3 q^2$$

$$= \frac{5!}{3!(5-3)!} \left(\frac{1}{2}\right)^3 \left(\frac{1}{2}\right)^2$$

$$= \left[\frac{5 \times 4 \times 3 \times 2 \times 1}{(3 \times 2 \times 1)(2 \times 1)}\right] \left(\frac{1}{8}\right) \left(\frac{1}{4}\right)$$

$$= 10 \times \frac{1}{8} \times \frac{1}{4}$$

$$= \frac{5}{16} = 0.3125$$

Example 26.4

Find out the combined probability in a test cross of heterozygous black individual (Bb x bb) that one will be black and one will be white offspring in a litter of two offspring.

Solution

There will be two ways to obtain one black and one white offspring in a litter of two offspring, with the probability of white as $q = ½$.

Ways	*Offspring Order*		*Probability*
	First	*Second*	
First	Black (p)	White (q)	$pq = ½ \times ½ = ¼$
Second	White (q)	Black (p)	$pq = ½ \times ½ = ¼$
		Combined probability	$= 2\,pq = 2 \times ½ \times ½ = ½$.

Similar results can be obtained with the help of genetic checker board as under –

Parents Bb × bb

Gametes B b b b

Progeny produced: (Bb and Bb) : (bb and bb)

Black : White (in equal ratio)

Example 26.5

Find out the combined probability of first two offspring being white in a test cross of heterozygous black individual (Bb x bb).

Solution

The probability of black offspring $(p) = ½$ and of white offspring $(q) = ½$. Thus, the combined probability of first two offspring being white is:

$$q \times q = q^2 = (½)^2 = ¼.$$

Example 26.6

From a cross of heterozygous parents (Bb), find out the combined probability -

(a) Of the first 3 offspring being alternately black – white – black or white – white – black

(b) Of being produced 2 black and one white among 3 offspring in any order.

Solution

The probability of black offspring (p) = ¾ and of white offspring (q) = ¼ because it is heterozygous mating.

(a) The probability of black-white-black offspring $= pqp = p^2q$

$$= \left(\frac{3}{4}\right)^2 \frac{1}{4} = \frac{9}{64}$$

The probability of white-white-black offspring $= q\,q\,p = q^2p$

$$= \left(\frac{1}{4}\right)^2 \frac{3}{4} = \frac{3}{64}$$

Therefore, the combined probability $= p^2q + pq^2 = pq\,(p + q) = pq$

$$= \frac{3}{4} \times \frac{1}{4} = \frac{3}{16}$$

(b) Taking the number of ways that 2 black and 1 white offspring be produced as:

Offspring Order			
I	*II*	*III*	*Probability*
Black	Black	White	$p^2q = \frac{9}{64}$
Black	White	Black	$p^2q = \frac{9}{64}$
White	Black	Black	$p^2q = \frac{9}{64}$
	Combined probability	$= 3(p^2q) = 3 \times \frac{9}{64} = \frac{27}{64}$	

Thus, in 3 ways, 2 black and 1 white offspring can be obtained with the total probability as $\frac{27}{64}$.

BINOMIAL DISTRIBUTION

Example 26.7

This can be made clear from the following example taking the birth of male and female children in two gestations with probability of boys as p = ½ and of girls as q = ½. There are 4 following possibilities (combinations) of birth of male and female calves in two gestations:

Possibilities	*First Gestation*	*Second Gestation*	*Probability*	
1	Male birth p	Male birth p	p^2	Both gestations had males,
2	Male birth p	Female birth q	pq	one boy: one girl
3	Female birth q	Male birth p	pq	" : "
4	Female birth q	Female birth q	q^2	Both gestations had females.
			$P^2 + 2pq + q^2$	

The results is same as obtained by the binomial expansion with n = 2 *i.e.* $(p+q)^2 = p^2 + 2pq + q^2$.

Example 26.8

The probability of any combination of male and/female calves in 3 gestations can be obtained from $(p + q)^3 = (p^2 + 2pq + q^2)(p + q) = p^3 + 3p^2q + 3pq^2 + q^3$. In this case there will be 8 combinations/ways for the birth of male and female calves in 3 gestations as:

Condition of each Term			*No. of Gestations*			*Probabilities*
Male	*Female*	*ways*	*1*	*2*	*3*	
3	0	1	Male	Male	Male	$p^3 = \left(\frac{1}{2}\right)^3 = \frac{1}{8}$
2	1	3	Male	Male	Female	
			Male	Female	Male	$3p^2q = 3\left(\frac{1}{2}\right)^2\left(\frac{1}{2}\right) = \frac{3}{8}$
			Female	Male	Male	
1	2	3	Male	Female	Female	
			Female	Female	Male	$3pq^2 = 3\left(\frac{1}{2}\right)\left(\frac{1}{2}\right)^2 = \frac{3}{8}$
			Female	Male	Female	
0	3	1	Female	Female	Female	$q^3 = \left(\frac{1}{2}\right)^3 = \frac{1}{8}$
						Total = $p^3 + 3p^2q + 3pq^2 + q^3 = 1.0$

Example 26.9

Consider a cross between two heterozygous black guinea pigs (Bb).

Find out that -

(a) In how many ways can 3 black and 2 white óffspring be produced,

(b) What is the probability from such a cross of obtaining 3 black and 2 white offspring in any order?

Solution

(*a*) No. of ways $=\left(\frac{n!}{s!f!}\right)={}^{n}C_{r}$

$$=\frac{n!}{r!(n\quad r)!} = \frac{5!}{2!(5\text{-}2)!}$$

$$=\frac{(5\times4\times3\times2\times1}{(3\times2\times1)(2\times1)}$$

$$=\frac{120}{12}=10$$

Where, n = No. of births,

s = r = no. of success = no. of getting 3 black offspring

f = n – s *or* n – r = no. of failure = no. of getting no black or no. of getting white offspring

(*b*) Probability = No. of ways x $p^s q^f$

$$=({}^{n}C_{r)}(p^{r}q^{n-r})$$

$$=\left(\frac{n!}{r!(n\quad r)!}\right)(p^{3}q^{2})$$

$$=\frac{5!}{(5\quad 2)!2!}=\left[\frac{(5\times4\times3\times3\times1}{(3\times2\times1)(2\times1)}\right]\left(\frac{3}{4}\right)^{3}\left(\frac{1}{4}\right)^{2}$$

$$=10\times\left(\frac{3}{4}\right)^{3}\left(\frac{1}{4}\right)^{2}=\frac{135}{152}=0.263$$

$P = \frac{3}{4}$ and

$q = \frac{1}{4}$ because the mating was among heterozygote parents.

The number of ways can be obtained by arranging the birth of black and white offspring in different order of combination.

	Offspring Order					
	I	*II*	*III*	*IV*	*V*	*Order combination for White*
1	white	white	—	—	—	1.2
2	white	—	white	—	—	1.3
3	white	—	—	white	—	1.4
4	white	—	—	—	white	1.5
5	—	white	white	—	—	2.3
6	—	white	—	white	—	2.4
7	—	whitw	—	—	white	2.5
8	—	—	white	white	—	3.4
9	—	—	white	—	white	3.5
10	—	—	—	white	white	4.5

Example 26.10

Find out the probability that in a sib ship of 5 offspring the number of males will be 3 and rest 2 will be females.

Solution

No. of ways $= ({}^{n}C_{r})$

$$= \left(\frac{n!}{r!(n \quad r)!}\right)$$

Probability $=$ No. of ways $\times$ $(p^{r} q^{n-r})$

$$= \left[\frac{(5\times4\times3\times2\times1}{(3\times2\times1)(2\times1)}\right] p^{3} q^{2}$$

$$= 10\left[\left(\frac{1}{2}\right)^{3}\left(\frac{1}{2}\right)^{2}\right] = 10\times\frac{1}{8}\times\frac{1}{4}$$

$$= \frac{5}{16} = 0.3125$$

Here, p =q = ½ = chance of male = chance of female birth.

Example 26.11

What is the probability that a mating Aa × aa will produce all Aa offspring in a sib ship of 6?

Solution

This mating (Aa × aa) will produce the Aa and aa offspring in 1:1 ratio and hence p = q = ½. Therefore,

$$\text{Probability} \quad = ({}^{n}C_{r})(p^{r}\, q^{n\ r}) = \left(\frac{n!}{s!f!}\right)(p^{s}\, q^{f})$$

$$= \left(\frac{n!}{r!(n\quad r)!}\right)(p^{6}\, q^{0})$$

$$= \left(\frac{6!}{(6\quad 0)!\,0!}\right)\left(\frac{1}{2}\right)^{6}\left(\frac{1}{2}\right)^{0}$$

$$= (1)\left(\frac{1}{2}\right)^{6}(1) = \frac{1}{64} = 0.015$$

TRINOMIAL DISTRIBUTION

Example 26.12

Find out the probability of 3 children of blood type M, 2 of blood type MN, and 1 of blood type N in a family of 6 children produced from marriage of parents both of which were MN blood type.

Solution

The heterozygous parents produce a genotype ratio of 1:2:1. Therefore, the frequency or the probability o 3 types of children will be –

P_1 = Probability of child being MM group = ¼ with their number = 3,

P_2 = Probability of child being MN group = ½ with their number = 2, and

P_3 = Probability of child being NN group = ¼ with their number = 1.

Total = 1.0 6.0

The combined probability will be obtained from the *trinomial formula* as –

$$P + q + r)^{3} \quad = \frac{n!}{[X!\,Y!\,Z!\,p^{X}\, q^{Y}\, r^{Z}]}$$

$$= \frac{6!}{3!\,2!\,1!\left(\frac{1}{4}\right)^{3}\left(\frac{1}{4}\right)^{2}\left(\frac{1}{4}\right)^{1}}$$

$$= \frac{6.5.4.3.2.1}{[3.2.1.2.1]\left(\frac{1}{64}\right)\left(\frac{1}{4}\right)\left(\frac{1}{4}\right)}$$

$$= 60\left(\frac{1}{1024}\right) = \frac{15}{256} = 0.058 = 5.8 \text{ per cent.}$$

Example 27.13

A sire and a cow both are polled but are heterozygous. They produced 4 calves. What is the probability that the calves include 1 female polled, 1 male horned and 2 female horned?.

Solution

The heterozygous parent produces 2 types of gametes each occurring with a probability of ½. The probability of producing polled calves is ¾ and of horned calves is ¼.

The probability of each of these calves phenotype is:

$$1 \text{ female polled} = \frac{1}{2} \times \frac{3}{4} = \frac{3}{8} = p$$

$$1 \text{ male horned} = \frac{1}{2} \times \frac{1}{4} = \frac{1}{8} = q$$

$$2 \text{ female horned} = \frac{1}{2} \times \frac{3}{4} = \frac{1}{8} = r$$

$$\text{Probability} = \frac{n!}{[X!\,Y!\,Z!\,p^X\,q^Y\,r^Z]}$$

$$= \frac{4!}{1!1\,2!\,2!\left(\frac{3}{8}\right)^1\left(\frac{1}{8}\right)^1\left(\frac{1}{8}\right)^2}$$

$$= \frac{103}{4096} = \frac{36}{102} = 0.00878 = 8.78 \text{ per cent.}$$

MULTINOMIAL DISTRIBUTION

Example 26.14

What is the probability from dihybrid cross (Horn and coat colour) of example 26.12 that out of 3 calves produced one will be male horned and red coloured and 2 will be female polled black colour ?.

Solution

Both are heterozygous for both the gene pairs and hence both will produce 4 types of gametes each occurring with probability of ¼. The following phenotypes will be produced:

Phenotypes	Probability
Polled Black	$\frac{9}{16}$
Polled red	$\frac{3}{16}$

Horned Black $\frac{3}{16}$

Horned red $\frac{1}{16}$

The probability of each of the 2 calves phenotypes are:

2 female polled black $= \frac{1}{2} \times \frac{9}{16} = \frac{9}{32}$

1 male horned red $= \frac{1}{2} \times \frac{1}{16} = \frac{1}{32}$

$$\text{Probability} = \frac{n!}{[X!\,Y!\,Z!\,p^X\,q^Y\,r^Z]}$$

$$= 10\left(\frac{3}{8}\right)^3\left(\frac{1}{8}\right)^2$$

$$= \frac{270}{32768} = 0.0082 = 8.2 \text{ per cent.}$$

Example 26.15

Find out the probability of the progeny with genotype aabb to be produced from the cross AaBb × Aabb.

Solution

The heterozygous will produce 4 types of gametes each occurring with a probability of ¼, whereas the other parent (Aabb) will produce 2 types of gametes each occurring with a probability of ½.Therefore, the combination of 2 gametes of ab genotype from two parents will occur with a probability of $\frac{1}{4} \times \frac{1}{2} = \frac{1}{8} = 12.5$ per cent.

Thus, the probability to have progeny of aabb genotype to be produced is 12.5 percent.

Example 26.16

Pollednes (P -) and black coat colour (B -) in cattle are dominant over horns (pp) and red coat colour (bb), respectively. What is the probability that the dihybrid cross will produce two polled black calves, assuming that 2 calves are indeed produced?.

Solution

Both the heterozygous parents will produce 4 types of gametes with equal probability of ¼. Since each type of gamete produced by the parents occurs with a probability of ¼, the combination of any two gametes will occur with a probability of 1/16 (= ¼ × ¼) because the production of gametes is an independent event. A polled black calve produced in any way of 9 ways:

Male Gametes	*Female Gametes*	*Genotype of Calf*
$\frac{1}{4}$ PB	$\frac{1}{4}$ PB	$\frac{1}{16}$ PPBB
$\frac{1}{4}$ PB	$\frac{1}{4}$ Pb	$\frac{1}{16}$ PPBb
$\frac{1}{4}$ PB	$\frac{1}{4}$ pB	$\frac{1}{16}$ PpBb
$\frac{1}{4}$ PB	$\frac{1}{4}$ pb	$\frac{1}{16}$ PpBb
$\frac{1}{4}$ Pb	$\frac{1}{4}$ PB	$\frac{1}{16}$ PPBb
$\frac{1}{4}$ Pb	$\frac{1}{4}$ pB	$\frac{1}{16}$ PpBb
$\frac{1}{4}$ pB	$\frac{1}{4}$ PB	$\frac{1}{16}$ PpBB
$\frac{1}{4}$ pB	$\frac{1}{4}$ Pb	$\frac{1}{16}$ PpBb
$\frac{1}{4}$ pb	$\frac{1}{4}$ PB	$\frac{1}{16}$ PpBb

The 9 separate ways of obtaining the genotype that produce a polled black calf are mutually exclusive. Therefore, the combined probability that the calf of this phenotype will be produced from dihybrid cross is obtained by adding all the 9 separate probabilities.

Now taking p as the frequency of polled black calves, q as for polled red, r for horned black, and s for horned red calves with their number to be produced being represented by W, X, Y and Z, respectively the probability that out of 2 births having polled black phenotype will be –

$$= \frac{n!}{[W!X!Y!Z!(p^W q^X r^Y s^Z)]}$$

$$= \frac{2!}{\left[2!0!0!0!\left(\frac{9}{16}\right)^2\left(\frac{3}{16}\right)^0\left(\frac{3}{16}\right)^0\left(\frac{1}{16}\right)^0\right]}$$

$$= 1\left(\frac{9}{16}\right)^2 = \frac{81}{256} = 0.316 = 31.6 \text{ per cent.}$$

Example 26.17

What is the probability that out of 5 calves there will be 3 calves with polled black phenotype and 2 will be of horned red phenotype from the mating of PpBb × ppBb?.

Solution

The heterozygous parent for 2 pairs of genes will produce 4 types of gametes occurring each with a probability of ¼ whereas the second parent (ppBb) will produce 2 types of gametes each with a probability of ½. The polled black calves will be produced in 3 ways out of 8 and hence the probability is $\frac{1}{8}+\frac{1}{8}+\frac{1}{8}=\frac{3}{8}$ whereas the horned red calves will be produced in only one way and hence the probability is $\frac{1}{8}$.

$$\text{Probability} = \frac{n!}{[W!X!Y!Z!(p^W q^X r^Y s^Z)]}$$

$$= \frac{5!}{\left[3!0!0!2!\left(\frac{3}{8}\right)^3\left(\frac{1}{8}\right)^3\left(\frac{1}{8}\right)^0\left(\frac{3}{8}\right)^0\left(\frac{1}{8}\right)^2\right]}$$

$$= 10\left(\frac{3}{8}\right)^3\left(\frac{1}{8}\right)^2 = \frac{270}{32768} = 0.0082 = 0.82 \text{ per cent.}$$

Example 26.18

In families of 5 children, find out the probability of getting

(a) 3 or more boys, (b) 3 or more boys or 3 or more girls,

(b) 2 or more boys or 2 or more girls, (d) oldest child is girl and the youngest is a boy,

(c) At least 1 boy, (f) one boy only, and (g) only one boy or only one girl.

Solution

Let p = probability of a boy = ½ and

q = probability of a girl = ½.

$(p+q)^5 =$	$p^5 +$	$5p^4q +$	$10p^3q^2 +$	$10\,p^2q^3 +$	$5pq^4 +$	q^5
Probability = of getting	(5 boys + & no girl)	(4 boys + &1 girl)	(3 boys + & 2 girls)	(2 boys + & 3 girls)	(1 boy + & 4 girls)	(no boy & 5 girls)
=	$(½)^5 +$	$(½)^4(½) +$	$(½)^3(½)^2 +$	$(½)^2(½)^3 +$	$(½)(½)^4 +$	$(½)^5$
=	$\frac{1}{32}+$	$\frac{5}{32}+$	$\frac{10}{32}+$	$\frac{10}{32}+$	$\frac{5}{32}+$	$\frac{1}{32}$

(a) $\frac{1}{32}+\frac{5}{32}+\frac{10}{32}=\frac{16}{32}=\frac{1}{2}$

(b) $\left(\frac{1}{32}+\frac{5}{32}+\frac{10}{32}\right)+\left(\frac{10}{32}+\frac{5}{32}+\frac{1}{32}\right)=\frac{16}{32}=\frac{32}{32}=1.0$

(c) $\left(\frac{1}{32}+\frac{5}{32}+\frac{10}{32}++\frac{10}{32}\right)+\left(\frac{10}{32}+\frac{10}{32}+\frac{5}{32}+\frac{1}{32}\right)\ \left(\frac{10}{32}+\frac{10}{32}\right)$

$=\frac{26}{32}+\frac{26}{32}-\frac{20}{32}=1.0$

This quantity 10/32 is included twice and hence $\frac{20}{32}$ will be deducted from $\frac{52}{32}$

(d)

(e) $\frac{31}{32}$ *i.e.* combined probability of first five terms by adding them

(f) $\frac{5}{32}$ *i.e.* equal to fifth term (One boy)

(g) $\frac{5}{32}+\frac{5}{32}=\frac{10}{32}$ *i.e.* sum of second and fifth term

Example 26.19

Sow and boar both heterozygous for dominant black produce 7 pigs. What is the probability that there will be:

(a) All black pigs, (b) All red pigs, (c) 2 black and 5 red pigs, (d) 4 black and 3 red pigs

(d) Rest of the phenotypes.

Solution

$(p + q)^7 = p^7 + 7p^6q + 21p^5q^2 + 35\ p^4q^3 + 35p^3q^4 + 21\ p^2q^5 + 7pq^6 + q^7$

The probability of black pigs = ¾ and of red pigs = ¼ for dominant allele Thus taking p as the frequency of black pigs = ¾ and q as that of red pigs = ¼. The answer can be obtained as:

(a) All black pigs = $p^7 = \left(\frac{3}{4}\right)^7$ = 0.1334 = 13.34 per cent

(b) All red pigs = $q^7 = \left(\frac{1}{4}\right)^7$ = 0.000061 = 0.006 per cent

(c) 2 black and 5 red pigs = $21p^5q^2\left(\frac{3}{4}\right)^2\left(\frac{1}{4}\right)^5$ = 0.0115 = 1.15 per cent

(d) 4 black and 3 red pigs = $35p^4q^3 = 35\left(\frac{3}{4}\right)^4\left(\frac{1}{4}\right)^3$ = 0.1730 = 17.30 per cent

(e) Probability of rest of the phenotypes -

$7p^6q$ = 0.3114 = 31.14 per cent

$21p^5q^2$ = 0.3114 = 31.14 per cent

$35p^3q^4$ = 0.576 = 5.76 per cent

$7pq^6$ = 0.00128 = 0.128 per cent

All = 78.17 per cent

Total of all = 0.99964 = 99.96 per cent.

Example 26.20

How often, in families of 8 children, will be all 8 be girl and all 8 are of the same sex *i.e.* either all boys or all girls.

Solution

$(p + q)^8 = p^8 + 8p^7q + 28p^6q^2 + 56\ p^4q^3 + 70p^4q^4 + 56\ p^3q^5 + 28p^2q^6 + 8\ pq^7 + q^8$

(a) All girls are represented by the binomial term of q^8

Where, q = ½ *i.e.* probability of girl

Thus, $q^8 = (½)^8 = \frac{1}{256}$ = 0.0035 = 0.39 per cent

(b) All girls = q^8 = 0.39 per cent

All boys = $p^8 = (½)^8 = \frac{1}{256}$ = 0.0035 = 0.39 per cent

Total = 0.78 per cent

Example 26.21

Black colour in Hampshire pigs is dominant over red. It is objectionable in purebred flock of black pigs to have red pigs. The probability of producing a red pig in a test cross (Bb × bb) is ½:

Parents	Bb		×	bb	
Gametes	B	b		b	b
Probability	½	½		½	½

Fertilization

Male gametes	Female gametes	
	b (½)	b (½)
B (½)	Bb (¼)	Bb (¼)

b (½)	bb (¼)	bb (¼)

Note: Figures in brackets are probabilities.

Thus ½ of the total pigs will be red (bb). Thus, the probability of producing red pig is 0.50. In this case, the probability of producing any number of black pigs would be $(½)^n$ where, n is the number of pigs produced. Thus, with the increase in number of mating the probability of producing red pig in subsequent mating will go on decreasing. Thus, if no offspring with recessive trait is produced out of 7 pigs, it shows that the individual under test is 99 per cent homozygous dominant: $(½)^7 =$ 0.007813 = 0.78 per cent. And if out of 10 pigs no red pig is born it then shows that individual under test is 99.9024 per cent homozygous dominant $(½)^{10} = 0.000976 =$ 0.0976 per cent probability.

Example 26.22

Black colour in Hampshire pigs is dominant over red. It is objectionable in purebred flock of black pigs to have red pigs. The probability of producing a red pig in a test cross (Bb x bb) is ½:

Parents	Bb		×	bb	
Gametes	B	b		b	b
Probability	½	½		½	½

Fertilization

Male gametes	Female gametes	
	b (½)	b (½)
B (½)	Bb (¼)	Bb (¼)
b (½)	bb (¼)	bb (¼)

Note: Figures in brackets are probabilities.

Thus ½ of the total pigs will be red (bb). Thus, the probability of producing red pig is 0.50. In this case, the probability of producing any number of black pigs would be $(½)^n$ where, n is the number of pigs produced. Thus, with the increase in number of mating the probability of producing red pig in subsequent mating will go on decreasing. Thus, if no offspring with recessive trait is produced out of 7 pigs, it shows that the individual under test is 99 per cent homozygous dominant: $(½)^7 =$ 0.007813 = 0.78 per cent. And if out of 10 pigs no red pig is born it then shows that individual under test is 99.9024 per cent homozygous dominant $(½)^{10} = 0.000976 =$ 0.0976 per cent probability.

Example 26.23

A multiple allelic system having 5 alleles affecting a trait is known. Find out the number of different mating possible.

Solution

No. genotypes possible = no. of homozygote + no.of heterozygote

$$= n + \frac{n!}{(n-r)!r!}$$

Where, n = total alleles = 5

r = no. of alleles forming a genotype = 2

$$\text{Genotypes} = 5 + \frac{5!}{3!2!}$$

$$= 5 + \frac{5.4.3.2.1}{3.2.1.2.1}$$

= 5 + 10 = 15

No. of different mating = no. of mating among homozygote + No. of mating among heterozygote

$$= 15 + \frac{15!}{13!2!}$$

$$= 15 + \frac{15.14.13!}{2.13!}$$

= 15 + (15 × 7) = 120

Example 26.24

Find out the number of genotypes produced and number of different kinds of mating with single locus two allelic system.

Solution

No. genotypes possible = no. of homozygote + no.of heterozygote

= no. alleles at locus + no.of ways of different combinations

$$= n + \frac{n!}{(n-r)!r!}$$

Where, n = no.of alleles at a locus

r = no. alleles forming a genotype

$$= 2 + \frac{2!}{(2-2)!2!} = 2 + \frac{2!}{0!2!} = 2 + 1 = 3$$

No. different mating = no. of mating among homozygote + No. of mating among heterozygote

$$= 3 + \frac{n!}{(n-r)!r!} = 3 + \frac{3!}{(3-2)!2!} = 3 + \frac{3.2.1}{1!2.} = 6$$

Chapter 27

Chi-Square (χ^2) Test

In Genetics are observed the results on certain character in terms of the number of individuals showing the particular phenotype of the character like horned and polled animals; birth of male of female calves; long and short hairs, all or none traits (threshold characters) like diseases resistance in animals falling all the animals in only two groups *viz.* healthy and sick or affected and not affected to a certain disease; or the animals falling in more than two groups for the character showing codominance controlled by single gene pair like yellow, cream and white hair colour in guinea pigs or epistasis controlled by more than one gene loci. In such cases the numbers of animals showing different phenotypes of a character are recorded. These numbers are called the observed frequencies. Now the question arises to test whether these observed frequencies are in accordance to the expectation of some hypothesis. The expected frequencies (number of animals) are estimated as per hypoyhesis. The difference between the observed and expected frequencies is called as the deviation. The deviation may be large or small.

The statistical technique used is the χ^2 test. This chi-square (χ^2) test is used to test the extent of deviation whether the deviations are within the limits of hypothesis or not. Thus, this χ^2 test is applied on the basis of frequencies for a qualitative trait to determine the degree of deviation between observed and theoretical expected frequencies so as to know/conclude whether the deviation between observed and expected frequencies is real due to some specific factor (large difference) or due to chance or chance error (small deviation). This χ^2 test is most commonly used non-parametric test (distribution free) in biological or genetic experiments.

The requirements to test the deviation in genotypic and phenotypic ratios are the hypothesis based on sampling theory, sample size (n), degree of freedom (n – 1), level of significance, and test of measurement, like χ^2 test.

27.1 HYPOTHESIS AND LEVEL OF SIGNIFICANCE

There is hypothesized probability in genetic ratios based on a large number of observations. However, some deviation from the expected ratios is observed because of limited ***sample size*** as well as by chance events and it is known as ***sampling error***. The hypothesis states that there is no difference between the observed and the expected results. The hypothesis is a statement under test and is called ***null hypothesis*** ($H_0 = \mu_1 = \mu_2$). The null hypothesis is usually framed in a negative fashion such as no variation/deviation between treatments or between observed and expected result, or there is no relation between two variables, *etc.*

The ***alternate hypothesis*** is $H_A: \mu_1 \neq \mu_2$. The ***composite hypothesis*** is one which does not specify distribution (mean, σ^2): $\mu_1 > \mu_2$, $\mu_1 < \mu_2$.

The null hypothesis is rejected which cannot be accounted for by chance (< 5 per cent of the time or cases) and such results are called significant (meaningful). This indicates that there are 5 per cent chances of discarding a valid hypothesis. The size of the discrepancy indicates whether the discrepancy (deviation) can commonly or only rarely be expected whereas the large discrepancy indicates that the fitness of observed results to those expected is poor *i.e.* the observed results fit better with expectation other than the proposed hypothesis. In case of small discrepancy the hypothesis is rejected which mean that the discrepancy is not significant whereas in case of large discrepancy the hypothesis is accepted which man that the deviation is significant.

Level of Significance

The level of probability which is considered small for rejecting the null hypothesis is called the *level of significance*. The results or the evidence for a real difference is said to be significant. Ordinarily a level of 0.05 is taken as small enough to indicate a significant result. If the probability attained is < 0.01 the results is stated to be highly significant. However, the level of significance provides the probability basis to reject hypothesis and do not make it sure whether the hypothesis is true or false. For instance, there is possibility for deviation even from a valid hypothesis, though it is fairly less *i.e.* less than 5 per cent of the time. The 5 per cent level of significance is considered as optimum/acceptable, 1 per cent level as low level and 10 per cent level as high level of significance.

Degree of Freedom

It is the number of independent variables (classes) which may take any value but the value of the last variable (class) is fixed by ΣX and the n – 1 or freely determined variables. Thus, the number of classes or variables minus one (n – 1) is the degree of freedom where n is the total number of classes or variables. For example, there are four phenotypic classes (4 – 1 = 3), the 3 of the phenotypic classes can be filled at random but the number in 4th class is governed by the total number of individuals observed/measured. Therefore, the degree of freedom is n – 1 = 4 – 1 = 3 in this case of 4 phenotypes. In two way classification when two factors are involved, the degree of freedom is (n-1)(m-1).

27.2 TEST OF MEASUREMENT – CHI SQUARE (χ^2) TEST

The χ^2 test is a *non-parametric test* as it is distribution free test. This χ^2 test is applied when the observed data is classified in the form of a frequency distribution based on some attribute (quality) of individuals rather than quantitative measurements and it is of interest to test whether the observed data are in agreement with certain theory (hypothesis) or when comparison is made with expectation and testing the independence of two traits.

The χ^2 statistic is computed as:

$$\chi^2 = \sum \frac{(0-E)^2}{E}$$

Where, O and E represent for observed and expected frequencies, respectively.

The E's are calculated on the basis of null hypothesis (H_0).

The calculated χ^2 is tested with theoretical χ^2 value at (n – k) degree of freedom

Where, n is the total number of classes and

k is linear restrictions.

27.3 USE OF χ^2 TEST

The χ^2 test has the following uses:

- To compare sample variance with the population variance as

  $$\chi^2 = \sum \frac{(X-\overline{X})^2}{\sigma^2}$$

  Where, χ represents the sample observations, and

  χ represents for sample mean.

- To test the homogeneity of several variances *i.e.* whether all the samples have been taken from the population of equal variance *i.e.* $\sigma^2_1 = \sigma^2_2 = \sigma^2_K$. This test is known as ***Bartlett test***.
- As a test of goodness of fit for testing whether a given sample has been taken for a specified population or distribution.
- To test the independence of attributes in contingency table.
- To test the homogeneity of several observed correlation coefficient,
- To analyze the genetic experiments for testing genetic hypothesis and to detect linkage
  - (i) Test of significance of ratio in a single factor segregation,
  - (ii) Testing homogeneity of several families in a single factor segregation,
  - (iii) Testing the significance of ratio in two factor analysis and thus to detect linkage.

27.4 COMPARISON WITH EXPECTATION

27.4.1 Distribution following Binomial Theorem

The sex ratio is normally expected to be 50:50. The interest is to test the hypothesis whether the distribution of males and females as a whole follow the normal expectation. The χ^2 test is used to test the normal expectation. This is done by obtaining the expected number of families based on the binomial distribution as –

$$\chi^2 = \sum \frac{(O_i - E_i)^2}{E_i}$$

And it is tested for n – 1 degree of freedom.

Where, n is the number of classes of different families having different combination of male and female children,

O_i is the observed number of families surveyed for sex ratio,

E_i is the expected number of families in different combination of male and female children.

Example 27.1

A total of 320 buffaloes each with 6 calves were examined for the number of male and females calves. The following are the results:

No. of buffaloes observed	6	33	71	99	69	37	5
No. of male calves	0	1	2	3	4	5	6
No. of female calves	6	5	4	3	2	1	0

Now the problem is to test whether this distribution indicates that male and female calves are occurring with equal frequency in the herd.

Solution

The probability of male calves = probability of female calves = ½. Here there are 7 different families of buffaloes and hence

$(p+q)^6$ =	p^6 +	$6p^5q$ +	$15p^4q^2$ +	$20p^3q^3$ +	$15\,p^2q^4$ +	$6pq^5$ +	q^6
Females =	6	5	4	3	2	1	0
Males =	0	1	2	3	4	5	6

$= (½)^6 + 6\,(½)^5\,(½) + 15(½)^4(½)^2 + 20\,(½)^3\,(½)^3 + 15\,(½)^2(½)^4 + 6(½)(½)^5 + (½)$

$= (½)^6 + 6\,(½)^6 + 15(½)^6 + 20\,(½)^6 + 15\,(½)^6 + 6(½)^6 + (½)^6$

and $(½)^6$ – 0.0156 multiplied by the respective coefficients, following results are obtained -

= 0.0156 +0.0937 + 0.2344 + 0.3125 + 0.2344 + 0.0937 + 0.0156

Expected no. of buffaloes with 6 female and 0 male calves = 0.0156 x 320 = 5

Expected no. of buffaloes with 5 female and 1 male calves = 0.0937 x 320 = 30

Expected no. of buffaloes with 4 female and 2 male calves = 0.2344 x 320 = 75

Expected no. of buffaloes with 3 female and 3 male calves = 0.3125 x 320 = 100

Expected no. of buffaloes with 2 female and 4 male calves = 0.2344 x 320 = 75

Expected no. of buffaloes with 1 female and 5 male calves = 0.0937 x 320 = 30

Expected no. of buffaloes with 0 female and 6 male calves = 0.0156 x 320 = 5

$$\chi^2 = \frac{(6-5)^2}{5} + \frac{(30-30)^2}{30} + \frac{(71-75)^2}{75} + \frac{(99-100)^2}{100} + \frac{(67-75)^2}{75} + \frac{(37-30)^2}{30} + \frac{(5-5)^2}{5}$$

$= 0.20 + 0 + 0.2133 + 0.01 + 0.48 + 1.6333 + 0$

$= 2.5366$ at $7 - 1 = 6$ degree of freedom.

The tabulated value at 6 d.f. is higher than the calculated χ^2 value. Therefore, the distribution is consistent with the assumption that male and female calves occur with equal frequency.

27.4.2 Testing Genetic Ratios

(i) Two Phenotypic Classes

$$\chi^2 = \frac{(m_2 a_1 - m_1 a_2)^2}{m_1 m_2 N}$$

Where, a_1 and a_2 are the no. of individuals observed in the two phenotypic classes,

m_1 and m_2 are the expected ratio of the two phenotypic classes,

$N = a_1$ and a_2.

However, the χ^2 can be calculated as $\chi^2 = \frac{(O-E)^2}{E}$

The expected frequencies (E) are obtained by multiplying the total number (N) with the expected ratio of that class.

Example 27.2

Test whether the observed frequencies 125 and 36 are in ratio of 3:1.

Solution

$$\chi^2 = \frac{(m_2 a_1 - m_1 a_2)^2}{m_1 m_2 N}$$

$$= \frac{(a_1 - 3a_2)^2}{3N}$$

$$= \frac{(125 - 3 \times 36)^2}{(3 \times 161)} = 0.5983$$

(ii) Three or more phenotypic classes:

$$\chi^2 = \sum \frac{(O-E)^2}{E}$$

The expected frequencies are calculated according to the expected ratios. The E are obtained by multiplying the total number (N) with the expected ratios of that class. This is applied for any number of classes *viz. 2, 3, 4, and more.*

Example 27.3

Short hairs in guinea pigs is a dominant trait controlled by the allele ***L*** and its recessive allele ***l*** produces long hair whereas the hair colour is governed by a pair of co-dominant alleles, YY produces yellow colour, YW cream colour and WW white colour. The two loci assort independently. The numbers of individuals obtained from a dihybrid cross (Ll YW x Llyw) were:

Short cream = 50; short yellow 22; short white = 24;

Long cream = 21; long yellow 7; and long white = 6. Total individuals = 130

Find out whether the observations agree with the expected genetic ratios.

Solution

The genetic ratios for phenotypic classes from this dihybrid cros will be 3:1 for hair length and 1:2:1 for hair colour. The expected frequencies will be:

Phenotype	*Expectation*	*Expected freq.*	*Observed Freq.*	*χ2*
Short yellow	$3:1 = \frac{3}{16} \times 130$	= 24	22	0.1667
Short cream	$3:2 = \frac{6}{16} \times 130$	= 49	50	0.0204
Short white	$3:1 = \frac{3}{16} \times 130$	= 24	24	0.0
Long yellow	$1:1 = \frac{1}{16} \times 130$	= 8	7	0.1250
Long cream	$1:2 = \frac{2}{16} \times 130$	= 16	21	1.5625
Long white	$1:1 = \frac{1}{16} \times 130$	= 8	6	0.5000
				Total χ^2 = 2.3746

The calculated χ^2 value is less than the tabulated vale at 5 d.f.Thus, the results did not differ significantly from the expectation.

27.4.3 Testing Homogeneity among Classes - or Experimental Conditions

When the variability between classes is high, the individual χ^2 test for different classes separately may not reflect common experimental conditions and thus pooling their results (Pooled χ^2) is not justified. Therefore a "***test of homogeneity***" is conducted to decide whether the separate samples or experimental conditions are uniform. This is done by two ways:

1st Method

The χ^2 due to heterogeneity is estimated by deducting the χ^2 for summed data (sum of all classes) from the total χ^2 obtained by summing the individual χ^2 values of all the classes. If this final value (χ^2 due to heterogeneity) is significant at n – 1 d.f., it then indicate that there are real differences between samples or experimental conditions or classes and so the data should not be pooled. This is applicable foe 2 x n contingency table.

2nd Method

The $$\chi^2 = \left[\frac{N^2}{C_1C_2}\right]\left[\sum\left(\frac{a_i^2}{R_i}\right) - \frac{C_i^2}{N}\right] \text{at } (n-1)\text{ d.f.}$$

Where, R_i is the total of ith row or set or class,

a_i is the number of observations in ith class 1,

b_i is the number of observations in ith set of column 2,

$C_1 = \Sigma\, a_i$ = the total number of observations of column 1 for all sets,

$C_2 = \Sigma\, b_i$ = the number of observations of column 1 for all sets or classes,

Example 27.4

In a herd of cattle sired by 10 sires, the total numbers of calves born sired by different sires are given below. Do the sires produced significantly different sex ratios (Male births).

Sire No. (Sets or Classes)	*Male Calves (a_i)*	*Female Calves (b_i)*	*Total Calves (R_i)*	*Individual χ^2 Value*
1	20	22	42	0.0952
2	25	25	50	0.0
3	30	20	50	1.8182
4	25	23	48	0.0833
5	15	13	28	0.1429
6	10	5	15	1.6667
7	18	9	27	3.0000

Sire No. (Sets or Classes)	*Male Calves (a_i)*	*Female Calves (b_i)*	*Total Calves (R_i)*	*Individual χ^2 Value*
8	20	12	32	2.0000
9	22	24	46	0.0870
10	10	8	18	0.2222
Total	195 ($C_1 = \Sigma a_i$)	166 ($C_1 = \Sigma b_i$)	361 (N)	9.1155 ($\Sigma \chi^2$)

χ^2 for all the 10 sires based on total no. of observations = 2.3296

The χ^2 heterogeneity is calculated by 2 methods as:

I Method: Difference method

The χ^2 heterogeneity is estimated by difference of χ^2 value ($\Sigma \chi^2$ - χ^2 for all sires). Thus, χ^2 heterogeneity = 9.1155 – 2.3296 = 6.7860. This χ^2 heterogeneity is 6.7860 is also non-significant which indicated that the sires do not differ for sex ratio.

II Method

$$\chi^2 = \left[\frac{N^2}{C_1C_2}\right]\left[\sum\left(\frac{a_i^{\ 2}}{R_i}\right) - \frac{C_i^{\ 2}}{N}\right] \text{at (n 1) d.f.}$$

$$\chi^2 = \left[\frac{(361)^2}{195\times166}\right]\left[\left(\frac{(20)^2}{42}\right)+.+\left(\frac{(10)^2}{18}\right)-\left(\frac{(195)^2}{361}\right)\right]$$

$$= \left(\frac{130321}{32370}\right)(106.69 - 105.33)$$

$$= 4.03 \times 1.36$$

$$= 5.48 \text{ at 9 d.f.}$$

This calculated χ^2 value (5.48) is also less than tabulated value of χ^2at 5 per cent (16.91) and at 1 per cent (21.66). Therefore, χ^2 heterogeneity is not significant which indicates that different sires do not differ significantly to produce male calf percentage (sex ratio).

27.4.4 Detection of Linkage: Two Factor Segregation

It is required to test whether two characters segregating separately agree with the respective expected ratios and whether they are segregating independently from each other or they are linked (associated or correlated). Considering the two characters segregating in the raio of r_1:1 and r_2:1, their joint segregation into 4 classes will be in the ratio of r_1r_2:r_1:r_2:1. For example, the two characters A and B are segregating in the ratio of 3:1 separately then their joint segregation will produce 4 classes in the ratio 9:3:3:1. The χ^2 test of association or independence or χ^2 due to linkage is applied to test whether the deviation from independence is significant or not. It the χ^2 test of association is significant then the deviation is purely due to linkage.

(i) F_2 DATA

The significant deviation from dihybrid ratio (9:3:3:1) indicate linkage. The deviation in dihybrid ratio can be tested as explained above. The χ^2 linkge can also be calculated as:

$$\chi^2\,(\text{Linkage}) = \frac{(a_1 + 3a_2 + 3a_3 + 9a_4)^2}{9N}$$

Where, $N = a_1 + a_2 + a_3 + a_4 = a + b + c + d$

$a_1 = AB$, $a_2 = aB$, $a_3 = Ab$, and $a_4 = ab$

A and B represent dominant phenotypes, and

a and b represent recessive phenotypes.

Example 27.5

Purple stem in tomato is a dominant character over its recessive character green stem. Another character hair of stem is a dominant character over hairless stem. In F2 population 400 plants were examined for both the characters with the following results:

	Hair on Stem (A)	*Hairless (a)*	*Total*
Stem : Purple (B)	200	90	***290***
Colour : Red (b)	100	10	***110***
Total	300	100	400

Find out whether (i) the purple – green ratio, and hairy – hairless ratio are compatible with expectation of 3:1 ratio, and (ii) the results are compatible with the hypothesis of independent assortment with no linkage.

Solution

The observations can be arranged as:

Hairless (A)	*Stem Colour (B)*	*Notations*	*Observed Frequencies*
Hairy (A)	Purple (B)	$AB = a = a_1$	200
	Green (b)	$Ab = c = a_2$	100
		Total	300
Hairless (a)	Purple (B)	$aB = b = a_2$	90
	Green (b)	$ab = d = a_4$	10
		Total	100

Hairless (A)	Stem Colour (B)	Notations	Observed Frequencies
	Purple	$a_1 + a_2$	290
	Green	$a_3 + a_4$	110
	Total	$a_1 + a_2 + a_3 + a_4$	400

χ^2 for stem colour $= \dfrac{(290-3\times110)^2}{3\times400}$

$= 1.333$ at 1 d.f.

χ^2 for stem hairness $= \dfrac{(300-3\times110)^2}{3\times400}$

$= 0$ at 1 d.f.

χ^2 (linkage) $= \dfrac{(200-3\times110-3\times90+9\times10)^2}{9\times400}$

$= 21.778^{**}$ at 1 d.f

Total $\chi^2 = 21.778 + 1.333 + 0.0 = 23.111$ at 3 d.f.

The χ^2 (total) can also be calculated by using the ordinary χ^2 formula:

$$\chi^2 = \sum\frac{(O_i - E_i)^2}{E_i}$$

The E_i are obtained as:

Purple hairy $= 400\times\dfrac{9}{16} = 225$

Purple hairless $= 400\times\dfrac{3}{16} = 75$

Green hairy $= 400\times\dfrac{3}{16} = 75$

Green hairless $= 400\times\dfrac{1}{16} = 25$

$$\text{Now}, \chi^2 = \sum\frac{(O_i - E_i)^2}{E_i} = 23.111 \text{ at 1 d.f.}$$

The total χ^2 obtained as $\sum\dfrac{(O_i - E_i)^2}{E_i}$ was partitioned into 3 parts *viz.* χ^2 due to stem colour, χ^2 due to hairyness, and χ^2 linkage.

The χ^2 values for the segregation of stem colour and for hairyness are non significant indicating that the two characters segregation is in agreement with 3:1

ratio. The χ^2 linkage was significant which indicated the strong evidence of linkage for gene loci for two characters. This is because significant departure from the expected F_2 ratio (9:3:3:1 indicates linkage. Thus, the two loci are linked/present on same chromosome.

(ii) Test Cross Data

In a similar way, the linkage may be detected by making the test cross as explained below:

Example 27.6

Taking the two characters of example of 27.28, the following results were obtained in a test cross producing 200 plants:

Phenotypes	*Observed Numbers*	*Total*
Hairy purple	82	
Hairy green	20	102
Hairless purple	13	
Hairless green	85	98

Test whether the two ratios separately are compatible with the expected ratio of test cross (1:1) and their joint ratio (1:1:1:1).

Solution

Observed ratio for hair and hairless = 102:98

Observed ratio for purple and green = 95:105

The expected ratios (E_i) are 50 for all the classes. Therefore,

$$\chi^2 = \sum \frac{(O_i - E_i)^2}{E_i}$$

$$= \frac{(82 \quad 50)^2}{50} + \frac{(20 \quad 50)^2}{50} + \frac{(13 \quad 50)^2}{50} + \frac{(85 \quad 50)^2}{50}$$

= 90.36** at 3 d.f. which is highly significant.

Now, this total χ^2 (90.36**) can be partitioned into 3 causes as under -

χ^2 Stem colour $= \frac{(95 \quad 105)^2}{200} = 0.50$

χ^2 hairness of stem $= \frac{(102 \quad 98)^2}{200} = 0.08$

χ^2 linkage $= \frac{(a_1 \quad a_2 \quad a_3 + a_4)^2}{N}$

$$= \frac{(82 \quad 20 \quad 13+85)^2}{200} = 89.78 ^{**}$$

Total χ^2

$$= 89.78 + 0.50 + 0.08 = 90.36^{**} \text{ at 3 d.f.}$$

The results indicate that the two ratios for both the characters are compatible with expected ratios of test cross (1:1) whereas the total χ^2 (90.36**) is highly significant indicating that the joint segregation does not follow the normal expectation of test cross (1:1:1:1). Thus, a strong evidence of linkage was observed. This was further confirmed from the significant value of linkage. Therefore, the two loci affecting two characters are linked being present on the same pair of chromosome.

27.5 TESTING THE INDEPENDENCE (ASSOCIATION OR CORRELATION)

There may be the following 3 types of observations arranged in 2 x 2 table, 2 x n table, and m x n table.

(1) 2 x 2 Table

The χ^2 is obtained as –

$$\chi^2 = \frac{(ad \quad bc)^2 N}{R_1 R_2 C_1 C_2}$$

Where, a = Phenotypic class showing both characters

b = Phenotypic class showing only first character

c = Phenotypic class showing second character

d = Phenotypic class showing recessive phenotype

$R_1 = a+b$; $R_2 = c+d$; $C_1 = a + c$; $C_2 = b + d$

Example 27.7

Tomar (1984) recorded abnormal births and retention of placenta in 452 buffaloes and arranged the data as under:

	Normal Births	*Abnormal Births*	*Total*
Placenta expelled	395	24	***419***
Placenta retained	25	8	***33***
Total	420	32	452

Find out whether the two disorders are independent.

Solution

$$\chi^2 = \frac{(ad \quad bc)^2 N}{R_1 R_2 C_1 C_2}$$

$$= \frac{(395 \times 8 \quad 25 \times 24)^2\, 452}{419 \times 33 \times 420 \times 32}$$

$$\frac{2560 \times 2560 \times 452}{419 \times 33 \times 420 \times 32}$$

$= 15.94^{**}$

This value of χ^2 is highly significant indicating the dependence or association or correlation between two characters.

This test of association is similar to the testing of homogeneity and to test linkage.

(2) 2 × n Table

The χ^2 of testing independence is similar to that the genetic ratios in 2 × n table.

$$\chi^2 = \left[\frac{N^2}{C_1 C_2}\right]\left[\sum\left(\frac{a_i^{\,2}}{R_i}\right) - \frac{C_i^{\,2}}{N}\right] \text{at (n} \quad \text{1) d.f.}$$

Example 27.8

In a herd of crossbred cattle comprising 5 genetic groups, the following results were obtained for type of calving (abnormal and normal):

Genetic Groups	*1*	*2*	*3*	*4*	*5*	*Total*
Animals with normal calving	189	230	226	265	310	1220
Animals with abnormal calving	11	20	24	35	40	130
Total animals	200	250	250	300	350	1350

Do the genetic groups differ significantly for the rate of abnormal calving?.

Solution

$$\chi^2 = \left[\frac{N^2}{C_1 C_2}\right]\left[\sum\left(\frac{a_i^{\,2}}{R_i}\right) - \frac{C_i^{\,2}}{N}\right] \text{at (n} \quad \text{1) d.f.}$$

$$\chi^2 = \left[\frac{(1350)^2}{130 \times 1220}\right]\left[\left(\frac{(11)^2}{200}\right) + \left(\frac{(20)^2}{250}\right) + \qquad + \left(\frac{(40)^2}{350}\right) - \left(\frac{(130)^2}{1350}\right)\right]$$

$= 11.49\ (13.16 - 12.52) = 7.35$ at 4 d.f.

This χ^2 value is non-significant indicating that the different genetic groups did not differ significantly for the rate of abnormal calving.

(3) m × n Table

The expected frequencies in 2 × 2, 2 × n, and m × n table can be obtained in the same way as shown below:

Expected frequencies $(X_{ij}) = \frac{C_j R_j}{N}$

Where, C_i is the total of ith column,

R_j is the total of jth row, and

N is the overall total.

$$\chi^2 = \sum \frac{(O_i - E_i)^2}{E_i} \text{ at } (m \quad 1) \text{ d.f.}$$

Example 29.9

In a study on incidence of mastitis and SNT gave the following data. Do the mastitis incidences differ in cows having different number of teat.

Teat no.	*Severe mastitis*	*Mild mastitis*	*Unaffected*	*Total*
4	19	16	1510	***1605***
5	13	13	162	***188***
6	15	14	189	***218***
Total	47	43	1921	2011

Solution

$E_{i's} =$ $1605 \times \frac{47}{2011} = 38$ $\quad 1605 \times \frac{43}{2011} = 34$ $\quad 1605 \times \frac{1921}{2011} = 1533$

$188 \times \frac{47}{2011} = 4$ $\quad 188 \times \frac{43}{2011} = 4$ $\quad 188 \times \frac{1921}{2011} = 180$

$218 \times \frac{47}{2011} = 5$ $\quad 218 \times \frac{43}{2011} = 5$ $\quad 218 \times \frac{1921}{2011} = 208$

$$\chi^2 \quad \frac{(O_i - E_i)^2}{E_i} \text{ at } (3 \quad 1)(3 \quad 1) \text{ d.f.}$$

$$\frac{(19-38)^2}{38} + \frac{(16-34)^2}{34} + ... + \frac{(189-208)^2}{208}$$

$= 100.16^{**}$ at 4 d.f.

This χ^2 value is highly significant indicating that the two characters are associated (correlated). The incidence of mastitis is significantly higher among cows having more than normal teats (SNT).

27.6 CORRECT USE OR LIMITATIONS OF CHI-SQUARE (X^2)

The following precautions or assumptions are necessary to use chi-square test (χ^2):

1. It is used on the number of observations and not on ratios or percentage obtained from data.
2. The sample should be larger (≥ 30).
3. It is not used when the $E_{i's}$ within any class is less than 5.
4. This test s based on a continuous distribution which is not found in genetic problems. Therefore, a correction is made for this lack of continuity before the test is applied as: $\chi^2 = \frac{(O_i - E_i - 0.5)^2}{E_i}$
5. The constraints if any are always linear.
6. The observations are independent.

Annexures

Annexure 14.1

Mechanisms Involved in Transition Mutation

The mutation inducing molecular mechanisms for the *transition mutations* in a polypeptide chain are *tautomerism, deamination, ionization,* and *inclusion of base analogs in place of normal bases*. These different mechanisms have been described here as under:

(1) Tautomerizationt of Nitrogenous Bases in DNA

Rearrangement in the distribution of hydrogen atoms in an organic molecule: The four nitrogen bases in DNA are present in common *stable forms* which are the ***keto*** form (C = O group) for one purine (Guanine) and one pyrimidine (Thymine) and the ***amino*** form (-NH_2 group) for one purine (Adenine) and one pyrimidine (Cytosine).

However, Watson and Crick also pointed out about the *non-static forms* (*unstable structures*) of the four nitrogen bases in DNA, known as ***enol*** (-OH) and ***imino*** forms (-NH group). These alternate forms (rare states) are called ***tautomers***. In describing the double helical structure of DNA, they also proposed the semi-conservative nature of replication based on specific base-pairing and a mechanism for explaining spontaneous mutation.

The mechanism of conversion of normal forms of bases (keto and amino forms) into alternate forms (enol and imino forms) is called ***tautomerism*** or *tautomerization* which occurs through rearrangement of electrons and protons in the molecules. The alternate forms (*tautomers*) of nitrogen bases are formed by the movement of the hydrogen atoms from one position to another position in a purine or pyrimidine. The transfer of hydrogen atoms occurs between the number 1 and number 6 positions. This ***shifting of hydrogen atoms*** from one position in an organic molecule to another position is called ***tautomeric shift***.

The tautomerization converts the stable amino group (-NH_2) of cytosine and adenine into unstable ***imino group*** (-NH) called imino tautamers whereas the guanine and thymine are converted from their stable keto form (– C=O group) into unstable ***enol state*** (-OH group) called enol tautomers.

The tautomeric shifts are rare but are also important in DNA metabolism from the point of changing the pairing potential of the bases. The change (shifting) in hydrogen atoms of bases between the positions results in changing their base-pairing potential and also causes mutation. A nitrogenous base in its rare or tautomeric state cannot pair with its normal partner as per the base pairing principle.

In case the DNA has a tautomer of adenine then during replication the adenine will pair with wrong partner, the cytosine instead of normal partner, the thymine. The newly introduced cytosine will pair with its normal partner guanine and not with thymine. Consequently the descendent strand (newly formed DNA strand) will have a exceptional base pair (G:C pair in place of A:T pair). This will change the genetic code, producing another protein and so the phenotypic expression of gene will be changed. This is called ***copy error*** and this state is not stable and hence the adenine is converted back to its common form in next replication of DNA and will pair with thymine. The cytosine induced into the complementary strand due to tautomeric shift in adenine will now pair with its normal partner guanine. Thus, A:T pair is converted into G:C pair and likewise G:C pair is converted into A:T pair. The mechanism of tautomerization for converting A:T pair to G:C pair and vice versa has been shown (after Burns, 1969) as below:

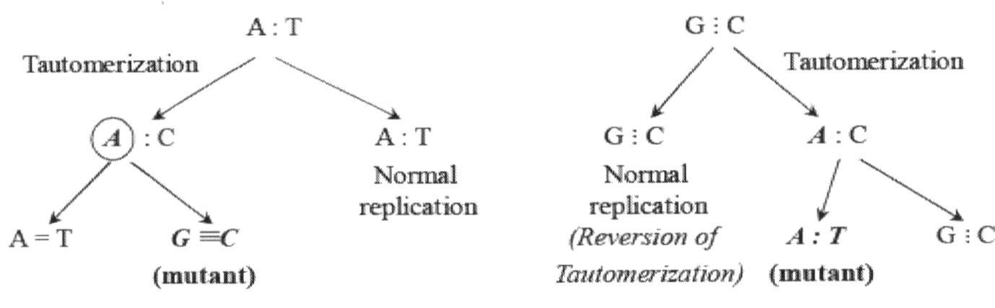

Figure 14.4: Conversion of A:T Pair to G:C and of G:C Pair to A:T Due to Tautomerization.

The tautomeric shift of bases results into mismatched and rare base-pairing of A:C [common amino form of A with rare imino form of C] and of G:T [common keto form of T with rare enol form of G] in place of normal A:T and G:C base-pairing with different stable forms (amino and keto). The rare base pairing also forms when T and A are in their rare enol and imino forms, respectively. This A:C and G:T base-pairing occurs when cytosine and guanine are in their rare imino and enol tautomeric forms, respectively. These mismatched base-pairs are segregated during subsequent replication producing an A:T to G:C or a G:C to A:T base-pair substitution. For example, G from its normal keto form undergoes a tautomeric shift to its rare enol form (G′) during DNA replication. The G′ shifts back to its more stable keto form (G). Therefore, the T incorporated opposite the enol form of G directs the incorporation of A during next DNA replication. This results from G:C to A:T base pair substitution. The tautomerization results into transition mutation.

Occasionally in adenine (A) a hydrogen atom involved in bonding with complementary strand can shift from amino group to the nitrogen in the ring. Similar happens with cytosine. The hydrogen atom of bases thymine and guanine (keto form) can shift from keto form to enol form.

The existence of a base in less stable tautomeric forms for a short time results into no change (no mutation) but the tautomeric shifts results into a mutation if a particular base either exists in rare less stable form during replication or induced into nascent DNA chain.

(2) Deamination of Nitrogen Bases in DNA

This is the replacement of amino group ($-NH_2$) of nitrogen bases by hydroxyl group ($-OH$): The oxidative deamination results to transitional mutations. The deamination occurs by the action of some chemical substances like nitrous acid and hydroxylamine.

(i) The ***nitrous acid*** **(HNO_2)** produces transitions in both the directions $(A:T \leftrightarrow G:C)$. Therefore, the mutations induced by nitrous acid are also induced back to wild type. The deamination by the action of ***nitrous acid*** (HNO_2) changes A, C, and G bases as:

- ☆ Adenine changes to hypoxanthine which exhibits bonding similarity with guanine. Thus, during DNA replication the hypoxanthine (after transforming into keto-tautomer) pairs with cytocine. This results A:T base pair to convert into G:C base pair.
- ☆ Cytocine is changed to uracil which pairs with adenine. Thus, during DNA replication the uracil will pair with adenine and the G:C pair is converted into A:T base pair, and
- ☆ Guanine is changed to xanthine which pairs by two hydrogen bonds with cytocine.

(a) Deamination of adenine (A)

Adenine + $HNO_2 \rightarrow$ Hypoxanthine

The adenine having-NH_2 group at number 6 carbon is deaminated (replaced by $-OH$ group) by nitrous acid to hypoxanthine has been shown (after Burns, 1969) as below:

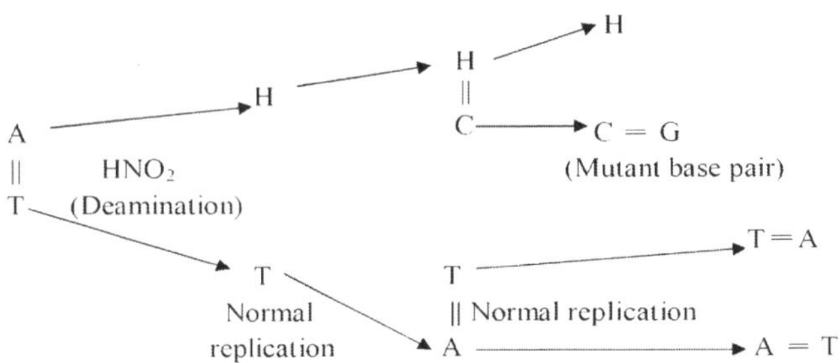

Figure 14.5 (i): Deamination Process by Nitrous Acid (HNO_2) for Adenine.

The ***adenine* (A)** is deaminated by the action of nitrous acid. This deamination changes the NH_2 group (amino) of adenine to OH group and the A is converted to *hypoxanthine* (H). The H behaves like G rather than A during replication. The H has thus the pairing property like that of G and hence it (H) will search/specify C and will pair with it (C). Thus, H specifies C, and C specifies G in next replication. The net result of deamination of A by nitrous acid is the conversion of A:T pairs to G:C (A to H to G). This change of A:T pair into G:C pair is transition of A:T to G:C. Therefore, the change brought by the action of nitrous acid is the transition mutation.

(b) Deamination of cytosine (C)

Cytosine + $HNO_2 \rightarrow$ Uracil

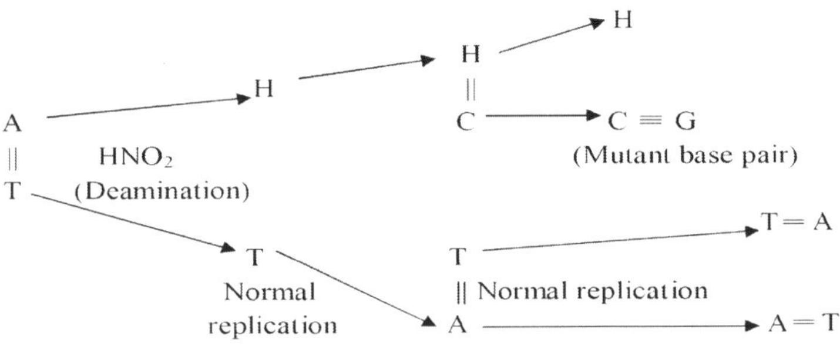

Figure 14.5 (ii): Deamination Process by Nitrous Acid (HNO_2) for Cytosine.

Similarly, the ***cytosine* (C)** is also deaminated by nitrous acid converting it (C) to uracil (U) which pairs with A instead of G. Thus, the U behaves like T rather than C during replication and hence pairs with A. Therefore, the net result of the deamination of C into U (after one cycle of DNA synthesis) is the change of G:C pair to A:T pair (C to U to T). This is also the transition of G:C pair to A:T pair and hence transition mutation.

(c) *Deamination of guanine*

Guanine + $HNO_2 \rightarrow$ Xanthine

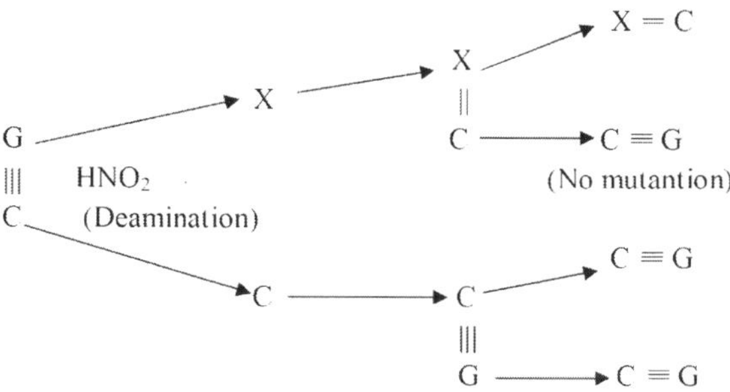

Figure 14.5 (iii): Deamination Process by Nitrous Acid (HNO_2) for Guanine.

The ***guanine* (G)** is deaminated of by nitrous acid producing xanthine which behaves like G and hence will base pair with C. Thus, it will lead no change in base pairing. The deamination of G is therefore not mutagenic.

(ii) Hydroxylamine and other compounds that seem to cause transition mutation are hydroxyl (OH) donors. The hydroxylamine is the most specific of all mutagens by adding OH group to the amino group of cytosine which then enables the base to undergo a tautomeric shift so that it can pair with adenine (A). The hydroxylamine is united with cytosine (C) producing hydroxyl-amino-cytosine and this changed cytosine (hydroxyl-amino-cytosine) then pairs with adenine (A) rather than guanine. Thus, during DNA replication it produces a change from C to A and introduces T:A. Therefore, it is transition mutation causing C:G to T:A.

The hydroxylamine introduces only one-way transition. This is because the transition so caused does not revert back. The transition from C:G to A:T (conversion of C:G pair to A:T base pair) by hydroxylamine has been shown (after Burns, 1969) as below:

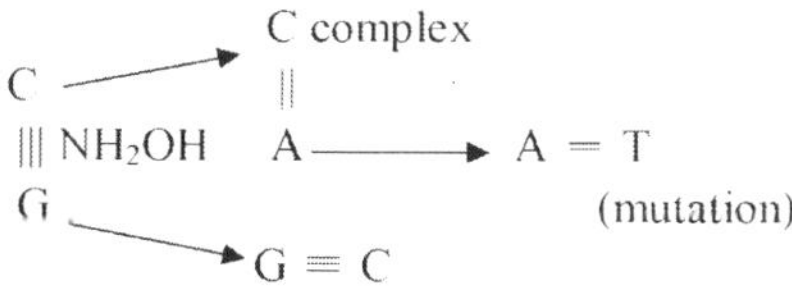

Figure 14.6: Mechanism of Transition from C:G to A:T by Hydroxylamine: Pairing of the Changed Cytosine to Adenine.

(3) Ionization of Nitrogenous Bases

The *ionization* of a base involves the ***loss of hydrogen*** which occurs at the time of DNA replication.

The hydrogen is lost from number 1 nitrogen of a nitrogenous base. The thymine in its ionized state pairs with normal guanine and ionized guanine pairs with normal thymine. The ionization results into transition mutation.

(4) Incorporation of Base Analogues in DNA – Unnatural Bases

The base analogues are certain chemical compounds which have molecular structure similar to the nitrogen bases found in nucleic acids but with some differences. The base analogues are derivatives of nitrogen bases of DNA, unnatural purines or pyrimidine bases, differ slightly from the natural bases, and they can be incorporated into nucleic acids. These are usually mutagenic. They are incorporated into DNA during replication due to their structure similar to bases but they increase the frequency of mis-pairing due to some differences in structure. Thus, during replication base analogues induce the transition mutations in both directions (A:T to G:C, and G:C to A:T).

The base analogues result into transition mutation. These base analogs are natural and also artificial.

The ***natural base analogues*** are:

- ☆ 5-methyl cytosine which occurs naturally in the DNA of wheat, grasses and many mammals (Doskocil and Sorm, 1962),
- ☆ 5-hydroxymethyl cytosine and 5-glucosyl hydroxymethyl cytosine which are present in *E. coli;*
- ☆ 5-hydroxymethyl uracil occurs in some viruses, and
- ☆ 6-methyl purine which is an adenine analogue and present in some bacteria.

The ***artificial base analogues*** most commonly used are

- ☆ 5-bromouracil and 5-iodouracil (structural analogue of thymine),
- ☆ 2-aminopurine (analogue of adenine),
- ☆ 2-bromo and 5-methyl cytosine (cytosine analogue).

The thymine analogues are incorporated in place of thymine replacing thymine in DNA replication while those of cytosine analogues are incorporated in place of cytosine and hence substitute cytosine during DNA replication.

(i) 5-bromouracil (BU)

The 5-***bromouracil*** (BU) or Bromodeoxyuridine (BudR) is the structural (chemical) analogous to the nitrogen base thymine (T). The bromine at the 5 position is similar to methyl group (- CH_3) at the 5 position in T. The 5-BU is incorporated into DNA during replication in place of thymine (T). The more common form of 5-BU is the keto form and its rare form is enol form or it may occur in ionized form. 5-Bu in its keto form pairs with adenine while it pairs with guanine in its rare enol form (short-lived changes to keto form). This enables BU to pair with G and changes the charge distribution increasing the frequency of tautomeric shifts. After tautomeric shift to its enol form, the 5-BU pairs with G. Thus, BU may be incorporated to its keto form as a pairing mate to A and then produce G:C substitution for the original A:T.

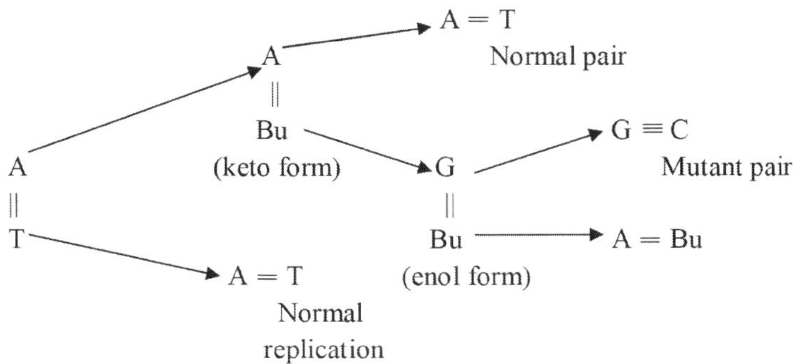

Figure 14.7 (i): Transition of A:T Base Pair to G:C by Keto Form of 5-BU.

The 5-BU may be incorporated in the enol form as a pairing mate with G and then converts to its keto form to produce an A:T substitution for the original G:C pair. This is the mistake of BU incorporation. The Bu is incorporated for C and then pairs with A. The 5-BU induces transitions in both directions $(A:T \leftrightarrow G:C)$. The most favourable direction is G:C to A:T transition mutation.

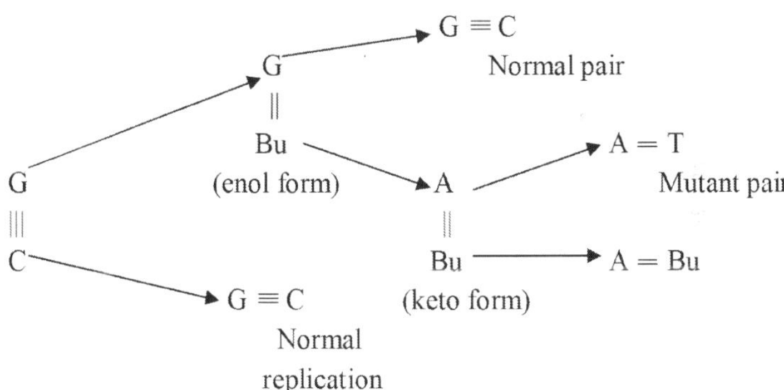

Figure 14.7 (ii): Transition of G:C Base Pair to A:T by Enol Form of 5-BU.

(ii) Aminopurine (AP)

The 2-*aminopurine* (AP) is an artificial base analogue of adenine and similar to 5-BU in its action but it is incorporated in DNA in place of A or G.

The 2-AP enables it to be incorporated as a substitute of A, but to pair subsequently with C or to pair initially with C and subsequently with T. The 2 AP pairs with C in imino form but it pairs with T in normal form. The favourable direction is A:T to G:C transition mutation.

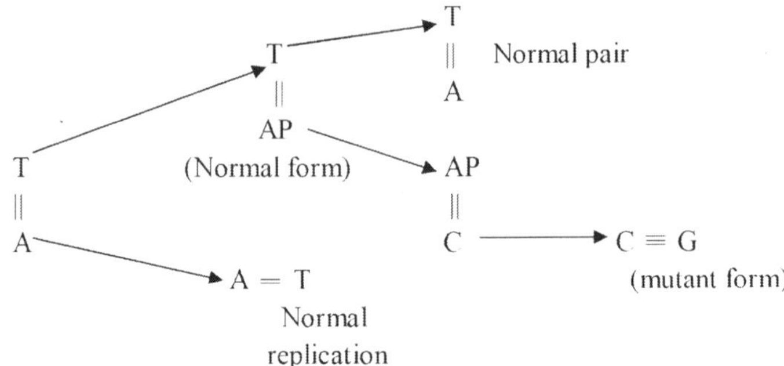

Figure 14.8 (i): Transition of A:T Base Pair to G:C by Base Analogue AP.

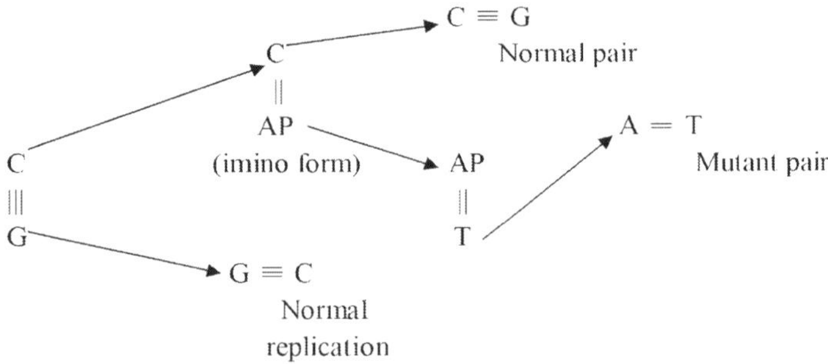

Figure 14.8 (ii): Transition of G:C Base Pair to A:T by Base Analogue AP.

Annexure 14.2

Mechanism of Transposition

The transposons have been categorized in three groups on the basis of the mechanism of transposition. The details are as under:

1. Cut-and-paste Transposition

This involves the excision of a transposable element (transposon) from its position in the chromosome and its insertion into another position on the same or different chromosome by the action of an enzyme called ***transposase***. This enzyme is encoded by the transposon itself. As the genetic element is cut physically (excised) at one site in a chromosome and pasted (inserted) into another site, so this mechanism of movement of the genetic element is called *cut-and-paste transposition.*

Such transposons following the cut-and-paste mechanism are found in both prokaryotes and eukaryotes. The examples of these transposons found in bacteria are *insertion sequences* (*IS elements*) and *composite transposons;* whereas those found in eukaryotes are the *P elements* and *hobo elements* (*Drosophila*); *sleeping beauty* (Salmon); *piggyback* (moth); and *Ac/Ds elements* (maize).

The different eukaryotic genetic transposable elements (transposons) which follow the cut-and-paste mechanism are Ac and Ds elements found in maize, and the P elements found in *Drosophila.*

The different transposons in bacteria are the *insertion sequences* (IS elements) which are simple and contain genes encoding proteins involved in transposition, and *composite transposons* which are complex and contain genes encoding products unrelated to the process of transposition. The bacterial transposons are demarcated by *terminal inverted repeats*. These repeats on inserting into a DNA molecule create a duplication of sequences at the insertion site, known as *target site duplication.*

(1.1) Ac and Ds Elements in Maize

B. McClintock discovered these transposable elements by studying chromosome breakage. She used the genetic markers that control the colour of maize kernels for detecting the breakage. The loss of particular marker (inferred from loss of colour of the *aleurone*, the outermost layer of the endosperm of maize kernels) indicated the loss of chromosomal segment on which the marker was located and thus the loss of marker indicated the breakage. She saw mosaic kernels in her experiment due to breakage at a particular site on chromosome 9. The chromosomal breaks producing factor was named by her as ***Ds***, for ***dissociation*** though this factor itself was unable to make breaks but it stimulates another factor, called ***Ac***, for ***activation***. The Ds element mediates chromosome breakage in response to the effect of another transposable element (Ac).

McClintock observed that Ac factor was not present in all the maize stocks but crossing the different stocks resulted in the combination of Ac with Ds in the cross and lead to chromosome breakage. She also found other breakages at different sites on chromosome 9 and also on other chromosomes. Since Ac was responsible for the breakage, the Ds factors were also involved. She proposed that Ds could be present at many different sites in the genome with its movement from one site to another (transposition). These Ac and Ds elements are structurally related to each other, belong to a family of transposons, both have multiple copies, both can move, can insert at many different sites, and alter or completely abolish the gene's function, thereby inducing mutations by inserting into genes. She also called these transposable elements as the ***controlling elements*** that are capable to influence the expression of a nearby gene.

The Ac/Ds elements are also found in other species including animals, like the *hobo* element found in some species of *Drosophila*.

The Ac elements contain 4563 np and bounded by inverted terminal repeats of 11 np long which are essential for transposition. Each of the Ac elements is also flanked by direct repeats of 8 np long which are created during insertion of the element into the chromosome. Therefore, the direct repeats are target site duplications rather than the integral part of the element. The Ds elements are structurally heterogeneous. However, both Ac and Ds elements contain the same inverted terminal repeats with variation in internal sequences and produces the following classes of Ds elements.

- Ds elements with missing of internal sequences: The loss of internal sequences from Ac elements produces some Ds elements. This loss may be caused due to incomplete DNA synthesis during replication or transposition.
- *Aberrant* Ds elements: These contain non-Ac DNA between their inverted terminal repeats (internal sequences) and hence these are unrelated to Ac DNA.
- *Double Ds* elements: One Ds element is inserted into another but in an inverted orientation and appears responsible to chromosome breakage.

The enzyme *transposase* encoded by Ac element is a *trans*-acting protein because it can diffuse through the nucleus, bind to a Ds element, and activate it. This *transposase* causes the activities of the Ac/Ds elements *viz.* excision and transposition, mutation and chromosome breakage, and interacts with sequences at or near the ends of Ac and Ds elements catalyzing their movement. This catalytic activity is abolished due to the deletions or mutations in the gene encoding the transposase and hence the Ds elements cannot activate themselves. But the presence of Ac element anywhere in the genome activates to the Ds elements.

(1.2) P Elements in *Drosophila*

These were found in *Drosophila* when Margaret and James Kidwell (1977) discovered an assortment of aberrant traits including frequent mutation, chromosome breakage, and sterility in the hybrids of some crosses. This syndrome of abnormalities was denoted by the term ***hybrid dysgenesis*** which has a Greek meaning "deterioration in quality". The hybrid dysgenesis is a syndrome of germ line abnormalities for which the transposable P elements are responsible. They took the dysgenic hybrids to classify *Drosophila* in two strains *viz.* P and M. The dysgenic hybrids were produced by crossing P and M strains provided the male parent belong to P strain whereas other crosses (P x P, M x M, and M x P) produced normal hybrids. Based on these findings, they concluded that P strain has genetic factors which are activated only if fertilizes the M strain ovum and induce mutations and chromosome breakage after activation.

Willium Eagels (1979) worked on dys-genesis induced mutations and found a reverse mutation to wild-type at a high rate. The instability strongly suggested the involvement of a transposon. Later on, the P strain was found to have the elements in multiple copies at different sites in the chromosome but these were not present in M strain. Therefore, this element was called the ***P element.*** These P elements are of variable size, the largest one having 2907 np including 31 np of terminal inverted repeats. The P element transposes to a new location in the genome when the gene present in the P element encodes an enzyme *transposase* which cleaves DNA near the end of a *complete* P element. But, some of the P elements are *incomplete* for the reason of deletion of some of their internal sequences and hence such incomplete P element lost the ability to produce the transposase. However, they contain the terminal and sub-terminal sequences recognized by transposase and hence these elements can be moved provided a transposase-producing complete element is present anywhere in the genome.

It is important to observe that hybrid dysgenesis is strictly germ-line phenomenon which means that P elements transpose only in germ line cells. This is due to the reason that somatic cells are unable to remove one of the introns from the P element's pre-mRNA. The P element activity within the germ line is regulated by small RNAs (piRNAs) derived from the P elements themselves.

(1.3) IS Elements in Bacteria

These are the transposons which reside in bacterial chromosomes and plasmids and can insert at many different sites in them. They are compactly organized containing short DNA sequences (800 – 1400 np) and the genes contained in them are only involved in regulating transposition. The IS elements are of many types and the bacterial chromosome may contain several copies of a particular type of IS element. The smallest element (IS1) is of only 768 np long, and 6to 10 copies of IS1 are present in *E. coli chromosome.* Each type is demarcated by short terminal sequences (identical or nearly identical) at its ends in inverted orientation to each other, called ***terminal inverted repeats***. These repeats have np ranging from 9 to 40 and are important in the transposition process because the mutation in these repeats lost the moving ability of repeat.

The transposition of IS element is mediated by an enzyme (*transposase*) encoded by the IS element itself. The enzyme binds at or near the ends of the element, cuts both strands of DNA, and excised the element from the chromosome or plasmid and inserted at a new position in the same or a different DNA molecule. The IS element in the F plasmid may pair and recombine with the same kind of IS element in the *E. coli* chromosome. The IS elements mediate recombination between non-homologous DNA molecules, *e.g.* between F factors and bacterial chromosomes. The smaller plasmid is integrated into the larger chromosome and produces a single circular molecule. The insertion of IS elements creates a duplication of part of the DNA sequence at that insertion site and locating one copy of the duplication on each side of the element. These duplicated or repeated sequences called ***target site duplications*** are short (2 to 13 np long) and arise from staggered cleavage of the DNA molecule.

Medical Significance of IS Elements

The IS Elements can mediate recombination between different DNA molecules. The bacterial plasmids spread the antibiotic resistant genes in the bacterial population. Thus, they can move genes from one bacterial cell to another and hence they have a medical significance. Such plasmids transferring the antibiotic resistance genes between bacteria are called ***conjugative R plasmids.*** These plasmids are formed by the successive integration of resistance genes by IS-mediated recombination. The IS elements mediate the recombination between two different plasmids. One plasmid may have a gene resistant to some antibiotics and this plasmid recombines with another plasmid (conjugative plasmid) that can be transferred between cells during conjugation. The IS 1 element present in both the plasmids mediates the recombination creating a large plasmid having gene resistant for antibiotic and the capability of transferring during conjugation. This process spread the antibiotic resistance gene between bacteria and hence the use of antibiotic as a treatment is not effective.

The conjugative R plasmids have two components *viz. resistance transfer factor* (RTF) and the R- *determinant.* The first component (RTF) has genes required for conjugative transfer between bacterial cells while the R- factor has antibiotic resistance gene(s). Some of such plasmids have genes resistant to several different antibiotics. As a result, the multiple drug resistance has been evolved in several species like *staphylococcus, Enterococcus, Neisseia, Shigella, and Salmonella* that are pathogenic to humans. Therefore, the pathogens have acquired resistance to several antibiotics and hence it has become difficult to treat many bacterial infections causing diseases like dysentery, T.B., and gonorrhoea.

(1.4) Composite Transposons in Bacteria

The composite transposons are formed by inserting two IS element near each other. Thus, the IS elements are part and flanking of these transposons. The composite transposons in the region between the IS elements contain genes which confer resistance to antibiotics and are not involved in transposition.

The region between the two IS elements is transposed by the joint action of elements. In this process the immobile DNA sequence is captured by two IS elements and gets the ability to become mobile. The examples of composite transposons are Tn9, Tn5, and Tn10. These transposons create target site duplications on inserting into DNA, like the IS elements do.

2. Replicative Transposition

This mechanism is based on a process that involves replication of the transposable element's DNA. This process is mediated by an enzyme ***transposase*** encoded by the element involving an interaction between the transposable element and the insertion site. The genetic element is replicated during the course of interaction.

The replicative transposons are found only in prokaryotes. The *example* is Tn3 element found in bacteria. These are large transposons found in bacteria and do not have IS Elements on their ends. The example is the ***Tn3 element*** which is a large replicative transposon of 4957 nucleotide pairs (np) long. The Tn3 element terminates in simple inverted repeats of about 38 to 40 np long instead of having the IS element at each of its end and creates target site duplication to insert into DNA. The Tn3 element has three genes (*tnpA, tnpR, and bla*) which encode a transposase, a resolvase/repressor, and beta lactamase. The beta lactamase provides resistance to the antibiotic ampicillin while other two proteins have their role in transposition.

The transposition of Tn3 is accomplished by the formation of a structure (*cointegrate*) between the donor and recipient plasmids. This is the fusion of two plasmids mediated by the enzyme *transposase* encoded by the gene *trpA* of T3 element. The donor plasmid has the transposable element (T3) whereas the recipient plasmid does not have the element but it has the insertion site into which the transposable element (T3) is inserted. The structure called ***cointegrate*** is formed after fusing DNA molecule of transposon into recipient plasmid. Tn3 element is replicated during this process of interaction and formation of cointegrate so that there is one copy of the Tn3 element at each junction in cointegrate. One copy of Tn3 is inserted at each point of fusing two plasmids. The *resolvase* encoded by the gene *tnpR* of T3 element resolves cointegrate between two Tn3 elements by mediating site-specific recombination. The donor and recipient plasmids separate from each other as two constituent plasmids, each one plasmid with a copy of Tn3.

3. Retrotransposition in Eukaryotes

This involves a mechanism that reverses the usual direction of flow of genetic information in cells. This means the information flows from RNA to DNA instead of the usual flow of the information from DNA to RNA. This process involves the insertion of copies of an element that were synthesized from the element's RNA and is called *retro-transposition*. The element's RNA is used by an enzyme (***reverse transcriptase***) as a template to synthesize DNA molecules that are inserted into new chromosomal sites. Thus, a retro-transposon produces RNA molecules that are reverse-transcribed into DNA molecules which are then inserted subsequently into new genomic position. In other words, the movement of these transposable elements depends on the reverse transcription of RNA into DNA. The ***retro*** is a Latin prefix meaning "backward". The ***reverse transcription*** has a crucial role in the life cycle of some viruses. The viral RNA being single-stranded is copied into double-stranded DNA on infecting a cell by the virus.

The retro-transposons are found only in eukaryotes. The retrotransposons utilize the enzyme reverse transcriptase to copy RNA into DNA which is subsequently inserted at different positions in genomic DNA. The retrotransposons are of the two categories *viz.* Retroposons and Retroviruslike elements.

The movement of some transposable genetic elements depends on the reversal in the flow of genetic information (reverse transcription of RNA into DNA). A transposable element (transposon) that creates new copies by reverse transcription of RNA into DNA is called ***retrotransposon.*** There are two classes of retrotransposons *viz. retroviruslike elements* and *retroposons.*

3.1 Retrovirus

The ***retrovirus*** is a virus that stores its genetic information in RNA and replicates by using reverse transcriptase to synthesize a DNA copy of its RNA genome. Any of the integrated retoviruses or the transposable element resembling retroviruses is called ***retroelement.*** An RNA virus was reported to cause tumour in chickens, cats, and mice and this lead to the discovery of retroviruses. David Baltimore and coworkers (1970) discovered an RNA dependent DNA polymerase, known as ***reverse transcriptase.*** This enzyme allows the virus to copy RNA into DNA (reverse transcription). Thus, reverse transcriptase catalyzes the synthesis of DNA using an RNA template.

The reverse transcription has resulted into many kinds of DNA sequences, including retroviruses. The retroviruses of many different types have been identified, like ***human immunodeficiency virus*** (HIV) which causes ***acquired immune deficiency syndrome*** (AIDS), a serious and lethal disease of immune system detected in the last quarter of the 20th century.

HIV's reverse transcriptase and other reverse transcriptases convert single-stranded RNA into double-stranded DNA which is then inserted anywhere in the chromosome of the infected cell with many copies of the viral genome. As a result the viral proteins are synthesized. The viral particles are extruded from the cell by a process of ***budding*** through the cell's membrane and infect other cells. This process replicates and disseminates the HIV's genetic material through a population of susceptible immune cells. The conversion of the viral RNA into viral DNA produces at both ends *of* the DNA molecules the signature sequences which are called ***long terminal repeats*** (LTR) and required for integration of the viral genome into DNA of the host cell. The integration of the viral DNA is catalyzed by an enzyme *integrase* which has endonuclease activity. The integrated HIV genome becomes a permanent part of the host genome and replicates like the host DNA

The retrovirus genomes are composed of single-stranded RNA having at least three genes named *gag, pol,* and *env*. These genes code for structural proteins, reverse transcriptase, and a protein embedded in the virus's lipid envelope, respectively. The human retrovirus HIV infects cells of the immune system causing life-threatening disease AIDS.

Retroviruslike Element

This element is a type of ***retrotransposon*** that resembles the integrated form of a retrovirus. These elements have genes homologous to *gag* and *pol*, but not to *env*. They vary in size and nucleotide sequence but they have the same basic structure of a central coding region flanked by long terminal repeats (LTR) for which these are sometimes called **LTR** ***retrotransposons***. The LTRs are of few hundred np long, oriented in the same direction, and each LTR is bounded by short, inverted repeats like those present in other types of transposons. The coding region contains small number of genes for their roles in the transposition process. The retroviruslike elements and the DNA forms of retroviruses inserted in cellular chromosomes are demarcated by LTR sequences.

The ***retroviruslike elements*** are *Ty 1* found in yeast (*Saccharomyces cerevisiae*); and *copia* and *gypsy* found in *Drosophila.*

- ☆ *Yeast* contains the retroviruslike element called *TY1* which is of about 5.9 kbp long and has about 35 copies. This element has LTRs of about 340 bp long and creates 5-bp target site duplication on being inserting into a chromosome. This element has only two genes (*TyA* and *TyB*) which produce viruslike particles.
- ☆ *Drosophila* also contains retroviruslike elements:
  - **(a)** One of the elements in *Drosophila* produces copious amounts of RNA and hence called *copia* whose structure is similar to Ty1 element of yeast.
  - **(b)** Another transposon in *Drosophila* is known as *gypsy*. This is larger than *copia* element. Both these elements present in *Drosophila* form viruslike particles.

3.2 Retroposon

This is a transposable element that creates new copies via reverse transcription of RNA into DNA but that lacks the long terminal repeat sequences (Non-LTR). These are DNA copies of polyadenylated RNA. These are large and widely distributed. The retroposons found in the genomes of *Drosophila* and human are discussed here.

(a) Retroposons in Drosophila Genome

The *retroposons* found in *Drosophila* are F, G, I elements, and telomeric retroposons. The retroposons are also called non-LTR retrotransposons which are large and widely distributed. The retroposons move through an RNA molecules (reverse transcribed into DNA), usually by a protein encoded by the elements themselves. On inserting into a chromosome, they create target site duplication but do not have inverted or direct repeats. They have at one end a A:T base pairs homologous sequence derived from reverse transcription of the poly(A) tail added near the 3′ end of the transposon RNA.

The *telomeric transposons* fill up again the DNA lost by incomplete chromosome replication, because the chromosome become shorter in each round of DNA replication due to movement of DNA polymerase only in one direction by adding nucleotides to the 3′ end of a primer which is usually the RNA. On removal of primer (RNA) a single-stranded DNA is left at the end of duplex and hence the deficient strand in the next round of replication produces a duplex shorter than the original. The chromosome lost the material from its end with the continuation of the process of replication of DNA.

A mechanism has been evolved in *Drosophila* for regenerating lost ends of chromosome. This function is performed by two different retroposons, called HeT-A and TART (telomere-associated retrotransposon) which are the components of telomeres of *Drosophila* chromosome. These two retroposons transpose preferentially to the ends of chromosomes by extending them by several kilo bases. However, the transposon sequences are lost again by incomplete DNA replication at the end and again these are restored through new transposition.

(b) Retroposons in Human Genome

The human genome has diverse array of transposons accounting for about 44 percent of human genome. The human DNA contains 33 percent retroposons of two classes (LINEs and SINEs), 8 percent retroviruslike elements, and 3 percent includes several families of genetic elements which are under the control of cut-and-paste mechanism. *Retroviruslike elements* derived sequences in human genome are more than 400, 000 which are mostly LTRs. Out of more than 100 different families of retroviruslike elements in human genome, only a few seem to be active transcriptionally.

The human genome contains two classes of transposable elements (retroposons). One class of sequences is known as the ***long interspersed nuclear elements* (LINEs)** and second most abundant class of transposable element is the ***short interspersed nuclear elements* (SINEs).**

The ***LINEs*** are families of long (6500 bp) moderately repetitive transposable elements in eukaryotes. The main element in *LINEs* class of sequences is the retroposon called L1 which is about 6 kb long, having internal promoter to be recognized by RNA polymerase II, and also having two open reading frames, *viz. ORF1* and *ORF2*. The ORF1 encodes a nucleic acid-binding protein while ORF2 encodes a protein with endonuclease and reverse transcriptase activities. The numbers of complete L1 elements in human genome vary from 3000 to 5000, in addition to more than 500, 000 L1 incomplete elements that are inactive transposionally. Each complete or incomplete L1 element is usually flanked by short target site duplication. Both the process of transcription of a complete L1 element into RNA and the reverse transcription of this RNA into DNA take place in the nucleus. The analysis of individuals with genetic diseases (*haemophilia* and *muscular dystrophy*) has revealed the transposed copies of certain complete L1 elements with low frequency. There are two other types of LINE sequences in human genome. These are L2 which has 315, 000 copies and L3 which has 37, 000 copies, but neither is active transpositionally.

The ***SINEs*** are families of short (less than 400 bp long, usually 150 – 300 bp) repetitive transposable elements of eukaryotes, do not encode proteins, and like all retroposons they have a sequence of A:T base pairs at one end. These are transposed involving reverse transcription of RNA, though the details of the process still unknown. However, it seems that SINEs depend on the LINEs to multiply and insert within genome. There are three families of SINEs in human genome (Alu, MIR, and Ther2/MIR3 elements), but only the Alu elements are transpositionally active and the best known SINE family.

Annexure 15.1

Causes of Cancer: Genetic Disease of Cell Division

The cancer is a group of diseases rather than a single disease and it can originate in many different tissues of the body. The speed of growth of different types of cancers is different from slow to aggressive and some respond to treatment while others do not.

The most frequent is lung cancer followed by prostate, breast, colorectal, bladder, lymphoma, melanoma, kidney, leukemia, endometrial, pancreatic, and thyroid, *etc.* The cells that divide actively are more prone to cancer, like the epithelial cells in the intestines, lungs, or prostate gland. The cells that typically do not divide like differentiated muscle or nerve cells develop rare forms of cancer. The techniques of molecular genetics have helped to devise new strategies for cancer therapy.

(1) Cancer in Relation to Cell Cycle

The different phases of cell division and the entry of a cell into different phases of cell cycle are under genetic control through the regulation of a mechanism (***checkpoint*** – *chapter 9*) that stops progression in the cell cycle until DNA synthesis is completed or damaged DNA is repaired. The checkpoints are regulatory mechanisms that are responsible for control and regulation of cell growth and differentiation. The most important checkpoint is the START.

The normal cells have a property of *"contact inhibition"* by which these cells in contact of other cells inhibit their uncontrolled growth. But some cells lost this property and hence they continue to divide forming to masses of cells called ***tumours***. These tumours may be benign or malignant. The benign and malignant tumours are both the result of uncontrolled cell division which is the underlying genetic change.

(i) The former type of tumour (***benign tumour***) is normally confined to its original location without invading the surrounding cells. Thus, these cells do not spread to other body parts and hence cause less damage.

(ii) The later type of tumour (***malingnant tumour***- harmful to life) is a mass of proliferating cells that are called *neoplastic* or *tumour cells* which grow rapidly and damage the neighbouring normal tissues. The cells from malignant tumour are detached, invade the surrounding tissues, and form a secondary tumour by spreading to other locations in the body. Such cells thus reaching distant sites through blood produce new tumour. These tumour cells have competition with the normal cells for nutrients due to their quick growth and division. This property or process of malignant tumours of spreading the cancer cells to unaffected organs is called ***metastasis*** (Greek word meaning to *change state*).

The checkpoint mechanism of controlling the growth and division of cells is deregulated due to some physical (radiation), chemical (mutagenic) or biological agents (certain types of viruses). These agents can transform normal cells into cancerous cells and these cancer causing agents are called ***carcinogens***.

(i) The *physical agents* are ionizing radiations (X-rays and gamma rays) and non-ionizing radiations (UV light) cause DNA damage results the normal cells to neo-plastic transformation.

(ii) The *chemical agents* (carcinogens) are present in tobacco smoke and cause lung cancer.

(iii) The *biological agents* are cancer causing viruses called ***oncogenic viruses*** or ***viral oncogens***.

(iv) The *dietary factors* (diet poor in fiber and rich in fatty foods) also increased the risk to develop cancer. This is because such diets may irritate the epithelial lining of the large intestine, causing loss of cells. Thus, there is a need of cell division in this tissue to replace the cells lost. This increases the chance of cancer-causing mutations.

(v) Some *genetic defects* due to gene mutation also cause deregulation of growth and division of normal cells.

The environmental forms of cancer also result from mutation in somatic cells. These somatic mutations are induced by environmental factors like tobacco smoking, chemical pollutants, ionizing radiations, UV light, excessive exposure to sunlight, and consumption of fatty foods containing little fibre. The environmentally induced somatic mutations are also frequently involved in the occurrence of hereditary forms of cancer.

The deregulation causes the failure of raising and lowering the abundance of the cyclin/CDK complexes. This may be the result of mutation in genes encoding the proteins (cyclins or CDKs), or affecting the formation or normal functioning of these complexes in any way. The cell cycle is deregulated by many types of genetic defects which ultimately cause the cells to become cancerous. This is because the genetic defects dysfunction the START checkpoint in mid-G_1 phase of cell division.

The START checkpoint prevents a cell from replicating damaged DNA. The cells with dysfunction of the checkpoint enter into S phase (synthetic) without repairing of their damaged DNA. The replication of unrepaired DNA accumulates in subsequent cell cycles. This accumulation further deregulates the cell cycle. This way a clone of cells becomes cancerous with a dysfunctional START checkpoint. Ultimately, *the cellular cycle of growth and division is unregulated in cancer.*

(2) Cell Death Phenomenon – Check on Cancer

There is a mechanism in the cells which is programmed itself in many species of animals. This mechanism disposes off the superfluous (useless or unnecessary) cells. Thus, it is called the *programmed cell death* which is fundamental and widespread phenomenon in animals. This programmed cell death is called ***apoptosis*** which is a Greek word meaning to "falling away".

The cell death phenomenon (*apoptotic mechanism*) is caused by proteolytic enzymes, called *caspases* which cleave the peptide bonds and make inactive the target proteins. The cleavage by this enzyme has a great impact on losing the integrity of the cells subjected to cleavage, fragmentation of their chromatin, bubbling of cytoplasm forming at their surfaces, and finally the cells start shrinking and disintegrating. Such integrated cells are engulfed by the scavenger cells of the immune system called as ***phagocytes*** and then destroyed. The programmed cell death is essential phenomenon due to the followings:

- ✰ This is essential for normal formation and function of organs by the cells otherwise the superfluous cells will impair the formation and function,
- ✰ The proliferation of unwanted cell gives rise to a clone that becomes cancerous by acquiring the ability to divide uncontrollably. Hence the programmed cell death stops the multiplication of abnormal cell and hence prevents the formation of a dangerous tumour (cancer).

(3) Genetic Cause of Cancer

The cancer is a genetic disease though environmental factors (physical, chemical and biological) are involved in many cancers. The cancer results from mutations in genes whose protein products are involved in the **regulation of cell cycle (growth and division).** Therefore, the mutation causes the biochemical processes to lead the unregulated proliferation of cells. The most peculiar characteristic of cancerous cells is that their growth is unregulated which results the cells to divide unstopped. These unstopped divided cells form tumour by piling up on top of each other.

The cancerous cells may be obtained either from a tumour and culturing *in vitro* or by treating normal cells to carcinogens. The normal cells in a culture form a single layer on surface of the culture medium while the cancer cells overgrow each other to form masses by piling up on the surface of the culture. This unregulated piling up of the cells is the result that the cancer cells do not respond to the chemical signals responsible to inhibit cell division. Moreover, the cancerous cells may synthesize unusual proteins which are displayed on their surfaces and also frequently have abnormal chromosome numbers (aneuploid).

Strong evidences in support of genetic basis of cancer:

- ☆ It is known that certain types of cancer are familial characters. A cancer of the eye (*retinoblastoma*) and some forms of *colon cancer* appear to be inherited as simple dominant conditions, though they show incomplete penetrance and variable expressivity.
- ☆ The chromosomal aberrations have shown association with certain types of cancer of WBC (*leukemias* and *lymphomas*).
- ☆ The cancerous state shows clonally inheritance on growing cancer cells in culture. The descendant cells are all cancerous because of the transmission of cancerous condition from each mother cell to its daughter cells during division.
- ☆ Some types of viruses induce the formation of tumours in experimental animals. This implies that cancerous state is produced by the proteins encoded by viral genes.
- ☆ The mutagens can induce cancer. The tumours can be induced in experimental animals by the mutagenic chemicals and ionizing radiation.

(4) Gene Mutation Causes CANCER

The use of molecular genetics technique in 1980s has discovered that cancer is caused by some genetic defects. The following two broad classes of genes on their mutation have been traced to develop the cancerous state. These are called *oncogenes* and *tumour suppressor genes.*

(I) Oncogenes

The *oncogene* is a Greek word meaning "tumour". The oncogenes are a class of genes which actively promote cell division. Some cancers are due to genes that have over-expression or abnormal activity of their mutant protein products. The genome of RNA viruses were first discovered to have *oncogenes* for inducing tumours in the vertebrate hosts. The *dominant gain-of-function mutations* in oncogenes cause cancer.

(i) Tumour-Inducing Retroviruses

Some viruses carry oncogenes that induce the formation of tumours in animals. The viral RNA after infecting host acts as template to synthesize complementary DNA which is catalyzed by an enzyme reverse transcriptase, for this reason these viruses are called retroviruses. These were first discovered by Peyton Rous (1910) to induce tumour or sarcoma in the connective tissue of chicken and hence called Rous sarcoma virus.

The RNA genome of this retrovirus has four genes *viz. Gag* (encodes capsid part), *pol* (encodes reverse transcriptase), *env* (encodes a protein of viral envelope), and *v-src* (encodes a protein kinase that insert into plasma membranes of infected cells). The ability of the virus to form tumour is conferred by only *v-src* gene as the tumour is not formed in case this gene is deleted from the virus.

There are other tumour-inducing retroviruses and at least 20 different viral oncogenes (denoted as *v-onc*) have been known now. These oncogenes have great role in regulating the expression of cellular genes, including the genes involved in the process of growth and division. The viral oncogene proteins are similar to cellular proteins involved in various regulatory activities like acting as signals, as receptors, as intracellular agents, and as transcription factors.

(ii) Proto-oncogenes

The cellular counterparts of the viral oncogenes (cellular homologues of viral oncogenes, called *proto-oncogenes* or normal *cellular oncogenes,* denoted *c-onc*) were later on discovered in many organisms. These cellular genes which are homologs to viral oncogenes can induce tumours on over-expressing or on mutating to produce abnormally active protein products. The viral oncogenes encode proteins that are similar to cellular proteins. The cellular homologue had helped to identify many of the cellular proteins encoded by viral oncogenes, *e.g.* the cellular homologue of the *v-src gene* was obtained from uninfected chicken cells. However, the homologue of *v-src* gene in chicken cells differs from *v-src* gene itself. There are about 11 introns in the chicken homologue of *v-src* gene but the introns are absent in *v-src* gene itself. The *c-oncs* do not induce tumours like *v-oncs* perhaps because *v-oncs* produce comparatively much more proteins. This excess supply of protein (kinase) upsets the delicate signalling mechanism controlling cell division, resulting unregulated growth.

(iii) Mutant Cellular Oncogenes

The mutation in proto-oncogenes actively promotes cell proliferation. The *c-oncs* has been found to induce cancer in human. This may be due to the upset of the biochemical balance within a cell. Human *bladder cancer* was first discovered due to mutant *c-onc.* However, the cause of cancer by these mutants was not found to oversupply of proteins but the valine-for-glycine substitution at position 12 impairs the ability of the mutant protein to hydrolyze one of its substrate (GTP). The mutant proteins transmit the signal to the nucleus causing the genes involved in cell division to be transcribed inappropriately and hence the cell division occurs in an uncontrolled way.

(iv) Chromosome Rearrangements Cause Cancer

Some of the chromosome rearrangements lead to cancer. This is because the breakpoints of chromosome rearrangement often put side by side a cellular oncogene to a promoter that stimulates the vigorous expression of the oncogene. The over-expression of gene product can lead to excessive cell division and growth. Most cancerous cells are aneuploid which deregulate the cell cycle. The aneuploidy may involve the loss of functional copies of tumour suppressor genes which would remove natural brakes on cell division, or the aneuploidy might involve the inappropriate duplication of proto-oncogenes which would increase the abundance of factors that promote cell division.

The chronic myelogenous ***leukemia*** (CML) in human is an example of cancer due to chromosome rearrangement 22 (reciprocal translocation between chromosome 22 and 9). This causes the WBC to become cancerous, possibly due to the involvement of the tyrosine kinase activity of the protein.

Another example of a WBC cancer is the ***lymphoma*** which is also associated to reciprocal translocation involving chromosome 8 and one of the three chromosomes (2, 14, and 22). The chromosome rearrangement may change the nature of protein products or enhance the expression of proto-oncogenes.

(II) Tumour Suppressor Genes - Anti-oncogenes

The cell cycle is regulated by normal alleles of genes and hence it is under genetic control. The normal genes that regulate cell cycle are called the tumour suppressor genes (***anti-oncogenes*)**. The mutant forms (alleles) of tumour suppressor genes are the second class of cancer producing/related genes. The mutant forms of these genes fail to repress (stop) cell division. However, the cancerous cell to achieve its full cancerous state needs additional mutations in genes that are involved in the stoppage of cell growth. Thus, there is inactivation of genes whose products have role in cell cycle regulation. The *recessive loss-of-function mutations* in tumour suppressor genes cause cancer.

(i) Two Mutations Theory (Two mutational hits)

The predisposition to develop cancer is due to mutation in the tumour suppressor gene. This is *loss-of-function mutation* which follows a dominant pattern of inheritance. Alfred Knudson (1971) proposed a theory that cancer develops only if a second mutation occurs in the somatic cells to knock out the function of the wild-type allele of the tumour suppressor gene. Thus, two mutations (loss-of-function) are required to develop mutation. This means the mutation is required in each of the two copies of the tumour suppressor gene. This is called *two mutational hits*.

Based on the pedigree analysis, about 40 per cent of the cases involve inherited mutation which predisposes the individual to develop cancer and rest 60 per cent of the cases are sporadic (non-inherited). Knudson explained the occurrence of a rare childhood cancer of eye (*retinoblastoma*) due to inactivation (by mutation) of both the copies of a particular gene that normally functions to suppress tumour formation in the eye. The retinoblastoma results from homozygosity for a loss-of-function (recessive) allele. The individuals homozygous for the wild-type allele of the RB gene develop retinoblastoma rarely. The individuals heterozygous for a mutant RB allele require only one somatic mutation to develop retinoblastoma. The sporadic occurrence of retinoblastoma (nonhereditary) develop tumour in only one eye because it has only one mutation (sporadic) whereas to develop tumours in both the eyes require two sporadic mutations in the same cell or cell lineage. On the contrary, the hereditary retinoblastoma develops tumours usually in both eyes.

The inherited cancers like retinoblastoma show a dominant pattern of inheritance. But the underlying genetic defect is a recessive loss-of-function mutation mostly the result of deletion. The heterozygous cell for such a mutation divides normally but the occurrence of second mutation turns the cell to be cancerous. If an individual inherits one mutation in RB gene, the individual is predisposed to develop retinoblastoma because a second mutation may occur any time during the formation of retina in either eye (retina has millions of cells). Thus, this predisposition shows a dominant pattern of inheritance.

The inherited and sporadic mutations spread through different modes *viz. Germ line* and *somatic tissue*. One of the two inactivation mutations in inherited cases is transmitted by germ cell while other inactivation mutation occurs during the course of development of somatic tissues of the eyes. On the contrary, both of the inactivating mutations occur during eye development in sporadic case.

(ii) Cellular Roles of Tumour Suppressor Proteins

A number of different inherited cancer syndromes have been identified but only 1 percent of all cancers are hereditary. The second important finding is that in nearly all of the inherited cases the underlying cancer causing defect is in a tumour suppressor gene instead in an oncogene. The protein products of these tumour suppressor genes function in a diverse array of cellular processes of their division, differentiation, apoptosis, and DNA repair. The *different tumour suppressor proteins* are as under:

- ☆ pRB is a RB gene product, essential for life, plays key role in regulation of the cell cycle, associated with retinoblastoma and other types of cancer (lung carcinomas, osteosarcomas, and carcinomas of bladder, cervical, prostrate), and is a 105-kilodalton nuclear protein;
- ☆ p53 is a 53-kilodalton tumour suppressor protein, 393 amino acid long transcription factor, encoded by a tumour suppressor gene (TP53), plays key role in cellular response to stress (in stress condition degradation of p53 decreases, it is phosphorylated, and converted into a stable and active form), induces cancers by certain DNA viruses, and associated with some syndrome (breast cancer). The gene TP53 that encodes p53 protein is most frequently mutated in human cancers. The p53 protein has no significant role in programmed cell death during embryogenesis;
- ☆ pAPC is a 310-kilodalton protein, 2843 amino acid long, and associated with an inherited condition leading to colorectal (large intestine) cancer. This protein has key role in regulating the renewal of cells in lining or epithelium of large intestine, and also regulate cell division;
- ☆ phMSH2 protein is human homologue of a DNA repair protein found in bacteria and yeast, associated with colorectal cancer;
- ☆ pBRCA1 is a 220-kilodalton polypeptide, the gene located on chromosome 17, and associated with breast cancer;
- ☆ pBRCA2 is a 384-kilodalton polypeptide, the gene is located on chromosome 13 and also associated with breast cancer. The mutation in tumour suppressor genes (pBRCA 1 and 2) is implicated in hereditary breast and ovarian cancer

In view of the above, the proteins encoded by tumour suppressor genes have important role in regulating the cell cycle but the mutational inactivation of various tumour suppressor genes is characteristic of most forms of cancer. Two mutations are required to remove both functional copies of a tumour suppressor gene in the cell. The tumour suppressor genes were discovered through their association with inherited cancers.

It can be concluded that a malignant tumour can be formed either due to the uncontrolled activation of a single proto-oncogene or to the inactivation of a single tumour suppressor gene. However, it is not such a simple because the genetic pathways to cancer are diverse and complex. The tumour formation, its growth, and metastasis (formation of secondary tumour) in most of the cancer cases is the result of accumulation of mutations in several different genes.

The following six peculiar characteristics of the pathways to malignant cancer have been proposed by Douglas Hanahan and Robert Weinberg:

- ☆ The cancer cells are self-sufficient to stimulate their growth and division,
- ☆ They are not sensitive to growth inhibiting signals,
- ☆ They escape from ***apoptosis*** (programmed cell death),
- ☆ They have potential to divide endlessly,
- ☆ They develop ways to nourish themselves, and
- ☆ They can invade other tissues (***metastasis***).

Diagnosis and Treatment of Cancer

More than million people in our country suffer from cancer and many of them die from cancer annually. Therefore early detection of cancer is must to treat this ailment successfully. The cancer may be detected on the basis of biopsy and histo-pathological studies of the tissue and blood, and the test of bone marrow for increased cell count in case of leukemia. The cancer of the internal organs can be detected by the techniques like *radiography* (use of rays), computed tomography (CT), and MRI (magnetic resonance imaging). Certain cancers are also detected by using the antibiotics against cancer-specific antigens. The genes with inherited susceptibility to certain cancers can be identified and detected by the techniques of molecular biology. The people having such genes susceptible to particular carcinogens are advised to avoid their exposure to such carcinogens like tobacco smoking in case of lung cancer.

The cancer is commonly treated by surgery, radiation therapy and immunotherapy separately or in combination of surgery, radiotherapy and chemotherapy. The radiotherapy involves irradiation of tumour cells. The cancerous cells are also killed by some chemotherapeutic drugs specific for particular tumours though these drugs have their side effect on the body of the patient like hair loss, anemia, *etc.* In addition to the above, some substances called biological response modifiers like α interferon are given to activate the immune system and destroying the tumour because the tumour cells are not detected and destroyed by immune system.

Annexure 19.1

Amino Acids: Structure and Polymerization

The amino acids are organic molecules containing an amino (NH_2) group and a carboxyl (COOH) group, and known as the building stones of proteins. The amino acids are formed of a set of three nucleotides each of which are composed of the nitrogen bases, a sugar and a phosphate (See chapter 15). Some of the amino acids are synthesized in the cell of a man but other amino acids are supplied from diet and called as essential amino acids.

There are 20 different amino acids. These 20 amino acids, necessary to form a protein molecule, are dispersed in the cell (cytoplasm). The different arrangements of these amino acids form the various types of proteins and a change of a single amino acid in a polypeptide chain can change the function of a protein.

The structure of different amino acids and their binding with each other to form proteins have been given here.

Structure of amino acids: Each of the 20 amino acids is commonly found in proteins (polypeptides) and each contain an *alpha carbon* to which the following four subunits (parts) are attached -

(*i*) *Carboxylic group* (C - OH) with a potential negative charge (C – O ⁻),
|| ||
O   O

(ii) Basic *amino group* (NH_2) with a potential positive charge (NH_3^+),

(iii) An H atom,

(iv) *Side group* (*subunit*) denoted by the letter R.

The first two subunits (free amino group and free carboxyl group) of amino acids are common to all the 20 amino acids, except proline. But the *side group* (R) of amino acids is different chemically (chemical diversity) for different amino acids. The amino acids differ from each other due to this subunit. The side group (R) varies from a single H atom (glycine) to a benzene ring (phenylalanine). These differences in side groups of amino acids are important to form amino acids of different size, to determine the charge of the amino acids, its relationship to water molecule, and its interaction with other amino acids. Therefore, this subunit of amino acids (R), having chemical diversity for different amino acids, provides the structural and functional diversity to proteins.

The common structure of all 20 amino acids indicating all the 3 parts (groups) can be represented as under:

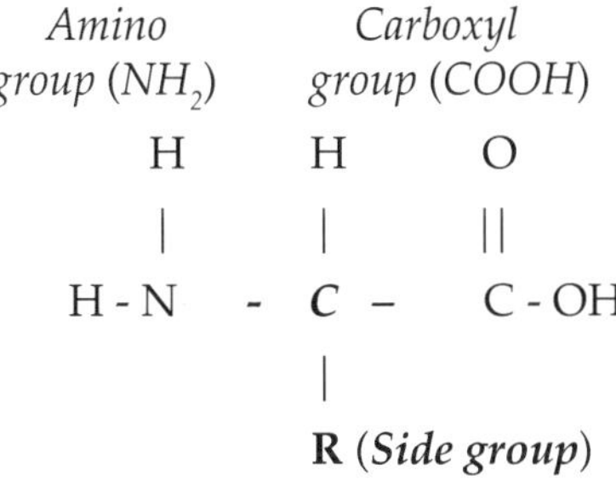

The side group (R) of different amino acids may be *aliphatic* (CH); *alcoholic (OH); carboxylic (COOH)* which are aspartic acid and glutamic acid; *aromatic* which contain *benzene* group (phenylalanine, tyrosine, and tryptophan); *phenolic* (one H of benzene is replaced by OH); *sulfur* containing *side group* (methionine and cysteine); or *basic* side group which contain additional NH group (lysine, arginine, and histidine).

Also the side group of different amino acids according to its nature may be broadly grouped into four types *viz.*

(i) *Acidic side groups* which are negatively charged (Aspartic acid, and Glutamic acid),

(ii) *Basic side groups* which contain additional NH group and are positively charged (Arginine, Lysine, and Histidine),

(iii) *Hydrophilic* or *polar sidegroups* (Asparagine, Cysteine, Glutamine, Serine, Threonine and Tyrosine), and

(iv) *Hydrophobic* or *Nonpolarside groups* (Glycine, Alanine, Valine, Leucine, Isoleucine, Proline, Phenylalanine, Tryptophan, and Methionine).

Polypeptides and Polymerization (Binding of Amino Acids and Peptide Bonds)

Two or more amino acids form a compound known as a ***peptide***. The peptide is a compound containing amino acids. This is also the breakdown or build up unit in protein metabolism. Long sequence of amino acids forms the ***polypeptide***. A polypeptide is a linear molecule with two or more amino acids and one or more peptide groups. Here at this point, it becomes important to know the numbers of polypeptides possibly to be formed and secondly the manner they are bound together.

The polypeptides vary in their length decided by the number of amino acids. For example, the protein *insulin* has a length of 51 amino acids whereas the *fibroin* (silk protein) has 1,000 amino acids. The numbers of different possible polypeptides are enormous as a result of the 20 amino acids combined in different combinations. The possible numbers of different amino acid sequences in a polypeptide to be formed will be equal to 20^n where n are the number of amino acids. Thus, a polypeptide having 100 amino acids will have 20^{100} different amino acid sequences. This number of amino acid sequences is too large to be accounted. So taking few numbers of amino acids, say only 7 amino acids in a peptide, the different amino acid sequences formed will be $20^7 = 1.28$ billion.

The amino acids are organic molecules. *Emil Fischer* made a classical contribution to show that the amino acids in polypeptide chain (protein molecule) are held together (bound or linked) covalently joined together by linkages, called *peptide bonds*. The ***peptide bond*** is a chemical bond holding amino acid subunits together in proteins. This binding forms a long polypeptide chain. The polypeptide chains are thus formed having as high as hundred or more amino acids. The ***peptide linkages*** connect the carboxyl radical of one amino acid with the amino group of another amino acid through loss of a molecule of water. There occurs a reaction between the amino group (NH_2) of one amino acid and carboxyl group (COOH, organic acid) of other amino acid to form each *peptide bond*. Thus, amino and carboxyl groups participate in formation of peptide bond during protein synthesis.

The process of linking the amino acids together is called *polymerization*. The term ***polymerization*** is used for chemical union of two or more molecules of the same kind to form a new compound having the same elements in the same proportions but a higher mol. Wt. and different physical properties. There are 20 amino acids which form polypeptide chains of different proteins. The polymerization to form protein needs catalytic agents. The catalytic agents in the living body are enzymes which are proteins too.

The binding of amino acids to each other (*polymerization*) in the formation of peptide through peptide bond involves elimination of a hydroxyl (OH) from the carboxyl group of one amino acid and hydrogen molecule (H) from amino group of another amino acid. The formation of ***dipeptide*** as a result of peptide bond between two amino acids resulting into the removal of water molecule (H_2O) has been shown as under -

$$\begin{array}{ccccc} \begin{matrix} \text{H} & \text{O} \\ | & || \\ H_2N-\text{C} - & \text{C}-\boldsymbol{OH} \\ | & \\ R_1 & \end{matrix} & + & \begin{matrix} & \text{H} & \text{O} \\ & | & || \\ \boldsymbol{H}-\text{N}- & \text{C}- & \text{C}-\text{OH} \\ | & | & \\ \text{H} & R_2 & \end{matrix} & \rightarrow & \begin{matrix} \text{H} & \boldsymbol{O} & \text{H} & \text{O} & \\ | & | & | & || & \\ H_2N-\text{C}- & \boldsymbol{C}-\boldsymbol{N}- & \text{C}- & \text{C}-\text{OH} & + H_2O \\ | & | & | & & \\ R_1 & \boldsymbol{H} & R_1 & & \end{matrix} \end{array}$$

Amino acid 1 Amino acid 2 ***Dipeptide*** ***Water***

The ***polypeptide*** chains are formed containing as many as a hundred or more amino acids. A protein may have one or more polypeptide chains reaching a molecular weight to 6,000,000 or more. The possible kinds of protein to exist depend upon the kind, sequence (order), relationship, and frequency of amino acids contained in the protein.

Annexure 19.2

Proteins Structure: Three-Dimensional Structure of Complex Molecule

Proteins

The proteins are major component of total mass of organisms after water. The total weight of living cells accounts by the water is about 70 per cent and the proteins constitute about 15 per cent of the wet weight of the cell. The proteins have vital role of the cells. Various proteins determine biological activities in an organism. Proteins make up body structures like organs and tissue, as well as control chemical reactions and carry signals between cells. If a cell's DNA is mutated, an abnormal protein may be produced, which can disrupt the body's usual processes and lead to a disease such as cancer. The proteins are of long chemical chains containing many amino acids. It is therefore important to know about proteins, particularly their structure.

The proteins are large macromolecules composed of polypeptides that are polymers of different amino acids. The amino acid sequence of each polypeptide is specified by the nucleotide sequence of a gene. The ***nucleotides*** as the repeating subunits form the nucleic acids (DNA or RNA) that are macromolecules. The *proteins* are thus ***polypeptides*** whereas the *nucleic acids* (DNA and RNA) are ***polynucleotides***.

The proteins synthesized in the cell are responsible for carrying out the development and all the life activities of an organism. The genes contain the instructions for the synthesis of these proteins. One or more chains of amino acids (constituents of protein) called as polypeptides, are contained by each of the protein. Each polypeptide has specific sequence of amino acids. The different polypeptide chains are formed by combining in myriad ways the 20 different kinds of naturally occurring amino acids to form different proteins. These polypeptide chains differ in their length of nucleotides sequences according to the protein they form.

The sequence of amino acids in the polypeptide chain within a gene is specified by a sequence of coding units, called ***codons*** which are triplets of adjacent nucleotides. Each codon (triplet nucleotide sequence) refers to the nucleotide sequence in mRNA and not in DNA. This codon specifies the incorporation of the indicated amino acid of polypeptide chain. Each gene has hundreds or even thousands of codons to specify the incorporation of an amino acid into a polypeptide. Thus, a polypeptide, considered as the gene's product, is synthesized under the direction of the information encoded within a gene.

Each of the estimated 20,000 to 25,000 genes in the human genome codes for an average of three proteins. The genes located on 23 pairs of chromosomes packed into the nucleus of a human cell, direct the production of proteins with the assistance of enzymes and messenger molecules. Specifically, an enzyme copies the information in a gene's DNA into a molecule called messenger ribonucleic acid (mRNA). The mRNA travels out of the nucleus into the cell's cytoplasm, where the mRNA is read by a tiny molecular machine called a ribosome, and the information is used to link together small molecules called amino acids in the right order to form a specific protein.

Protein Structure

The proteins are the polymers of amino acids. However, the proteins instead of being building up by one kind of *monomer* (constituted of only one amino acid), they are built from 20 different *amino acids* forming the polypeptide chains in different combinations of amino acids.

The proteins have complex three-dimensional structures which have 4 different levels of structural organization. The complex three-dimentional structures allow in part the vast functional diversity to proteins. The 4 levels of organization of protein structure are primary, secondary, tertiary, and quaternary structures as given below:

Primary Structure

This level of structure of a polypeptide is its amino acid sequence forming a polypeptide. This is specified by the nucleotide sequence of a gene. The primary structure of polypeptide determines the secondary, tertiary, and quaternary structures of proteins.

Secondary Structure

This level of structure of polypeptide is formed by the spatial organization of adjacent amino acids in the segments of a polypeptide. There are two most common types of secondary structure in proteins. These are α *helices* and β *sheets.* These two structures are maintained by hydrogen bonding between peptide bonds. α- *helix* is a rigid structure. In this α *helix* structure, each peptide bond is hydrogen bonded between amino acids 3 to 4 residues away. The amino acid *proline* cannot be present within α *helix* due to rigid structure of α *helix*. In case of β *sheet* a polypeptide folds back upon itself which may occur repeatedly sometimes.

Tertiary Structure

This structure of a polypeptide is defined by the overall folding of the complete polypeptide in three-dimensional space and this is called the ***conformation***. The folding of most of the polypeptides is spontaneous in a specific conformation as per direction of their primary structures. It happens in most of the cases that all the information required to determine the shape lies in the primary structure of the protein whereas in some cases the protein folding interacts with proteins. These interacting proteins called ***chaperones*** help nascent polypeptides fold into their proper three-dimensional structures.

The hydrophilic amino acids are located on the surface of proteins but the hydrophobic interact themselves in the interior surface. This tertiary structure is maintained by relatively weak non-covalent bonds, with only exception of covalent bonds of disulfide (S – S) bridges which form between cysteine residues. The different non-covalent bonds (interactions) involved are:

- *Ionic bonds* (These occur between side chains of amino acids with opposite charges *viz.* lysine and glutamic acid),
- *Hydrogen bonds* (These are between electronegative atoms having a partial negative charge and hydrogen atoms having electropositive charge),
- *Hydrophobic interactions* (These are associations of nonpolar groups with each other when present in aqueous solutions due to insolubility in water), *and*
- *Van der Waals interactions* (These occur between atoms when they are placed closely to each other).

Quaternary Structure

This level of structure indicates the association of two or more polypeptides in a protein. It is important to note that the quaternary structure does not exist in all the proteins but only in those which contain more than one polypeptide. Therefore, the haemoglobin is a good example of quaternary structure. Haemoglobin is a tetrameric compound having 4 polypeptide chains (2 chains of α-globin and 2 chains of β-globin) beside 4 iron-containing hem groups.

Annexure 19.3
One Gene-One Polypeptide Concepts

A gene's nucleotide sequence specifies a polypeptide's amino acid sequence. Before discussing this mechanism it is better to understand the relation between genes and their polypeptide products. The classic genetic studies regarding the one gene-one enzyme versus one gene-one polypeptide, and the co-linearity between gene and polypeptide are important here to mention.

(i) One Gene-One Enzyme versus One Gene-One Polypeptide

Beadle George and B. Ephrussi (1937) in conducting experiments on eye colour mutants in *Drosophila* identified the genes responsible for the synthesis of the specific eye pigments. This indicated that metabolic pathways catalyzed by enzyme are controlled by genes.

Beadle and Tatum, Edward (1941) extended this work on *neurospora crassa* (Bread mould) which could be grown on minimal medium containing inorganic salts, simple sugar and biotin (vitamin), which must be capable to synthesize all the other essential metabolites like purines, pyrimidine, amino acids, and other vitamins, *de novo* and the biosynthesis of these growth factors must be genetically controlled. They presumed that the mutants produced for the genes biosynthesizing the essential metabolites will require additional growth factor. They identified the mutants that could not grow on minimal medium but required for their growth the complete medium supplemented with all the amino acids, purines, pyrimidines, and vitamins as well as those mutant strains that could grow on media supplemented with each of the growth factors separately. Thus, each mutant strain produced required one growth factor and hence they concluded that one mutation resulted in the loss of one enzyme activity. The *one gene – one enzyme* concept was thus proposed.

However, it was known subsequently that many enzymes and structural proteins are heteromultimeric, having two or more different polypeptide chains encoded each by a separate gene. For example, haemoglobin in humans and tryptophan synthetase enzyme are heterotetrameric proteins, each of the two containing 2 α and β chains of polypeptides. Likewise, the DNA polymerase III and RNA polymerase II in *E. coli* contain many different polypeptide subunits, each encoded by a separate gene. These findings modified the earlier concept of one gene-one enzyme proposed by Beadle and Tautam into the new concept of *one gene-one polypeptide.*

(ii) Co-Linearity of Gene with Polypeptide Chain

The colinearity is a relationship in which the units in one molecule occur in the same sequence as the units in another molecule which they specify, *e.g.* the nucleotides in a gene are collinear with the amino acids in the polypeptide encoded by that gene. Crick (1958) proposed that DNA determine the sequence of amino acids in a polypeptide. This relationship between the gene and the polypeptide indicate that they are both linear structures. The gene is a sequence of nucleotides and the polypeptide is a sequence of amino acids. Consequently, a linear sequence of nucleotides should determine a specific amino acid and this relationship should be specified by the genetic code, and secondly a mutational change in a particular position of the nucleotide sequence should produce a change in a corresponding linear position in the amino acid sequence. Thus, the nucleotide and amino acid sequences should be co-linear and hence a genetic map of nucleotide changes should correspond with a mutational map of amino acid changes.

The powerful evidence of co-linearity between gene and its polypeptide product has been demonstrated by the studies made by Sarabhai and coworkers (1964) on co-linearity of the gene with the polypeptide chain on a number of different T4 mutants and by Yanofsky, C. and coworkers (1967) using the A polypeptide chain of the tryptophane synthetase enzyme of *E. coli.* The observations of these studies indicated that the sequences of nucleotide pairs in a gene and the amino acids in its polypeptide products are collinear.

Annexure 19.4

Roles of different Components in Protein Synthesis

The process of translation (protein synthesis) is very complex and hence requires the functioning of a large number of macromolecules. These include the followings:

(i) Ribosome required in synthesizing a polypeptide,

(ii) Polypeptides (over 50) and RNA molecules (3 to 5 types) transcribed from DNA templates and present in each ribosome. The mRNA molecule provide specifications for the amino acid sequences of the polypeptide,

(iii) tRNA molecules (40 to 60) to function as adaptor molecule by mediating the incorporation of proper amino acids into polypeptides in response to codons (nucleotide sequences) in mRNAs,

(iv) Enzymes to activate amino acids, called ***aminoacyl-tRNA synthetases*** (at least 20, one for each amino acid). This enzyme catalyzes the formation of high energy bonds between amino acids and tRNA molecules. The aminoacyl-tRNA synthesis involves the activation of the amino acid, using energy from ATP.

(v) Soluble proteins (numerous) involved in the process of 3 stages of polypeptide chain initiation, elongation and termination.

(i) Ribosomes

The location, structure, and function of ribosomes have been given in chapter 9 (Animal Cell – structure and division).

The ribosomal RNA (rRNA) molecules are transcribed from a DNA template, like mRNA. The synthesis of rRNA in eukaryotes occurs in the nucleolus (component of nucleus with its main function of synthesis of rRNA and their assembly into ribosomes) and catalyzed by RNA polymerase I. The RNA precursors are produced by the transcription of rRNA genes. The rRNA precursors are much larger than the RNA molecules found in ribosomes and are processed post-transcriptional to produce the mature rRNA molecules.

In mammals, the rRNA gene transcript is a 45S precursor which on endonucleolytic cleavage produces 5.8S, 18S, and 28S rRNAs whereas a separate gene transcript on its post-transcriptional processing produces the 5S rRNA. In *E. coli,* the rRNA gene transcript is a 30S precursor which produces on endonucleolytic cleavage the 5S, 16S, and 23S rRNA plus one 4S tRNA molecule. Besides the posttranscriptional cleavage of rRNA precursors, many of the nucleotides in rRNA are methylated posttranscriptionally to protect rRNA molecules from degradation by ribonucleases.

There are present a large number of ribosomes in each cell. Therefore, there are multiple copies of the genes for rRNA in the genomes of all organisms.

- ✰ In *E.coli,* there is distribution of 7 rRNA genes among 3 sites on the chromosome, and
- ✰ In eukaryotes, 100 to 1000 of copies of rRNA genes are present.

The 5.8S-18S-28S rRNA genes exist in tandem arrays in the NOR (nucleolar organizer regions) of the chromosomes of eukaryotes. The NOR in eukaryotes are located on different chromosomes, *viz.* on chromosome 6 in maize, on sex chromosomes in *Drosophila,* and on short arms of chromosomes 13, 14, 15, 21, and 22 in humans.

The 5S rRNA genes in eukaryotes are highly redundant (plenty or excessive) like 5.8S-18S-28S rRNA genes. They are distributed among many chromosomes instead of NOR.

Each Ribosome has three tRNA Binding Sites

The positions of these three tRNA binding sites at the 50S-30S interface and relative positions of the rRNAs as well as ribosomal proteins have been shown by X-ray crystallography. The three tRNA binding sites on ribosome are -

- ✰ ***Aminoacyl site*** (A site): This site binds the incoming aminoacyl-tRNA, the tRNA carrying the next amino acid to be added to the growing polypeptide chain. This binding site at ribosome contains the aminoacyl-tRNA.
- ✰ ***Peptidyl site*** (P site): This site binds the tRNA to which the growing polypeptide chain is attached, and
- ✰ ***Exit site*** (E site): This is the ribosome binding site that contains the free tRNA prior to its release or this site binds the departing uncharged tRNA.

The aminoacetyl-tRNA binding sites are largely located on the 50S subunit while the mRNA molecule is bound to the 30S subunits. The mRNA codon which is part of the binding site provides the specificity for the aminoacyl-tRNA binding in each site. This specificity for the aminoacyl-tRNA binding in the sites (A, P. and

E) changes with the movement of ribosome along an mRNA or with the shuttling of mRNA across the ribosome as different mRNA codon moves into register in the binding sites. Thus, the ribosomal binding sites by themselves (without mRNA) are capable of binding any aminoacyl-tRNA.

A molecule that can bind to another molecule in or on cells is called ***ligand.*** A molecule that can accept the binding of a ligand is called ***receptor.***

(ii) Transfer RNA

The tRNA molecules are transcribed from genes (DNA) in the form of larger precursor molecules that undergo posttranscriptional processing of cleavage, trimming, methylation, and so on like rRNAs. The tRNA molecules contain several unusual nucleosides (inosine, pseudouridine, dihydrouridine, 1-metyhul guanosine, and others) that are not present in the primary tRNA gene transcripts, but produced posttranscriptional and by enzyme-catalyzed modifications of the 4 nucleosides incorporated into RNA during transcription. These tRNA molecules are required for the translation of a coded mRNA message into a sequence of amino acids in a polypeptide. The specifications for each polypeptide are encoded in an mRNA molecule.

There is no direct interaction between the amino acids and the nucleotide triplets (codon) in mRNA. Considering this fact, Crick, Francis (1958) proposed the idea of an adaptor molecule to mediate the specification of amino acids by codons in mRNA during protein synthesis. Such adaptor molecules were identified as RNA molecules which were small (4S containing 70-95 nucleotides long) and called first as soluble RNA but subsequently as transfer RNA (tRNA) molecules. The tRNA molecules contain a triplet nucleotide sequence (the ***anticodon***) which is complementary to and base-pairs with the codon sequence in mRNA during translation. Each of the 20 amino acids has one to four tRNA.

The tRNA though small but must have specificity. They must respond to the correct codons and hence should have the correct anticodon sequences. They must be activated with the correct amino acids and hence should have been recognized by the correct enzyme (aminoacyl-tRNA synthetase). They must function as adaptors and hence should bind to the appropriate sites on the ribosomes.

The mRNA transmits the code, received from DNA for a certain protein, to the ribosomes in the cytoplasm. Amino acids are present in the cytoplasm but these are not in the active form as such and hence they do not take part in protein synthesis. These amino acids need ***activation*** which is done through ATP. The amino acids of the cytoplasm are selected and their sequence to form a protein molecule is encoded in the base sequence of mRNA. This requires the help of another type of RNA, called tRNA.

The tRNA found in the cytoplasm identifies amino acid through anticodon corresponding to the codon in the mRNA molecule and transfers it to the ribosomes. The nucleotide triplets in the tRNA molecules are called *anticodons.* In other words, the amino acids are brought to the ribosome by their appropriate tRNA to be incorporated in to protein. The tRNA identifies a particular amino acid by means of anticodon which corresponding the codon of the mRNA. The tRNA carries this amino acid to the ribosome along the mRNA molecule. The different amino acids are bound together to form molecules in the ribosomes as per the code sent by mRNA. Different kind of tRNAs are present in the cytoplasm and recognize certain amino acids, assemble them in the sequence specified by the DNA molecule (gene). The different codes are sent by DNA to form different proteins in the ribosomes.

The *first step* in incorporating an amino acid in to a protein involves the amino acid attachment to its correct tRNA. The nucleotide sequence of mRNA determines the type and sequence of amino acids in a protein chain, but the amino acid themselves do not interact with the mRNA. The amino acids are attached to the tRNAs by high-energy bonds (symbol ~) between the carboxyl group of the amino acids and the 3′-hydroxyl termini of the tRNA.

Secondly, the tRNA (adaptor or acceptor or soluble RNA) take up proper activated amino acids from cytoplasm and transfer them to the mRNA. One end of tRNA molecule contains anticodon and the other end makes an attachment with one of the appropriate amino acid to involve in protein synthesis. With the movement of molecules of tRNA with attached amino acid along the molecule of mRNA, the amino acids are placed in position to be connected together to form a chain of protein. After attaching the amino acid to each other, the tRNA molecules are free from mRNA and from amino acids.

The ***interaction between mRNA and tRNA*** takes place only on the ribosomes. The ATP provides the energy required for the reaction involved between amino acid and tRNA. The amino acid is first activated by ATP to form *amino acid adenylate* after which reacts with tRNA to form *amino-acyl tRNA.* When the ribosome reaches the mRNA the translation of the nucleotide code into amino acid sequence is complete. Thus, it is a two steps process *viz. amino acid activation* and *transfer of activated amino acids to tRNA.*

(a) Amino Acid Activation

The activation is controlled by specific enzymes. Each amino acid has its own specific enzyme, in general. At least 20 different tRNA molecules and 20 different enzymes (aminoacyl-tRNA synthetase) are required for 20 amino acids. The activation or charging of amino acids by the tRNA is a two step process. The enzyme, aminoacyl-tRNA-synthetase, catalyses the reaction of a specific amino acid with ATP and forms the aminoacyl-adenosine monophosphatase (AMP) and pyrophosphatase.

Aminoacyl – tRNA synthetase

Amino acid + ATP----------------------------------amino acid ~ AMP + pyrophosphate

The amino acid + AMP are referred to as an activated amino acid which is linked to adenosine by a phosphatase ester bond and is now raised to an energy level whereby it can react with its tRNA.

(b) Transfer of Activated Amino Acid to tRNA

The enzyme bound activated amino acids aminoacyl adenylates become attached with their tRNA molecule.

Aminoacyl – tRNA synthetase

Amino acid ~ AMP + tRNA-------------------------------------Amino acid ~ tRNA + AMP

Following amino acid activation and binding to tRNA, the charge tRNA diffuses to the ribosome, where actual assembly into polypeptide chains takes place. The process of the sequential incorporation of amino acid into proteins by peptide bond formation is completed.

Annexure 23.1

Biological Tools Used in Recombinant DNA Technology

The technique of synthesizing the recombinant DNA requires some tools which are biological in nature. These are the

- ☆ Enzymes,
- ☆ Vector DNA (vehicle) –plasmid or phage, and
- ☆ Passenger DNA (DNA for transfer).

The use of DNA (as vehicle or passenger) often requires the isolation of DNA from the cell. A segment of DNA, the *lac gene* of *E. Coli* (which enables the bacterium to utilize lactose) was isolated and purified by Beckwith and co-workers.

1. Enzymes

There are some specific enzymes used in synthesizing recombinant DNA (genetic engineering). These enzymes are lysing enzymes, cleaving enzymes, synthesizing enzymes, joining enzymes, alkaline phosphatises.

(*i*) ***Lysing enzymes*** – used to open up the cells to get DNA for genetic experiments. The bacterial cell wall is dissolved commonly by the ***lysozyme***.

(*ii*) ***Cleaving enzymes*** – used to break DNA molecules and such enzymes are:

- ☆ *Exonucleases* – which cut off nucleotides from 5′ or 3′ ends of DNA molecule,
- ☆ *Endonucleases* – which cleave DNA duplex at any point (middle part) except the ends, and

☆ *Restriction endonucleases* – which cleave DNA duplex at specific points in a manner that single-stranded free ends projects (called sticky ends) from each fragment of DNA duplex. These are called sticky because they can join similar complementary ends of DNA fragment from other organism. Arber (1962) found restriction endonuclease in bacteria. The colon bacterium *E. Coli* has Restriction endonuclease – 1 (ECO R-1) which recognizes the base sequence GAATTC in DNA duplex and cleaves its strands between G and A.

(*iii*) **Synthesizing enzymes** – play a role in the synthesis of DNA strands on suitable templates and are of 2 types –

☆ *DNA polymerases* – which help in the synthesis of complementary DNA strands on DNA templates, and

☆ *Reverse transcriptases* – which help in the synthesis of complementary DNA stranda on RNA templates.

(*iv*) ***Joining enzymes*** – help in sealing gaps in DNA fragments which are otherwise joined by complementary base pairing, *e.g. Tu ligases.*

(*v*) ***Alkaline phosphatise*** – which cut off phosphate group from the 5′ end of linearized circular DNA to check its re-circularization.

2. Vector (Vehicle or Carrier) DNA

It is the DNA which is used as a carrier for transferring a fragment of foreign DNA into a suitable host. The vector DNAs are of two types –

(*i*) ***Plasmid DNA*** – The plasmids were discovered by William Hays and Josua Lederberg (1952) in bacteria. The plasmid DNAs are circular molecules, are shorter (about one-tenth) than the chromosomal DNA, and carry genes for sexuality, antibiotic resistance, and for other traits but not for any vital function for which the bacterium can survive without its plasmids. The following features of plasmids make them suitable for use as vehicle DNA:

☆ The plasmids can replicate independently like the chromosomal DNA,

☆ Known to move around freely in the bacterial world,

☆ Can be easily isolated and transferred,

☆ May pick up genes from one bacterium and transfer those genes into another bacterium,

☆ Can be easily isolated and transferred because they are not a part of the main genome, and

☆ Retain their characters after combining with foreign DNA.

For having the above characteristics of gene transfer, the asexually multiplying bacteria have variability.

(*ii*) ***Bacteriophage DNA***: This DNA has its phage DNA, sheath, head, collar, tail, core, tail plate, and tail fibre. These are viruses which parasitize (attack) bacteria and kill them, have their DNA suitable for use as vehicle

DNA. The DNA of Simiann virus (SV 40) is used as a vector (vehicle) to transfer genes in mammals.

3. Passenger DNA

It is the DNA which is transferred from one organism to another in combination with the vehicle DNA. The followings are 3 types of DNA that are used as passenger:

(*i*) ***Complementary DNA*** (*cDNA*) – which is synthesized on RNA template with the help of reverse transcriptase enzyme, The DNA strand is isolated from the RNA-DNA complex by using alkaline phosphatise enzyme. A cDNA is then synthesized on the isolated single-stranded DNA template with the help of DNA polymerases. This formed cDNA duplex can be joined to vehicle DNA to introduce into a host.

(*ii*) ***Synthetic DNA*** (*sDNA*) – which is synthesized with the help of DNA polymerases on DNA template or from free nucleotides with or without a template as:

- ☆ *Synthesis of DNA on template*: Kornberg and co-workers (1962) were successful to synthesize DNA from a mixture of deoxyribonucleoside triphosphate, DNA polymerase enzyme, metal ions, and a segment of viral DNA as a primer. This synthetic DNA had biological activity and on introducing this DNA into bacteria coded for the formation of virus particles similar to that from which was taken the primer DNA (a short nucleotide sequence with a reactive 3′ OH that can initiate DNA synthesis along a template).
- ☆ *Synthesis of DNA without template*: He was Khurana, H. (an Indian Chemist) and his co-workers (1965) who produced the first synthetic DNA purely chemically. They synthesized the gene coding for *alanine-tRNA* of yeast which required only 77 bp and whose base sequence was known at that time. They obtained full sequence of the gene by synthesizing the short segments with sticky ends and joining them later. The segments were synthesized by stepwise condensation between the hydroxyl (OH) group at the 3′ position of the first or receiving nucleotide and phosphate (PO_4) group at the 5′ position of the second or incoming nucleotide. The di-, tr-, and polynucleotides of specific nucleotides were in this way synthesized and ultimately formed the DNA segments. However, this synthesized gene did not function.

Another gene coding for *tyrosine-tRNA* of *E. Coli* was also synthesized by Khorana and co-workers (1973). The synthesis was made in 4 segments which were joined to complete the gene. However, this gene lacked the initiator and terminating codon and hence was not functional in the beginning. But this group of workers was successful to synthesize a complete *tyrosine tRNA gene* which functioned on being introduced along with a phage DNA into *E. coli*.

(*iii*) ***Random DNA*** – which is small fragments formed by breaking an entire chromosome of an organism with the help of *restriction endonuclease,* each segment is then joined to a suitable vehicle DNA to form recombinant DNA of different nature, and transferred to a host organism.

Annexure 23.2
Restriction Endonuclease

The growth of bacteriophage in *E. coli* in the year 1963 was found restricted by two enzymes which were isolated. It was observed that one of the two enzymes added the methyl group to DNA while the second enzyme cut the DNA. This second enzyme was called ***restriction endonuclease***.

Hamilton Smith and Daniel Nathans (1970) discovered that ***restriction endonuclease*** is a special class of enzymes. They shared the 1986 Nobel Prize in physiology or Medicine with Werner Arber for his pioneer research work leading to the discovery of restriction enzymes.

The first *restriction endonuclease* isolated and characterized was restriction endonuclease – Hind II. It was found that the functioning of this Hind-II depended on a specific DNA nucleotide sequence and it always cut DNA molecules at a particular point after recognizing the specific sequence of 6 base pairs and this sequence is called *recognition sequence for this enzyme* (*Hind – II*). Now a many restriction enzymes (about 900 or more) have been isolated from more than 230 strains of bacteria with their peculiarities to recognize different recognition sequences.

The ***endonuclease*** is an enzyme that breaks strands of DNA at internal positions. Some endonucleases are involved in recombination of DNA. The ***restriction enzyme*** is an endonuclease that recognizes a specific short sequence in DNA and cleaves the DNA molecule at or near that site. The ***restriction endonucleases*** are enzymes that cleave DNA molecules in a sequence-specific manner such that all of the fragments produced have the same nucleotide sequence at their ends. A fragment of DNA produced by cleaving a DNA molecule with one or more restriction endonucleases is called ***restriction fragment***. A DNA sequence that is cleaved by a restriction enzyme is called ***restriction site.*** The regions in the DNA that are highly susceptible to digestion with endonuclease are called ***hypersensitive sites.***

Why the Name Restriction Endonuclease

The *endon is Greek* word meaning *'within'*. The endonucleases are the enzymes that make internal cuts (cleavage) in DNA molecules. Some of the endonucleases make the random cuts in DNA molecules whereas the restriction endonucleases make site-specific internal cuts. The specific nucleotide sequences where the restriction endonucleases cleave the DNA molecules are called restriction sites. Thus, such enzymes which make internal cuts at specific sites in DNA molecules, irrespective of the source of DNA, are called restriction endonucleases. This is a special class of enzyme on which rests the ability to clone and sequence any gene (DNA sequence) from any species. The restriction endonucleases are used in genetic engineering in forming the recombinant DNA molecules composed of the DNA from different genomes/sources.

The restriction enzymes are a large class of enzymes that are called *nucleases.* The nucleases are of the following ***two types***:

- ✰ Endonucleases – which make cuts at specific positions within the DNA, and
- ✰ Exonucleases – which remove nucleotides from the ends of the DNA.

Nomenclature of different Restriction Endonucleases

Different microorganisms produce different restriction endonucleases which recognize different nucleotide sequences in DNA. There is a definite pattern of nomenclature of these restriction endonucleases obtained from different microorganisms. This pattern of nomenclature is to take the first letter of the genus and first two letters of the species producing that enzyme. In addition a letter of the strain is appended to the name of the restriction endonuclease if the enzyme is produced by a specific strain. Moreover, the first restriction endonuclease identified from a bacterial strain is designated as I, the second enzyme as II, and so on. Thus, if an enzyme is designated as *E.co R I,* it indicates that the enzyme is produced by *Escherichia coli strain RY 13.* The Roman numbers (I, II) following the names indicate the order of their isolation from that bacterial strain.

The restriction endonucleases which cleave the DNA molecules at many different DNA sequences are available and hundreds of them have been purified and characterized.

Recognition Sequences and Cleavage Sites of different Restriction Endonucleases

Some of the restriction endonucleases with their names, sources (microorganisms producing them), and recognition sequences and sites have been given here below:

Enzyme	*Source (Microorganism)*	*Recognition Sequence and Cleavage Sites*		
AvaI	*Anabaena*	5′-C/Py.CGPuG-3′	= 5′-C	+ 5′-PyCGPuG-3′
	variabilis	3′-GPu GCPy/C5′	= 3′-GPuGCPy-5′	C-5′
AluI	*Arthrobacter*	*5′-AG./CT-3′*	= *5′-AG-3′*	+ *5′-CT-3′*
	luteus	3′-TC/GA-5′	= 3′-TC-5′ 3′-GA-5′	
BamHI	*Bacillus*	*H 5′-G/GA.TCC-3′*	= *5′-G*	+ *5′-GATCC-3′*
	amyloliquefaciens	3′-CCT AG/G-5′	= 3′-CCTAG-5′ G-5′	
Bgl II	*Bacillus*	5′-A/GA.TCT-3′	= 5′-A	+ 5′-GACT-3′
	globigli	3′-TCT AG/A-5′	= 3′-TCTAG-5′ A-5′	
ClaI	*Caryophanon*	5′-AT/C.GAT-3′	= 5′-AT	+ 5′-CGAT-3′
	latum	3′-TAG C/TA-5′	= 3′-TAGC-5′ TA-5′	
EcoRI	*Escherichia coli*	*5′-G/AA.TTC-3′*	= *5′-G*	+ *5′-AATTC-3′*
	RY13	3′-CTT AA/G-5′	= 3′-CTTAA-5′ G-5′	
Eco RII	*E.coli R245*	*5′-/CCA.(T)GG-3′*	= *5′-*	+ *5′-CCA(T)GG-3′*
		3′-GGT (A)CC/-5′	= 3′-GGT(A)CC-5′ -5′	
HincII	*Haemophilus*	5′-GTPy./PuAC-3′	= 5′-GTPy-3′	+ 5′-PuAC-3′
	influenza Rc	3′-CAPu PyTG-5′	= 3′-CAPu-5′ 3′-PyTG-5′	
HindIII	*Haemophilus*	5′-A/AG.CTT-3′	= 5′-A	+ 5′-AGCTT-3′
	influenza Rd	3′-TTC GA/A-5′	= 3′-TTCGA-5′ A-5′	
Hinfl	*Haemophilus*	*5′-G/A.NTC-3′*	= *5′-G*	+ *5′-ANTC-3′*
	influenza Rd	3′-CTN A/G-5′	= 3′-CTNA-5′ G-5′	
HpaI	*Haemophilus*	*5′-GTT./AAC-3′*	= *5′-GTT*	+ *5′-AAC-3′*
	parainfluenzae	3′-CAA/TTG-5′	= 3′-CAA-5′ TTG-5′	
HpaII	*Haemophilus*	5′-C/C.GG-3′	= 5′-C	+ 5′-CGG-3′
	parainfluenzae	3′-GG C/C-5′	= 3′-GGC-5′ C-5′	
Nla III	*Neisseria lactamica*	5′-CA.TG/-3′	= 5′-CATG	+ 5′- -3′
		3′-/GT AC-5′	= 3′- -5′ GTAC-5′	
Not I	*Nocardia otitidis*	*5′-GC/GG.CCGC-3′*	= *5′-GC*	+ *5′-GGCCGC-3′*
		3′-CGCC GG/CG-5′	= 3′-CGCCGG-5′ CG-5′	
Pst I	*Providencia stuartii*	*5′-CTG.CA/G-3′*	= *5′-CTGCA-3′* + *G-3′*	
		3′-G/AC GTC-5′	= 3′-G 3′-ACGTC-5′	
Sac I	*Streptomyces*	*5′-GAG.CT/C-3′*	= *5′-GAGCT*	+ *C-3′*
	achromogenes	3′-C/TC GAG-5′	= 3′-C 3′-TCGAG-5′	
Sau 3A	*Staphylococcus*	3A 5′-/GA.TC-3′	= 5′-	+ 5′-GATC-3′
	aureus	3′-CT AG/-5′	= 3′-CTAG-5′ -5′	
Taq I	*Thermus*	5′-T/C.GA-3′	= 5′-T	+ 5′-CGA-3′
	aquaticus YT I	3′-AGC/T-5′	= 3′-AGC-5′ T-5′	

Dots (.) indicate the axis of dyad symmetry in each *palindromic* recognition sequence (palindromes). The DNA sequences have the same reading in opposite directions from dot (.),

Pu = purine, Py = pyrimidine, N = any of the four bases,

The oblique line (/) indicates the position of each bond cleaved,

The cuts are staggered as well as blunt.

Special Features of Restriction Endonucleases

The restriction endonucleases are of great value to the microorganism that produces them and show other features:

(i) Protection of the Genetic Material of Bacteria

The restriction endonuclease has a biological function to protect the genetic material of bacteria from invasion by foreign DNAs, such as DNA molecules from another species or viral DNA. The restriction endonucleses are thus believed to provide a kind of the *immune system* to their producing organism by protecting their genetic material from invasion of foreign DNAs from viruses or other pathogens or the environment DNA which could be taken by microorganism.

The restriction endonuclease protects all cleavage sites in the DNA of an organism from being cleaved, otherwise the organism will suicide by degrading its own DNA. The protection of endogenous cleavage sites is accomplished in many cases by ***methylation*** of one or more nucleotides in each nucleotide sequence which is recognized by the organism's own restriction endonuclease. The site-specific methylases produced by the organism catalyzes the methylation to occur rapidly after replication. A foreign DNA molecule is cleaved by each restriction endonuclease into a fixed number of DNA fragments depending on the number of restriction sites in the particular DNA.

(ii) Palindrome DNA Sequences

The functioning of each restriction endonuclease is such that it inspects the length of a DNA sequence and finds its specific recognition sequence. It then binds to DNA and cut each of the two strands of the double helix at specific points in their sugar-phosphate backbones. More interestingly, the restriction endonucleases commonly recognize ***palindrome*** DNA sequences (nucleotide-pair sequences with same forward or backward read from a central axis of symmetry) like ***AND DNA, MALAYALAM, MADAM***. Thus, palindrome means that the same word is read in both directions and the palindrome in DNA is a sequence of base pairs that reads same on the two strands on keeping same the orientation reading, *e.g.* the following sequences reads the same on the two strands in 5′ to 3′ direction which is also true if read in opposite direction (3′ to 5′):

5′........GAATTC................GAATTC........3′

3′........CTTAAG................CTTAAG........5′

(iii) Two Types of Cuts

The restriction endonucleases make two types of cuts. These are the ***staggered cuts*** which are formed by cleaving the two complementary strands at different points. The staggered cuts produce DNA segments with complementary single-stranded ends due to the palindromic nature of restriction sites. The second type is the ***blunt cut*** which is formed when the restriction endonucleases cut both strands of double helix at the same point (place).

The cleaving of the following DNA molecule with staggered cut can be shown as -

5′........GAATTC................GAATTC........3′

3′........CTTAAG................CTTAAG........5′

The above DNA molecule with staggered cut with *E.coli* will be as under -

5′........G	+ AATTC................G	+ AATTC........3′
3′........CTTAA	G................CTTAA	G........5′

(iv) Position of Cut

The restriction enzyme cut the DNA strand a little away from the centre of the palindrome sites but between the same two bases on the opposite strands, leaving single stranded part at the ends on each strand and these are sticky ends (overhanging stretches) which facilitate the action of the enzyme DNA ligase. These are called sticky because they form hydrogen bonds with their complementary cut counterparts.

(v) Same Kind of Cuts

The resultant DNA fragments produced, after cutting by the same restriction enzyme, have the same kind of 'sticky ends' which can be joined together end to end using DNA ligases.

(vi) Hydrogen Bonding and Rejoining of DNA Fragments

The DNA fragments so produced have complementary single-stranded termini and so they will hydrogen bond with each other and can be rejoined under renaturation conditions by the enzyme DNA ligase to reform the missing phosphodiester linkages in each strand.

(vii) Random Pairing of Base Pairs

The sequence of base pairs along a DNA molecule occurs strictly at random. The frequency of a specific (restriction enzyme recognition) sequence of the length depends on the number of base pairs. For example, the frequency of a specific sequence of the length with 3 and 4 base pairs will be as:

$(\frac{1}{4})^3 = 1/64$ for 3 base pairs, and

$(\frac{1}{4})^4 = 1/256$ for 4 base pairs.

Annexure 23.3

Plasmid, Phage or Viral Chromosome

A ***vector*** is a *plasmid, phage or viral chromosome* that may be used to construct recombinant DNA molecules for introduction into living cells. A plasmid capable of replicating in two different organisms, such as yeast and *E. coli,* is called ***shuttle vector.***

The ***cloning vector*** is a small, self-replicating DNA molecule - usually a plasmid or viral chromosome – into which foreign DNAs are inserted in the process of cloning of desired genes or DNA sequences. A cloning vector has three essential components -

- ☆ An origin of replication – a sequence to start replication, any piece of DNA can replicate within the host cells on joining this sequence, andis responsible to control the number of copies of linked DNA.
- ☆ A dominant selectable marker gene – an antibiotic-resistance gene that confers drug resistance to the host cell bacterium because the *E. coli cells* do not have resistance against any of the antibiotics like *ampicillin, tetracycline, kanamycin, chloramphenicol.* The vector requires a selectable marker (antibiotic resistant gene) to help in identification and elimination of non-transformants and selectively allowing the growth of transformants. When the transformed cells are spread on agar plates containing ampicillin (for example), only the transformed cells grow but the untransformed recipient cells do not grow and hence die. The transformed cells are selected in the presence of ampicillin due to ampicillin resistance gene. Thus, the ampicillin resistant gene in this case is called a ***selectable marker.***

  This is the process of ***transformation*** by which a piece of DNA is introduced in a host bacterium. The most useful selectable markers for

E. coli are the genes encoding resistance to antibiotics like *ampicillin, tetracycline, kanamycin, chloramphenicol.*

- ☆ Cloning sites: One unique restriction endonuclease cleavage site which is present only once in a region of the vector that does not disrupt either the origin of replication or the selectable marker gene. The vector needs to have recognition site for the commonly used restriction enzyme to link alien DNA. The presence of more than one site generates many fragments which in turn complicate the gene cloning.

Modern cloning vectors, instead of having only one unique restriction cleavage site, have a ***multiple cloning site* (*MCS*)** or polycloning site or ***polylinker.*** This is a cluster of unique cleavage sites for a number of different restriction endonuclease in a nonessential region of the vector into which the foreign DNA can be inserted. The utility of a vector, with more restriction endonuclease cleavage sites, is greater for cloning a wide variety of different restriction fragments.

Most of the cloning vectors are derived from plasmids or bacteriophage chromosomes. Many of them are modified versions of plasmids, the extra-chromosomal, double-stranded circular DNA molecule of bacteria. Many plasmids carry antibiotic-resistance genes which are ideal selectable markers. The plasmids are of limited size ranging from about 1 kb (1, 000 base pairs) to over 200 kb and many replicate autonomously. Therefore, the plasmid vectors have a limitation of accepting small foreign DNA inserts of about 10 – 15 kb. The ***plasmids*** and ***phagemids*** have the maximum insert size of 15 kb whereas the ***phage lambda*** has 23 kb capacity of maximum insert.

Vectors which Accept Large Size DNA Inserts

Geneticists have evolved vectors that may replicate in the presence of very large DNA inserts and hence the capacity of the vectors to accept large size DNA inserts has been increased. The new vectors to accept large size DNA inserts have been constructed by combining components from viruses and plasmids. These are as under:

(i) ***Phagemids***: These are cloning vectors that contain components derived from both phage chromosome (M 13) and parts of plasmids, and have the maximum insert size of 15 kb.

(ii) ***Cosmids*** contains the cohesive ends of lambda in plasmids, and has maximum insert size of 44 kb. These are cloning vectors that are hybrids between phage lambda chromosome and plasmids,

(iii) ***Bacterial artificial chromosome*** (BACs): These are cloning vectors that combine *multiple cloning sites* (*MCS*) and selectable marker genes with essential components of bacterial fertility (F) factor, and have the capacity of accepting 300 kb foreign DNA inserts,

(iv) ***Phage P1 artificial chromosomes* (*PACs*)** combine MCS and selectable marker gene with phage P1 chromosome and accept 300 kb DNA inserts.

(v) ***Yeast artificial chromosomes* (*YACs*)** are linear cloning vectors (mini chromosomes) containing essential parts of yeast chromosomes – the

origin of replication, centromere, and telomeres along with a selectable marker and a MCS. This vector may accept much larger foreign DNA inserts of 200 to 500 kb in size.

Characteristics of Sophisticated Vectors (BACs, PACs and YACs)

(i) The sophisticated vectors (BACS, PACs, and YACs) which accept much larger DNA inserts (300 – 600 kb) have made easier to conduct research on large genes and chromosomes, *e.g.* the gene for human dystrophin which is a protein that links filaments to membranes in muscle cells, has a length of over 2000 kb.

(ii) The BACs and PACs are less complex and hence easy to construct and work with compared to YACs. Moreover, these two vectors replicate in *E.coli* like plasmid vectors and hence they have replaced YAC vectors.

(iii) The PACs permit negative selection against vectors lacking foreign DNA inserts. They contain the *sac*B gene of *Bacillus subtilis* and this gene encodes the enzyme *levan sucrase* which catalyzes the transfer of fructose groups to various carbohydrates and this enzyme is lethal to *E.coli cells* in 5 per cent sucrose containing medium. The insertion of foreign DNA in a *Bam* HI restriction site in the gene inactivates the *sac* B gene and hence used to select vectors containing DNA inserts. Therefore, the 5 per cent sucrose containing medium divides the cells either to grow or not. This medium permits to grow only those cells which contain vectors with DNA inserts and the cells containing vectors lacking DNA inserts are lysed in the first hour of their growth in 5 per cent sucrose medium. Consequently, all the surviving cells contain vectors with DNA inserts located within the *sac* B gene - inserts that eliminate levan sucrose activity.

(iv) The BAC and PAC vectors can be used to produce ***shuttle vectors*** by their modification so as the shuttle vectors can replicate both in *E.coli* and in mammalian cells. The shuttle vector contains the *sac* B gene which permits positive selection of cells carrying vectors with DNA inserts plus the origin of replication and the gene encoding nuclear antigen 1 of the Epstein-Barr virus which makes easier the replication of the vector in mammalian cells. The puromycin-resistance gene has also been added in this shuttle vector for which the mammalian cells carrying the vector are selected on puromycin containing medium.

Annexure 23.4

Sources and Procedures to obtain Isolated Gene

The identification and isolation of the desired gene (DNA fragment or DNA insert) for cloning may be done either by isolating from DNA libraries of an organism (cDNA library and genomic library), or synthesizing the gene chemically or enzymatic, or by amplification of genes either *in vivo* (cloning vectors) or *in vitro* (PCR technique):

23.4.1. ISOLATION OF DESIRED GENE (DNA FRAGMENTS)

The DNA can be isolated either from an organism or from DNA libraries.

(1) Isolation of DNA from Organism

This is accomplished by opening (breaking) the cell (enclosing the DNA) with enzyme, digestion by restriction endonuclease, and separation (isolation) of DNA fragments by gel electrophoresis.

(*i*) *Cell opening by enzyme for DNA isolation in purified form*: The DNA is enclosed within the membrane and hence it requires opening the cell by its breaking so as to release the DNA out of cell. This is done by treating the cell (bacteria/plant/animal) with enzyme like *lysozyme* (bacteria), *cellulase* (plant cells), *chitinase* (fungus). After opening the cell, the proteins (histones) interwoven with DNA molecules are removed by treatment with protease and other molecules are removed by appropriate treatments. The treatment by the addition of chilled ethanol precipitates out the purified DNA which can be seen as collection of fine threads in the suspension.

(*ii*) *Digestion (cutting) of DNA by enzyme to get DNA fragments*: The purified DNA molecules are incubated with the enzyme restriction endonuclease under appropriate conditions for the enzyme. This called as digestion. The enzyme cuts the DNA at specific sites and the DNA fragments (pieces) are produced.

(*iii*) *Isolation of DNA* fragments: The technique of *gel electrophoresis* is used to separate (isolate) the DNA fragments. These DNA fragments are negatively charged molecules and hence can be isolated by forcing them to move towards the anode (positive electrode) under an electric field through a medium (*agarose gel* extracted from sea weeds) which provides a sieving like effect to resolve (isolate/separate) the DNA fragments according to their size. The small size DNA fragments move farther. Further only the digested set of DNA fragments can migrate while the undigested ones cannot.

The separated/isolated DNA fragments can be seen after their staining with *ethidium bromide* followed by exposure to UV radiation because the DNA fragments cannot be seen without staining in visible light. The bright orange colour DNA bands can be seen. The separated bands of DNA are cut out from agarose gel and extracted from the gel piece, the process called as elution. The purified DNA fragments are then used in constructing recombinant DNA by joining them with cloning vectors.

(2) Isolation of DNA from DNA Libraries

The DNA libraries can also be constructed in two ways either having complete sets of genomic DNA sequences (genomic libraries) or DNA copies of mRNAs in an organism (cDNA libraries). These DNA libraries provide the desired gene for cloning.

(*i*) ***cDNA library:*** The cDNA is the complementary DNA produced by using mRNA as a template. Therefore, cDNA is a collection of bacterial transformants or phage lysates in which each mRNA (isolated from an organism or tissue) is represented as its cDNA insertion in a plasmid or phage vector. However, the RNA of any type can be used to produce cDNA. The enzyme reverse transcriptase which is RNA-dependent DNA polymerase is used to produce the DNA copy of RNA molecule. This enzyme was discovered by Temin and Baltimore (1970) from avian mycloblastosis virus (AMV) and it is similar in reaction to DNA polymerase.

The complementary DNA (cDNA) libraries can be more easily used to identify the expressed DNA sequences from non-expressed sequences. The nucleotide-pair sequences of genomic DNA clones and cDNA clones of specific genes of higher plants and animals have the most frequent observing difference. Most genes of higher animals and plants contain non-coding intron (intervening) sequences which remain present in the genomic clones but these introns are not present in cDNA clones. This is because cDNAs are synthesized using mRNA templates and the intron sequences are removed during the processing of primary transcripts to produce mature mRNAs.

(*ii*) ***Genomic library:*** A genomic library has essentially all of the DNA sequences in the genome. Thus, a genomic library is a collection of plasmid clones or phage virus containing recombinant DNA molecules. The entire genome of the organism concerned is represented by the sum total of all the DNA inserts in this collection. Hundreds of thousands of different recombinant clones are contained in genomic libraries in case of large genomes. The construction of a genomic DNA library (DNA clones containing the entire genome) is useful in gene cloning from an organism.

Usually in preparing the genomic libraries, the DNA of an organism is first isolated by digesting it with a restriction endonuclease and inserting the DNA fragments into an appropriate cloning vector. The DNA fragments with staggered cuts can be ligated directly into vector DNA molecule cut with the same enzyme. In this case, the foreign DNA inserts can be excised (cut) from the vector DNA by cleavage with the restriction endonuclease. The recombinant DNA molecules (after ligating the genomic DNA fragments into vector DNA) are introduced into host cells for amplification by replication *in vivo.* The *E.coli* is treated with chemicals or with a short impulse of electricity to make the bacteria permeable to DNA. The selection of transformed cells is done based on their growth in the medium.

The individual chromosomes of an organism are also sometimes isolated based on their size and DNA content and used to construct chromosome-specific DNA libraries. Such chromosome specific libraries help to search a gene known to be located on a particular chromosome, particularly in case of large genomes like that of humans. These libraries are used to identify the individual genes or DNA sequence after their amplification by replication.

Screening DNA Libraries to Identify the Gene of Interest

The DNA libraries (cDNA or genomic libraries) can be screened to identify and obtain the desired gene or other DNA sequences of interest for its cloning. Two procedures of either the genetic complementation (genetic selection) or hybridization to labelled nucleic acid probes containing sequences of known function are used.

(a) Genetic Selection

It is a simple and most efficient procedure to identify and cloning genes. This procedure requires preparing a genomic library in an expression vector such as Blueprint using DNA from resistant strain and screening the library for resistant gene by transforming sensitive *E.coli cells* with the clones in the library and plating the transformed cells on medium containing the resistant strain. Only the cells transformed with the resistant gene will produce colonies in the medium containing resistant drug.

This can be understood by taking the example of the *Salmonella typhimurium* gene responsible for resistance to penicillin. This gene (*pen*) can be easily cloned. The penicillin-sensitive *E. coli* cells transformed with the recombinant DNA clones in the library are grown on penicillin containing medium. These are only transformed cells with *pen* gene which will grow in the presence of penicillin.

This procedure of screening has some limitations. The first is that this method of screening the eukaryotic clones in *E. coli* is restricted to cDNAs from which the intron sequences have already been excised. Secondly, this method depends on the correct transcription of the cloned gene in the new host. This method works well with prokaryotic genes in prokaryotes and likewise the eukaryotic genes in eukaryotic organisms. Therefore, this method of complementation screening is used to screen eukaryotic DNA libraries using the *S. cerevisiae.*

(b) Molecular Hybridization (in situ colony or plaque hybridization)

The labelled nucleic acid probes containing sequences of known function is used to screen genomic DNA libraries for isolating the specific genes. The RNA transcript of genes can be easily isolated from the concerned cells in which the major product of the gene is produced *viz.* the RBC are highly specialized cells for the synthesis and storage of haemoglobin and the chicken oviduct cells synthesize the ovalbumin. Therefore, the RNA transcripts of the globin and ovalbumin genes can be easily isolated from reticulocytes and oviduct cells, respectively. The RNA transcripts can be used to synthesize radioactive cDNAs which in turn can be used to screen genomic DNA libraries by either procedure of hybridization.

The ***colony hybridization*** is used with plasmid and cosmid vectors based libraries whereas the ***plaque hybridization*** is used with phage lambda vector based libraries.

See **annexure 23.6** for ***in situ colony hybridization.***

23.4.2. GENE SYNTHESIS

The base sequence of the gene based on codons for the amino acids can be deducted from either the amino acid sequence of protein or the base sequence of mRNA produced by the gene. Though some problem may arise in degeneration of gene tic code, but the functional sequence of the gene is a better choice. After knowing the base sequence of a gene, the same base sequence of a polynucleotide (desired gene) can be synthesized either by chemically or by enzymatic synthesis as:

(i) Chemical Synthesis of Gene

The chemical synthesis of a gene needs chemical reagents in completing the different approach of this process. The different approaches differ to protect the OH groups of the phosphate residues. These approaches are:

(*a*) *Phosphodiester method* of chemical synthesis of gene was invented in 1970 by *Khorana and Co-workers* for the synthesis of gene of *alanine* (suppressor) tRNA and to synthesize the gene for *tyrosine* (suppressor) tRNA of *E. coli* by Brown and co-workers. This approach suitably protects 3′ and 5′ OH groups of the deoxy-ribose of nucleosides by selectively unblocked for joining of the additional nucleotides.

(*b*) *Phosphotriester method* of chemical synthesis of gene involves the following steps:

- ☆ The *stepwise addition of protecting groups* (amino group and 5′OH group) of mononucleotides and oligo-nucleotides to all the four deoxy-ribonucleosides. The amino group (NH_2) of deoxy-adenosine and deoxy-cytidine are protected by Benzoate (Benzoylation) and the NH_2 group of deoxy-guanosine is protected by isobutyryl group (*isobutyration*).
- ☆ There is also stepwise *removal of protecting group* for all these three deoxy-nucleosides by a process of mild alkaline hydrolysis. The amino groups of fourth deoxy-nucleoside of DNA (*i.e.* thymidine) neither require any protection nor any removal of protecting group. The hydroxyl group (5′ OH) of deoxy-ribose is protected by dimethoxytrityl [DMTr or $(MeO)_2$] and this protecting group is removed or freed through gentle acid hydrolysis by benzene sulfonic acid ($ZnBr_2$).
- ☆ The above two steps (stepwise *addition of protecting groups viz.* amino group and 5′OH group by suitable chemical reagents) and (*their removal by suitable hydrolysis process*) are common for both phosphor-triester as well as phosphate trimester method as described below. The phosphor-triester method also follows the following 7 steps –
- ☆ The 3′OH in *Phospho-triester method* is coupled with a suitable phosphor-rylating agent like p-chlorophenyl-phospho-dichloridate and the phosphate residue having a free OH group accepts any nucleotide or oligonucleotide with a free 5′ OH group. The protected nucleotides in this way have phosphor-diesters to serve as the 5′-terminus residue in oligonucleotide synthesis.
- ☆ There is further modification of such protected and phosphorylated nucleotides to become suitable for joining to the OH group of 3′ phosphate residue (of such nucleotides) which is blocked by a suitable agent like β-cyano-ethanol after which the 5′ OH is made free by mild acid hydrolysis to remove the $(MeO)_2Tr$. This results phosphor-triester nucleotides having a free 5′ OH.
- ☆ There is mixing of a desired diester nucleotide free OH at 3′ phosphate residue with the desired trimester nucleotide and an agent that promote their coupling is added to the mixture. The coupling is promoted by arylsulfonyl compounds (tri-iso-propylbenzene-sulfonyl chloride, TPS). This yields a fully protected dinucleotide which is removed (either fully or selectively) and used as the starting material in constructing the large molecules.
- ☆ The hydrolysis with an acid like benzene-sulfonic acid or $ZnBr_2$ selectively removes the 5′ OH of a dinucleotide whereas the OH group of 3′ phosphate is removed by preferential removal of the cyano-ethyl ester through tri-ethylamine.

- ☆ The coupling together the two di-nucleotides (one with a free 5′ OH and second with a free OH at 3′ phosphate) produce tetra-nucleotide and so on.
- ☆ After each addition to the growing chain requires essentially the tedious purification to remove the uncoupled mononucleotides/ oligonucleotides.
- ☆ The solid support *e.g.* controlled pore glass beads, for fixing the first nucleotide is used to eliminate the tedious purification and some other problems. It is better to fix 3′OH compared to fix the 5′OH. An ester is formed between the 3′OH and a carboxyl group (COOH) for fixing on a solid support. There is then addition of nucleotides with protected 5′OH one by one and coupled to growing chain. Mild acid hydrolysis is used to make free the 5′OH of the growing chain in between each addition.

(*c*) *Phosphite triester method* involves the following steps:

- ☆ The nucleosides with protected bases and 5′OH groups are used as the *basic materials*.
- ☆ The 3′OH of the terminal nucleotide is *fixed to a solid support* and then 5′OH is *removed by gentle acid hydrolysis*.
- ☆ The subsequent nucleotides are used as 3′-phosphoramidities (stable and efficient *coupling agents*) which are easily produced by coupling the nucleotides with di-iso-prophyl-ammonium-tetrazolite.
- ☆ Now added the desired nucleotide 3′-phosphoramidities and is activated by adding of tetrazole. The product produced is a phosphite which is oxidized to phosphate by iodine (I_2) and remains as a triester.
- ☆ There is removal of 5′OH of the second nucleotide, addition of the third desired nucleotide 3′-phosphoramidite, joining to growing chain, and thus elongating the oligo-nucleotide chain.
- ☆ The chain is removed from the solid support by alkaline hydrolysis after final removal of various protective groups.

(ii) Enzymatic Synthesis of Gene (DNA)

The enzymatic synthesis of short oligonucleotides of defined sequence is simple compared to chemical methods, especially in case of availability of automated systems of *gene machines*. This does not requires any protective groups but the reactions are limited and difficult to control.

Bacterial enzyme is used in this approach. The enzymatic process is completed in following steps:

- ☆ The enzyme is polynucleotide phosphorylase specific for ribonucleotides but the rate of polymerization by this enzyme becomes slow for deoxyribonucleotides in case Mg^{2+} is replaced by Mn^{2+} in reaction mixture.
- ☆ This enzyme does not require a template.

- ☆ This enzyme uses the de-oxyribo-nucleoside diphosphates as *substrate* and a *primer* at least 3 nucleotides long.
- ☆ One or two nucleotides at a time are added to the primer and to the growing chain by this enzyme.

23.4.3 GENE AMPLIFICATION (MULTIPLICATION OR CLONING) PROCEDURE

The desired gene or other DNA sequences can be obtained by its amplification either *in vivo* (cloning vectors) or *in vitro* by P. C. R. as:

A chromosome segment carrying the gene of interest is produced and then introduced into an appropriate host cell. This is a two stage process. The first stage is the incorporation of the desired gene into a small self-replicating chromosome. This involves the *production of recombinant DNA molecule* by joining of two or more DNA molecules of different origin. For example, a human gene is inserted into an *E.coli* plasmid or other self-replicating mini-chromosome. The second stage is the *gene cloning* in which the recombinant DNA molecule is introduced in an appropriate host cell (*E.coli* cells - *in vivo*) where it replicates to produce many identical copies for further use (biochemical analysis).

(1) Amplification of Desired Gene in Cloning Vector (*in vivo* amplification)

The amplification requires that one of the parental DNAs of the recombinant DNA molecule is capable of self-replication. The gene or DNA sequence is inserted into a specially chosen cloning vector. The insertion of foreign DNA insert in the vector is indicated by inactivation of the function of the vector at the site where the foreign DNA has been inserted. For example, the bluescript is a phagemid vector with multiple cloning sites (MCS) and contains many unique restriction enzyme cleavage sites, two distinct origins of replication, and a good selectable marker. This marker gene makes the host bacterium resistant to ampicillin. An enzyme (β-galactosidase) encoded by a gene in this vector catalyzes a step in the catabolism of lactose. Insertion of foreign DNA segment in one of the restriction sites in the MCS disrupts the function of the vector (plasmid) and hence the enzyme β-galactosidase which catalyzes one step in lactose catabolism in inactivated. This inactivation is a test to determine the insertion of foreign DNA insert into the plasmid (vector). The disfunctioning of the enzyme β-galactosidase is indicated that the cells containing active β-galactosidase produce blue colonies on agar medium but the cells lacking the enzyme β-galactosidase activity produce white colonies on plates.

(2) Amplification of Desired Gene by PCR (*in vitro* amplification)

The DNA sequence of interest is synthesized and amplified a million-fold or more in just a few hours *in vitro*. The *in vitro* synthesis uses two sets of primers. The one is the small chemically synthesized oligonucleotides that are complementary to the regions of DNA and the second is the special heat stable DNA polymerase (isolated from a bacterium, *Thermus aquaticus*) without using cloning vectors or host cells. This enzyme DNA polymerase remains active during the high temperature induced denaturation of double stranded DNA molecule. The enzyme extends the primers using the nucleotides provided in the reaction and the genomic DNA as template. This procedure is called ***polymerase chain reaction* (*PCR*).**

The PCR is a powerful tool of gene amplification (multiplication) million times. The PCR does not require cloning the sequence by replication *in vivo* and hence the PCR technique has replaced the earlier *in vivo* amplification protocol. This PCR technique has its limitation that it can be used only when nucleotide sequences flanking (on either side of) the gene or DNA sequence of interest are known.

See ***annexure*** 23.7 for details of PCR technique.

Annexure 23.5

Techniques of DNA Transfer (Integration)

The recombinant DNA molecule is a **vector** (See ***annexure** 23.3*) into which the desired DNA fragment has been inserted for its cloning in an appropriate host (Bacterium). The recombinant DNA molecule contains a gene from one organism joined to regulatory sequences from another organism. Such a gene is called ***chimeric gene.*** The vectors containing DNA segments for cloning are called ***DNA inserts*** **(*chimeric vectors*)** or ***cloning vectors*** which are introduced into a suitable organism, usually a bacterium (called as host). This process is called ***transformation.***

The DNA from one organism to another is transferred by the techniques of *transformation* and *transduction*.

(A) Transformation

The *genetic transformation* is the genetic change of an organism brought about by the incorporation of foreign DNA into cells. The phenomenon of bacterial transformation was discovered by Griffith (1928) in *Diplococcus pneumonia.* This refers to the genetic change in the properties of one bacterium mediated by soluble DNA from another bacterium. This is a process of taking up DNA by a cell from another, incorporates it into its own DNA, and finally expresses the trait coded by the incoming DNA.

The gene transfer may take place from one bacterium to another, or it may be plasmid mediated gene transfer, and also chromosome-mediated gene transfer.

(*i*) *Transformation from one bacterium to another*: Avery Oswald, Macleod Colin and Macrathy Maclyn (1944) repeated Griffith's experiment (1928) on pneumonia causing bacteria (*Pneumo-coccus*). They showed that one type of this bacterium can be transformed into another type *in vitro* and thus concluded that DNA is the transforming substance which could bring about transformation of avirulent bacteria (Type II R cells in pneumococci) into virulent form (Type III S cells). This is done by treating the growing culture of one type with a purified DNA from the other.

(*ii*) *Plasmid - mediated gene transfer*: The insulin gene from rat DNA is transferred to *E. Coli* with a plasmid. This is done by isolating the plasmid of bacterium and insulin gene of rat DNA and sliced with restriction endonuclease to produce complementary sticky ends in both DNA segments. The complementary pairing of the plasmid DNA and rat DNA segments results at sticky ends, the gaps are sealed with ligase, and a circular DNA containing two DNA's segments is formed. This recombinant DNA (hybrid plasmid) replicates when introduced into a bacterium.

This technique has also been applied to introduce into the bacterium *E. Coli* the different genes of different species (somatostatin hormone gene of sheep, ribosomal gene of toad, and globulin gene of rabbit). Although the recombinant DNA so formed was transcribed in the bacterium but failed in protein synthesis (translation). Recently it has been reported by Walter Gilbert that small amount of *proinsulin* (different from insulin) was produced in the bacteria containing rat insulin gene.

Human hormone somatostatin which is a brain hormone having a role in regulation of growth was produced by Herbert Boyer in *E. Coli*. He showed the working of a foreign gene into a host. The somatoatatin hormone is now being manufactured using this technique by an American company for research work. This hormone is of known base sequence and of shorter length having 18 amino acids formed by 54 nucleotides. The synthesized somatostatin gene was inserted into a plasmid and transferred into *E. Coli K–12* which produced a protein from which somatostatin was excised.

(*iii*) *Chromosome- mediated gene transfer*: Chinese hamster (small rat-like rodent) chromosome at metaphase stage isolated by Mc Bride (1973) was placed in a nutrient mixture having mutant mouse cells which took it. It was partly lysed by lysosome and a segment was integrated into genome. This chromosome segment of hamster produced an enzyme (HPRT) in mouse cell but the mutant mouse lacks that enzyme (HPRT) which enables cells to grow in artificial medium.

(B) Transduction

This is the transfer of DNA from one organism to another and it is the phage DNA-mediated gene transfer. The transduction may take place from bacteria to bacteria (See ***section 12.10.3***), from bacteria to human cells, and also from man to man.

(*i*) *Transduction from bacterium to bacterium*: The phenomenon of the transfer of DNA from one bacterium to another by *bacteriophage* was discovered by Lederberg and Zinder (1952) in *Salmonella typhimurium*. This process neither require cell contact nor sensitive to DNase for degradation of DNA. The bacterial DNA is injected by a phage into a bacterium, but it does not replicate. Some viruses are gene-specific for transduction like some lambda bacteriophages transduce the *lac gene* of *E. Coli* into haploid cells of tomato. Thus, the use of specialized viruses seems possible to transduce normal genes into the cells of the mutant individuals.

(*ii*) *Transduction from bacteria to human cells*: The transfer of a gene from the bacterium (*E. coli*) into cultured human cells through an intermediate virus (bacteriophage DNA) was reported by Merill, Geier and Petricciani (1971). That man was unable to produce the enzyme β-galactosidase required for lactose (milk sugar) digestion. The enzyme deficient human cells survived in the culture through many divisions due to the presence of *gal gene* of *E. Coli* which synthesizes the β-galactosidase. The daughter cells were found to have normal enzyme and were able to produce the required enzyme. This was an evidence of entering of bacterial *gal gene* into human cells with bacteriophage DNA and that it was found functioning. Therefore, the replication and transcription of bacterial DNA in the human cells may be carried out and it has shown the possibility to transmit the genes of an organism into another by using viruses as vector or vehicle DNA (transmitters).

(*iii*) *Transduction from man to man*: The virus SV 40 infects humans and it has been found to transfer a DNA segment from one host (man) to another.

Annexure 23.6

In situ Colony or Plaque Hybridization

In situ Hybridization

Mary Lou Pardue and Joseph Gall (1969) developed the technique to hybridize radioactive single strands of DNA with complementary strands of DNA in chromosomes on glass slides. This technique, called *in situ* hybridization, was used to determine the chromosomal locations of repetitive DNA sequences. ***In situ*** is a Latin word meaning *"in its original (natural) place"*; refers to experimental treatments performed on cells or tissues rather than on extracts from them. The hybridization is the formation of hybrid duplex molecules by the base pairing of complementary strands of DNA or RNA.

***In situ* hybridization** is a method of determining the location of specific DNA sequences in chromosomes by hybridizing labelled DNA or RNA to denatured DNA in chromosome preparations and visualizing the hybridized probe by autoradiography or fluorescent microscopy. The procedure of *in situ* hybridization involves the following steps:

- ☆ Spreading mitotic chromosomes on a glass slide,
- ☆ Denaturing the DNA in the chromosomes by exposure to alkali (0.07 N NaOH) for a few minutes,
- ☆ Rinsing with buffer to remove the alkaline solution,
- ☆ Incubating the slide in hybridization solution containing radioactive copies of the nucleotide sequence of interest,
- ☆ Washing off the radioactive strands that have not hybridized with complementary sequences in the chromosome,

- Exposing the slide to a photographic emulsion that is sensitive to low-energy radioactivity,
- Developing the autoradiograph, and
- Superimposing the autoradiograph on a photograph of the chromosomes.

In situ or ***cytological hybridization*** is used to locate specific genes in chromosomes, especially in giant chromosomes. This requires a radioactive clone (representing a gene) most often labelled cDNA copies of the mRNA produced by the gene, is used as probe. The location of specific sequences in particular band of salivary gland chromosome of *Drosophila* was known. This method is also used to detect the virus in the cells and tissues for disease diagnosis.

The first *in situ* hybridization experiment showed that the satellite DNA sequence of the mouse is present in heterochromatin regions flanking the centromere. The mouse genome contains about 10^6 copies of this satellite DNA sequence which is about 400 np long, making about 10 percent of the mouse genome. The satellite DNA sequences are usually not transcribed.

FISH (Fluorescent *in situ* hybridization)

The FISH is the *in situ* hybridization when performed by using a DNA or RNA probe coupled to a fluorescent dye (or antibodies tagged with fluorescent compounds). The ***FISH*** has been used to demonstrate the presence of the repetitive sequence TTAGGG in the telomeres of human chromosome.

Chromosome painting is a variant of ***FISH***. This involves the painting of chromosomes with different colours by using DNA hybridization probes labelled with fluorescent dyes that emit light of different wave lengths. The chromosome painting has been used for comparative genome analyses to study the organization and evolution of chromosomes and to demonstrate the conserved linkage relationship of genes in species where high-density maps are available.

Colony Hybridization

This technique is a form of ***in situ hybridization***. Colony hybridization is a screening procedure to identify the bacterial colonies in a plate which contain a specific DNA sequence. The bacterial cells to obtain these colonies are the transformed cells into which the desired sequence was introduced through genetic engineering and the desired sequence is represented by the probe used in hybridization. The procedure involves the transfer of the colonies formed by transformed cells onto nylon membranes, hybridization with a radioactively labelled DNA or RNA probe, and autoradiography. Thus, a radioactive cDNA is used as a hybridization probe. The steps involved in screening DNA libraries by colony hybridization are as:

- Synthesis of radioactive cDNA using purified mRNA as template,
- Incubate the plate bacteria carrying the recombinant DNA molecule on agar medium till colonies are formed.
- Transfer of colonies onto nylon membrane,

- ☆ Use the labelled DNA or RNA as a probe for hybridization to denatured DNA from colonies grown on nylon membranes. The DNA from the lysed cells is bound to the membrane before hybridization so that it does not come out,
- ☆ The membranes are washed thoroughly with buffered salt solutions to remove non-hybridized cDNA,
- ☆ Expose to X-ray film to detect the presence of radioactivity on the membrane. The presence of radioactivity is indicated by a dark spot (radioactive spots) on autoradiogram. The colonies containing DNA sequences complementary to the radioactive cDNA produce radioactive spots on the autoradiograph. Thus, the colonies whose DNA hybridizes with the probe show the radioactive spots which are detected by autoradiography, and
- ☆ Colonies containing DNA of interest are picked up from agar medium and used to purify DNA clones having the genes or DNA sequence of interest. Thus, the recombinant DNA is isolated.

Annexure 23.7

Amplification of DNA Sequence or Desired Gene *In vitro*: Polymerase Chain Reaction

The PCR technique is *in vitro* process to amplify the specific DNA sequence. This method was devised by Kary Mullis (1985) who received the 1993 Noble Prize in Chemistry for developing this technique. The *in vitro* is a Latin word meaning "within glass". This refers to biological processes made to occur experimentally outside the organism in a test tube or other container. On the contrary, the word used is the *in vivo* which means (Latin language) "within the living organism".

This (PCR) assay is a procedure involving multiple cycles of denaturation, hybridization to oligonucleotide primers (primer annealing), and polynucleotide synthesis that amplifies (extends) a particular DNA sequence by DNA polymerase. The PCR allows amplifying any sequence to high copy numbers in short time period with high accuracy and specificity, like a ***'Xerox machine'***.

It is a simple ingenious primer mediated enzymatic method of amplifying short, specific segments of longer DNA or cDNA template. The PCR technique is the *in vitro* amplification (enzymatic synthesis of DNA) of particular DNA sequences or loci, with the help of specifically or arbitrarily chosen oligonucleotide sequences (primers) and thermostable DNA polymerase enzyme. This technique is extremely powerful and generates microgram (µg) quantities of DNA copies of desired DNA (or RNA) segment in few hours. The technique involves the use of synthetic oligonucleotides complementary to known sequences flanking the sequence of interest to prime enzymatic amplification of the intervening segment of DNA in the test tube (*in vitro*).

The amplified fragments are separated electrophoretically and banding patterns are detected by different methods as staining and autoradiography.

The conventional technique before the development of PCR technique was time consuming which used to require the cloning of target sequence, its isolation, amplification in the host cell and purifications.

Principle

This technique is a chain reaction. A small fragment of the specific DNA part of interest is identified. This serves as the template for producing primers to initiate the reaction. The DNA polymerase has the ability to synthesize new strand of DNA complementary to the offered template strand and hence there is an exponential amplification of a DNA fragment. Repeatedly adding of DNA polymerase was required before the thermostable DNA polymerase.

Steps in PCR

The PCR involves three- temperature cycles of heating and cooling the tubes containing the reaction mixture and repeated for 30 to 40 cycles. The process of PCR is completed in three steps, each replicated many times. The three steps involved are denaturation, annealing and extension:

(*i*) *Denaturation of DNA sequence* (heating of DNA mixture) of interest for amplification, being heated to 92-95° C for about 15 seconds, and separates two strands of target DNA.

(*ii*) *Annealing of denatured DNA* to chemically synthesized oligonucleotide primers (with sequences complementary to sites on opposite sides of the DNA segment of interest) by incubating them together at 50 – 60° C for 30 seconds. The temperature of reaction mixture is cooled to this temperature at which primer anneals with complementary sites on the single stranded DNA molecule.

(*iii*) *Enzymatic replication of the DNA segment* (using the DNA polymerase between the sites complementary to the oligonucleotide primers). The primer provides the free 3′ – OH required for covalent extension while the denatured DNA provides the required template function. In this final step, the temperature is raised to 72 °C for 60 seconds at which the DNA polymerase (enzyme) extends the primers and produces complementary copy of each DNA strand.

PCR Requirements

The basic PCR set up requires:

- Taq polymerase, buffer solution, loading buffer, electrophoresis buffer, agarose powder, gel casting trays, electrophoresis chamber, ethidium bromide, nuclease free water,
- DNA template that contains the DNA to be amplified
- The PCR uses two oligonucleotide primers. They hybridize to opposite strands (one forward primer and one reverse primer which is

complementary to the 3′ ends of each of the sense and anti-sense strand of the DNA target). These are the primers of specific sequences targeted to a particular region of a genome or primers of arbitrary sequences. Thus, the PCR based methods are ***sequence specific PCR assays*** and the ***arbitrary PCR assays***. The arbitrary primers can be purchased from commercial companies, have the benefit of not requiring prior genetic or biochemical information, amplify several anonymous polymorphic discrete DNA fragments and produces multiple arbitrary amplicon profiling (MAAP) which includes RAPD, Arbitrary Primer PCR (AP-PCR) and DNA amplification fingerprinting (DAF). The AFLP (Amplified fragment length polymorphism) is an intermediate technique between RFLP and RAPD.

The polymerization is done at 70-72° C for 1.5 minutes. The products so formed from first cycle of replication are subjected to denaturation, annealing to oligonucleotide primers, and replicating again by DNA polymerase. This procedure involving all the three steps is repeated many times till the desired quantities are obtained.

It is of interest that the amplification occur geometrically *viz.* one double DNA helix yield 2 double helices after one cycle of replication, 4 after two cycles, 8 after three cycles, 16 after four cycles, 1024 after 10 cycles, and so on. In this way, more than a billion copies of the DNA sequence are produced after 30 cycles of amplification.

The PCR has become the method of choice of people. The entire amplification (enzymatic synthesis of DNA) is performed *in vitro* as opposed to standard cloning procedure. It is especially valuable because the reaction is highly specific, easily automated, very quick process (completed in few hours), requires very little amount of biological material (0.5 µg of DNA or RNA) and can amplify the template DNA many thousand or million times (Between 10^6 and 10^{12} times).

Improvement in PCR was made with the discovery of heat-stable polymerase enzyme. Earlier the DNA polymerase I of *E. coli* was used as the replicase in performing the PCR and its fresh dose was required to be added at step 3 of each cycle of replication because this enzyme is heat-inactivated during the denaturation step. Later, heat-stable DNA polymerase isolated from thermophilic bacterium, *Thermus aquaticus*, called ***Taq polymerase*** was discovered. The DNA polymerase *T. aquaticus* is stable at high temperature and remains active even after DNA denaturation (heating) and hence avoid the need to add new DNA polymerase after each cycle. This technique relies on thermal cycling, consisting of cycles of repeated heating and cooling of the reaction for DNA melting and enzymatic replication of the target gene or DNA fragment.

However, the use of *Taq polymerase* has increased the frequency of replication errors.

- ☆ The first is that this enzyme does not contain a built-in 3′...... 5′ proofreading activity. The PCR is performed using heat-stable polymerase like *Pfu (Pyrococcus furiosus) or Tli (Thermococcus litolaris)* that have 3′...... 5′ proof reading activity.

- Secondly, the *Taq polymerase* amplifies long tracts of DNA inefficiently, greater than a few thousand nucleotide pairs.
- Thirdly, the PCR cannot efficiently amplify the DNA fragments longer than 35 kb. The *Tfl* from *Thermal flavus* is used in place of *Taq* polymerase in amplifying the long DNA segments. The *Tfl* polymerase can amplify DNA fragments up to about 35 kb in length.

Variants of PCR

The following need based modifications from time to time have been used in basic PCR method. These are as under:

- *Multiple PCR* – which uses more than one pair of primers so as several segments of target DNA or different target present in the sample are amplified in the same reaction. This variant approach increases the chance of primer-dimers and other non-specific droducts that may interfere to the amplification of specific products. Moreover, the multiple primer pair may compete with each other in the reaction and hence the concentrationof individual primer pair is to be amplified with different efficiencies,
- *Nested PCR* – is used to increase the specificity of DNA amplification by reducing background due to non-specific amplification of DNA. When two sets of primers are used in two successive runs of PCR, the second set indent to amplify a secondary target within the product of first run. There is semi nested PCR when when either primer of primary set was used with corresponding new primer for second amplicon.
- *Competitive PCR* – used for quantification of DNA present in the sample using real time PCR by co-amplifying with target DNA a competitor internal standard. The target is quantified from the melting curves of the target and the competitor.
- *Quantitative PCR* – is also used to measure the quantity of a PCR product, preferably real-time). It is better method to quantitative measurement starting amounts of DNA, cDNA or RNA. This method is used to know whether a DNA sequence is present in a sample and number of its copies in the sample. This method uses fluorescent dyes like SYBR Green and fluuorophore-containing DNA probes such as *TaqMan Probe, molecular beacons, scorpion probes, etc.*
- *Hot-start PCR* – which caused reduction of non-specific amplification because dsDNA is denatured by heating the sample at its denaturation temperature followed by reducing the temperature suddenly to 55 °C at which primer and taq polymerase is added. This method of hot-start and cold-finish PCR is achieved with new hybrid polymerases that are inactive at ambient temperature but activated at elongation temperature.
- *Touchdown PCR* – used to reduce nonspecific amplification. There is high annealing temperature in earliest step and the temperature is decreased in increment for every subsequent set of cycles.This high temperature results

greater specificity for primer binding and lower temperature allow more efficient amplification from the specific products of initial cycle.

- *PCR-RFLP* – An organism may be differentiated through RFLP by analysis of patterns derived from cleavage of their DNA from a set of restriction enzyme (RE). The length of the fragment produced differ when DNA is digested with RE if two organisms differ in the distance between sites of cleavage of a particular RE. The species and even the strain can be differentiated from another based on similarity of the patterns generated. The RFL analysis distinguishes the PCR product for SNP by designating primers that will introduce or destroy a restriction site for one of the allele.

Applications of PCR

PCR is a common and often indispensible process.

- This technique is used in medical and biological research labs for gene cloning in recombinant DNA technology.
- The PCR process can be used to amplify a specific gene in different individuals of a species and even in different somatic or germ cells when very small amounts of DNA are available. The PCR by amplification of specific gene can be used to know the mutational changes in individuals, cells or gametes.
- The PCR helps to prenatal diagnose the inherited human diseases when very small amounts of fotal DNA is available. Hence, it is more important in disease diagnosis and population genetics
- This technique has also its application in forensic cases to identify a person using DNA isolated from very small tissue samples. The DNA sequences can be obtained from minute amounts of DNA isolated from a few drops of blood, semen or hairs by using the PCR procedure. Therefore, PCR is important in DNA *profiling* (*fingerprinting*) in legal matters where identity of a person is uncertain.
- The PCR can be used to know transgenesis (transfer of genes) in case if the amplification occurs which occurs only in the presence of the transgene. The amplified DNA is detected as a band on the electrophoresis gel. The PCR technique is quick and uses no radioactivity, but ethedium bromide is used in staining for detection of DNA band produced by amplification. On the other, use of nucleic acid hybridization techniques (Colony, dot blot, southern and northern hybridization) for this purpose is time taken and also use radioactivity.

Annexure 23.8

PROBE: Suitably Labelled Nucleic Acid Molecule of 15-30 Bases Long

The ***probe*** is a piece of suitably *labelled nucleic acid molecule* which can be used to detect another nucleic acid molecule that has a homologous sequence by complementary base pairing. The probe is a small nucleotide sequence of 15 – 30 bases long and is capable of hybridizing with its complementary chain sequence consisting of complementary DNA (cDNA) or chemically synthetic sequences or genome fragments having complete or partial gene or intergenic sequences.

Both the DNA and RNA are used as probes. The RNA probes are ordinarily single stranded. *The* denatured double stranded DNA molecules can also be used. Further, the probes may be single locus or multilocus. The single stranded DNA probes *more convenient and preferable.* The single locus probes (SLPs) are mostly used in DNA profiling. The SLPs detect two DNA bands amongst DNA fragments separated by size one band corresponding to each allele at the locus.

The cDNA is the DNA copy of a mature mRNA. It is not a naturally occurring molecule of a cell but obtained artificially by enzymatic synthesis in an *in vitro* system.

Purpose of Using Probes

The nucleic acid probes are used for the following purposes:

- ☆ For screening of gene libraries,
- ☆ For mutation analysis (detection of mutation),
- ☆ Diagnosis of infectious diseases, and
- ☆ For DNA based markers in gene mapping.

Probe Preparation

There are a number of ways to obtain probes. Some of them are given here. The mRNAs are naturally single stranded and they can be used as probes that are highly purified. Three types of DNA probes are available. These are

- ☆ Cloned cDNA or *genomic fragments,*
- ☆ *Synthetic oligonucleotides,* and
- ☆ *PCR generated probes.*

The several ways of preparation of probes of different types of probes are as -

- ☆ Cloning of the corresponding DNA sequences (***cloned cDNA***) may be done by inserting into a special vector like *p*GEM. This vector has a different and specific prokaryotic promoter on the two ends of the DNA insert. In order to obtain RNA molecules complementary to either one of the strand of the DNA insert, the recombinant DNA after linearizing is transcribed with appropriate prokaryotic polymerase.
- ☆ The ***double stranded probes*** may be obtained as DNA segments isolated from the genome of an organism or cDNA molecules prepared from mRNAs can be cloned in *E. coli*.
- ☆ The cloning the concerned DNA segment in a vector like phage M13 vectors of *E. coli* may be prepared as ***single stranded DNA probes***. The probes complimentary to either of the strand of the cloned DNA segment will be obtained from different recombinant clones of this vector. Limiting the copies of mRNA by reverse transcriptase to only one strand can be used to prepare the single strand DNA probes.
- ☆ ***PCR generated probes, called asymmetric PCR*** can be obtained by generating single stranded copies of a DNA sequence.
- ☆ ***Synthetic oligonucleotides*** can be prepared easily for use as probes in case of the known base sequence of DNA to be detected or of RNA produced by it. The amino acid sequence of a small segment up to 5 amino acids can be used to detect the base sequence of a part of gene after mRNA sequence based on base pairing principle. This can be shown as under:

Amino acid sequence in a polypeptide:	trp.	glu.	Met.	Lys.	Met
mRNA base sequence:	UGG	GAA	AUG	AAA	AUG
DNA base sequence:	ACC	CTT	TAC	TTT	TAC

However, the degeneration of genetic code (one amino acid is coded by two or more codons) makes it impossible to know the exact base sequence of the gene. The problem of degeneracy is tackled by synthesizing a mixture of oligonucleotides having all the possible base sequences based on the degenerate code.

Labelling of Probes

The radioactive labels like ^{32}P or non-radioactive labels like biotin, digoxigenin can be used for the labelling of the probes. Some non-radioactive probes can be stored at -20° C for long period of time compared to radioactive probes which have short half-life of radioisotopes and hence can be used shortly after they are prepared.

(*i*) The nucleic acids can be ***radioactively labelled*** by the following approaches:

- ***Nick translation*** (*oldest method of nucleic acid labelling* and is still most commonly used to label radioactive or non-radioactive labelling, for double DNA strand molecule),
- Primer extension,
- RNA polymerase based method,
- End labelling by DNA sequencing, and
- Direct labelling methods. Direct labelling a nucleotide labelled with ^{32}P is provided during production of the probe to include this radioactive nucleotide in the probe.

(*ii*) The ***non-radio active labelling*** of nucleic acids has the following approaches:

- Labelling with biotin: These biotin labelled probes are prepared by nick translation by use of biotin conjugated (biotinylated) nucleotides. These probes are hybridized with the nucleic acid fixed to a solid support and washing off the non-hybridized probes. The hybridized samples are detected by the development of blue colour following a series of cytochemical reactions. This approach is faster than radioactive probes which require autoradiography but its filter (solid support) cannot be reused and the nucleic acid is fixed to it for hybridization with other probes while radioactive probes are easily washed under high pH which favours denaturation and the same filter can be used.
- Labelling with dioxigenin (plant derived chemical): It may be used in nick translation to produced digoxigenin labelled probes
- Labelling with fluorescent molecules: The nucleotides may also be conjugated with other legends that produce detectable signals (fluorescence, enzyme activity).

Application of Probes

The probes allow reliable efficient detection of nucleic acid sequence complementary to used probes and hence have varied applications

- Identification of the recombinant clone carrying the desired DNA insert. This is the most critical step in DNA cloning when southern, northern, colony, dot blot hybridization techniques are used.
- Confirmation of the integration of a DNA insert in the host genome (Southern hybridization) and its expression in transformed cells (Northern hybridization).

- ✰ Determination of embryo sexing can be done using PCR. Thus in case of IVF the sex of the embryo can be determined using Y chromosome-specific primers before their implantation in uterus
- ✰ In DNA finger printing process
- ✰ To studty DNA polymorphism
- ✰ Development of RFLP maps
- ✰ To determine the location of specific sequence in specific chromosome (*in situ hybridization*)caused by parasites, pathogens or defective virus
- ✰ The PCR with DNA technology can be used to estimate the frequency of recombination between specified genes by DNA amplification of individual sperms and this frequency is used to construct linkage maps which not possible in higher species like man.
- ✰ The physical location of genes on chromosomes can be determined for the micro-dissected segments of chromosomes like those of salivary glands chromosome of *Drosophila* using the PCR.

Annexure 23.9

Autoradiography

The autoradiography is a technique to detect and localize radioactive isotopes (to examine the distribution of radioactivity) in cytological preparations or macromolecules (DNA, RNA, proteins, chromosomes) by exposure to a photographic emulsion that is sensitive to low-energy radiation. The emulsion contains silver halides that produce silver grains on exposing to the charged particles emitted during the decay of radioactive isotopes. This technique works on the principle of photography which makes a picture of the scene or a target. Autoradiography prepares an image of the location of radioactivity (***radioactive isotopes*** – an unstable isotope, a form of an atom that emits ionizing radiation) in the macromolecules, cells, or tissues. The difference in the two techniques is that the film of a camera is sensitive to visible light while the film used for autoradiography is sensitive to radioactivity.

Annexure 23.10

Electrophoresis

The agarose and acrylamide gels separate the polynucleotide chains or DNA strands (DNA molecules) on the basis of their size and conformation (length in nucleotides in terms of the numbers of nucleotide pairs). This is because the DNA chains have essentially constant charge per unit mass - one negative charge per nucleotide.

The chains with less numbers of nucleotides migrate the largest distance during electrophoresis. The passage of large size molecules in the gel (Agarose or acrylamide) are retarded more than small molecules. Linear DNA molecules with difference in their length by one nucleotide can be separated by the *polyacrylamide gel* electrophoresis for chains up to a few hundred nucleotides long.

The *agarose gels* are better molecular sieves for large molecules in terms of the number of nucleotides whereas for separating small size DNA molecules the *acrylamide gels* are better.

The agarose gel electrophoresis is used in biochemistry, molecular biology, and clinical chemistry to separate a mixed population of DNA proteins in a mixture of agarose. The charged molecules migrate either to positive or negative pole on the basis of their charge on placing them in an electric field. The proteins may be separated by charge and or size. The nucleic acids have a consistent charge imparted by their phosphate back bone, migrate towards anode, and are separated based on their length. Agarose gels got more popularity for their use due to their easy casting in the shape of thin slab and suitability for separating larger DNA. Mostly the agarose gels between 0.7 to 2 per cent are dissolved in a suitable electrophoresis buffer. The separated DNA can be seen under UV light after staining with ethidium bromide and can be extracted from gel using commercial kit.

Annexure 23.11

Somatic Cell Hybridization

Different types of somatic cells are fused together. The result cell is called hybrid cell. In general the human fibrocytes or leucocytes are fused with mouse cell lines. The mixing can be done of human and mouse cells or cells of any two mammalian species or of the same species. Spontaneous cell fusion occurs at a very low rate (10^{-6}). The addition of of ultraviolet inactivated Sendalby (parainfluenza) virus or a chemical called PEG (Polyethylene glycol) can increase the rate by 100 to 1000 times. This is because the properties of plasma membrane of cells after adherence of these agents are changed to facilitate the fusion. This fusion result in the production of hybrid cell with two nuclei and subsequently both these nuclei are also fused in a single nucleus of the hybrid cell.

The hybrid cells are very useful in the following cases:

- ☆ For gene or chromosome mapping, based on fusion of human and mouse somatic cells.
- ☆ For production of monoclonal antibodies, This is done by hybridoma production which is the hybrid cells between an immortalized cell and an antibody producing lymphocyte,
- ☆ For studying the control of cell division and gene expression
- ☆ For investigating mlignant transformation, and
- ☆ For obtaining viral replication.

Annexure 23.12

Enzyme Linked Immune-Sorbent Assay (ELISA)

The antibody antigen reaction is highly specific to produce an antigen-antibody complex. This means an antibody reacts only with the region of an antigen for which it is specific. A *precipitate* is formed by ag-ab complex on reacting soluble proteins with an antibody while ag-ab complex agglutinates in case of particulate antigens. This can be written as: Soluble protein + antibody = precipitate; particulate antigen + antibody = agglutinates. In each case, the quantity of antigen or antibody involved in the interaction is known by the amount of ag-ab complex formed or by the rate of its formation. For this purpose the following various assays are as

- ☆ Gel reactions: Western blotting, immuno-electrophoresis, rocket electrophoresis,
- ☆ Precipitin reaction,
- ☆ Agglutination reactions
- ☆ Labelled antibody techniques: Direct or primary method, indirect or secondary method.

The indirect method of labelled antibody is further divided as:

- ☆ Radio-immune assay (RIA),
- ☆ *Enzyme linked immune-sorbent assay* **(ELISA),**
- ☆ Fluorescent labels,
- ☆ Electron dense labels
- ☆ Nonspecific binding to immunoglobulin, and
- ☆ Flow cytometry.

ELISA Procedure

There are two approaches of this ELISA procedure. The two methods are called as DAC ELISA and DAS ELISA. Both the approaches include two reactions (primary and secondary).

(i) DAC (Direct Antigen Coating) ELISA

The primary reaction is the formation of antigen-antibody complex. This includes the *immobilization of the concerned antigen* on the surface of a test tube or ELISA plates having small wells at uniform intervals. The antibody specific to antigen is added so as to react with the absorbed antigen. The molecules of un-reacted antibody are washed away.

The secondary reaction includes the addition into the vessel an anti-immunoglobulin (an antibody that reacts with all the antibodies) and allows the reaction wth the already formed antigen-antibody complex. The anti-Ig binds to the antibody component of the antigen-antibody complex. The ant-Ig is linked and labelled with an enzyme molecule without impairing the anti-Ig activity. Now, the un-reacted anti-Ig is washed away and substrate of the enzyme is added along with the necessary reagents. The enzyme activity develops the purple colour.

The colour intensity which is proportional to the enzyme concentration is used to know the quantity of antigen or antibody or simply to detect their presence. For this a computerized ELISA reader may be used. This procedure is called direct antigen coating (DAC) ELISA. This estimates the amount of specific antibody present in the antiserum used for the primary reaction.

(ii) DAS (Double Antibody Sand-witch) ELISA

The second approach of ELISA procedure includes the *immobilization of an unlabelled antibody* specific to the antigen in a microtitter well. The antigen is added to react with the immobilized antibody to form antigen-antibody complex. A second antibody specific to the antigen and labelled with an enzyme is added to react with the antigen-antibody complex. The antigen should have at least two accessible binding sites for antibodies – one each for the immobilized antibody and for the labelled antibody. The enzyme substrate is added after washing out the unreacted antibodies and the colour change is measured. This procedure is called double antibody sandwich (DAS) ELISA and is used for the detection or quantitative assay of the antigen of interest.

The enzymes used for labelling of antibodies are horseradish peroxidase, alkaline phosphatase, β-galactosıdase, lactoperoxidase, *etc.*

Annexure 23.13
Nick Translation

The nick is a point in one strand of a double-stranded DNA molecule at the site of breaking the phosphodiester bond. This nick moves (translate) along the DNA duplex as a result of the action of *E.coli* DNA polymerase I so as to add new nucleotides to the free 3′ OH group. Thus, this process is called nick translation which is different from protein synthesis.

The technique of nick translation for labelling of nucleic acid is old one, but still most commonly used, quite flexible for probe size, specific activity and concentration, suited for the production of large quantities of probes for use in multiple hybridization reactions and/or where a high probe concentration is required.

For labelling the DNA preparation is treated with DNase I for short time for inducing the nicks randomly in DNA molecules and each nick contains a free 3′OH group. The nicked sample of DNA is subjected to *E. coli* DNA polymerase I. This adds new nucleotides successively to the free 3′OH group. With the synthesis of new DNA segment, the existing homologous strand in the duplex is progressively displaced and digested away by the 5′ to 3′ exonuclease activity of the enzyme. This reaction radiolabels one of the deoxynucleoside triphosphates with ^{32}P but more or even all the four nucleotides could be labelled. These are then incorporated into the newly synthesized segment. It has the sequence same to that replaced because this segment is synthesized by complementary base-pairing.

This process moves (translates) the nick along the DNA duplex due to the activities of *E. coli* DNA polymerase I and hence called nick translation. The process of nick translation can be used with a variety of labels to generate probes suitable for most hybridization applications. This has been used to generate probes with high enough specific activity to detect single copy genes on Southern blots of mammalian DNA.

Annexure 23.14
Dot Blot Technique

The presence of a given sequence of DNA/RNA in the non-fractioned DNA (not subjected to gel electrophoresis) is detected by this technique. A single test – run is required to test the sample DNAs from several tissues/individuals. The presence of sequence being transferred in a number of suspected transgenic individuals and the presence of the specific mRNA in several individuals or tissues of an individual can be detected.

The procedure of dot blot involves the transfer of sample DNAs or RNAs from different individuals or tissues on to a nitrocellulose filter in the form of dots. A single filter is used to dot blot several samples. A sample DNA or RNA is the total DNA or RNA extracted from an individual or a tissue.

The DNA is denatured first and then the filter is baked at 80°C to fix the DNA firmly onto the filter. The filter is now pretreated to prevent nonspecific binding of the probe to the filter). The pre-treatment is the treating of the baked membrane with a solution containing 0.2 per cent each of Ficoll (artificial polymer of sucrose) supplemented with an irrelevant nucleic acid, *e.g.* tRNA. The pre-treatment is essential because single-stranded DNA has a high affinity for nitrocellulose filter membrane (though RNA does not have this property of affinity). The same retreatment is done in southern hybridization.

The filter is now treated with radioactive single-stranded DNA probe for hybridization. The free probe is removed by repeatedly washing the filter. The dots having DNA or RNA sequence hybridize with radioactive probes and are detected by autoradiography. The extent to which DNA or RNA is represented in the sample corresponds fairly with the intensity of dot in the autoradiograph.

The dots in the autoradiograph denote the individuals or tissues in which the DNA or RNA sequence corresponding to the probe is represented. Southern hybridization is used for the dot blot positive individual (in case of transgenic individuals) to derive more correct information about the presence and location of the sequence integrated into the genome.

Subject Index

D

E

F

G

H

Q

R

S

T

U

V

W

X

Y